**FOR
REFERENCE ONLY**

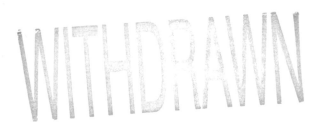

ATLAS OF GENERAL SURGICAL TECHNIQUES

ATLAS OF GENERAL SURGICAL TECHNIQUES

Courtney M. Townsend, Jr., MD

Professor
John Woods Harris Distinguished Chairman
Department of Surgery
Robertson-Poth Distinguished Chair in General Surgery
The University of Texas Medical Branch
Galveston, Texas

B. Mark Evers, MD

Director, Lucille P. Markey Cancer Center;
Professor and Vice-Chair for Research
University of Kentucky Department of Surgery;
Markey Cancer Center Director Chair;
Physician-in-Chief, Oncology Service Line
University of Kentucky Healthcare
Markey Cancer Center
Lexington, Kentucky

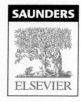

SAUNDERS
ELSEVIER

1600 John F. Kennedy Blvd.
Ste 1800
Philadelphia, PA 19103-2899

Library of Congress Cataloging-in-Publication Data

Atlas of general surgical techniques / [edited by] Courtney M. Townsend Jr., B. Mark Evers. -- 1st ed.

p. ; cm.

Includes bibliographical references and index.

ISBN 978-0-7216-0398-8 (hardcover : alk. paper) 1. Surgery--Atlases. I. Townsend, Courtney M. II. Evers, B. Mark, 1957-

[DNLM: 1. Surgical Procedures, Operative--methods--Atlases. WO 517 A8797 2010]

RD41.A782 2010

617.0022'3--dc22

2009049217

Acquisitions Editor: Judith Fletcher
Developmental Editor: Kristina Oberle
Publishing Services Manager: Julie Eddy
Senior Project Manager: Laura Loveall
Design Direction: Louis Forgione
Artwork: Michael A. Cooley
        Mike de la Flor
        Peggy Firth
        Victoria Heim
        Alexandra Hernandez
        Lauren Shavell
        Jennifer Smith
        Gina Urwin
        Electronic Publishing Services Inc., NYC

Printed in the United States

Last digit is the print number: 9   8   7   6   5   4   3   2   1

CONTRIBUTORS

Carlos A. Angel, MD, FACS
Associate Professor
Department of Surgery
University of Missouri—Columbia
Columbia, Missouri

Valerie P. Bauer, MD
Assistant Professor
Department of Surgery
The University of Texas Medical Branch
Galveston, Texas

Edward Y. H. Chan, MD
Surgical Resident
Department of Surgery
Mount Sinai School of Medicine
New York, New York

Celia Chao, MD
Assistant Professor
Department of Surgery
The University of Texas Medical Branch
Galveston, Texas

Charlie C. Cheng, MD
Assistant Professor
Department of Vascular Surgery
The University of Texas Medical Branch
Galvaston, Texas;
Assistant Professor
Department of Vascular Surgery
Mainland Medical Center
Texas City, Texas

Dai H. Chung, MD
Professor and Vice-Chair
Department of Pediatric Surgery
Vanderbilt University Medical Center
Nashville, Tennessee

Concepcion Diaz-Arrastia, MD
Associate Professor and Director
Division of Gynecologic Oncology
Department of Obstetrics and Gynecology
Baylor College of Medicine
Houston, Texas

B. Mark Evers, MD
Director, Lucille P. Markey Cancer Center;
Professor and Vice-Chair for Research
University of Kentucky Department of Surgery;
Markey Cancer Center Director Chair;
Physician-in-Chief, Oncology Service Line
University of Kentucky Healthcare
Markey Cancer Center
Lexington, Kentucky

James J. Gallagher, MD
Assistant Professor of Surgery
Department of Surgery
Weill Medical College;
Assistant Attending Surgeon
Department of Surgery
New York Presbyterian Hospital
New York, New York

Dennis C. Gore, MD
Professor
Department of General Surgery
The University of Texas Medical Branch
John Seely Hospital
Galveston, Texas

Baiba J. Grube, MD, FACS
Associate Professor
Department of Surgery
Yale University School of Medicine
New Haven, Connecticut

Kristene K. Gugliuzza, MD, FACS
Professor, Departments of Surgery and Pediatrics
Alonzo Alverly Ross Centennial Chair in General
  Surgery
Program Director, General Surgery Residency
Director, Kidney and Pancreas Transplant Program
  in the UTMB Texas Transplant Center
Scholar, John P. McGovern Academy of Oslerian
  Medicine
The University of Texas Medical Branch
Galveston, Texas

David N. Herndon, MD
Chief of Staff
Director of Research
Shriners Hospitals for Children—Galveston;
Professor of Surgery
Jesse H. Jones Distinguished Chair in Burn Surgery
The University of Texas Medical Branch
Galveston, Texas

Glenn C. Hunter, MD, FRCSC, FACS
Professor
Department of Surgery
University of Arizona;
Staff Surgeon
Department of Surgery
Southern Arizona VA Healthcare Service
Tucson, Arizona

Margie A. Kahn, MD
Associate Professor
Department of Obstetrics and Gynecology
Tulane University School of Medicine
New Orleans, Louisiana

Lois A. Killewich, MD, PhD
Professor and Chief, ad Interim
Section of Vascular Surgery
Department of Surgery
The University of Texas Medical Branch
Galveston, Texas

Thomas D. Kimbrough, MD
Professor
Department of Surgery
The University of Texas Medical Branch
Galveston, Texas

Tien C. Ko, MD
Jack H. Mayfield, MD Distinguished Professor in
    Surgery
Vice Chairman for Harris County Hospital District
The University of Texas Health Science Center at
    Houston
Chief of Surgery at Lyndon B. Johnson General
    Hospital
Houston, Texas

Jacqueline A. Lappin, MD, FRCSI, FACS
Assistant Professor of Surgery and Director of
    Pancreas Transplantation
Department of Surgery
University of Texas Health Science Center and
    Memorial Hermann Hospital;
Assistant Professor of Surgery
Department of Surgery
St. Luke's Episcopal Hospital and Texas Children's
    Hospital
Houston, Texas

Jong O. Lee, MD
Assistant Professor
Department of Surgery
The University of Texas Medical Branch;
Staff Surgeon
Shriners Hospitals for Children—Galveston
Galveston, Texas

David B. Loran, MD
Thoracic, Vascular, and General Surgery
Meadville Medical Center
Meadville, Pennsylvania

William J. Mileski, MD, FACS
Professor
Chela and Jimmy Storm Distinguished Professor
Chief of Trauma Services
Department of Surgery
The University of Texas Medical Branch
Galveston, Texas

William H. Nealon, MD
Professor and Vice Chairman
Department of Surgery
Vanderbilt University;
Associate Surgeon-in-Chief
Department of Surgery
Vanderbilt University Hospital
Nashville, Tennessee

Colin D. Pero, MD
Clinical Assistant Professor
Department of Otolaryngology—Head and Neck
    Surgery
University of Texas Southwestern Medical School
Dallas, Texas;
Department of Otolaryngology—Head and Neck
    Surgery, Facial Plastic and Reconstructive Surgery
Baylor Regional Medical Center
Plano, Texas

Anna M. Pou, MD, FACS
Professor and Program Director
Otolaryngology—Head and Neck Surgery
Louisana State University Health Sciences Center,
    New Orleans
New Orleans, Louisana

Lori Cindrick Pounds, MD, FACS RVT
Peripheral Vascular Associates
San Antonio, Texas

Taylor S. Riall, MD, PhD
Associate Professor
Department of Surgery
The University of Texas Medical Branch
Galveston, Texas

Arthur P. Sanford, MD, FACS
Associate Professor
Department of Surgery
Loyola University Medical Center
Maywood, Illinois

Michael B. Silva, Jr., MD
The Fred J. and Dorothy E. Wolma Professor of
    Vascular Surgery
Professor of Radiology
Director
Texas Vascular Center;
Department of Vascular Surgery
The University of Texas Medical Branch
Galveston, Texas;
Department of Vascular Surgery
Mainland Medical Center
Texas City, Texas

Courtney M. Townsend, Jr., MD
Professor
John Woods Harris Distinguished Chairman
Department of Surgery
Robertson-Poth Distinguished Chair in General
    Surgery
The Unversity of Texas Medical Branch
Galveston, Texas

Michael D. Trahan, MD
Surgeon
Martha Jefferson Surgical Associates
Charlottesville, Virginia

Kenneth J. Woodside, MD
Assistant Professor of Surgery
Division of Transplant and Hepatobiliary Surgery
Department of Surgery
University Hospitals Case Medical Center
Cleveland, Ohio

Joseph B. Zwischenberger, MD
Johnson-Wright Professor and Chairman
Department of Surgery
University of Kentucky College of Medicine
Lexington, Kentucky

PREFACE

"An education in medicine involves both learning and learning how; the student cannot effectively know, unless he knows how."

—EXCERPT FROM ABRAHAM FLEXNER, "Medical Education in the United States and Canada," 1910.

The fundamental core knowledge of general surgery remains the cornerstone of all surgical disciplines. Over the last decades, we have witnessed a proliferation of surgical specialties. The majority of graduating residents elect to pursue additional training in highly specialized fields of surgery. However, a sound foundation in general surgical techniques and principles is critical for success in these areas. Therefore, an atlas describing common general surgical procedures in a clear and concise fashion is an essential complement to current surgical textbooks to ensure that the student not only "learns how" but, most importantly, "knows how." With that said, putting together a surgical atlas is a daunting challenge. Coordinating schedules of busy surgeons and medical illustrators is, at times, akin to herding cats. So, why expend the time and effort to put this together?

For one, we have been privileged to edit the *Sabiston Textbook of Surgery* for the last three editions. This text provides a comprehensive compendium on the physiology, diagnosis, and treatment of surgical diseases, yet we are limited in the ability to describe the operative procedures in any detail. A good textbook must provide the basic knowledge to ensure that the student "learns" the material. However, it is vastly different from an atlas which teaches the student "how." Textbooks that have tried to be a comprehensive text as well as an atlas have usually failed on both accounts. Therefore, this surgical atlas series provides an important and necessary complement to the *Sabiston Textbook of Surgery* (Saunders).

The illustrations have been meticulously drawn by medical illustrators who share the same philosophy of art design. Illustrations are drawn in detail from the perspective of the operating surgeon, yet the drawings are simple enough that the reader is not distracted with extraneous colors or overly complicated design. The essential steps of the procedure are illustrated with an emphasis on surgical anatomy. Each concludes with three to five "pearls" or pitfalls from master surgeons with years of experience. Recognizing that many general surgical procedures are now performed laparoscopically, we have illustrated steps of both the open and the minimally invasive techniques where applicable. Except for the approach and the instruments, the basic tenets of the dissection and attention to detail are common to both techniques.

Finally, we were inspired to produce this atlas series based on our interactions over the years with numerous talented and hard-working surgical residents who need a concise reference to study and review prior to entering the operative suite. This atlas is meant to provide these trainees with the essential steps in performing common general surgical procedures. We recognize that the atlas is not all-inclusive. In the interest of space, we have omitted some procedures which are less commonly performed by the general surgeon in practice. However, we believe that this atlas provides a great start.

COURTNEY M. TOWNSEND, JR., MD
B. MARK EVERS, MD

ACKNOWLEDGMENTS

We would like to recognize the invaluable contributions of publication coordinators Karen Martin, Steve Schuenke, Eileen Figueroa, and administrator, Barbara Petit. Their dedicated professionalism, tenacious efforts, and cheerful cooperation are without parallel. They accomplished whatever was necessary, often on short or instantaneous deadlines, and were vital for the successful completion of the endeavor.

Our authors, all respected authorities in their fields and busy physicians and surgeons, did an outstanding job in sharing their wealth of knowledge.

We would also like to acknowledge the professionalism of our colleagues at Elsevier: Developmental Editor, Kristina Oberle; Publication Service Manager, Julie Eddy; Project Manager, Laura Loveall; Designer, Louis Forgione; and Publishing Director, Judith Fletcher.

Contents

HEAD AND NECK AND ENDOCRINE PROCEDURES

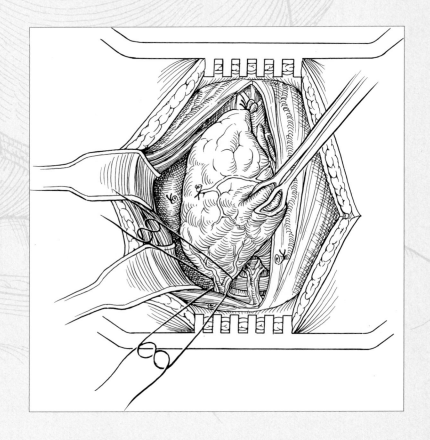

CHAPTER 1

THYROIDECTOMY (LOBECTOMY, SUBTOTAL RESECTION, TOTAL THYROIDECTOMY)

B. Mark Evers

STEP 1: SURGICAL ANATOMY

- ◆ A comprehensive understanding of the anatomy of the neck is critical before undertaking surgical procedures on the thyroid.

- ◆ **Figure 1-1** demonstrates key anatomic structures that must be considered with thyroidectomy.

- ◆ **Figure 1-2** demonstrates the relationship of the thyroid gland with the underlying trachea and esophagus and also demonstrates the usual anatomic location for the recurrent laryngeal nerve in the tracheoesophageal groove.

STEP 2: PREOPERATIVE CONSIDERATIONS

- ◆ The indications for thyroid resection include the following:
  - ◆ A solitary thyroid nodule usually with fine needle aspiration (FNA) indicative of a suspicious lesion or cancer;
  - ◆ A multinodular goiter with continued enlargement and symptoms ranging from dysphagia, choking, pain, or cosmetic concerns;
  - ◆ Occasionally hyperthyroidism particularly if radioiodine ablation or antithyroid medications are contraindicated.

- ◆ Thyroid resections range from lobectomy and isthmusectomy, subtotal thyroid resection, or total thyroidectomy.

- ◆ Decisions regarding the extent of resection are operator dependent and can be controversial.

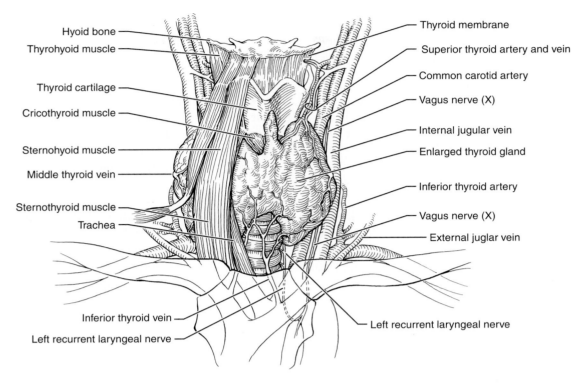

Hyoid bone
Thyrohyoid muscle
Thyroid cartilage
Cricothyroid muscle
Sternohyoid muscle
Middle thyroid vein
Sternothyroid muscle
Trachea
Inferior thyroid vein
Left recurrent laryngeal nerve

Thyroid membrane
Superior thyroid artery and vein
Common carotid artery
Vagus nerve (X)
Internal jugular vein
Enlarged thyroid gland
Inferior thyroid artery
Vagus nerve (X)
External juglar vein
Left recurrent laryngeal nerve

FIGURE 1–1

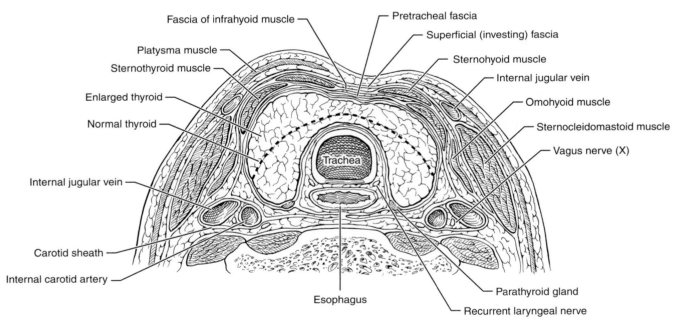

Fascia of infrahyoid muscle
Platysma muscle
Sternothyroid muscle
Enlarged thyroid
Normal thyroid
Internal jugular vein
Carotid sheath
Internal carotid artery
Esophagus

Pretracheal fascia
Superficial (investing) fascia
Sternohyoid muscle
Internal jugular vein
Omohyoid muscle
Sternocleidomastoid muscle
Vagus nerve (X)
Trachea
Parathyroid gland
Recurrent laryngeal nerve

FIGURE 1–2

STEP 3: OPERATIVE STEPS

1. INCISION

- Proper positioning of the patient is critical for adequate exposure of the thyroid gland. This is normally accomplished by hyperextension of the neck using a rolled sheet between the shoulder blades. The head is then supported with a foam rubber doughnut-shaped ring. In addition, the patient is placed in the semierect (semi-Fowler) position **(Figure 1-3)**.

- The incision must be carefully planned to allow optimal access to the thyroid gland, as well as to provide a cosmetically acceptable scar. The incision line is normally approximately two fingerbreadths above the sternal notch, placed to conform to Langer's lines. The incision should be symmetrical and extend equidistant from the midline and have a gentle upward curve. Some surgeons use a heavy silk suture to outline the incision site by compressing the suture on the neck **(Figure 1-4)**.

- The incision extends through the subcutaneous tissue; the platysma muscle is divided using the electrocautery **(Figure 1-5)**.

- Flaps are then mobilized superiorly and inferiorly using the cautery, as well as blunt dissection, just deep to the platysma muscle. The superior flap is extended to the level of the thyroid cartilage and the inferior flap extends to the clavicular heads and suprasternal notch **(Figure 1-6)**.

2. DISSECTION

- A Mahorner retractor is used to retract the skin flaps. The dissection then proceeds in the midline raphe, which provides a bloodless plane for the separation of the strap muscles **(Figure 1-7)**.

- Continuing in the midline, the loose pretracheal fascia is incised using sharp dissection or the electrocautery **(Figure 1-8)**.

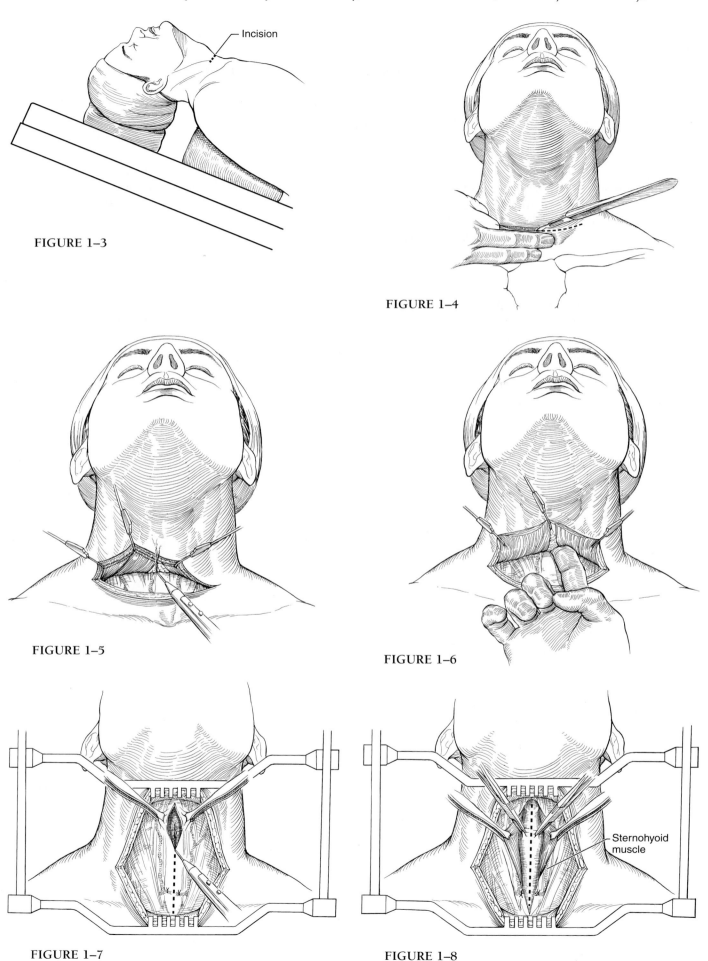

FIGURE 1–3

FIGURE 1–4

FIGURE 1–5

FIGURE 1–6

FIGURE 1–7

FIGURE 1–8

- ◆ The thyroid lobe is further exposed by mobilizing the strap muscles away from the lobe using a combination of sharp and blunt dissection **(Figure 1-9)**.

- ◆ A small Richardson retractor is then placed under the strap muscles, retracting them laterally **(Figure 1-10)**.

- ◆ Occasionally, for large bulky thyroid lesions, better exposure of the thyroid lobe can be obtained by dividing the strap muscles, which are then approximated at the end of the procedure. If transection of the strap muscles is necessary, this should be performed superiorly to minimize denervation, because both of these muscle groups are innervated from a caudal direction through the ansa hypoglossi nerves **(Figure 1-11)**.

- ◆ The thyroid lobe is grasped with Babcock forceps (shown) and retracted gently toward the midline to expose the middle thyroid vein, which is ligated using either 3-0 or 4-0 silk suture and divided. This allows further mobilization of the lobe and identification of the parathyroid glands, as well as the recurrent laryngeal nerve **(Figure 1-12)**.

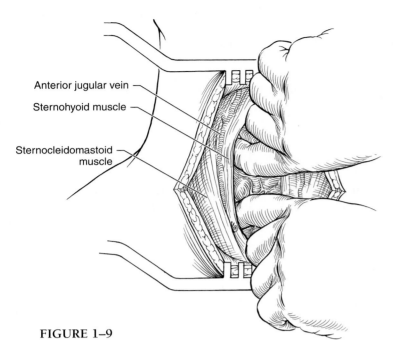

Anterior jugular vein

Sternohyoid muscle

Sternocleidomastoid
muscle

FIGURE 1–9

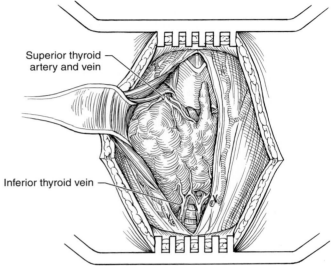

Superior thyroid
artery and vein

Inferior thyroid vein

FIGURE 1–10

Sternohyoid
muscle

FIGURE 1–11

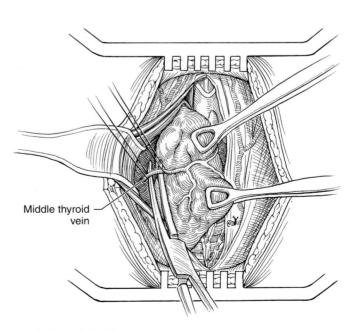

Middle thyroid
vein

FIGURE 1–12

◆ The thyroid gland is regrasped with the Babcock clamp and retracted downward to expose the superior pole vessels, including the branches of the superior thyroid artery. The external branch of the superior laryngeal nerve courses along the cricothyroid muscle just medial to the superior pole vessels. Therefore, to avoid injuring this nerve, which controls tension of the vocal cords, the superior pole vessels are divided individually as close as possible to the thyroid gland **(Figure 1-13)**.

◆ Next, the Babcock clamp is repositioned to grasp the thyroid lobe so that the inferior thyroid veins can be exposed and ligated as they enter the thyroid gland. Occasionally, a venous plexus (i.e., thyroid ima) is noted in the midline position over the trachea and entering the isthmus. These vessels are likewise carefully ligated and divided, avoiding injury to the trachea **(Figure 1-14)**.

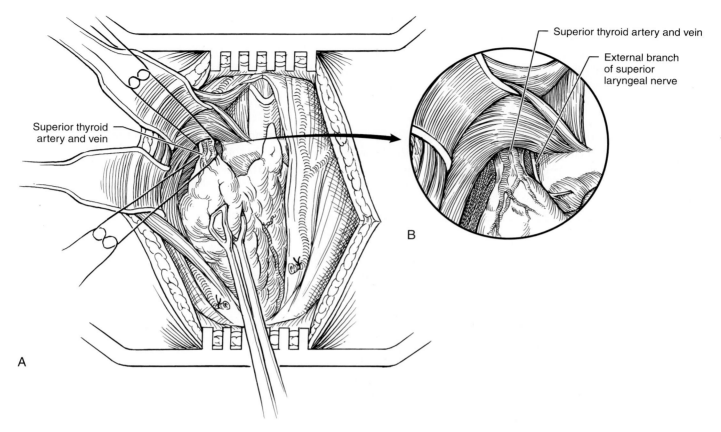

Superior thyroid artery and vein

External branch of superior laryngeal nerve

Superior thyroid artery and vein

B

A

FIGURE 1–13

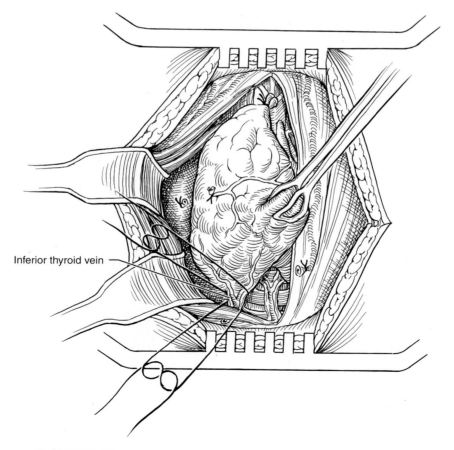

Inferior thyroid vein

FIGURE 1–14

◆ As the thyroid lobe is retracted medially, gentle dissection is performed to expose the parathyroid glands, inferior thyroid artery, and recurrent laryngeal nerve. The recurrent nerve usually passes behind the inferior thyroid artery in the tracheoesophageal groove but can occasionally lie anterior to the artery. The nerve is best found by careful dissection just inferior to the inferior thyroid artery **(Figure 1-15)**.

◆ At this point, the nerve can then be traced upward and its position in relation to the thyroid can be determined. Parathyroid glands that lie on the thyroid surface can be mobilized with their vascular supply and thus preserved **(Figure 1-16)**.

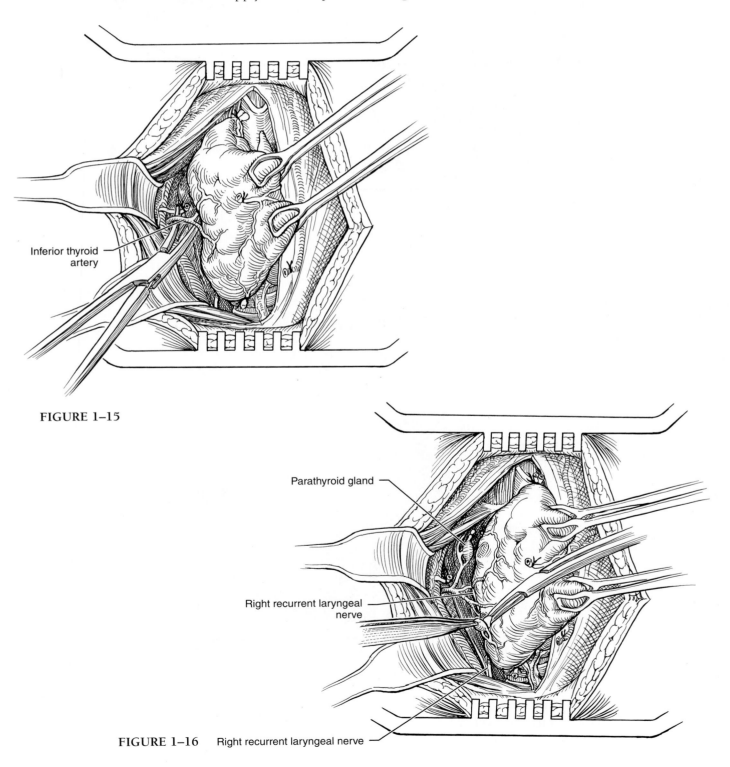

Inferior thyroid artery

FIGURE 1–15

Parathyroid gland

Right recurrent laryngeal nerve

FIGURE 1–16   Right recurrent laryngeal nerve

◆ The branches of the inferior thyroid artery are divided at the surface of the thyroid gland and individually ligated using 3-0 or 4-0 sutures. The connective tissue (ligament of Berry), which tethers the thyroid gland to the tracheal rings, is then carefully divided by sharp dissection. There are usually several small accompanying vessels, which must be individually ligated after careful dissection, because the recurrent nerve is closest to the thyroid at this point and most vulnerable. Division of the ligament allows the thyroid to be mobilized medially **(Figure 1-17)**.

◆ Dissection of the thyroid from the trachea can then be performed with the electrocautery by division of the loose connective tissue between the structures **(Figure 1-18)**.

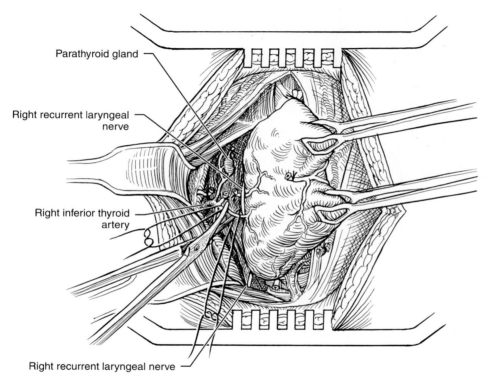

Parathyroid gland

Right recurrent laryngeal nerve

Right inferior thyroid artery

Right recurrent laryngeal nerve

FIGURE 1–17

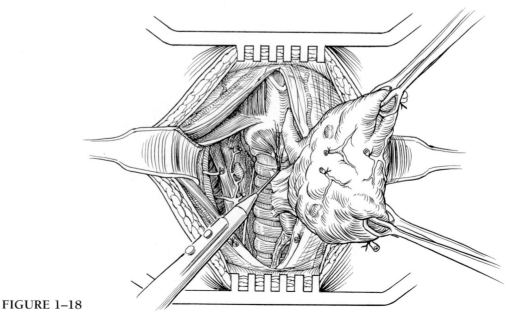

FIGURE 1–18

◆ If lobectomy is indicated, then the isthmus is clamped using a Kocher or tonsil clamp **(Figure 1-19, A)**, divided, and oversewn with an interlocking continuous 3-0 Vicryl suture **(Figure 1-19, B)**.

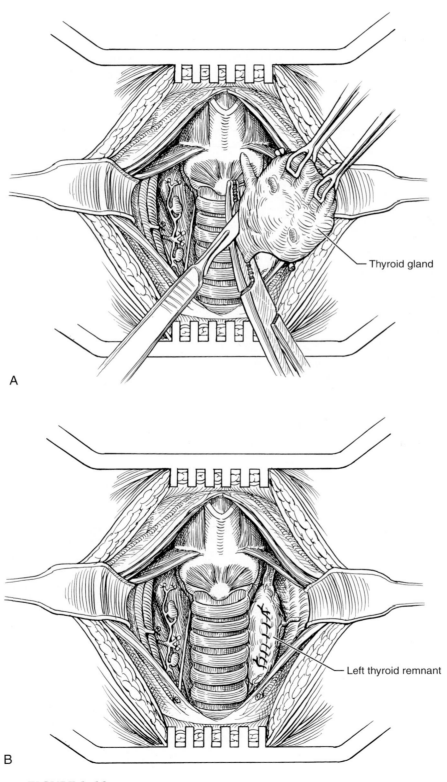

Thyroid gland

A

Left thyroid remnant

B

FIGURE 1–19

◆ If total thyroidectomy is indicated, the operation is continued in a similar fashion on the other side to remove the thyroid gland in toto (**Figure 1-20, A**) and to preserve both the parathyroid glands and the recurrent laryngeal nerves (**Figure 1-20, B**).

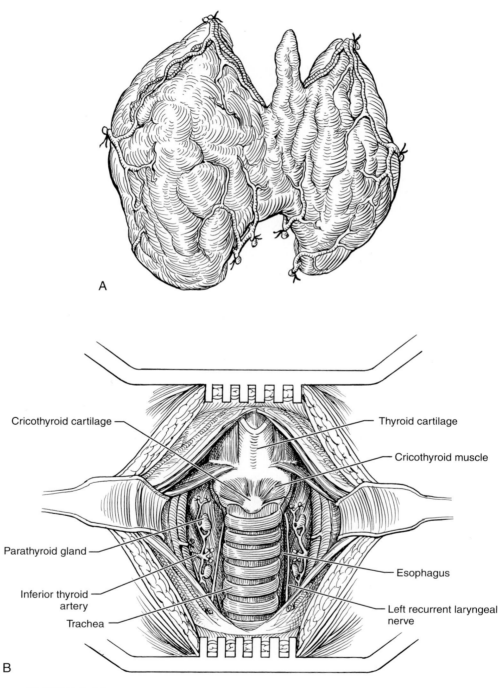

A

Cricothyroid cartilage

Thyroid cartilage

Cricothyroid muscle

Parathyroid gland

Esophagus

Inferior thyroid artery

Left recurrent laryngeal nerve

Trachea

B

FIGURE 1–20

◆ Some surgeons prefer to perform a subtotal resection if operating for benign disease, thus preserving the parathyroid glands and not dissecting in the area of the recurrent laryngeal nerves. The line of resection on the thyroid lobe to preserve this rim of thyroid tissue overlying the parathyroid glands is shown in **Figure 1-21, A.** The remnant thyroid tissue is illustrated in **Figure 1-21, B.**

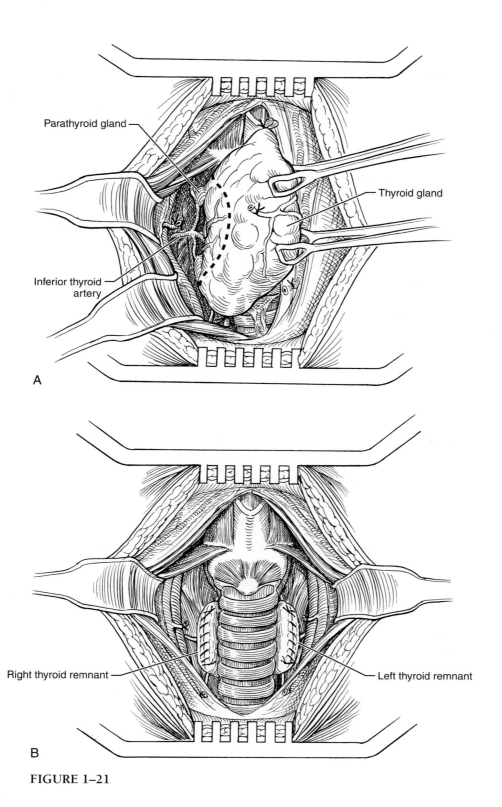

FIGURE 1–21

3. CLOSING

- Once resection is completed and hemostasis is ensured, closure is performed by first reapproximating the strap muscles at the midline using interrupted 3-0 Vicryl sutures **(Figure 1-22)**.

- The platysma muscle is likewise reapproximated using interrupted 3-0 Vicryl sutures **(Figure 1-23)**.

- Finally, the skin is reapproximated with a subcuticular stitch of 4-0 Monocryl suture **(Figure 1-24)**.

STEP 4: POSTOPERATIVE CARE

- Although once routinely placed after thyroid resection, drains are seldom indicated.

- One of the most immediate postoperative complications can be wound hematoma, which occurs in a small percentage of patients. It is more common in those patients who are taking anticoagulant medications or nonsteroidal anti-inflammatory drugs (NSAIDs) or who have had total thyroidectomy.

- A small hematoma in this location can severely compromise respirations and should be immediately evacuated either in the operating room or, if this is not possible, at the bedside.

- Injury of a recurrent laryngeal nerve can lead to hoarseness; bilateral injury of the recurrent laryngeal nerves may result in paralysis of both vocal cords, which would require reintubation and possibly tracheostomy.

- Postoperative hypoparathyroidism is usually a transient phenomenon that is relatively rare but occurs more often after total thyroidectomy. Calcium replacement and possibly vitamin D may be required to maintain adequate serum calcium levels.

- In an uncomplicated thyroid lobectomy, patients may be discharged on the same day as surgery.

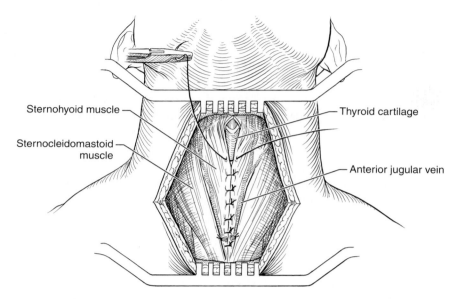

Sternohyoid muscle

Sternocleidomastoid muscle

Thyroid cartilage

Anterior jugular vein

FIGURE 1–22

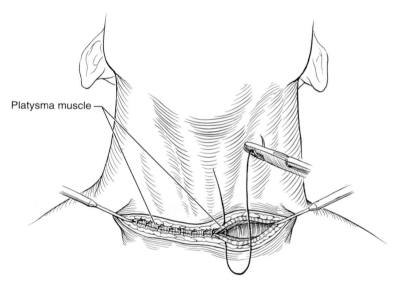

Platysma muscle

FIGURE 1–23

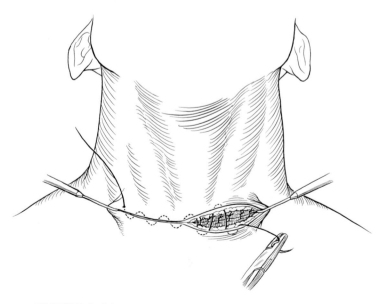

FIGURE 1–24

STEP 5: PEARLS AND PITFALLS

- The most dreaded complication of thyroid resection is damage to the recurrent laryngeal nerve. It is imperative to identify the nerve throughout its course in the neck to avoid injury.

- During thyroidectomy, the recurrent laryngeal nerve is at greatest risk of injury at the ligament of Berry, during ligation of branches of the inferior thyroid artery, or at the thoracic inlet.

- In most patients, the dissection can be carried out entirely through the cervical incision. In the rare patient, a partial median sternotomy may be required for anterior mediastinal lesions that cannot be safely mobilized through the cervical incision. This possibility should be anticipated by preoperative physical examination.

SELECTED REFERENCES

1. Hanks JB: Thyroid. In Townsend CM Jr (ed): Sabiston Textbook of Surgery: The Biological Basis of Modern Surgical Practice, 17th ed. Philadelphia, Saunders, 2004, pp 947-983.
2. Wong CKM, Wheeler MH: Thyroid nodules: Rational management. World J Surg 2000;24:934-941.
3. Schlumberger MJ: Papillary and follicular thyroid carcinoma. N Engl J Med 1998;338:297-306.
4. Clark OH: Surgical anatomy. In Braverman LE, Utiger RE (eds): Werner and Ingbar's The Thyroid, 7th ed. Philadelphia, Lippincott-Raven, 1996, pp 462-468.

CHAPTER 2

MODIFIED RADICAL NECK DISSECTION PRESERVING SPINAL ACCESSORY NERVE

Anna M. Pou

STEP 1: SURGICAL ANATOMY

- ◆ Modified radical neck dissection (MRND) is a modification of the radical neck dissection described by Crile in 1906. It includes the en bloc removal of all node-bearing tissues in the anterior and posterior cervical triangles, the tail of the parotid gland, the submandibular gland, and cervical sensory nerves with sparing of one of all of the following structures: the sternocleidomastoid (SCM) muscle, the internal jugular vein (IJV), and the spinal accessory nerve (SAN).

- ◆ A comprehensive understanding of all neck anatomy is critical and cannot be overestimated **(Figure 2-1).** The SCM muscle was removed to show underlying structures (see Figure 2-1, B).

- ◆ Key structures include the platysma muscle, SCM muscle, anterior and posterior bellies of the digastric muscle, posterior belly of the omohyoid muscle, trapezius muscle, marginal mandibular branch of the facial nerve, brachial plexus, phrenic nerve, hypoglossal nerve, SAN, thoracic duct, and contents of the carotid sheath.

- ◆ The SAN lies lateral to the IJV in 70% of patients, lies medial to the IJV in 27%, and passes through the IJV in 3% of cases.

- ◆ The platysma is dehiscent in the lower anterior midline of the neck and posteriorly in the area of the external jugular vein and the greater auricular nerve.

- ◆ The levels of the neck must be understood before the start of the operation. Lymph nodes are contained in seven levels of the neck, which are defined by certain anatomic boundaries:
  - ◆ Level IA: The submental (triangle) is formed by the anterior bellies of the digastric muscle and the hyoid bone.
  - ◆ Level IB: The submandibular (triangle) is formed by the anterior and posterior bellies of the digastric muscle and the body of the mandible superiorly.
  - ◆ Level II: The upper jugular extends from the level of the skull base superiorly to the level of the hyoid bone inferiorly and to the posterior border of the SCM muscle. It is divided into Levels IIA and IIB by the SAN. Level IIA is located anterior to the SAN and Level IIB is located posterior to the SAN.

- Level III: The mid-jugular extends from the hyoid bone superiorly to the level of the cricoid cartilage inferiorly and to the posterior border of the SCM muscle.
- Level IV: The lower jugular extends from the level of the cricoid superiorly to the clavicle inferiorly and to the posterior border of the SCM muscle.
- Level V: The posterior triangle (spinal accessory and transverse cervical) is bounded by the anterior border of the trapezius muscle posteriorly, the posterior border of the SCM muscle anteriorly, and the clavicle inferiorly. Sublevel VA (spinal accessory nodes) is separated from VB (nodes following the transverse vessels) by a horizontal plane marking the inferior border of the anterior cricoid arch.
- Level VI: Contains the prelaryngeal (Delphian), pretracheal, and paratracheal (anterior central compartment) nodes and extends from the hyoid bone superiorly to the suprasternal notch inferiorly and laterally to the medial border of the carotid sheath bilaterally.
- Level VII: The upper mediastinal is inferior to the suprasternal notch in the superior mediastinum.

STEP 2: PREOPERATIVE CONSIDERATIONS

- Neck dissections are often done in conjunction with resection of the primary tumor. In this case, the neck incision may be modified to include resection of both nodal disease and the primary tumor. A tracheotomy may also be necessary.

- Indications for MRND with preservation of the SAN include the following:
  - The presence of a clearly defined plane between the SAN and tumor
  - Bulky nodal disease (stage N2, N3)
  - Persistent or recurrent nodal disease following radiation/chemoradiation therapy

- Preoperative counseling must include the possibility of sacrifice of cranial nerves if involved with tumor, as well as the resulting deficits.

- Two units of packed red blood cells are typed, screened, and held for transfusion if necessary.

- Perioperative antibiotics are given if the upper aerodigestive tract is to be entered to resect the primary tumor.

- The patient's airway should be discussed with the anesthesiologist before surgery. The presence of a primary tumor, laryngeal edema, or effects of previous radiation therapy may dictate fiber-optic intubation or awake, local tracheotomy.

- The proximity of nodal disease to the carotid sheath must be assessed for resectability. Carotid artery balloon test occlusion is performed if there is suspicion of carotid artery invasion. This will determine risk of cerebrovascular accident (CVA) if the carotid artery is resected. Carotid artery resection with or without reconstruction using saphenous vein graft is typically not considered except in radiation failures and recurrent disease.

- The surgeon must be able and prepared to modify the surgical plan and the order in which various steps are performed if the tumor dictates such.

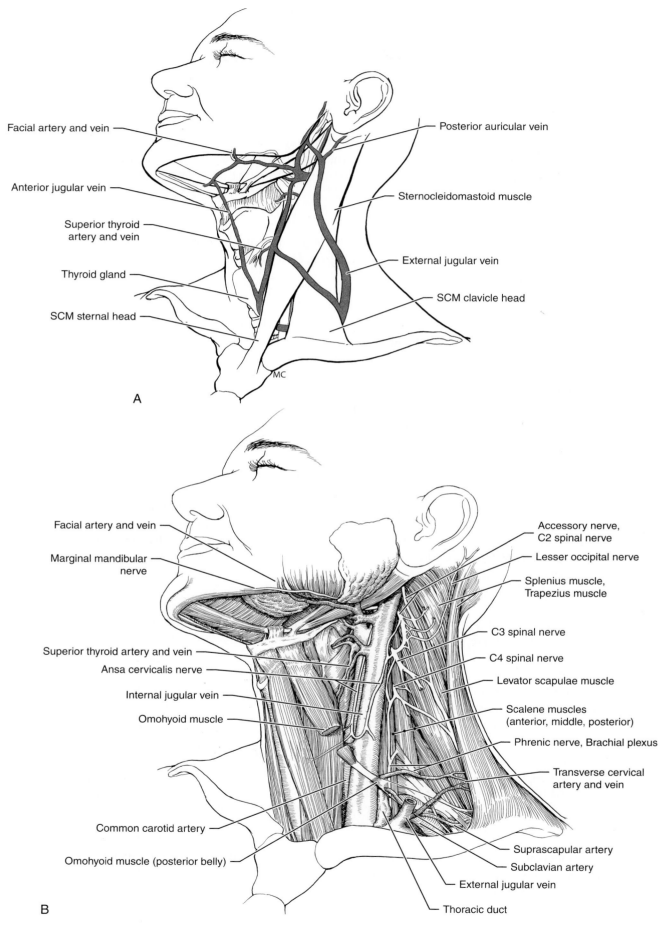

Facial artery and vein

Anterior jugular vein

Superior thyroid
artery and vein

Thyroid gland

SCM sternal head

Posterior auricular vein

Sternocleidomastoid muscle

External jugular vein

SCM clavicle head

A

Facial artery and vein

Marginal mandibular
nerve

Superior thyroid artery and vein

Ansa cervicalis nerve

Internal jugular vein

Omohyoid muscle

Common carotid artery

Omohyoid muscle (posterior belly)

Accessory nerve,
C2 spinal nerve

Lesser occipital nerve

Splenius muscle,
Trapezius muscle

C3 spinal nerve

C4 spinal nerve

Levator scapulae muscle

Scalene muscles
(anterior, middle, posterior)

Phrenic nerve, Brachial plexus

Transverse cervical
artery and vein

Suprascapular artery

Subclavian artery

External jugular vein

Thoracic duct

B

FIGURE 2–1

STEP 3: OPERATIVE STEPS

1. INCISION

- Following oral endotracheal intubation or tracheostomy, the patient is placed supine. The neck is extended using a shoulder roll, and the head is stabilized using a doughnut cushion. The ipsilateral arm is tucked and the bed is turned with the operative field facing out (away from the anesthesiologist).

- Following induction of general anesthesia, muscle relaxants are not used. This allows testing of cranial nerves with a nerve stimulator. This must be communicated to the anesthesiologist.

- The surgical site is sterilely prepped with betadine from the level of the lower lip to right above the nipples, including the lower face, earlobe, and posterior neck. The prep is extended across the midline of the neck. If the primary tumor is to be resected, this area is also sterilely prepped in continuity with the neck and chest.

- The sterile drapes surrounding the head and neck field are stapled or sutured to the patient.

- There are many options for skin incisions, with the most commonly used ones seen here (**Figure 2-1, C** [half H], **Figure 2-1, D** [modified Schobinger], **Figure 2-1, E** [hockey stick]). The incision chosen depends on tumor location, including the primary tumor, and surgeon preference. I prefer the hockey stick incision that slightly crosses midline (See Figure 2-1, E) to avoid dropping a limb. If a limb is dropped, the trifurcation should be placed posterior to the carotid artery. In the event of skin necrosis, the carotid artery would not be exposed with this design.

- The incision is outlined on the neck using a sterile marking pen. The mastoid tip and suprasternal notch are used as a reference.

- The skin and subcutaneous tissue are injected with 1% lidocaine with 1:100,000 epinephrine to obtain hemostasis.

- The superior and inferior skin flaps are raised in a subplatysmal plane to the level of the mandibular body and the clavicle, respectively. The posterior aspect of the superior flap is raised in a plane lateral to the external jugular vein, great auricular nerve, and tail of the parotid (**Figure 2-2**). Medially, the skin flap is elevated slightly past the midline.

- If a tracheotomy is present, care must be taken not to violate the tracheotomy incision. If this does occur, the tracheotomy incision must be separated from the remainder of the neck incision to prevent contamination with air and mucus. This is done by sewing the subcutaneous tissue surrounding the tracheotomy site to the strap muscles.

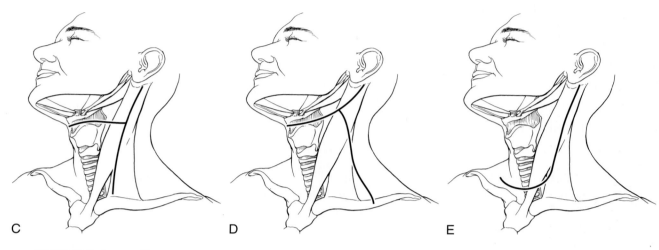

FIGURE 2–1, cont'd

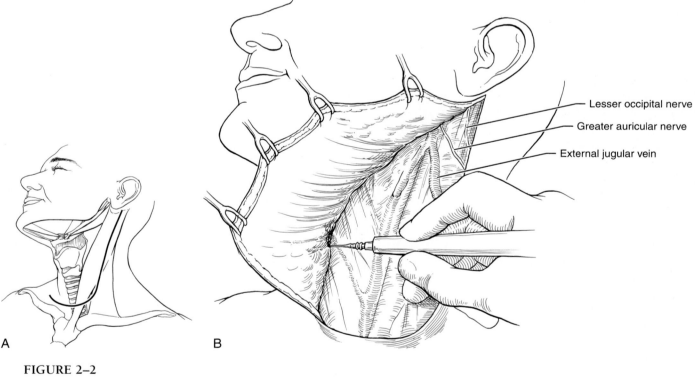

Lesser occipital nerve

Greater auricular nerve

External jugular vein

FIGURE 2–2

◆ The superior and inferior skin flaps are secured to the drapes using 2-0 silk stick ties and hemostats. During the dissection, retraction of the skin flaps should occasionally be released to prevent venous congestion of the flaps.

◆ The posterior skin flap can be elevated at this time or after the level I nodal dissection is complete. I prefer the latter.

2. DISSECTION

◆ The superficial layer of the deep cervical fascia overlying the submandibular gland is incised 1 cm anterior and 1 cm inferior to the angle of the mandible. The marginal mandibular nerve will be found in this location. It lies lateral to the facial vessels. The nerve is sharply dissected from the underlying tissue and elevated superiorly together with the fascia **(Figure 2-3)**. This is necessary in order to dissect the prevascular facial nodes.

◆ An Allis clamp is placed on the fibro-fatty tissue in the midline submental area lying between the anterior bellies of the digastric muscle. This tissue is dissected in an inferior and posterior direction, exposing both anterior muscle bellies and the central portion of the mylohyoid muscle. The nerve and vessels to the mylohyoid are ligated. This tissue is left attached to the hyoid bone **(Figure 2-4)**.

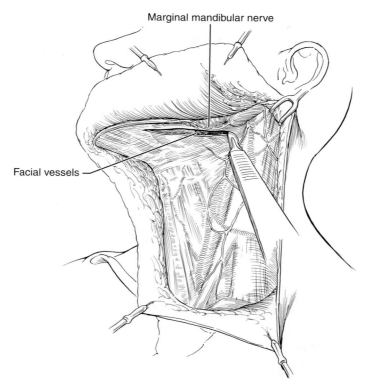

Marginal mandibular nerve

Facial vessels

FIGURE 2–3

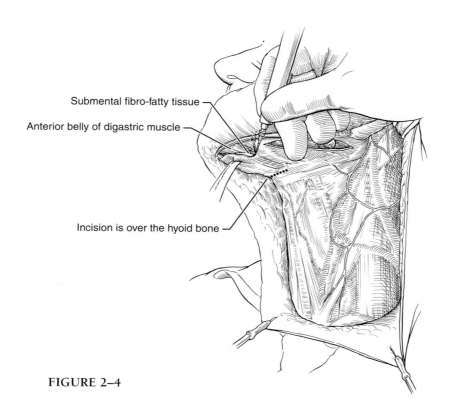

Submental fibro-fatty tissue

Anterior belly of digastric muscle

Incision is over the hyoid bone

FIGURE 2–4

- The periosteum overlying the inferior border of the mandibular body is incised with electrocautery, and the tissue in the submandibular triangle is retracted inferiorly. The facial vessels are ligated at the lower border of the body of the mandible **(Figure 2-5)**.

- The posterior border of the mylohyoid muscle is identified during this dissection **(Figure 2-6)**.

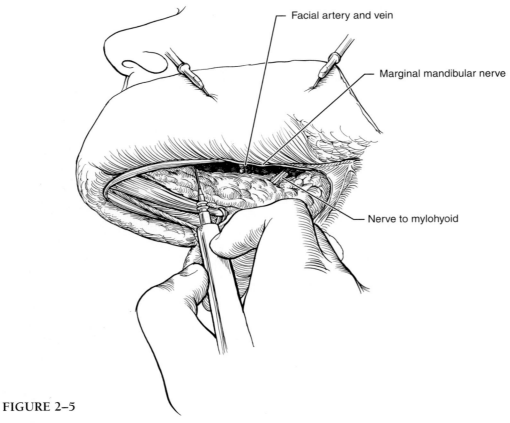

Facial artery and vein

Marginal mandibular nerve

Nerve to mylohyoid

FIGURE 2–5

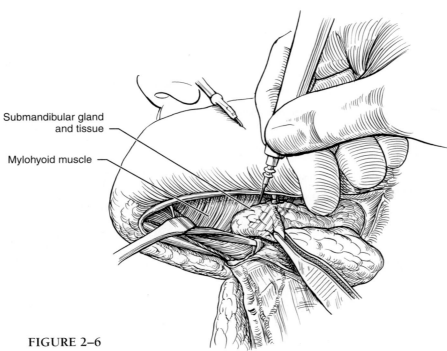

Submandibular gland and tissue

Mylohyoid muscle

FIGURE 2–6

◆ An Army-Navy retractor is placed under the posterior aspect of the mylohyoid muscle, and it is retracted cephalad. The lingual nerve, submandibular ganglion, and submandibular duct are identified **(Figure 2-7, A).**

◆ A clamp is placed below the submandibular ganglion, and the postganglionic fibers are transected and ligated. This releases the lingual nerve **(Figure 2-7, B-C).**

◆ The submandibular duct is located medial to the ganglion; it is transected and ligated (Figure 2-7, B-C).

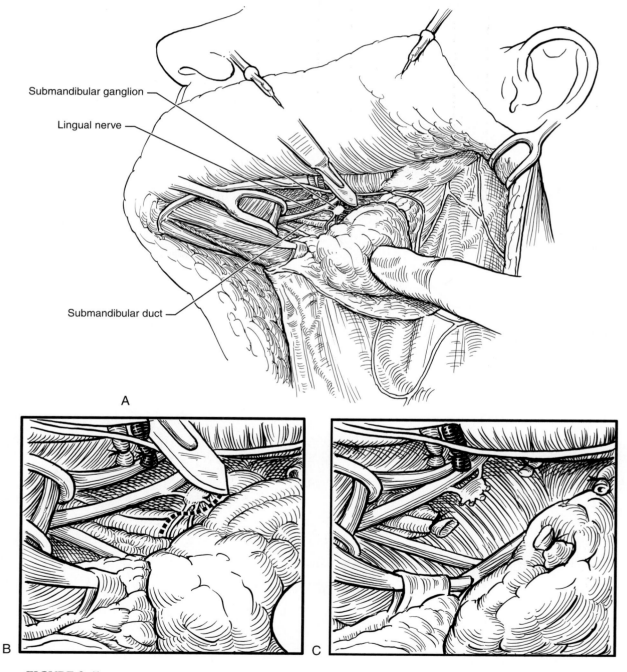

Submandibular ganglion

Lingual nerve

Submandibular duct

A

B

C

FIGURE 2–7

◆ Inferior retraction of the submandibular contents reveals the facial vessels as they cross the superior aspect of the posterior belly of the digastric muscle. The vessels are clamped, transected, and ligated. The posterior belly of the digastric muscle is isolated in its entirety. This muscle belly provides a landmark for levels I and II and the carotid sheath. The contents of the submental and submandibular triangles, including the prevascular nodes, are pedicled at the level of the hyoid bone **(Figure 2-8)**.

◆ Attention is now directed to the posterior skin flap. Elevation of the flap proceeds in a subcutaneous plane until the anterior border of the trapezius muscle is reached **(Figure 2-9)**. The platysma is deficient in this area, and care must be taken to not "button hole" the skin flap by dissecting too superficially or to injure the SAN by dissecting too deeply; the SAN lies superficial in the posterior triangle. The use of electrocautery may stimulate the SAN and cause the shoulder to "jump."

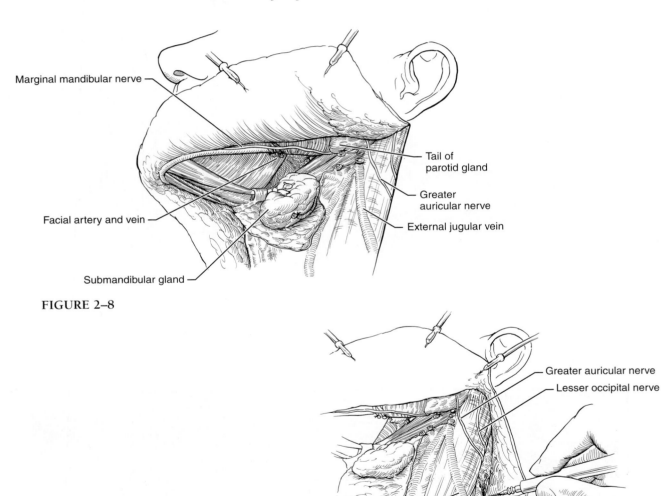

FIGURE 2–8

FIGURE 2–9

◆ The SAN is identified in the posterior triangle as it enters the trapezius muscle. A spreading technique using a fine hemostat or Metzenbaum scissors is used to dissect the soft tissue and fascia overlying the nerve. The nerve is traced as it passes from the trapezius muscle to the SCM muscle (**Figure 2-10**).

◆ The SAN exits the SCM muscle and dissection continues anteriorly and superiorly to the skull base, transecting the overlying muscle with the nerve constantly in view. This divides the SCM muscle in two (**Figure 2-11**). The posterior belly of the digastric muscle is retracted superiorly for exposure of the nerve and the IJV at the skull base. The relationship of the SAN to the IJV is noted during this dissection.

◆ The nerve is sharply dissected from the underlying tissue. The branch to the SCM muscle must be divided to mobilize the nerve. A nerve hook or vein retractor can be used to retract the nerve as it is being skeletonized to minimize trauma.

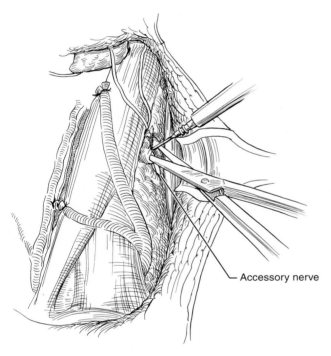

— Accessory nerve

FIGURE 2–10

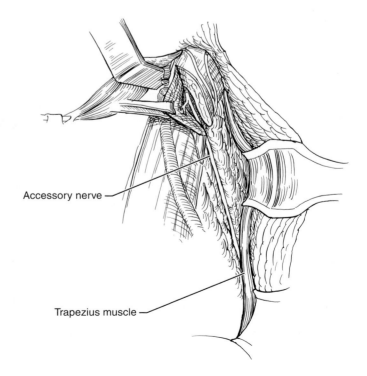

Accessory nerve —

Trapezius muscle —

FIGURE 2–11

- The IJV at the skull base is isolated circumferentially from the surrounding tissue so that it can be ligated at a later time.

- The sternal and clavicular heads of the SCM muscle are transected one fingerbreadth above the clavicle **(Figure 2-12)**. Upward traction is placed on the muscle with a sponge, and the layers of the muscle are carefully transected so as not to injure the contents of the carotid sheath that lie immediately deep to the muscle.

- Once the SCM muscle is divided inferiorly, the posterior belly of the omohyoid muscle is visualized. The tissue overlying the muscle posteriorly is incised **(Figure 2-13)**.

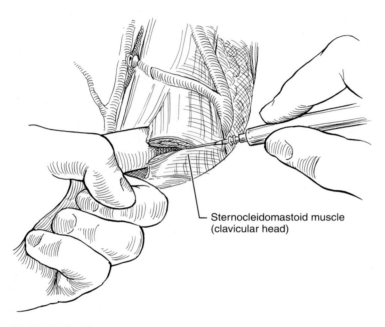

Sternocleidomastoid muscle
(clavicular head)

FIGURE 2–12

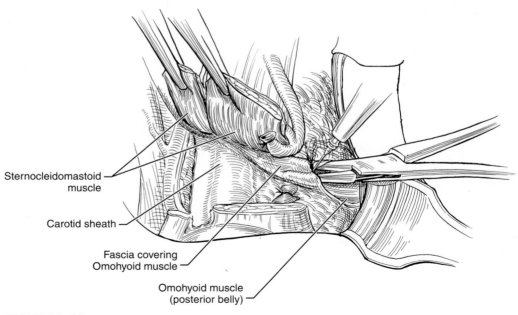

Sternocleidomastoid
muscle

Carotid sheath

Fascia covering
Omohyoid muscle

Omohyoid muscle
(posterior belly)

FIGURE 2–13

◆ The muscle belly itself is transected near its origin at the scapula (**Figure 2-14**) and elevated anteriorly to its attachment at the hyoid bone. The anterior jugular veins will be encountered at this point and should be ligated. This defines the anterior limit of the neck dissection.

◆ The fascia underlying the posterior belly of the omohyoid muscle is incised horizontally. The supraclavicular fat pad is then opened using blunt dissection exposing the brachial plexus and phrenic nerve, which lies on the surface of the anterior scalene muscle (**Figure 2-15**). The dissection should not continue until the brachial plexus and phrenic nerve are identified, because injury to these structures can be catastrophic. The transverse cervical vessels will also be seen in this area. It is not always necessary to divide these vessels.

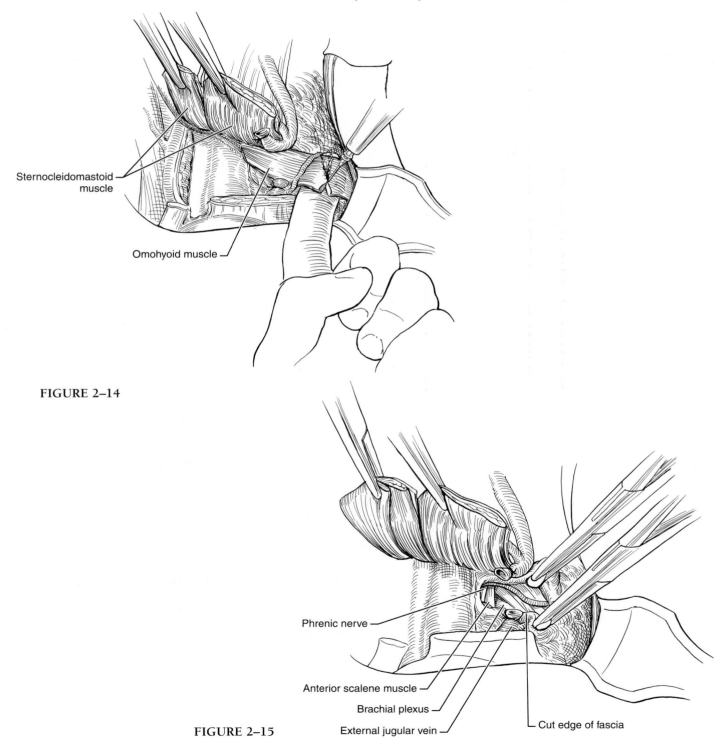

FIGURE 2–14

FIGURE 2–15

◆ The fibro-fatty tissue between the brachial plexus and the anterior border of the trapezius muscle (supraclavicular fat pad) is clamped and ligated. The brachial plexus must be directly visualized while the clamps are being placed. This tissue can be bluntly dissected using a finger. This area is known as the "bloody gulch," and bleeding will occur if the tissue is not ligated (**Figure 2-16**).

◆ Dissection is then carried superiorly along the anterior border of the trapezius muscle until the SAN is encountered. The SAN is retracted anteriorly to avoid injury during this dissection. The SCM muscle is transected just inferior to the mastoid tip, and the fascia is incised at its posterior aspect (**Figure 2-17**). This allows the specimen to be retracted medially.

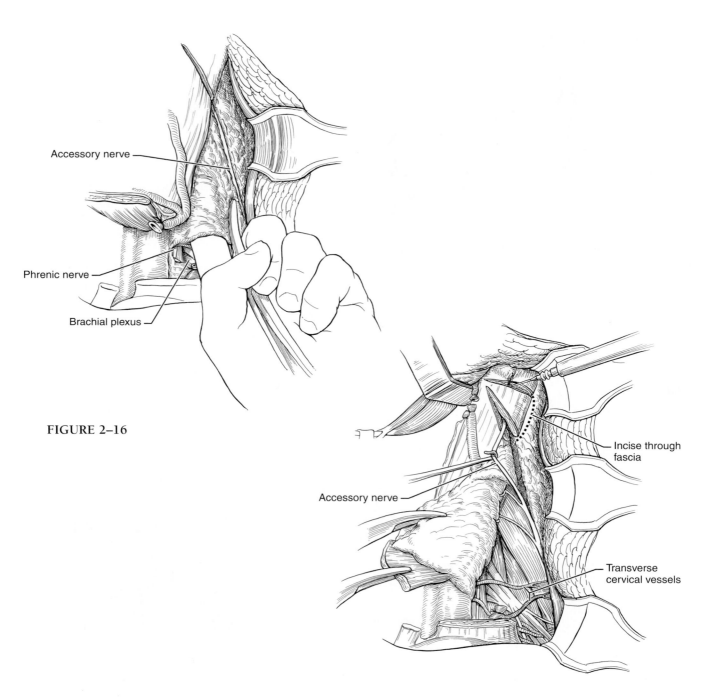

FIGURE 2–16

FIGURE 2–17

◆ The specimen, including the fibro-fatty and lymphatic tissue in level V, as well as the superior aspect of the SCM muscle, is dissected in a posterior to anterior direction. The specimen is passed underneath the SAN, gently retracting the SAN laterally **(Figure 2-18)**.

◆ The deep limit of dissection is the fascia of the deep cervical muscles; the dissection proceeds along the medial aspect of the levator scapulae and the scalene muscles. The rootlets of the cervical plexus are exposed. The cutaneous branches are transected and removed with the specimen. Care must be taken to preserve the nerve supply to the posterior compartment musculature and the contributions to the phrenic nerve. This is done by transecting the cervical rootlets approximately 1 cm anterior to the takeoff of the phrenic nerve, that is, "high" in the specimen. Vessels typically accompany the rootlets and should be controlled using bipolar cautery or suture ligation. In addition, care must be taken to avoid direct injury to the phrenic nerve by lifting it off the anterior scalene muscle with the specimen **(Figure 2-19)**.

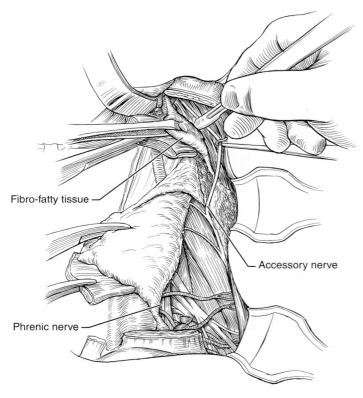

Fibro-fatty tissue

Accessory nerve

Phrenic nerve

FIGURE 2–18

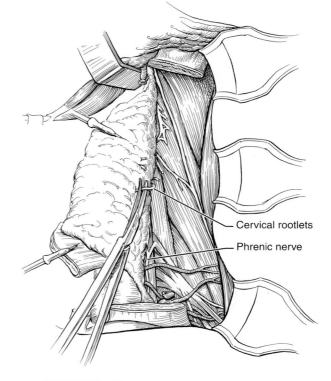

Cervical rootlets

Phrenic nerve

FIGURE 2–19

◆ Mobilization of the specimen continues until the IJV is exposed in its full length **(Figure 2-20)**.

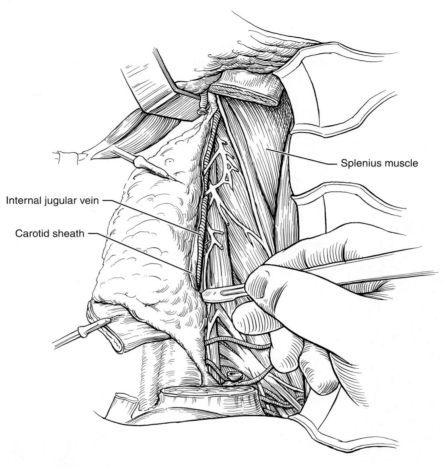

Splenius muscle

Internal jugular vein

Carotid sheath

FIGURE 2–20

◆ At this time, the IJV and the lymphatic pedicle containing the thoracic duct (accessory duct on the right) are isolated and ligated. When clamping these structures, care is taken to avoid dividing the vagus nerve (**Figure 2-21, A**).

◆ Careful circumferential dissection of the IJV inferiorly is done both sharply and bluntly to avoid injury to the vein itself, the carotid artery, the sympathetic chain, and the vagus and phrenic nerves. The proximal end of the vein is doubly clamped, and a single clamp is placed on the distal end. The vein is transected between the second and third clamps, and the proximal end is ligated using a 2-0 silk tie and a 2-0 silk suture ligature. The other end is ligated with a single 2-0 silk tie (**Figure 2-21, B**).

◆ The thoracic duct can typically be seen at the lower lateral aspect of the IJV. It is very thin walled, and extreme care in isolating the lymphatic pedicle is necessary to avoid inadvertent injury with chyle leak. The lymphatic pedicle is isolated and ligated (**Figure 2-21, C**). A Valsalva maneuver at this time will assess for a leak.

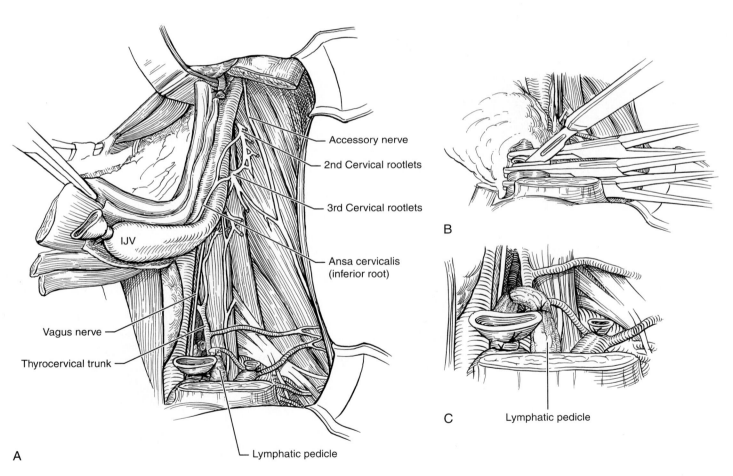

FIGURE 2–21

◆ The dissection now proceeds in a cephalad direction in a plane between the IJV and the carotid sheath. The dissection also proceeds medially and superiorly along the anterior belly of the omohyoid muscle. The hypoglossal nerve (located approximately 2 cm superior to the carotid bifurcation) and the descendens hypoglossi branch are visible in the course of dissection. Following the descendens hypoglossi branch superiorly will help in identification of the hypoglossal nerve. Retraction of the posterior belly of the digastric muscle is needed for visualization **(Figure 2-22)**.

◆ The ranine veins lie lateral to the hypoglossal nerve and require ligation to avoid meddlesome bleeding. Ligation of these vessels is done with the hypoglossal nerve under direct visualization to avoid inadvertent injury to and/or transection of the nerve.

◆ The surgical specimen is now pedicled on the upper end of the IJV. The specimen is flipped into its anatomic position, and the IJV is doubly clamped, transected, and ligated using a 2-0 silk tie **(Figure 2-23)**.

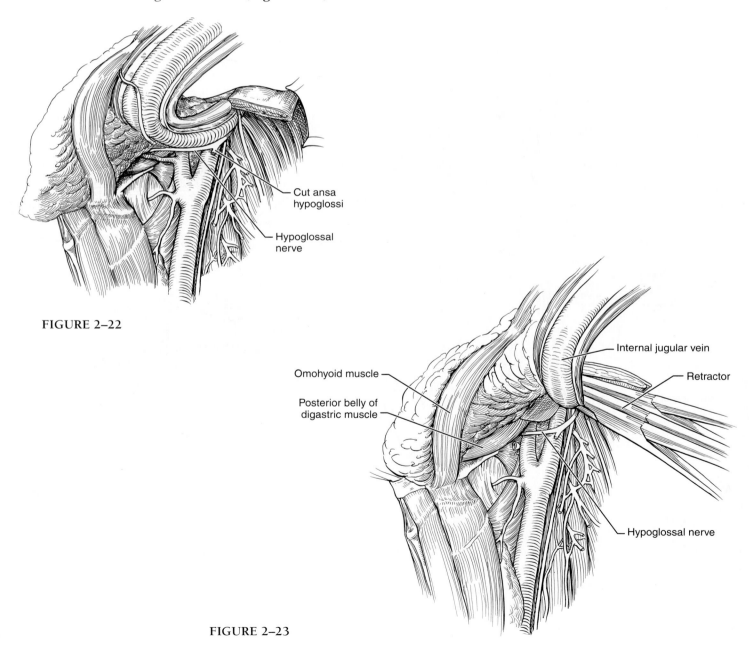

Cut ansa
hypoglossi

Hypoglossal
nerve

FIGURE 2–22

Omohyoid muscle

Posterior belly of
digastric muscle

Internal jugular vein

Retractor

Hypoglossal nerve

FIGURE 2–23

◆ As seen here, the SCM muscle, IJV, omohyoid muscle, and nodal levels 1-5 have been removed, preserving the SAN **(Figure 2-24).**

◆ The surgical specimen is removed from the surgical field, and each level of nodal dissection is labeled for the pathologists.

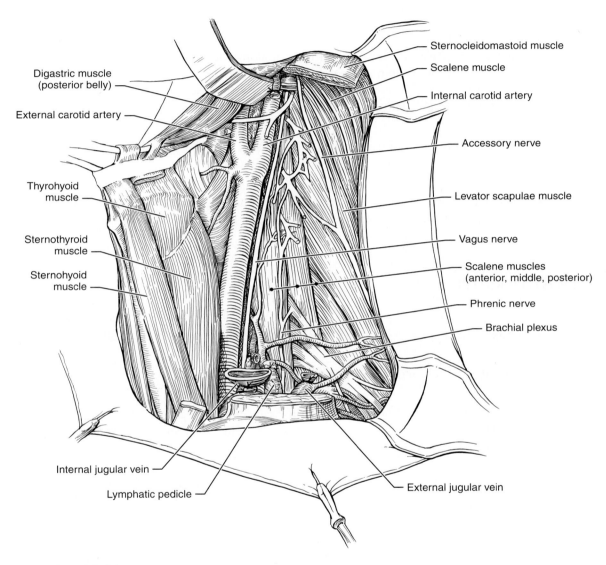

Digastric muscle (posterior belly)

External carotid artery

Thyrohyoid muscle

Sternothyroid muscle

Sternohyoid muscle

Internal jugular vein

Lymphatic pedicle

Sternocleidomastoid muscle

Scalene muscle

Internal carotid artery

Accessory nerve

Levator scapulae muscle

Vagus nerve

Scalene muscles (anterior, middle, posterior)

Phrenic nerve

Brachial plexus

External jugular vein

FIGURE 2–24

3. CLOSING

- A Valsalva maneuver is performed to check for a chyle leak.

- Meticulous hemostasis is obtained.

- The wound is copiously irrigated with normal saline.

- Two 10-mm Jackson-Pratt drains are placed into the wound through separate stab incisions; one is placed posteriorly in the neck along the trapezius muscle and the other is placed anteriorly in the neck, parallel to the strap muscles. To prevent suction on the carotid artery, the drains may be loosely sewn to the fascia of the deep muscles of the neck using an absorbable suture to hold them in place.

- The incision is closed in two layers; the platysma is tightly closed using an absorbable stitch, and the skin is closed using surgical staples or suture.

- Antibiotic ointment only is applied to the incision. A pressure dressing is not applied (my preference), because this increases risk of IJV occlusion in the contralateral neck.

STEP 4: POSTOPERATIVE CARE

- Perioperative antibiotics are given for 24 hours only if the upper aerodigestive tract was entered.

- Head of bed is elevated to 45 degrees to reduce edema.

- Neck drains are placed on low continuous wall suction for 2 days, then switched to bulb suction. The nursing staff is required to "strip" the drains every shift to prevent occlusion of the drain from fibrinous debris.

- Neck incision is cleaned twice daily (bid) and as needed (prn) with half-strength hydrogen peroxide and saline. Following this, antibiotic ointment is then applied to the neck incision bid. This is discontinued after 3 days.

- Drains are individually removed when output is 20 mL or less per 24 hours.

- Routine tracheotomy care is performed if one is present (see Chapter 5).

- Physical therapy is initiated following drain removal. Exercises for range of motion in neck and upper extremities and strengthening exercises for upper extremities are ordered.

- Speech and swallowing evaluation is particularly important for patients who underwent tracheotomy, resection of the primary tumor, and/or previous radiation therapy.

- Staples are removed on postoperative day 7. If the patient has previously received radiation therapy, the staples remain for 10 to 12 days.

STEP 5: PEARLS AND PITFALLS

- Posterior belly of the digastric muscle is considered the "resident's friend"; there are no important structures lateral to it, and the contents of the carotid sheath are deep to it. This is a very important landmark.

- The omohyoid muscle lies lateral to the carotid sheath, brachial plexus, and phrenic nerve. It is also considered the "resident's friend" and is a very important landmark.

- The skin flaps in a previously irradiated patient should be raised sharply, or a Shaw knife should be used to decrease chance of skin necrosis.

- The marginal mandibular nerve is most commonly injured where it courses near the angle of the mandible.

- If there is a question intraoperatively as to whether the tumor can be dissected off of the carotid artery, proximal and distal control of the vessel should be obtained and vessel loops placed before dissection of the area in question.

INTRAOPERATIVE COMPLICATIONS

- "Button hole" of posterior skin flap

- Injury to brachial plexus (sensory and motor deficits in upper extremity) and cranial nerves: marginal mandibular (weakness in lower lip), hypoglossal (weakness/atrophy hemitongue), vagus (aspiration, dysphonia), phrenic (elevated hemidiaphragm, respiratory compromise), and spinal accessory (shoulder droop, chronic pain)

- Injury to cervical sympathetic chain (Horner syndrome)

- Chyle leak: If this occurs, the thoracic duct is ligated and fibrin glue and Gelfoam are placed over the repair. Loupe magnification is helpful in this situation.

- Laceration of the IJV: Small laceration of the vein can typically be repaired with a vascular suture of 6-0 nylon. If the laceration is too large to repair, the vein is sacrificed. This causes a problem in the case of bilateral neck dissections only if the contralateral IJV must be sacrificed because of tumor. If laceration of the vein occurs at the skull base, bleeding can be stopped by packing the area with Gelfoam and applying pressure or suturing the stump to the digastric muscle. If laceration occurs near the thoracic inlet, the assistance of a thoracic surgeon may be necessary to control the bleeding, and an air embolus may occur.

- Injury to the subclavian vein

- Air embolus through open cervical veins is rare ("gurgle" heard via precordial stethoscope and blood pressure drops). If this occurs, the patient is immediately placed in the left lateral position and the central line is aspirated. If a central line is not present, one should be immediately placed. If there is no time, direct left ventricular puncture should be attempted.

◆ Hemorrhage resulting in transfusion

◆ Bradycardia due to carotid dissection/retraction: If this occurs, all dissection stops and 1% plain lidocaine is injected into the adventitia in the area of the carotid bulb.

◆ CVA: Many patients with head and neck cancer also suffer from atherosclerotic disease, with plaque noted in the carotid arteries on preoperative imaging. Careful retraction of the carotid artery during neck dissection will lessen the risk of an embolic event and CVA.

◆ Carotid artery injury resulting in CVA or death: This type of injury is rare and can occur when tumor is closely dissected from the artery, or when the artery is ectatic in its course (particularly in the elderly).

POSTOPERATIVE COMPLICATIONS

◆ Hematoma

◆ Seroma

◆ Visible scar on neck

◆ Blood loss anemia

◆ Wound infection

◆ Chyle fistula: Milky drainage in the suction bulb or high output drainage is indicative of a chyle leak. Drain fluid can be sent for triglyceride level if necessary to confirm the diagnosis. This is treated with a pressure dressing and a medium-chain triglyceride diet. Intravenous hyperalimentation may be necessary. If high output continues, neck exploration is indicated.

◆ Weakness and chronic shoulder pain

◆ Skin flap necrosis, with or without carotid artery exposure

◆ If the carotid artery is exposed, immediate coverage using a flap is mandatory to prevent carotid "blowout." A pectoralis major myocutaneous flap is typically used.

◆ Carotid blowout: This occurs when the carotid artery becomes exposed because of skin necrosis or if it is bathed with saliva from a fistula that develops following resection of the primary tumor. The ABCs of resuscitation are as follows: If the patient is stable, a bilateral carotid artery arteriogram is obtained and the artery may be embolized or stented radiographically. An unstable patient is taken immediately to the operating room for ligation of the carotid artery. Carotid blowout is often preceded by a "herald" bleed. A herald bleed is manifested by sudden onset of bright red blood coming from the neck wound or the tracheotomy site that is brief in duration. This is a warning and allows the surgeon time to assess the carotid artery system via arteriogram.

◆ Persistent/recurrent tumor

SELECTED REFERENCES

1. Eibling DE: Neck dissections. In Myers EN (ed): Operative Otolaryngology Head and Neck Surgery. Philadelphia, Saunders, 1997, pp 676-718.
2. Peters GE, Price JC, Johns ME: Cervical lymphadenectomy. In Johns ME, Price JC, Mattox DE (eds): Atlas of Head and Neck Surgery. Philadelphia, BC Decker, 1990, pp 378-411.
3. Crile G: Excision of cancer of the head and neck with special reference to the plan of dissection based on 132 operations. JAMA 1906; 47:1780.
4. Head and neck sites. In Greene FL, Page DL, Fleming ID, et al (eds): AJCC Cancer Staging Manual, 6th ed. New York, Springer, 2002, pp 17-22.
5. Martin H, Del VB, Ehrlich H, Cahan WG: Neck dissection. Cancer 1951; 4:441.

CHAPTER 3

PARATHYROIDECTOMY

B. Mark Evers

STEP 1: SURGICAL ANATOMY

- A comprehensive understanding of the anatomy of the neck is critical (see Figure 1-1). In addition, a thorough knowledge of the embryology and development of the parathyroid glands is important to understand where in the neck or mediastinum the parathyroid gland may lie, based on normal embryologic descent of the superior and inferior glands.

- Whereas bilateral neck explorations are still being performed for hyperparathyroidism, more endocrine surgeons are choosing to localize the abnormal gland before surgery as a result of improvements in imaging techniques over the past decade. Several noninvasive preoperative localization modalities are available including Technetium-99m sestamibi scintigraphy, ultrasonography, computed tomography (CT), magnetic resonance imaging (MRI), and most recently, four-dimensional CT and positron emission tomography. These studies have been used with great success for parathyroid localization preoperatively. This allows for more directed operation and a smaller incision. **Figure 3-1** illustrates an abnormally enlarged right inferior parathyroid gland.

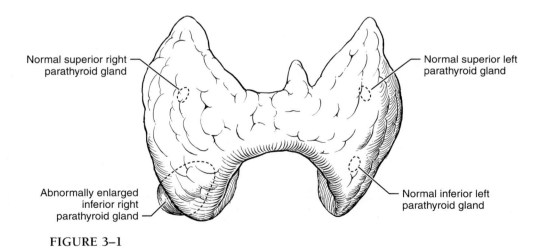

Normal superior right parathyroid gland

Normal superior left parathyroid gland

Abnormally enlarged inferior right parathyroid gland

Normal inferior left parathyroid gland

FIGURE 3–1

STEP 2: PREOPERATIVE CONSIDERATIONS

- Criteria for surgical referral, as noted by the National Institutes of Health workshop in 2002, include: serum calcium concentration greater than 1 mg/dL above the upper limits of normal, 24-hour urinary calcium greater than 400 mg, creatinine clearance reduced by greater than 30% in comparison with age-matched subjects, bone density greater than 2 standard deviations below peak bone mass, all individuals with hyperparathyroidism and age younger than 50 years, and patients for whom medical surveillance is either undesirable or impossible. In addition, all patients who are symptomatic from their hypercalcemia should be referred for surgical management.

- Preoperative localization is imperative before primary exploration if unilateral exploration is desired. As noted previously, this can be accomplished by one of several noninvasive techniques.

STEP 3: OPERATIVE STEPS

1. INCISION

- Proper positioning of the patient is critical for adequate exposure. This is normally accomplished by hyperextension of the neck using a rolled sheet between the shoulder blades. The head is supported with a foam rubber doughnut-shaped ring. In addition, the patient is usually placed in the semierect (semi-Fowler) position **(Figure 3-2)**.

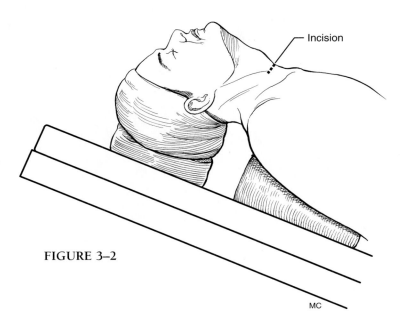

FIGURE 3–2

◆ If unilateral dissection is planned, the incision can be smaller than required for bilateral exploration. The incision extends through the subcutaneous tissue, and the platysma muscle is divided using electrocautery **(Figure 3-3)**. Flaps are then mobilized superiorly and inferiorly using the cautery, as well as blunt dissection, just deep to the platysma muscle **(Figures 3-4 and 3-5)**. The flaps do not need to be extended superiorly and inferiorly as one would do for a thyroid resection, but only enough to allow adequate exposure and placement of retraction.

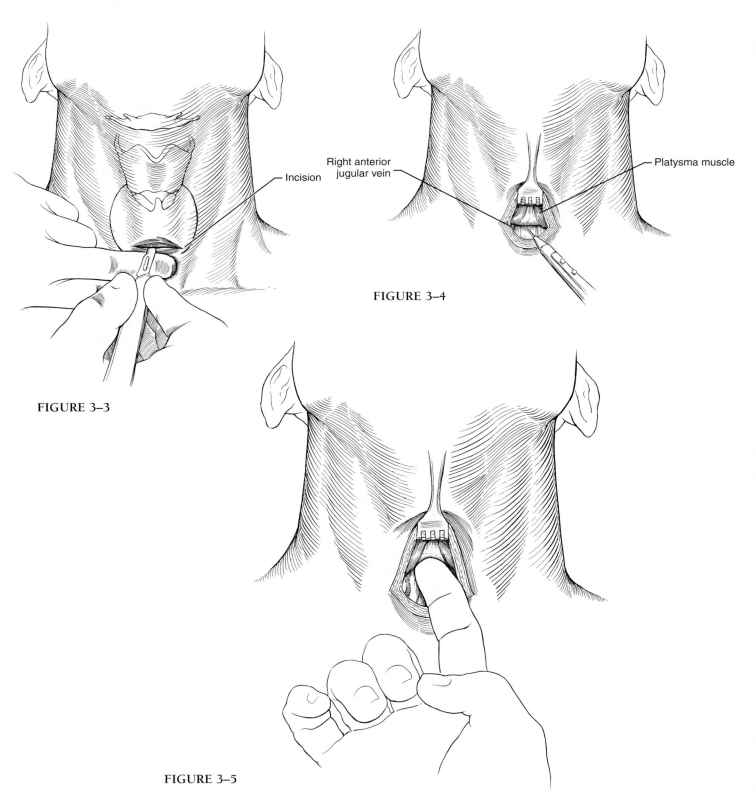

Incision

Right anterior jugular vein

Platysma muscle

FIGURE 3–4

FIGURE 3–3

FIGURE 3–5

2. DISSECTION

◆ A self-retaining retractor is used to retract the skin flaps. The dissection then proceeds in the midline raphe, which provides a bloodless plane for the separation of the strap muscles **(Figure 3-6).**

◆ As noted in **Figure 3-7,** the parathyroid adenoma has been localized preoperatively to the right inferior location. In this situation the right inferior pole of the thyroid gland is identified and this portion of the gland is gently mobilized.

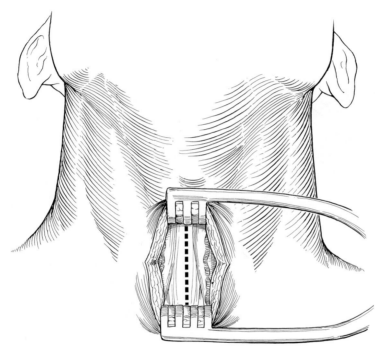

FIGURE 3–6

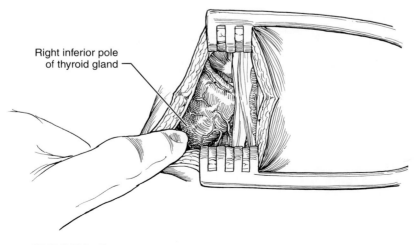

Right inferior pole of thyroid gland

FIGURE 3–7

◆ The parathyroid adenoma is now mobilized, with care taken to preserve the recurrent laryngeal nerve and minimize manipulation of the tumor during ligation of the end artery (**Figure 3-8**).

◆ If the adenoma is adherent to the thyroid gland, a pledget of gauze is effective in gently teasing the adenoma away from the thyroid (**Figure 3-9**).

◆ Once the parathyroid adenoma is mobilized, care is taken to ensure that the vascular supply is isolated and secured with either clips or ties, and the gland is then completely excised (**Figure 3-10**). If a unilateral exploration had been undertaken with preoperative localization, then many endocrine surgeons will obtain a rapid parathyroid hormone (PTH) assay to confirm the adequacy of resection.

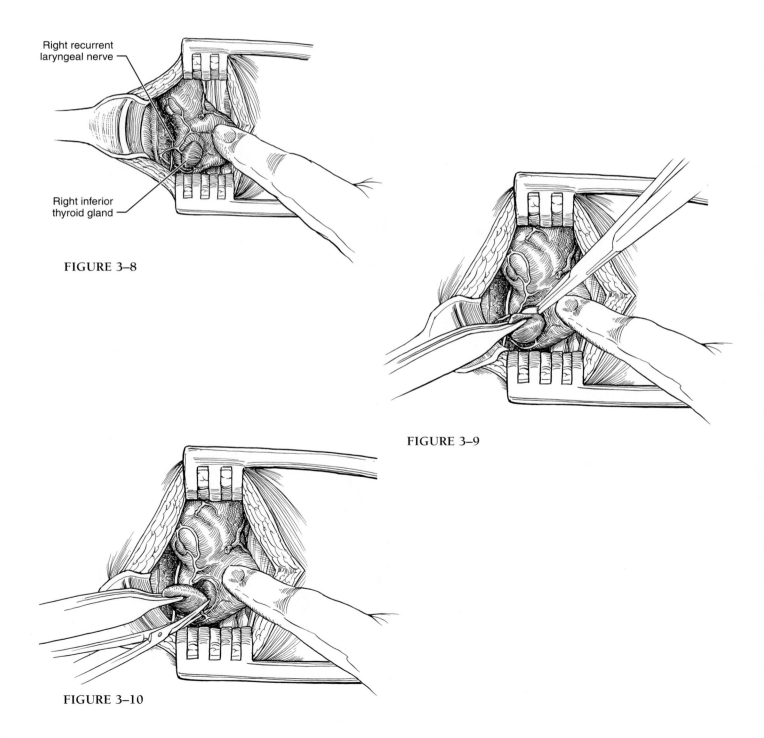

Right recurrent laryngeal nerve

Right inferior thyroid gland

FIGURE 3–8

FIGURE 3–9

FIGURE 3–10

◆ If the operation being performed was for parathyroid gland hyperplasia, then a total parathyroidectomy would be performed with autotransplantation of a portion of one of the glands into, most commonly, the forearm or the sternocleidomastoid muscle. The gland to be transplanted is minced into 1-mm pieces, and 12 to 18 pieces are embedded in well-vascularized muscle and marked with a stitch or clip **(Figure 3-11)**.

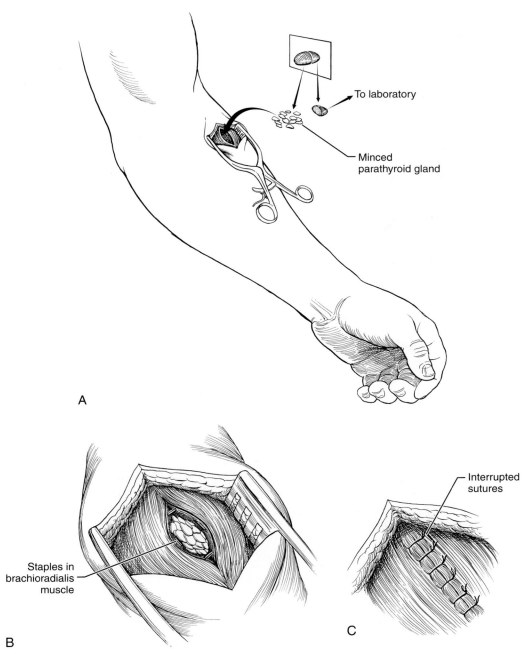

FIGURE 3–11

3. CLOSING

♦ Once the procedure is completed and hemostasis is ensured, closure is performed by first reapproximating the strap muscles at the midline using interrupted 3-0 Vicryl sutures **(Figure 3-12).**

♦ The platysma muscle is likewise reapproximated using interrupted 3-0 Vicryl sutures **(Figure 3-13).**

♦ Finally, the skin is reapproximated with a subcuticular stitch of 4-0 Monocryl suture **(Figure 3-14).**

STEP 4: POSTOPERATIVE CARE

♦ Operative complications are similar to those of thyroid surgery and include injury to the recurrent laryngeal nerve, hematoma, and wound infection. The risk for these complications is theoretically less when exploration is confined to one side of the neck.

♦ Most patients undergoing a minimally invasive parathyroidectomy are discharged on the day of surgery. They are monitored carefully as outpatients, and serum calcium and intact PTH levels are measured within the first week of follow-up.

STEP 5: PEARLS AND PITFALLS

♦ With better radiographic localization techniques, many endocrine surgeons are opting to perform preoperative localization combined with intraoperative PTH assessment in the management of patients with parathyroid adenomas. Rather than using general anesthesia, some surgeons are advocating cervical blocks, which can be performed by the surgeon before the procedure.

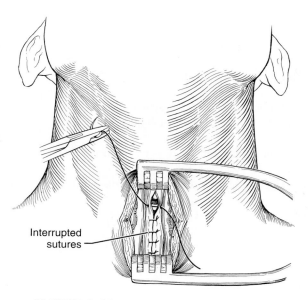

Interrupted sutures

FIGURE 3–12

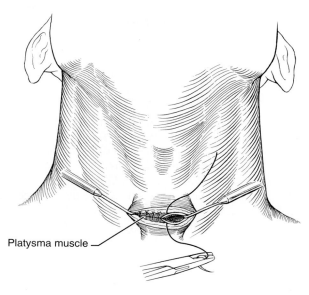

Platysma muscle

FIGURE 3–13

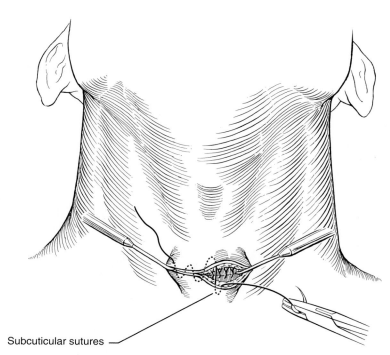

Subcuticular sutures

FIGURE 3–14

SELECTED REFERENCES

1. Akerström G, Malmaeus J, Bergström R: Surgical anatomy of human parathyroid glands. Surgery 1984;95:14-21.
2. Bilezikian JP, Potts JT Jr, Fuleihan EH, et al: Summary statement from a workshop on asymptomatic primary hyperparathyroidism: A perspective for the 21st century. J Clin Endocrinol Metab 2002;87: 5353-5361.
3. Boggs JE, Irvin GL, Molinari AS, et al: Intraoperative parathyroid hormone monitoring as an adjunct to parathyroidectomy. Surgery 1996;120:954-958.
4. Roman SA, Sosa JA, Mayes L, et al: Parathyroidectomy improves neurocognitive deficits in patients with primary hyperparathyroidism. Surgery 2005;138:1121-1128.
5. Udelsman R, Donovan P: Remedial parathyroid surgery: Changing trends in 130 consecutive cases. Ann Surg 2006;243:471-479.

CHAPTER 4

PAROTIDECTOMY

Anna M. Pou and Colin D. Pero

STEP 1: SURGICAL ANATOMY

- ◆ Identification and preservation of the facial nerve and its branches is key to successful parotid surgery.

- ◆ The anatomic landmarks that are used include the following **(Figure 4-1)**:
  - ◆ The mastoid process with the insertion of the sternocleidomastoid (SCM) muscle
  - ◆ Posterior belly of the digastric muscle
  - ◆ Tragal pointer
  - ◆ Temporoparotid fascia
  - ◆ Tympanomastoid fissure
  - ◆ Styloid process

- ◆ The parotid gland is anatomically composed of one lobe with an accessory lobe along Stensen's duct. The plane of the facial nerve divides the gland into lateral and deep lobes for surgical purposes.

- ◆ The deep lobe is located along the posterior border of the ascending mandibular ramus or adjacent to the masseter muscle along the ramus.

STEP 2: PREOPERATIVE CONSIDERATIONS

- ◆ Patients with parotid masses commonly present with painless, slowly enlarging preauricular or upper cervical masses.
  - ◆ Deep lobe masses may appear as lateral oropharyngeal masses.
  - ◆ Tail of parotid masses can be mistaken for a cervical node.
  - ◆ Facial nerve paresis/paralysis, pain, rapid growth, firm mass, presence of multiple paraglandular and upper cervical palpable lymph nodes, lack of mobility, and skin involvement are suggestive of malignancy.

- ◆ Most parotid tumors are located in the tail (80%), and 80% of all parotid tumors are benign (pleomorphic adenoma most common type).

- If malignancy or deep lobe involvement is suspected, imaging should be obtained.

- Fine needle aspiration is 94% sensitive, 97% specific, and 95% accurate in diagnosis of parotid masses. Inconclusive lymphoid cells do not exclude lymphoma. Fine needle aspiration is useful for preoperative counseling.

- Open biopsy is not recommended because of the risk of implantation of malignant cells and possible injury to the facial nerve. Open biopsy is indicated when malignancy is suspected (facial nerve paralysis, skin involvement) and diagnosis cannot be confirmed with fine needle aspiration.

- If tumor is believed to be malignant, preoperative counseling should include possible facial nerve sacrifice, neck dissection, reconstruction of the facial nerve, and possible facial reanimation surgery.

- Indications for lateral lobectomy include the following:
  - Benign or malignant tumor (exceptions include benign lymphoepithelial cysts and parotid lymphoma)
  - Refractory sialolithiasis, sialoadenitis (chronic parotitis), and chronic sialorrhea; some authors advocate total parotidectomy for chronic parotitis
  - As part of lymph node dissection for other head and neck primary tumors, primarily cutaneous malignancies of the face and scalp
  - Excision of first branchial cleft cyst involving parotid gland

- Although superficial parotidectomy is performed for tumors located in the lateral lobe of the parotid, most authors now recommend excision of the tumor with a healthy cuff of normal gland, particularly if the tumor is located in the tail.

- Enucleation of benign tumors is to be condemned. This increases risk of facial nerve injury, unacceptable risk of tumor recurrence, and increased difficulty of facial nerve preservation with repeat excision.

- Total parotidectomy with facial nerve preservation is indicated for tumors arising from or extending to a plane deep to the facial nerve and for all medium- to high-grade malignant tumors, regardless of location.

- Radical parotidectomy (total parotidectomy with facial nerve sacrifice) is indicated in cases of malignant involvement of the main trunk of the facial nerve.

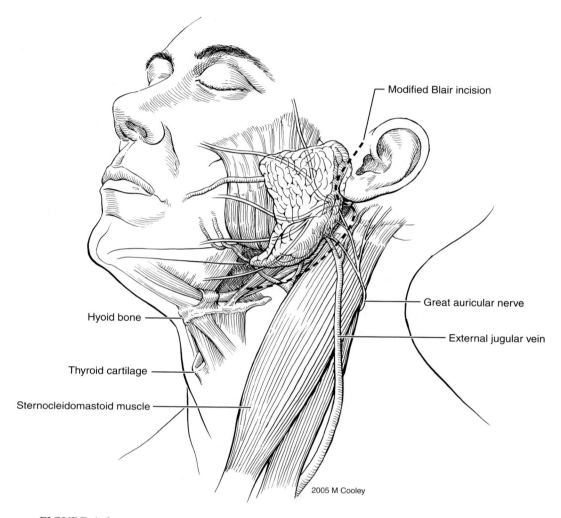

Modified Blair incision

Great auricular nerve

External jugular vein

Hyoid bone

Thyroid cartilage

Sternocleidomastoid muscle

2005 M Cooley

FIGURE 4–1

STEP 3: OPERATIVE STEPS

1. INCISION

◆ General endotracheal anesthesia without the use of muscle relaxants is preferred so that facial nerve function can be monitored during the surgery.

◆ The patient is placed supine, with the head at the top of the table and the ipsilateral shoulder as close to the edge of the operating table as possible. A shoulder roll is used to extend the neck, and the head is supported with a foam rubber doughnut-shaped ring.

◆ The ear, neck, parotid gland, corner of mouth, and corner of eye are exposed so that facial nerve function can be monitored. The cornea of the exposed eye is protected by suturing the eyelid shut using 6-0 silk suture. A small Tegaderm dressing can be used in lieu of this stitch.

◆ A modified Blair incision (standard parotidectomy incision) is outlined using a sterile marking pen. The incision is made in a relaxed preauricular skin crease, curves around the lobule toward the mastoid tip and then anteriorly along a natural skin crease, curving approximately 2 fingerbreadths below the angle of mandible (see Figure 4-1). The skin incision inferiorly remains supraplatysmal to prevent injury to the peripheral nerve branches. The only visible portion of the skin incision after healing occurs is along the upper neck incision. If a neck dissection or mastoidectomy is required for malignant tumors, the incision must be modified accordingly.

◆ The anterior skin flap is raised sharply in a supraplatysmal plane, above the parotid fascia, to the anterior border of gland. The subcutaneous fat is elevated with the skin flap. The posterior skin flap is then elevated, exposing the anterior border of the SCM muscle and the mastoid process **(Figure 4-2).** Not shown here, the lobule is retracted posteriorly using a 2-0 silk suture to visualize the mastoid tip and cartilaginous ear canal.

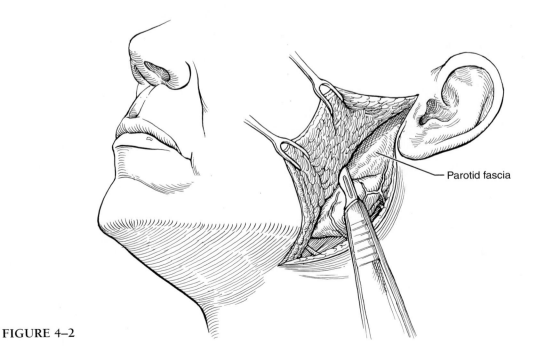

Parotid fascia

FIGURE 4–2

2. DISSECTION

♦ For a parotidectomy to be performed safely, wide exposure and knowledge of important anatomic landmarks are key.

♦ The operation begins in the plane deep to the tail of the parotid. The fascia along the anterior border of the SCM muscle is incised, exposing the muscle toward the level of the mastoid process. Electrocautery can be used in this dissection **(Figure 4-3)**.

♦ The great auricular nerve and external jugular vein are identified at this time. If the nerve has multiple branches, the posterior branch is preserved to maintain sensation to the external ear. Maximal nerve length is dissected in the event that it is needed for a facial nerve graft (see Figure 4-3).

♦ As the dissection proceeds anteriorly, the tail of the parotid is dissected from the SCM muscle and mastoid process, and the posterior belly of the digastric muscle is exposed. The gland is retracted using an Allis clamp or hemostats (see Figure 4-3).

♦ The posterior belly of the digastric muscle is further exposed toward its origin by retracting the SCM muscle posteriorly and both sharply and bluntly dissecting the tissue overlying the muscle (see Figure 4-3).

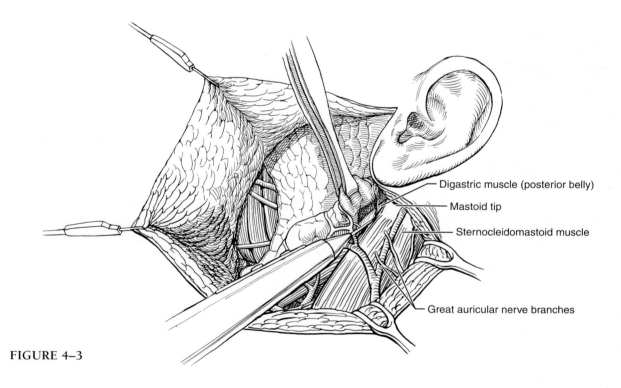

Digastric muscle (posterior belly)

Mastoid tip

Sternocleidomastoid muscle

Great auricular nerve branches

FIGURE 4–3

◆ The posterior aspect of the gland is now dissected from the external auditory canal. The parotid tissue is carefully bluntly and sharply dissected from the ear canal using a fine curved hemostat or scissors and bipolar cautery to maintain hemostasis. It is critical to maintain absolute hemostasis in order to identify the facial nerve trunk without injury **(Figure 4-4)**.

◆ Once the parotid gland is freed from its fibrous attachments, blunt dissection along the ear canal perichondrium using a finger will allow the surgeon to palpate the bony-cartilaginous junction of the ear canal, the tympanomastoid fissure, and the tragal pointer (see Figure 4-4).

◆ The main trunk of the facial nerve is now close by. It is approximately 1 cm deep to the tip of tragal pointer (anterior and inferior), 6 to 8 mm below the end of the tympanomastoid fissure (groove palpated separating the mastoid tip from the tympanic portion of the temporal bone), and just above and on the same plane as the attachment of the digastric muscle in the digastric groove.

◆ The remaining bridge of parotid tissue located between the superior border of the posterior belly of the digastric muscle and the external auditory ear canal is now dissected. The mobilized portions of the parotid gland are retracted anteriorly, putting the residual parotid tissue on stretch. A retractor is placed so that the posterior belly of the digastric muscle is also exposed during this dissection. This tissue is bluntly and sharply dissected, layer by layer, to expose the junction of the superior aspect of the posterior belly of the digastric muscle and the tympanomastoid fissure. The tips of the dissecting instrument face upward and dissection is done along a broad front (see Figure 4-4).

◆ Once the temporoparotid fascia, which runs from the tympanomastoid fissure to the gland, is transected, the parotid tissue is released and the facial nerve will be easily identified (see Figure 4-4).

◆ The nerve stimulator should be used only if there is a question as to the identity of the main trunk of the facial nerve (see Figure 4-4).

◆ Following identification of the main trunk, dissection proceeds in a plane superficial to the nerve. A curved hemostat or scissors, with tips facing upward, is used to spread the tissue immediately superficial to the nerve, keeping the nerve under direct vision at all times. The main trunk is dissected anteriorly until the pes anserinus is reached. The upper (zygomaticotemporal) and lower (cervicofacial) divisions are identified **(Figure 4-5)**.

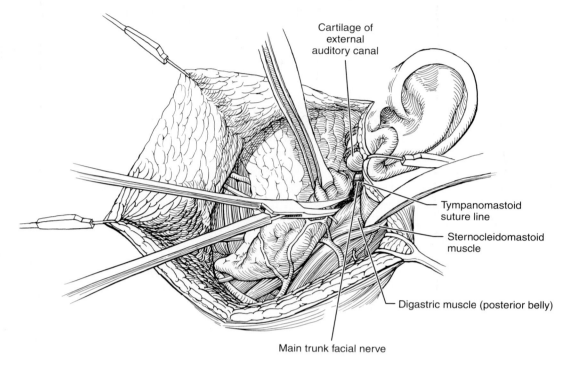

Cartilage of
external
auditory canal

Tympanomastoid
suture line

Sternocleidomastoid
muscle

Digastric muscle (posterior belly)

Main trunk facial nerve

FIGURE 4–4

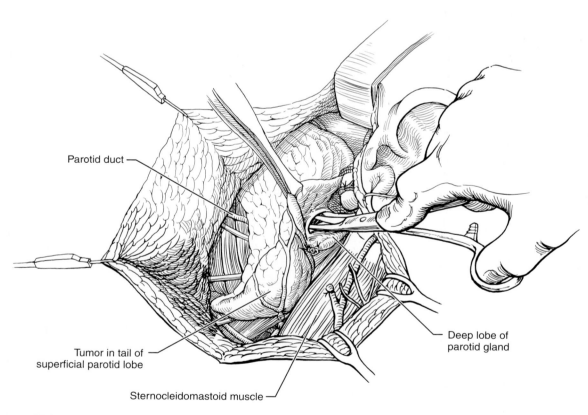

Parotid duct

Tumor in tail of
superficial parotid lobe

Sternocleidomastoid muscle

Deep lobe of
parotid gland

FIGURE 4–5

◆ Dissection of individual facial nerve branches to the periphery of the gland is performed in an orderly fashion. Dissection can proceed from inferior to superior or superior to inferior, depending on tumor location **(Figure 4-6)**.

◆ A fine curved hemostat or scissors is used to dissect just on top of the nerve, elevating the parotid tissue off the nerve. The instrument is opened, spreading the parotid tissue and exposing the nerve. The tissue is cut in a horizontal plane parallel to the nerve. If the nerve is not visualized, do not cut the tissue! Once a nerve branch is completely exposed, the surgeon again returns to the major division where he or she was working and the next nerve branch in sequence is exposed. This is done until all the branches are exposed and the gland is removed. The parotid tissue is retracted forward using Allis clamps and other retractors during this dissection (see Figure 4-6).

◆ In this example, the benign tumor is located in the tail of the parotid. The branches of the lower division are dissected and the tumor is removed with a large cuff of parotid tissue. Care should be taken to avoid injury to the marginal mandibular branch when ligating the posterior facial vein. In addition, the "flanking maneuver" (swinging around the tail of the parotid) should also be avoided because it may also result in injury to the marginal mandibular branch (most common site of injury). A complete superficial parotidectomy with dissection of all of the upper division nerve branches is unnecessary in this case **(Figure 4-7)**.

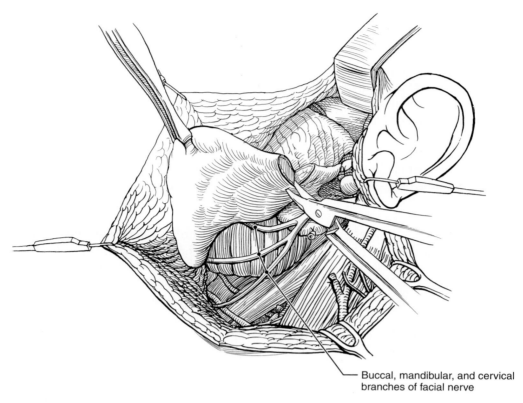

Buccal, mandibular, and cervical branches of facial nerve

FIGURE 4–6

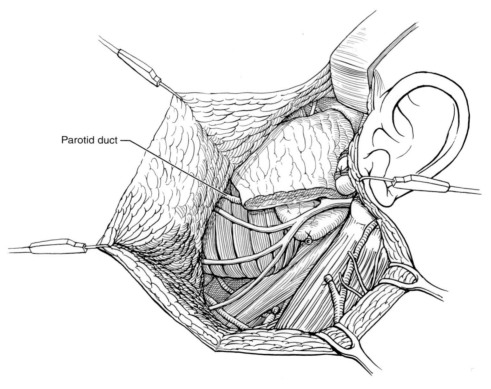

Parotid duct

FIGURE 4–7

3. DEEP LOBE PAROTIDECTOMY

- All branches of the upper and lower divisions of the facial nerve are systematically dissected, and the entire lateral lobe of the parotid is removed when the tumor located in the lateral lobe dictates it and in cases in which a total parotidectomy is required (deep lobe tumor, malignancy, chronic parotitis). The superficial lobe is sent as a separate specimen **(Figure 4-8)**.

- Stensen's duct is transected at the anterior border of the gland and ligated. Care is taken not to injure the buccal branch of the nerve that runs parallel to Stensen's duct (see Figure 4-8).

- To remove the deep lobe of the parotid, the surgeon very delicately and meticulously dissects the main trunk of the facial nerve and its branches to free them from the deep lobe.

- After each branch is completely freed from the deep lobe, the surgeon uses gentle retraction using a vein retractor, nerve hook, or very small vessel loops to lift the nerves, allowing blunt and sharp dissection and mobilization of the deep lobe. Excessive retraction of the nerves will result in a stretch injury (see Figure 4-8).

- The gland may be dissected from the stylohyoid and stylopharyngeus muscles. During dissection of the deep lobe the following vessels may be encountered: the superficial temporal vessels, the internal maxillary artery (running deep to mandibular ramus), the occipital artery, the posterior auricular artery, and the pterygoid plexus of veins. Bleeding can be substantial, and patience must be used in identifying and controlling the bleeding vessel to avoid inadvertent injury to the nerve **(Figure 4-9)**.

- Removal of the deep lobe may be accomplished inferior to, superior to, or between facial nerve branches (see Figure 4-9).

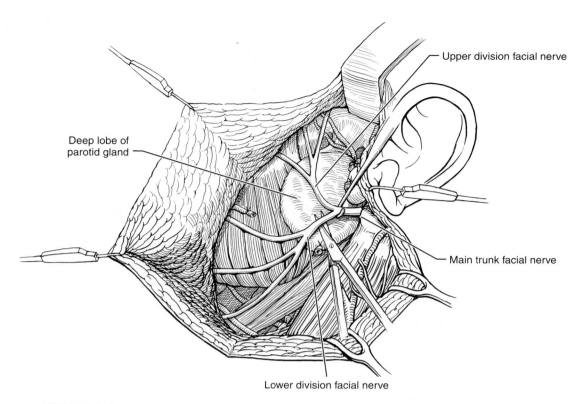

Upper division facial nerve

Deep lobe of parotid gland

Main trunk facial nerve

Lower division facial nerve

FIGURE 4–8

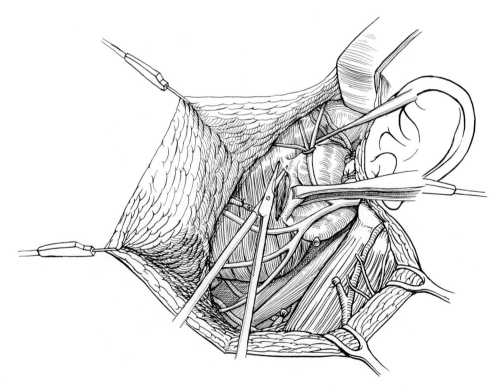

FIGURE 4–9

◆ A thin layer of masseter muscle (margin) is removed when dealing with recurrent benign tumors, and a larger margin or the entire muscle is removed if the lesion is malignant **(Figure 4-10)**.

◆ Stensen's duct is followed through the buccinator muscle to the mucosa in cases of chronic and recurrent sialadenitis associated with sialolithiasis (stones).

4. RADICAL PAROTIDECTOMY

◆ Radical parotidectomy (total parotidectomy with facial nerve sacrifice) is indicated in cases of malignant involvement of the main trunk of the facial nerve. Sacrifice of one or all of the peripheral nerve branches without sacrifice of the main trunk is indicated when the nerve branches are involved but the main trunk is not.

◆ Intraoperative frozen section analysis are performed on all proximal and distal nerve stumps to ensure negative margins. The branches are tagged with a fine suture so that they may be easily located intraoperatively for facial nerve grafting.

◆ Mastoidectomy may be necessary to obtain clear proximal facial nerve margins.

◆ The great auricular or sural nerve can be used to reconstruct the facial nerve. The main trunk and the marginal mandibular, buccal, and temporal branches are reconstructed to restore oral competency and eye closure. However, reconstruction of the facial nerve branches anterior to lateral canthus is not required.

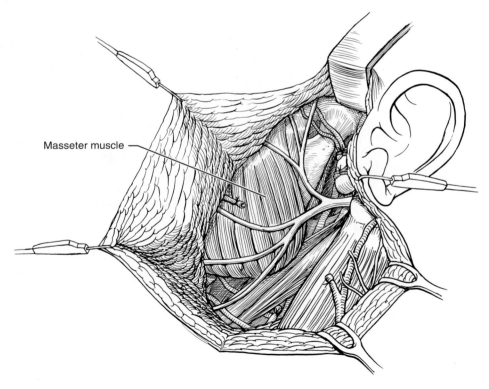

Masseter muscle

FIGURE 4–10

5. CLOSING

- The main trunk of the facial nerve is stimulated (0.5 mA) to prove that all branches are intact before the wound is closed. If some or all of the branches do not respond to stimulation, careful inspection to ensure anatomic integrity of nerve is performed.

- The skin is closed in two layers using fast absorbing versus monofilament suture. Care is taken to accurately reapproximate the lobule.

- A 10-mm Jackson-Pratt drain is placed via a separate stab incision in the postauricular area. Care is taken to avoid placement of the drain next to the nerve.

- A figure-of-eight pressure dressing is placed around the neck, face, and head.

STEP 4: POSTOPERATIVE CARE

- Facial nerve function is evaluated as soon as the patient is awake and cooperative.

- If facial nerve paresis or paralysis is noted, steroids may be given only if the facial nerve is known to be intact. If it is possible that the main trunk or nerve branch was transected during surgery, immediate exploration and repair of nerve must be performed.

- Pressure dressing is removed the next morning.

- Closed suction drain is removed when output is less than 15 to 30 mL over 24 hours.

- If eye closure is poor (neuropraxia, nerve sacrifice), saline drops are used multiple times per day, and Lacri-Lube and eye taping are prescribed nightly to prevent exposure keratitis.

STEP 5: PEARLS AND PITFALLS

- A nerve integrity monitor and magnification (loupe or microscope) may be used to aid in facial nerve identification and preservation, particularly in reoperations and cases of chronic infection with scarring.

- Overuse of the facial nerve stimulator can cause neuropraxia.

◆ If the tumor location precludes identification of the main trunk of the facial nerve using standard techniques, the main trunk can be identified using retrograde dissection along the temporal, buccal, or marginal mandibular branch (most common) or via mastoidectomy.

◆ Parotid specimen and/or lymph nodes are sent for intraoperative frozen section analysis if malignancy is suspected.

◆ The posterior auricular artery or its branch can cross the main trunk of the facial nerve and cause significant bleeding and inadvertent injury to the nerve if not properly identified and ligated.

◆ Facial paralysis or paresis can result from aggressive dissection or inadvertent injury of the nerve. Recovery of facial nerve paresis/paralysis can occur over 3 to 4 weeks if neuropraxic injury and up to 1 year if axon death has occurred.

◆ Hematoma formation, manifested by acute postoperative pain, swelling of flap, and oozing from wound, demands reexploration and evacuation. Hematoma can cause airway compression if significant. Extreme care must be taken to avoid injury to the exposed facial nerve.

◆ Skin flap necrosis is rare but can occur in heavy smokers and in the postauricular area when the skin flap is too thin and the skin incision is made at an acute angle.

◆ Frey's syndrome (gustatory sweating) is associated with sweating in the area of skin overlying the parotid bed. Most patients have this to some degree, and it is typically subclinical. It occurs because of the aberrant regrowth of parasympathetic motor fibers from the auriculo-temporal nerve into the sympathetic nerve fibers controlling sweat glands. Raising thicker subcutaneous flaps may reduce its occurrence. Medical therapy includes topical scopolamine. Surgical remedies are rarely successful (dermal graft, tympanic neurectomy).

◆ Postoperative sialocele or salivary fistula (salivary drainage from wound) is rare and can usually be successfully managed with aspiration and compression dressings. Atropine-like drugs may be beneficial.

SELECTED REFERENCES

1. Johnson JT: Parotid. In Myers EN, Carrau RL (eds): Operative Otolaryngology: Head and Neck Surgery, 1st ed. Philadelphia, Saunders, 1997, pp 504-518.
2. Olsen KD: Parotid superficial lobectomy. In Bailey BJ, Calhoun KH, Coffey AR, Neely JG: Atlas of Head & Neck Surgery—Otolaryngology. Baltimore, Lippincott-Raven, 1996, pp 2-11.
3. Lore JM, Medina J: The parotid salivary gland and management of malignant salivary gland neoplasia. In Lore JM, Medina J (eds): An Atlas of Head and Neck Surgery, 4th ed. Philadelphia, Saunders, 2005, pp 861-891.
4. Olsen KD: Superficial parotidectomy. Oper Tech Gen Surg 2004;6:102-114.
5. Shah JP, Patel SG: Salivary glands. In Shah JP, Patel SG (eds): Head and Neck Surgery and Oncology, 3rd ed. Edinburgh, Mosby, 2003, pp 439-474.

CHAPTER 5

TRACHEOTOMY

Anna M. Pou

STEP 1: SURGICAL ANATOMY

- The following landmarks are useful in performing a tracheotomy or cricothyroidotomy (**Figure 5-1**):
  - Hyoid bone
  - Thyroid notch
  - Cricoid cartilage
  - Sternal notch

- The thyroid isthmus overlies the anterior trachea at the level of the first tracheal ring.

- See Figure 1-2 for demonstration of the relationship of the trachea to the thyroid gland, esophagus, and great vessels in the neck.

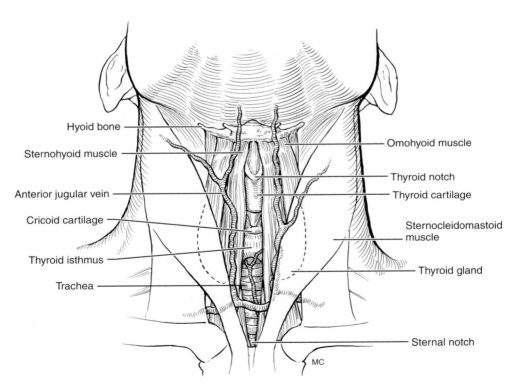

Hyoid bone

Sternohyoid muscle

Anterior jugular vein

Cricoid cartilage

Thyroid isthmus

Trachea

Omohyoid muscle

Thyroid notch

Thyroid cartilage

Sternocleidomastoid muscle

Thyroid gland

Sternal notch

MC

FIGURE 5–1

STEP 2: PREOPERATIVE CONSIDERATIONS

- Indications:
  - Respiratory failure with ventilator dependence
  - Airway obstruction: edema, trauma, tumor, hematoma

- Status of cervical spine:
  - If status of cervical spine is in question, seek neurosurgical clearance before extending the neck.
  - In patients with a cervical spine injury, the neck remains in a neutral position and the head and neck are stabilized with sandbags.

- If the patient has had a previous tracheotomy, the operative report is reviewed with attention to the level of the tracheotomy and the presence of anatomic abnormalities.

- A vertical, rather than horizontal, skin incision is useful in the following cases: (1) redo tracheotomies, because it gives a larger area of exposure, which is helpful when dealing with scar tissue; (2) in patients whose landmarks are not easily palpated; and (3) in infants and children.

- Local, awake tracheotomy should be considered in patients with laryngeal obstruction (edema, tumor) who are not in acute airway distress and who are determined to be difficult fiber-optic intubations.

- "High" tracheotomies are performed in patients with laryngeal carcinoma so that maximal tracheal length can be preserved for stoma construction in the event a total laryngectomy is required for treatment.

- The size of the tracheotomy tube is decided preoperatively (a size 6 cuffed tube is usually placed in a woman, and a size 8 cuffed tube is usually placed in a man). An extended-length tracheotomy tube may be necessary in patients with large necks and should be available in the operating room before the tracheotomy is performed.

- The cuff of the tracheotomy tube is tested before use.

- The surgeon and anesthesiologist discuss the surgical plan preoperatively; the airway is shared by both parties.

STEP 3: OPERATIVE STEPS

1. INCISION

- The patient is placed supine. The neck is extended using a shoulder roll and the head is stabilized using a doughnut cushion.

- The anesthesiologist should be at the head of the table to maintain control of the airway.

- The surgical site is sterilely prepped with betadine and draped in such a manner that the anesthesiologist has easy access in the event reintubation becomes necessary.

- Using a sterile marking pen, the surgeon outlines the previously mentioned landmarks on the neck and a 2-cm horizontal skin incision 2 fingerbreadths above the sternal notch **(Figure 5-2).**

- The skin incision and subcutaneous tissues are injected with 1% lidocaine with 1:100,000 epinephrine.

- The skin incision is made using a no.10 scalpel blade and extends through the underlying subcutaneous tissues (see Figure 5-2).

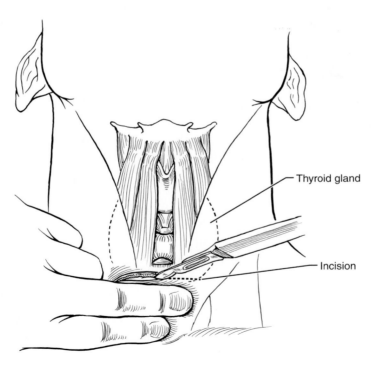

FIGURE 5–2

2. DISSECTION

◆ The superior and inferior skin flaps are retracted **(Figure 5-3)**.

◆ A vertical incision is made in the midline fascia between the strap muscles. This is usually a bloodless plane (see Figure 5-3).

◆ The strap muscles and, typically, the anterior jugular veins are retracted laterally (see Figure 5-3).

◆ The dissection proceeds vertically in the midline through the pretracheal tissue and fat. The lateral retractors are placed deeper in the wound as the dissection proceeds to a deeper level.

◆ The cricoid cartilage and thyroid isthmus are encountered **(Figure 5-4)**.

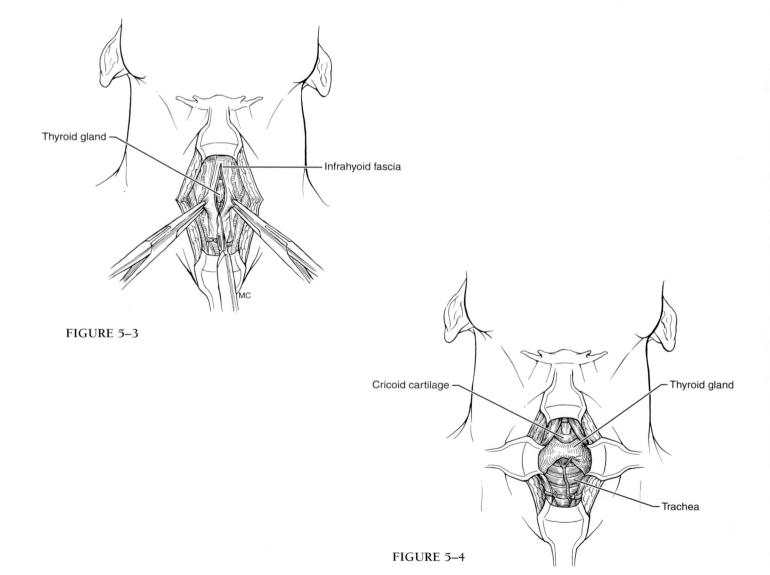

FIGURE 5–3

FIGURE 5–4

◆ The isthmus is retracted superiorly using an Allis clamp (**Figure 5-5, A**).

◆ If the isthmus is difficult to retract, it is transected. A horizontal incision is made in the anterior suspensory ligament of the thyroid, which is between the inferior edge of the cricoid cartilage and the isthmus. A curved hemostat is used to dissect the thyroid isthmus from the anterior surface of the trachea (**Figure 5-5, B**), and the thyroid isthmus is transected using electrocautery. Care is taken to not violate the anterior surface of the trachea or to pass the hemostat deep to the cricoid cartilage.

◆ The pretracheal tissue is palpated in this area for a "high-riding" innominate artery before the tracheotomy incision is made.

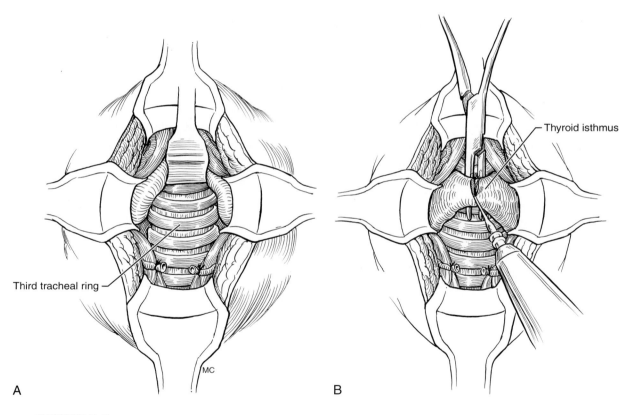

A   B

FIGURE 5–5

◆ The anterior surface of the trachea is further cleaned; the tracheal fascia is incised vertically in the midline and bluntly dissected laterally.

◆ A 2-mL injection of 4% lidocaine plain is given intraluminally. This is especially important in awake patients to prevent coughing and anxiety while placing the tracheotomy tube.

◆ Before entering the airway, the surgeon notifies the anesthesiologist and the scrub nurse so that the remainder of the procedure can proceed in a highly organized fashion. All necessary instruments and the previously tested tracheotomy tube should be readily available and placed in the order of need on the Mayo stand.

◆ The anesthesiologist untapes the endotracheal tube (ETT), holds it in place, and waits for instructions from the surgeon. All extraneous noise in the room should cease.

◆ A horizontal incision (5 to 8 mm in length) is made directly above the tracheal ring of choice (second, third, or fourth) using a no. 15 scalpel blade, taking care not to puncture the cuff on the ETT **(Figure 5-6, A).**

◆ The incision continues in a manner necessary to remove an anterior portion of the ring (Figure 5-6, B). An alternative method is to perform a broad, inferiorly based, U-shaped flap extending the length of one tracheal ring (Figure 5-6, C).

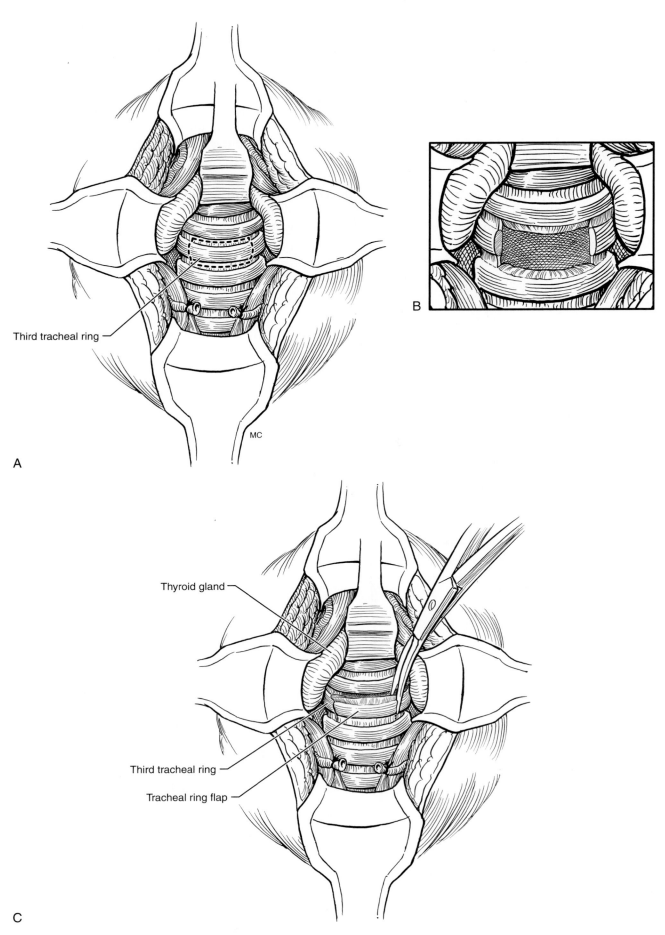

Third tracheal ring

MC

A

B

Thyroid gland

Third tracheal ring

Tracheal ring flap

C

FIGURE 5–6

◆ The trachea is delivered into the wound and stabilized using the retractors already in place or a cricoid hook **(Figure 5-7)**. (The thyroid isthmus was removed in the figure for visualization of the underlying cricoid cartilage.)

◆ A 2-0 silk suture is placed through the inferior and superior tracheal rings, from outside to inside the lumen. The needles are removed and the sutures are not cut; the ends are brought out through the wound and can be used for retraction **(Figure 5-8)**.

◆ The ETT is now withdrawn under direct visualization. The cuff is deflated and ventilation is stopped. The surgeon instructs the anesthesiologist to slowly withdraw the ETT until the tip is seen immediately above the tracheotomy incision and no farther.

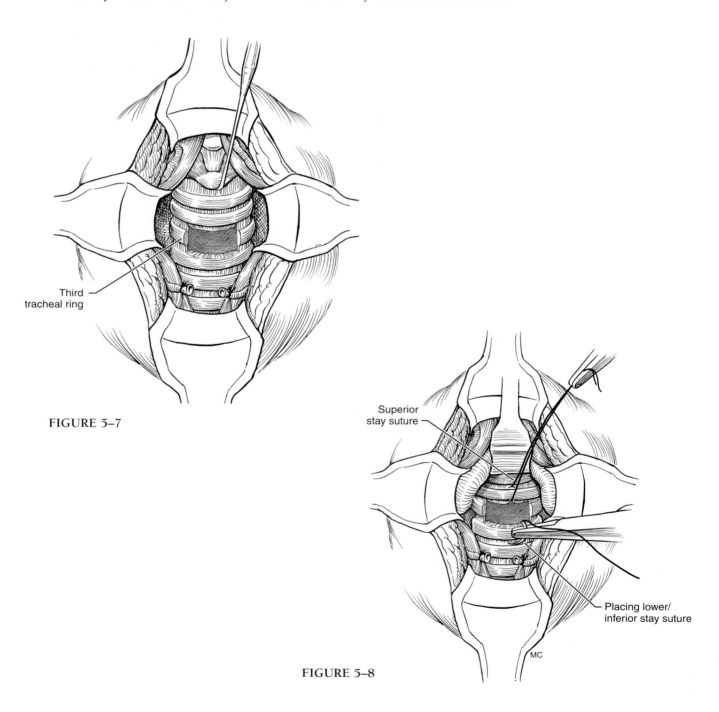

Third tracheal ring

FIGURE 5–7

Superior stay suture

Placing lower/ inferior stay suture

MC

FIGURE 5–8

◆ The surgeon places the tracheotomy tube (with obturator in place) into the airway under direct visualization. The tube is introduced at a right angle and then turned inferiorly **(Figure 5-9)**.

◆ Once the tube is in place, the obturator is removed, the inner cannula is placed, the cuff is inflated, and the anesthesia circuit is hooked to the tracheotomy tube. The return of carbon dioxide following ventilation is confirmed, and the chest is auscultated for the presence of bilateral breath sounds. Confirmation is required before completely removing the ETT from the airway.

◆ Tracheotomy ties are placed around the neck, and the flanges of the tracheotomy tube are also sewn to the skin as an extra precaution to prevent accidental decannulation **(Figure 5-10)**.

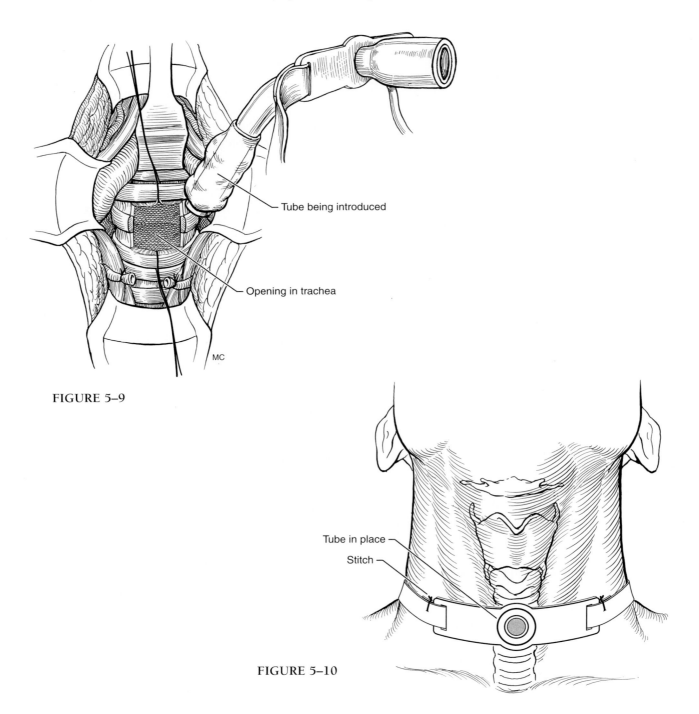

Tube being introduced

Opening in trachea

MC

FIGURE 5–9

Tube in place

Stitch

FIGURE 5–10

3. CLOSING

- Not applicable.

STEP 4: POSTOPERATIVE CARE

- The "stay sutures" are taped to the inferior and superior skin flaps, respectively. The pieces of tape have "Do Not Remove" written on them so that these sutures can be used to retract the trachea in the event of accidental decannulation.

- Postoperative orders should include the following:
  - Tracheal suctioning every shift and as needed (prn). Patient may require tracheal suctioning every hour in the immediate postoperative period. Preoxygenation with 100% oxygen may be necessary.
  - Saline irrigation is used before suctioning to lubricate the trachea and suction catheter and to thin secretions in selected patients (copious, thick secretions).
  - The inner cannula must be changed/cleaned every shift and prn.
  - Continual humidification via a tracheotomy collar to prevent mucous plug and obstruction of inner cannula with dried secretions.

- Gauze dressing is placed under the tracheotomy flange to keep the area clean. Care is taken not to dislodge the tube when changing this dressing.

- Regarding ventilator-dependent patients, the tracheotomy tubing is stabilized to prevent subglottic and/or tracheal stenosis and accidental dislodgment of the tube.

- The cuff pressure should be minimal to prevent tracheal necrosis and resultant subglottic and/or tracheal stenosis.

- Tracheotomy care is taught to the patient and his or her caregiver(s) as soon as possible.

- The "stay sutures" are removed on postoperative day 5.

- Speech pathology is consulted to address speech and swallowing problems associated with tracheotomy.

STEP 5: PEARLS AND PITFALLS

- Complications include the following:
  - Injury to the esophagus or great vessels intraoperatively. This is rare but can occur in operative fields filled with scar tissue or tumor and in emergent cases.
  - Pneumothorax

- Bleeding: cut edge of thyroid or trachea (early); tracheo–innominate artery fistula (late)
- Infection: tracheitis
- Mucous plug
- Accidental decannulation (may result in death)
- Aspiration

- In morbidly obese patients, pretracheal fat is excised to decrease the amount of subcutaneous tissue lying between the cervical skin incision and the tracheotomy. In rare patients, submental skin and fat must be excised before the tracheotomy to prevent obstruction of the tracheotomy tube postoperatively by soft tissue.

- A saline-filled syringe with a small-gauge needle can be used to localize the trachea in a badly scarred neck (previous surgery, infection, radiation therapy, or a combination). The needle is placed in the presumed tracheal lumen and the plunger is withdrawn. The presence of air bubbles in the syringe confirms the location of the tracheal lumen.

- If there is difficulty placing the tracheotomy tube, the anesthesiologist is instructed to advance the ETT and resume ventilation. The cuff of the ETT should be past the tracheotomy incision so that air does not escape from the wound.

- If it is difficult to place the tracheotomy tube and the ETT cannot be advanced distal to the tracheotomy site, a small ETT (size 4 or 5) can be placed through the tracheotomy incision to ventilate the patient. Troubleshooting can then commence with the patient under stable conditions.

- When a local awake tracheotomy is performed, the patient's face is left undraped (a towel is placed over the chin) to allow the anesthesiologist access for mask ventilation and emergent intubation.

SELECTED REFERENCES

1. Myers EN: Tracheostomy. In Myers EN (ed): Operative Otolaryngology: Head and Neck Surgery. Philadelphia, Saunders, 1997, pp 575-585.
2. Morris WM: Cricothyroidotomy. In Lore JM, Medina J (eds): An Atlas of Head and Neck Surgery, 4th ed. Philadelphia, Elsevier, 2005, pp 82-83.
3. Tracheostomy. In Lore JM, Medina J (eds): An Atlas of Head and Neck Surgery, 4th ed. Philadelphia, Elsevier, 2005, pp 1015-1023.
4. McWhorter AJ: Tracheotomy: Timing and techniques. Curr Opin Otolaryngol Head Neck Surg 2003;11:473-479.

CHAPTER 6

CRICOTHYROIDOTOMY

Anna M. Pou

STEP 1: SURGICAL ANATOMY

- The following landmarks are useful in performing a tracheotomy or cricothyroidotomy (**Figure 6-1**):
  - Hyoid bone
  - Thyroid notch
  - Cricoid cartilage
  - Sternal notch

- The thyroid isthmus overlies the anterior trachea at the level of the first tracheal ring.

- The relationship of the trachea to the thyroid gland, esophagus, and great vessels in the neck are demonstrated in Figure 1-2.

STEP 2: PREOPERATIVE CONSIDERATIONS

- Indications:
  - Acute airway obstruction above the level of the cricoid cartilage (glottis, supraglottis)
  - Elective procedure following median sternotomy

- The surgeon must be prepared to perform this procedure with the patient in a semirecumbent or sitting position.

- Because of the emergent nature of this procedure, the surgeon must maintain calm and remain in charge. This rarely takes place in the operating room.

- Necessary instruments include good lighting.

- Small endotracheal tubes (ETTs) should be available. A small ETT is placed to prevent fracture of the cricoid cartilage.

- See tracheotomy procedure (Chapter 5).

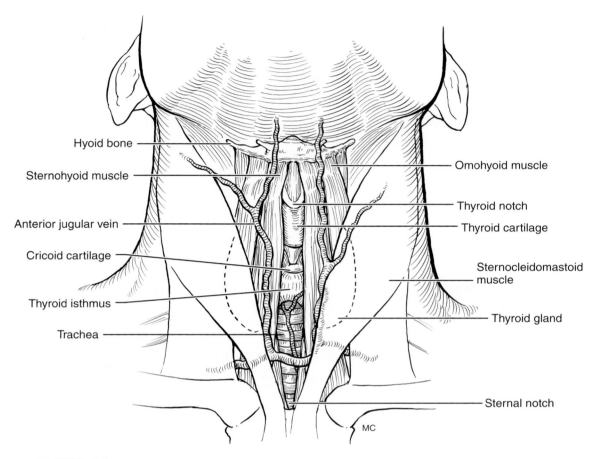

Hyoid bone

Sternohyoid muscle

Anterior jugular vein

Cricoid cartilage

Thyroid isthmus

Trachea

Omohyoid muscle

Thyroid notch

Thyroid cartilage

Sternocleidomastoid muscle

Thyroid gland

Sternal notch

MC

FIGURE 6–1

STEP 3: OPERATIVE STEPS

1. INCISION

♦ The patient is placed supine. The neck is extended using a shoulder roll, and the head is stabilized using a doughnut-shaped cushion.

♦ The anesthesiologist is positioned at the head of the table.

♦ The patient's neck is cleaned with betadine and draped in sterile fashion if patient is stable.

♦ The landmarks in the neck are palpated and the skin overlying the cricothyroid (CT) membrane is marked using a sterile marking pen.

♦ The skin and subcutaneous tissue is anesthetized with 1% lidocaine with 1:100,000 epinephrine.

♦ The skin overlying the CT membrane is "put on stretch," with the surgeon using the nondominant hand, and a horizontal skin incision is made using a no. 15 scalpel blade **(Figure 6-2, A)**. A vertical, rather than horizontal skin incision, is useful in patients whose landmarks are not easily palpated due to trauma, hematoma, or obesity **(Figure 6-2, B)**.

2. DISSECTION

♦ Using an index finger, the surgeon palpates the CT membrane in the wound **(Figure 6-2, C)**.

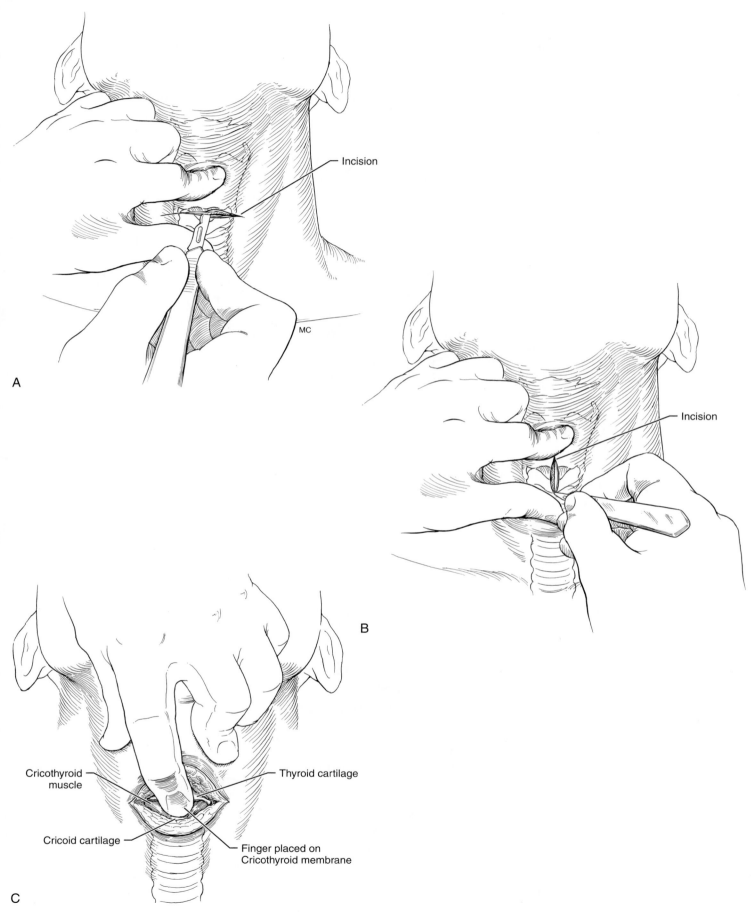

A

B

C

Incision

MC

Incision

Cricothyroid
muscle

Thyroid cartilage

Cricoid cartilage

Finger placed on
Cricothyroid membrane

FIGURE 6–2

- The CT membrane is cut horizontally using a no. 15 scalpel blade (**Figure 6-3**).

- A hemostat is placed in the CT membrane and the tissue is spread open (**Figure 6-4**).

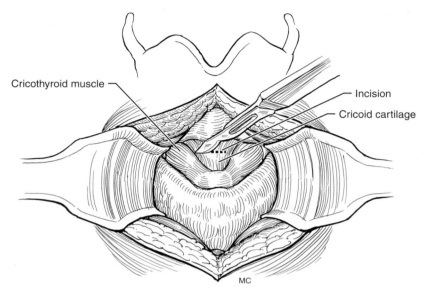

FIGURE 6–3

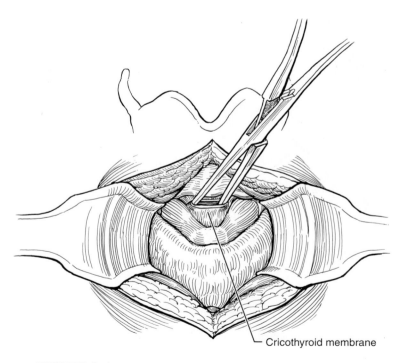

FIGURE 6–4

- A small ETT is placed in the incision (**Figure 6-5**).

- Placement is confirmed with the return of CO_2 and the auscultation of bilateral breath sounds.

- The tube is secured.

3. CLOSING

- Not applicable.

STEP 4: POSTOPERATIVE CARE

- The cricothyroidotomy is converted to a formal tracheotomy as soon as possible.

- See tracheotomy procedure (Chapter 5).

- If the previously described process is delayed, the ETT is replaced with a small tracheotomy tube.

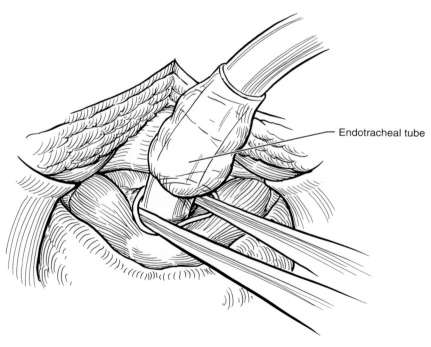

Endotracheal tube

FIGURE 6–5

STEP 5: PEARLS AND PITFALLS

- Complications:
  - Subglottic stenosis
  - Chondritis
  - Bleeding
  - Cricoid fracture

- If the landmarks are nonpalpable or there is a hematoma present, a vertical midline incision is made to gain wider exposure (see Figure 6-2, C). This incision can be extended if necessary.

SELECTED REFERENCES

1. Myers EN: Tracheostomy. In Myers EN (ed): Operative Otolaryngology: Head and Neck Surgery. Philadelphia, WB Saunders, 1997, pp 575-585.
2. Morris WM: Cricothyroidotomy. In Lore JM, Medina J (eds): An Atlas of Head and Neck Surgery, 4th ed. Philadelphia, Elsevier, 2005, pp 82-83.
3. Tracheostomy. In Lore JM, Medina J (eds): An Atlas of Head and Neck Surgery, 4th ed. Philadelphia, Elsevier, 2005, pp 1015-1023.
4. McWhorter AJ: Tracheotomy: Timing and techniques. Curr Opin Otolaryngol Head Neck Surg 2003;11:473-479.

CHAPTER 7

THYROGLOSSAL DUCT CYST

Dai H. Chung

STEP 1: SURGICAL ANATOMY

- The thyroglossal duct is a persistent remnant of the thyroid gland's embryologic descending tract from the floor of the pharynx to its final position in the neck. Thyroglossal duct cysts occur most commonly in the midline, just inferior to the level of the hyoid bone.

STEP 2: PREOPERATIVE CONSIDERATIONS

- The exact location of the thyroid gland should be determined clinically, because aberrant ectopic thyroid tissue may be mistaken for a thyroglossal cyst.

- When a thyroglossal cyst is infected, it should be first treated with antibiotics and/or surgical drainage before complete excision.

- Imaging studies are not necessary (unless clinical examination findings are suspicious for aberrant ectopic thyroid).

STEP 3: OPERATIVE STEPS

1. INCISION

- This operation (Sistrunk procedure) is performed with the patient under general anesthesia.

- The patient is positioned supine and the neck is hyperextended by placing a shoulder roll.

◆ A transverse skin incision is made over the cyst; however, caution should be used to avoid making a skin incision over the main prominence of the cyst, well away from the hyoid bone (**Figure 7-1**).

◆ The subcutaneous dissection through the platysma is carried out using scissors and cautery. Deep cervical fascia is cut in the midline to expose the cyst (**Figure 7-2**).

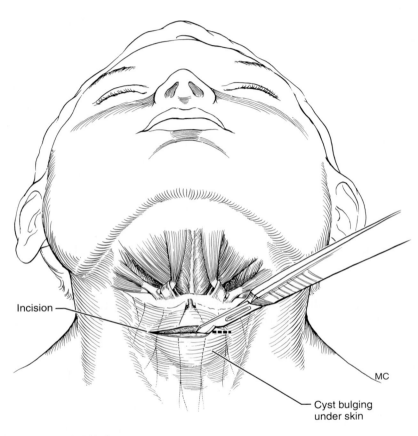

Incision

MC

Cyst bulging under skin

FIGURE 7–1

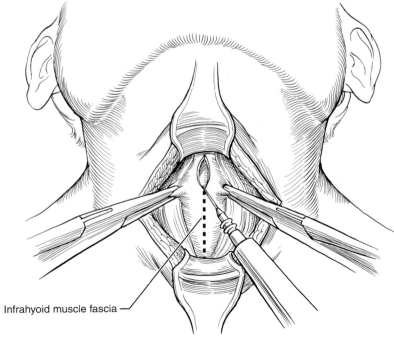

Infrahyoid muscle fascia

FIGURE 7–2

2. DISSECTION

◆ The cyst is dissected away from surrounding superficial attachments and followed between the sternohyoid muscles to the hyoid bone **(Figures 7-3 and 7-4)**. The central portion of the hyoid bone is freed from strap muscle attachments (sternohyoid muscle inferiorly and mylohyoid, geniohyoid muscles superiorly). After freeing up the posterior plane of the hyoid bone from the thyrohyoid membrane, the surgeon resects the central portion (1 to 1.5 cm) of the hyoid bone along with the thyroglossal duct attachment **(Figure 7-5)**.

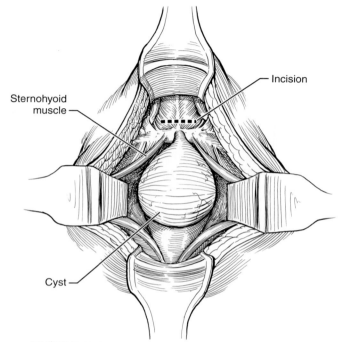

FIGURE 7–3

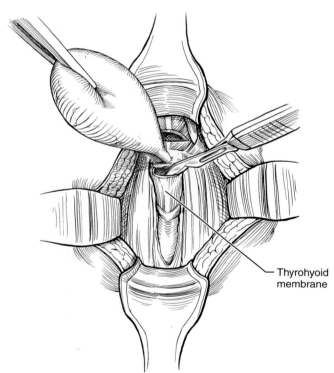

FIGURE 7–4

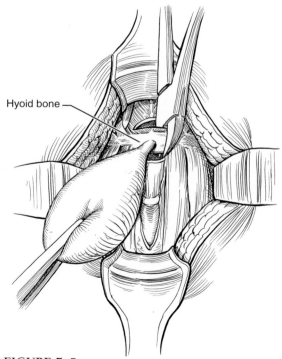

FIGURE 7–5

◆ The dissection is continued caudally toward the base of the tongue (**Figure 7-6**) and the remaining duct is ligated with absorbable sutures (**Figure 7-7**).

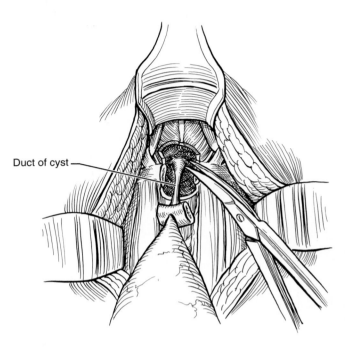

Duct of cyst

FIGURE 7–6

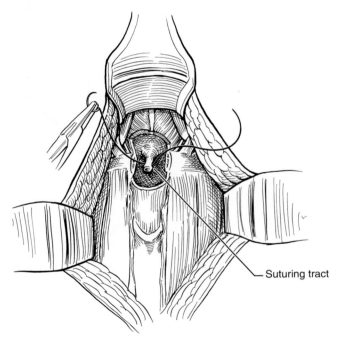

Suturing tract

FIGURE 7–7

3. CLOSING

- After meticulous hemostasis, including at the cut ends of the hyoid bone, fascia is approximated in the midline using 3-0 polyglycolic acid sutures. After approximation of platysma using 4-0 polyglycolic acid sutures, subcuticular skin closure is performed. No drain is used.

STEP 4: POSTOPERATIVE CARE

- This procedure is routinely performed as an outpatient procedure.

STEP 5: PEARLS AND PITFALLS

- Resection of the central portion of hyoid bone with the thyroglossal duct specimen is essential.

- Meticulous hemostasis must be achieved before wound closure to avoid postoperative hematoma.

- Rule out presence of aberrant ectopic midline thyroid gland.

SELECTED REFERENCES

1. Foley DS, Fallat ME: Thyroglossal duct and other congenital midline cervical anomalies. Semin Pediatr Surg 2006;15:70-75.
2. Bratu I, Laberge JM: Day surgery for thyroglossal duct cyst excision: A safe alternative. Pediatr Surg Int 2004;20:675-678.
3. Ostlie DJ, Burjonrappa SC, Snyder CL, et al: Thyroglossal duct infections and surgical outcomes. J Pediatr Surg 2004;39:396-399.
4. Sistrunk WE: The surgical management of cysts of the thyroglossal tract. Ann Surg 1920;71:121-123.

CHAPTER 8

ADRENALS—ANTERIOR, POSTERIOR (OPEN AND LAPAROSCOPIC)

Michael D. Trahan

STEP 1: SURGICAL ANATOMY

- Successful adrenalectomy requires a precise knowledge of the anatomy of the retroperitoneal space, the anatomic relationships of the adrenals to the surrounding structures, and the differences in the blood supply to the two glands (**Figure 8-1**).

- The arterial supply to the adrenal glands enters the perimeter of the gland originating from multiple sources including the inferior phrenic and renal arteries and directly from the aorta. These are named the superior, inferior, and middle adrenal arteries, respectively.

- The right adrenal vein is very short and enters the vena cava on its posterior lateral aspect. This vein does not necessarily get longer as an adrenal mass gets bigger. A large mass can make identification of the vein very difficult and potentially hazardous. Great care should be used to get control of this structure early in the dissection to avoid catastrophic hemorrhage on the posterior aspect of the vena cava.

- The left adrenal vein is longer than the right. It is joined by the left inferior phrenic vein before it drains into the left renal vein.

STEP 2: PREOPERATIVE CONSIDERATIONS

- The indications for adrenalectomy include:
  - Select adrenal cancers
  - All biologically active adrenal masses
  - Adrenal metastases
  - Incidentally found masses more than 4 to 5 cm
  - Primary adrenal hyperplasia

- The choice of surgical approach (open vs. laparoscopic, anterior vs. posterior) depends on a number of factors including surgical training/experience, pathology, and presence of contraindications to laparoscopic surgery.

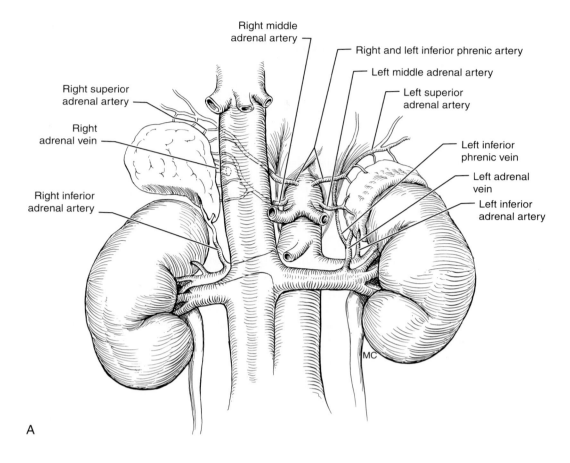

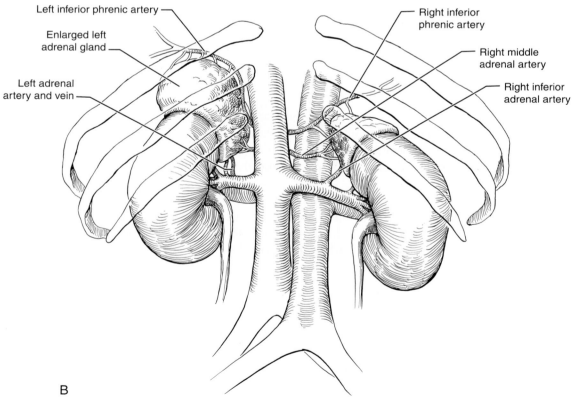

FIGURE 8–1

- Unilateral adrenalectomy is perfectly suited for the laparoscopic approach because of the small size of most adrenal masses and the large incision necessary for open excision.

- Resection of an adrenal cancer should include en bloc resection of involved organs. Such an extensive resection is best performed with an open approach.

- Patients with pheochromocytomas must be medicated preoperatively with phenoxybenzamine (alpha blocker) for 7 days or longer to control hypertension. If tachycardia is present once the blood pressure is controlled, a beta blocker is added for another 5 days before operation.

- A stress dose of glucocorticoids should be given preoperatively to all patients with hypercortisolism.

- Routine prophylaxis against deep venous thrombosis and pulmonary thromboembolism is standard of care.

- Preoperative intercostal nerve blocks or placement of an epidural catheter should be considered for the open approaches to help with postoperative pain control.

STEP 3: OPERATIVE STEPS

1. INCISION

- Unilateral adrenalectomy is approached laparoscopically in most cases. The patient is placed in the lateral decubitus position with the table flexed. The open flank incision in the lateral decubitus position or the posterior approach in the prone position is favored for larger masses (>10 cm), which have a higher malignant potential.

- Bilateral adrenalectomy is often approached through a midline or bilateral subcostal incision with the patient in the supine position. The laparoscopic approach can be used, but the patient usually must be repositioned into the contralateral decubitus position after the first side is complete.

- Four ports are usually sufficient for the laparoscopic approach. The size of the trocars will depend on the size of the available instrumentation (scopes, clipping device, right-angle dissector, liver retractor, retrieval bag) and the size of the lesion.

- The incision for the posterior approach is along the ipsilateral 12th rib with the patient appropriately padded in the prone, jackknife position **(Figure 8-2)**.

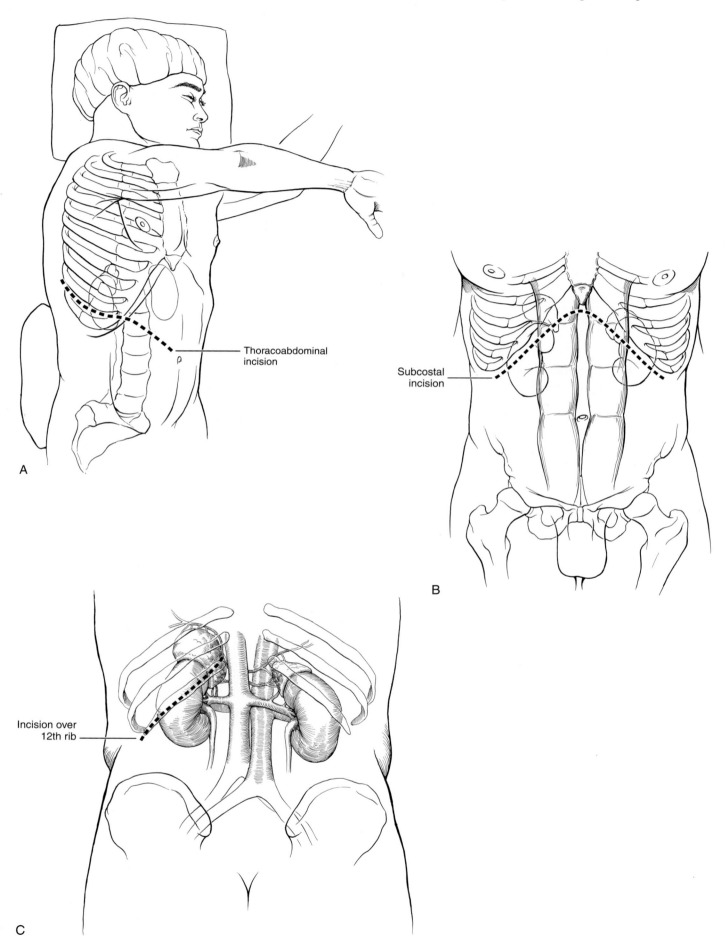

Thoracoabdominal incision

Subcostal incision

Incision over 12th rib

A

B

C

FIGURE 8–2

2. DISSECTION

Laparoscopic Adrenalectomy

◆ The first port (12 mm) is placed using a trocar with internal visualization or by open technique just below the ipsilateral costal margin in the anterior axillary line.

◆ A 12-mm port is placed higher along the costal margin at least a handbreadth from the first. Two 5-mm ports are placed lower along the costal margin down to the posterior axillary line. The left colon will need to be mobilized before the most posterior port can be placed for left-sided operations.

Left-Sided Laparoscopic Operation

◆ The splenic flexure and some of the descending colon need to be mobilized using a combination of sharp and blunt dissection with care used to stay anterior to the kidney. The hook cautery or ultrasonic dissector is used to accomplish this. The spleen and tail of the pancreas are then mobilized by dividing the splenorenal ligament. Gravity will help these organs fall medially and out of the dissection field **(Figure 8-3)**.

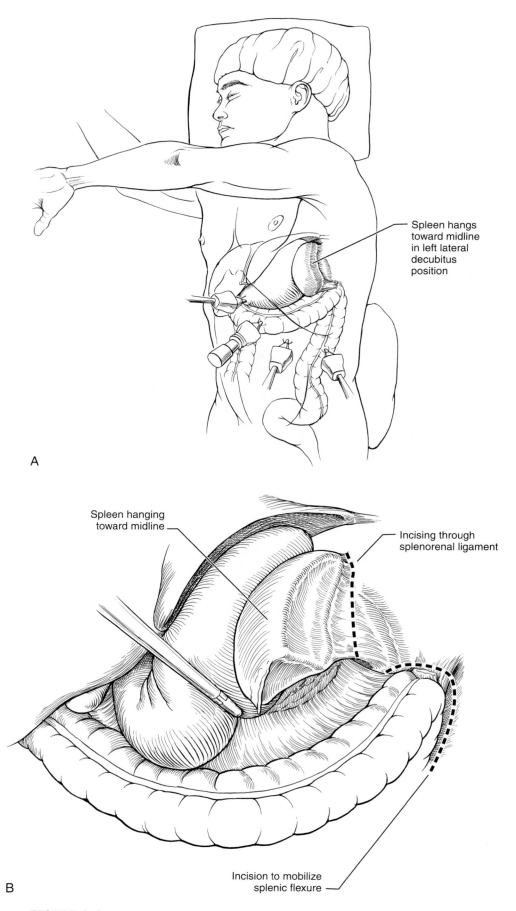

Spleen hangs
toward midline
in left lateral
decubitus
position

A

Spleen hanging
toward midline

Incising through
splenorenal ligament

Incision to mobilize
splenic flexure

B

FIGURE 8–3

◆ Dissection medially between the adrenal gland and the superior pole of the kidney will reveal the adrenal vein, which should be clipped and divided early in the operation **(Figure 8-4).**

◆ The remainder of the gland's blood supply and attachments can be effectively divided with the ultrasonic dissector. Occasionally a larger blood vessel may be encountered that warrants more secure ligation with clips. The inferior phrenic vein enters the left adrenal vein medially and can be a source of troublesome bleeding if not identified and controlled.

◆ The entire gland is then placed in a retrieval bag and removed after slightly enlarging one of the port sites.

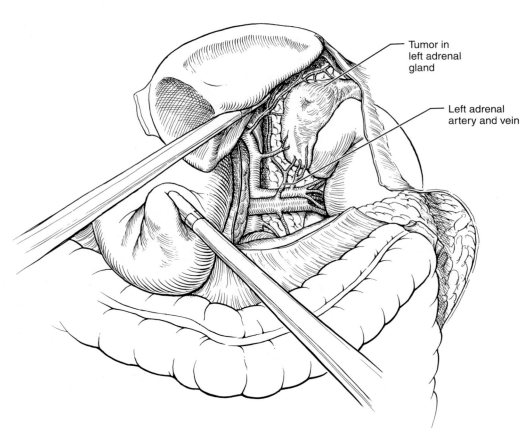

Tumor in
left adrenal
gland

Left adrenal
artery and vein

FIGURE 8–4

Right-Sided Laparoscopic Operation

◆ The triangular ligament of the right hepatic lobe is divided, and gravity retracts it medially usually without the need for a specific liver retractor. At this time the adrenal gland is usually easily identified above the kidney and lateral to the vena cava **(Figure 8-5).**

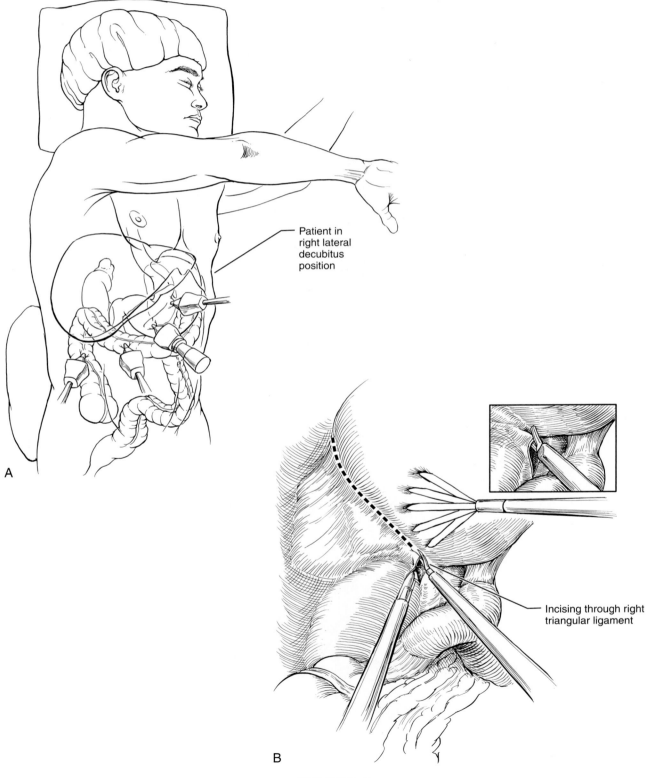

Patient in
right lateral
decubitus
position

A

Incising through right
triangular ligament

B

FIGURE 8–5

◆ Identification of the adrenal vein is then pursued at the lateral aspect of the vena cava with lateral displacement of the adrenal gland. A right-angle dissector is very useful here. Once identified, the vein is clipped and divided **(Figure 8-6)**.

◆ The remainder of the blood vessels and attachments are easily controlled and divided with the ultrasonic dissector **(Figure 8-7)**. This dissection progresses medial to lateral, so the lateral attachments provide lateral retraction until the completion of the mobilization.

◆ Once liberated from its attachments, the gland is placed in a retrieval bag and removed.

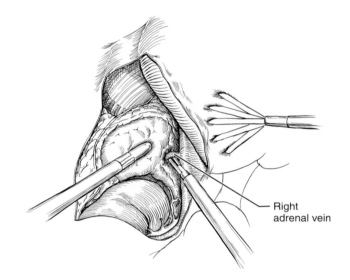

Right
adrenal vein

FIGURE 8–6

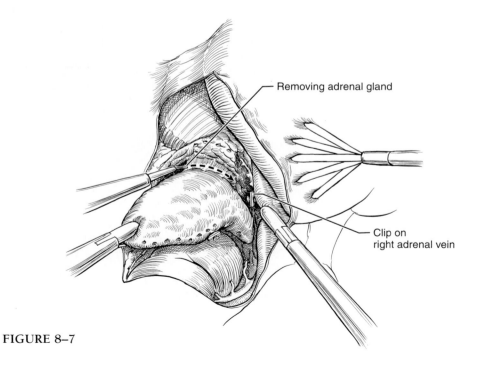

Removing adrenal gland

Clip on
right adrenal vein

FIGURE 8–7

Left-Sided Anterior Open Approach

◆ One approach to left adrenalectomy is full mobilization of the splenic flexure and splenorenal ligament as described in the laparoscopy section.

◆ Another approach is through the lesser sac. After the abdominal incision of choice is made, the lesser sac is opened by incision of the greater omentum at the insertion onto the left side of the transverse mesocolon (**Figure 8-8**).

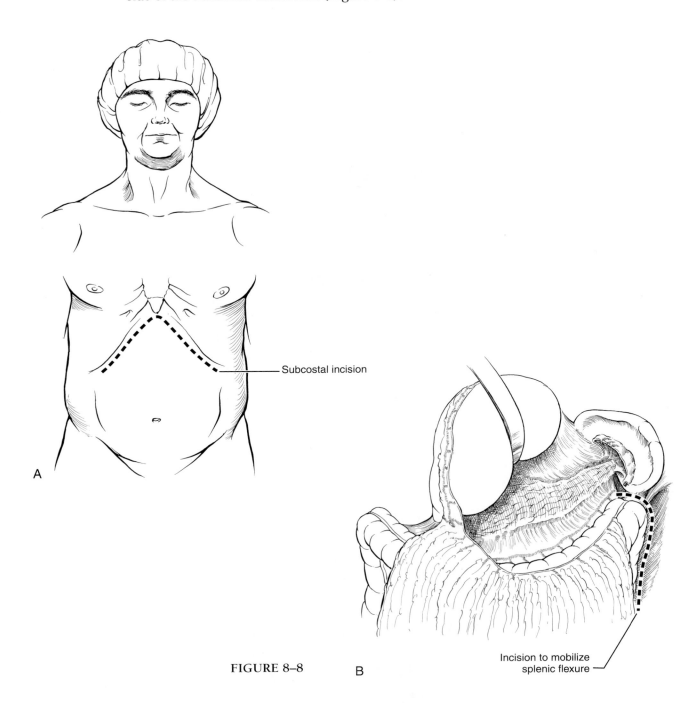

Subcostal incision

A

Incision to mobilize
splenic flexure

FIGURE 8–8   B

◆ The peritoneum below the tail of the pancreas is incised so that the tail of the pancreas can be retracted superiorly **(Figure 8-9)**.

◆ The peritoneum covering the left renal vein is opened, and the left adrenal vein is identified on the superior aspect of the left renal vein lateral to the aorta. The left renal vein is ligated and divided **(Figure 8-10)**.

◆ The blood vessels and tissues around the perimeter of the adrenal gland are divided using a combination of blunt and sharp dissection and suture ligation when needed. This dissection proceeds from medial to superior, then lateral, and finally inferior.

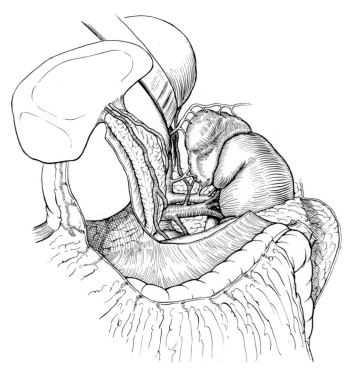

FIGURE 8–9

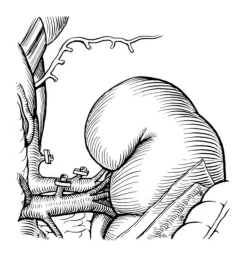

FIGURE 8–10

Right-Sided Anterior Open Approach

◆ The right lobe of the liver is retracted superiorly, or the triangular ligament is incised to retract the liver medially. The kidney, vena cava, and adrenal mass should be visualized behind the peritoneal covering. Occasionally, a Kocher maneuver may be performed to provide better exposure.

◆ The peritoneum just lateral to the vena cava is incised. Dissection in the plane between the vena cava and the adrenal gland will expose the right adrenal vein, which should be ligated and divided at this time **(Figure 8-11)**.

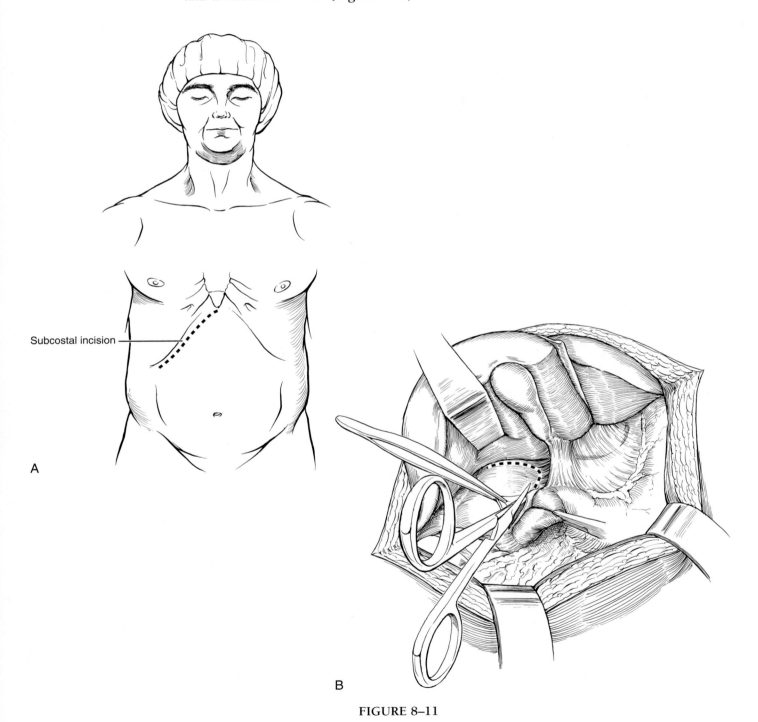

Subcostal incision

A

B

FIGURE 8–11

◆ The remaining attachments of the adrenal gland should be divided around its perimeter **(Figure 8-12)**. Occasionally, for larger tumors, a large feeding vessel may be encountered, which may require ligation, but most of this mobilization can be done with the ultrasonic dissector.

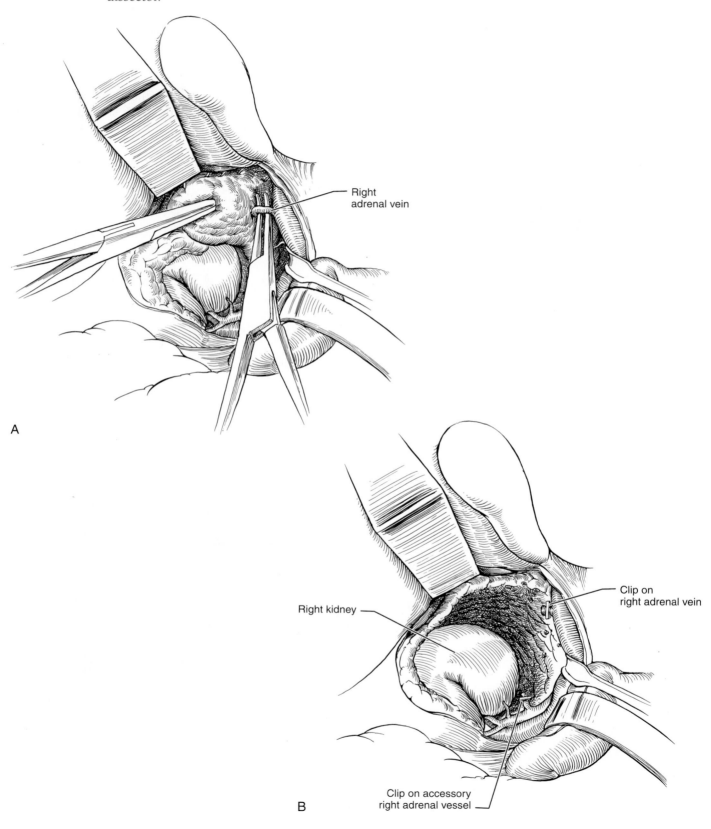

FIGURE 8–12

Posterior Open Approach

◆ The posterior approach requires appropriate positioning and padding of the patient in the prone position.

◆ The incision over the 12th rib is deepened to the level of the periosteum, which is then incised. The 12th rib is resected as far medially as reachable. A self-retaining retractor is placed to provide exposure **(Figure 8-13)**.

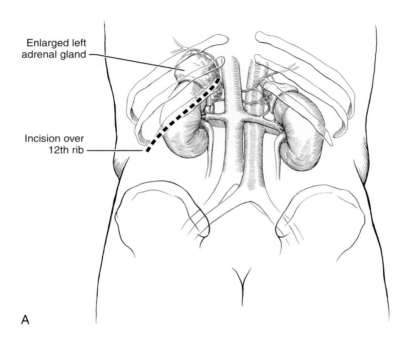

Enlarged left
adrenal gland

Incision over
12th rib

A

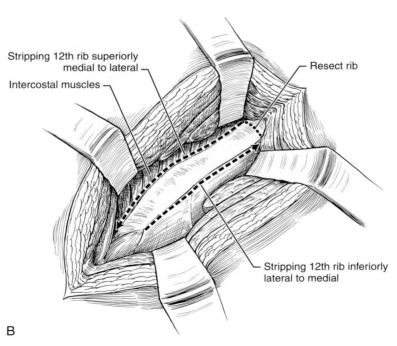

Stripping 12th rib superiorly
medial to lateral

Intercostal muscles

Resect rib

Stripping 12th rib inferiorly
lateral to medial

B

FIGURE 8–13

◆ The intact pleural membrane is carefully dissected from its attachments to the diaphragm, and the diaphragm may need to be incised radially along the line of its fibers. Care is taken to avoid injury to the intercostal nerve, especially during subsequent retraction **(Figure 8-14).**

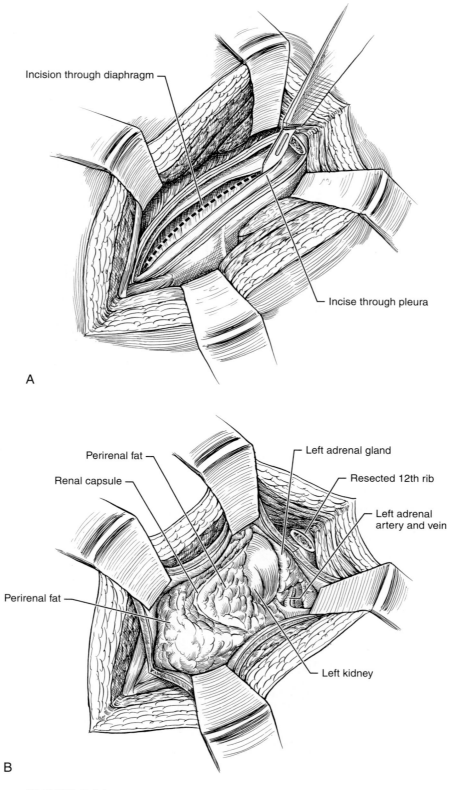

Incision through diaphragm

Incise through pleura

A

Perirenal fat

Renal capsule

Perirenal fat

Left adrenal gland

Resected 12th rib

Left adrenal artery and vein

Left kidney

B

FIGURE 8–14

◆ The fascia enveloping the kidney and adrenal gland (Gerota's fascia) is incised. A retractor placed medially and beneath Gerota's fascia and the diaphragm provides exposure while the fat and adrenal gland are swept inferiorly **(Figure 8-15).**

◆ As with the other adrenalectomy techniques, the dissection should be aimed at careful identification, ligation, and division of the adrenal vein early. However, the small adrenal arteries should be ligated as they are encountered on the way to the vein. For a left adrenalectomy, the left adrenal vein may not be visible until the gland is mobilized circumferentially.

◆ The remaining attachments are divided and the entire gland is removed.

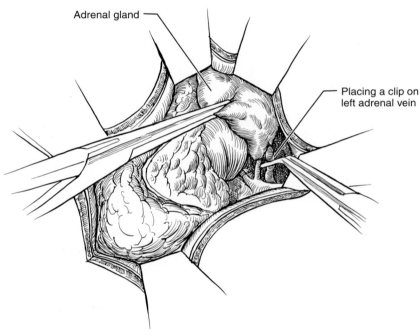

FIGURE 8–15

3. CLOSING

◆ Port sites up to and including 12 mm do not need fascial closure if dilating tip trocars are used in place of cutting trocars. For cutting trocars, all port sites larger than 5 mm should be closed using a laparoscopic suture passer.

◆ Standard closure of the incision after the open approaches should be tailored to the surgeon's preference.

◆ For the posterior approach, the diaphragm is closed with interrupted, horizontal mattress polypropylene sutures. The pleural membrane should then be inspected for holes, and if present, a small caliber drainage tube should be placed before the hole is sutured closed. The remaining layers are closed with absorbable suture.

STEP 4: POSTOPERATIVE CARE

◆ Pain management for laparoscopic adrenalectomy is with oral analgesics, whereas the open approaches typically require intravenous narcotics.

◆ The diet should be advanced as tolerated, with the expectation that the anterior open approaches may result in some degree of postoperative ileus.

◆ The most common complications are the result of injury to adjacent structures. Adrenal vein, vena cava, liver, and kidney injuries result in life-threatening bleeding during the operation or more subtle bleeding with the development of a hematoma postoperatively. A missed thermal or retractor injury to the intestines will cause sepsis in the first week after the operation.

◆ Acute adrenal insufficiency should be suspected in patients developing hemodynamic instability postoperatively. Prompt recognition and treatment with steroids are critical to avoid a potentially fatal outcome.

◆ Glucocorticoid stress doses are tapered postoperatively for patients with cortisol-secreting tumors but should be administered until the function of the hypothalamic-pituitary-adrenal axis is confirmed with an adrenocorticotropic hormone (ACTH) suppression test.

◆ Patients having bilateral adrenalectomy should have life-long replacement of glucocorticoids and mineralocorticoids.

STEP 5: PEARLS AND PITFALLS

- The appropriate preoperative preparation of the patient with a pheochromocytoma cannot be overstated. Failure to follow the sequence of alpha blockade followed by beta blockade can lead to hemodynamic catastrophe.

- Even with the appropriate preparation, patients with pheochromocytomas may have wide fluctuations in blood pressure as the adrenal gland is manipulated intraoperatively. Early control of the adrenal vein and appropriate hemodynamic monitoring and intervention are keys to minimizing this complication. Careful attention to fluid management should continue into the postoperative period.

- Manipulation should be by grasping the tissue around the adrenal glands or pushing it to the side, and dissection of the adrenal glands should be extracapsular. Lacerations of the gland will cause bleeding, which compromises adequate visualization and/or causes spillage of potentially malignant cells.

SELECTED REFERENCES

1. Bravo EL: Pheochromocytoma: Diagnosis, localization and management. N Engl J Med 1984;311: 1298-1303.
2. Gagner M: Laparoscopic adrenalectomy. Surg Clin North Am 1996;76:523-537.
3. Prinz A: A comparison of laparoscopic and open adrenalectomies. Arch Surg 1995;130:489-492.

THE BREAST

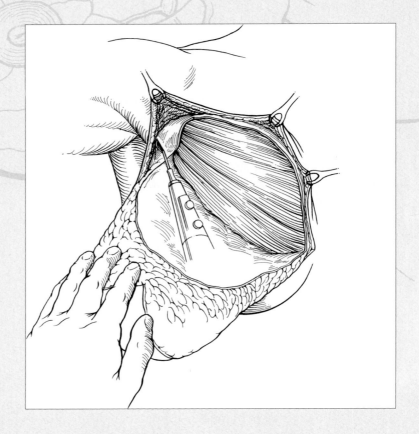

CHAPTER 9

WIDE LOCAL EXCISION

Baiba J. Grube

STEP 1: SURGICAL ANATOMY

- ◆ The breast is an organ that is composed of lobes, ducts, fibrous stroma, ligaments, adipose tissue, nerves, blood vessels, and lymphatics. The nipple-areolar complex is a specialized structure containing elements of skin epithelium, sweat and sebaceous appendages, and ductal epithelium with a nerve supply from branches of the second to sixth intercostal nerves.

- ◆ The breast parenchyma is organized into lobes that have a central duct, peripheral branching ducts, and glandular tissue.

- ◆ The lobes are variable in size, shape, and extent of branching.

- ◆ Ducts from different lobes are not constructed in wedge-like radial fashion but may lie over or under one another in an overlapping manner like intertwining roots.

- ◆ Most experts believe that ducts from one lobe do not anastomose with ducts of another lobe, but this is still an area of investigation.

- ◆ The nonuniform distribution of lobe anatomy influences the ability to map the breast parenchyma and has implications for surgical resection. Most tumors are localized and limited in extent, with a smaller percentage distributed segmentally and a minor number coursing in an irregular intertwined pattern.

- ◆ The peripheral ducts terminate in five to nine central ductal orifices in the nipple.

- ◆ Breast cancer is primarily a disease that begins in the terminal duct lobular units.

- ◆ Definition of terms for breast conservation:
  - ◆ Lumpectomy, tylectomy, wide local excision, partial mastectomy, or segmental mastectomy are roughly synonymous terms referring to the removal of a cancer through a small incision on the breast with a rim of normal healthy breast tissue, leaving the majority of normal breast tissue undisturbed. In most cases the nipple-areolar complex is left intact.

- Quadrantectomy usually refers to a wider excision that resects a quadrant of breast tissue, sometimes associated with the resection of redundant skin.
- Lumpectomy is combined with sentinel node biopsy and/or axillary dissection for an invasive cancer (see Chapters 10 and 11).
- Lumpectomy is usually followed by radiotherapy.

- Randomized trials have demonstrated that patients who undergo lumpectomy, axillary staging, and radiotherapy have the same overall survival as those who have modified radical mastectomy.

STEP 2: PREOPERATIVE CONSIDERATIONS

- In a well-screened population, breast cancer is commonly identified as a nonpalpable mammographic abnormality. Interval cancers may occur in a well-screened population, especially in patients who are *BRCA1* and *BRCA2* gene mutation carriers. A clinician experienced in breast disease may also palpate small breast cancers.

- Preoperative evaluation of a screen-detected nonpalpable abnormality or palpable lesion requires diagnostic mammograms. Additional images may include magnification and exaggerated and medial-lateral views. Other imaging modalities such as ultrasound and magnetic resonance imaging (MRI) may provide detailed information to map the area involved with tumor.

- A pathologic diagnosis of an image-detected abnormality or a palpable abnormality is obtained by fine needle aspiration, core biopsy, or excisional biopsy. The preferred method is a core biopsy, which allows for receptor analysis and permits discussion of treatment options.

- Selection of a surgical option for local control of breast cancer is a complex decision, based on the tumor features, breast size, location, associated medical problems, and individual choice. Interdisciplinary discussion with radiation oncologists, medical oncologists, and plastic surgeons in addition to the oncologic surgeon provides a comprehensive understanding of the options available to the patient.

- Lumpectomy with axillary staging may be an alternative procedure to a modified radical mastectomy for many women, especially in the current era of mammographic screening, identification of earlier stage disease, and the use of induction chemotherapy to reduce the size of the primary tumor.

- Lumpectomy is followed by breast radiotherapy.
  - Whole breast irradiation may be given with or without a boost to the site of the tumor.
  - Accelerated partial breast radiotherapy is a recent approach that limits the radiation to a smaller field, delivering a higher dose over a shorter period of time.

- Evaluation of the primary lesion and the planned procedure should be reviewed with the radiologist and the radiation therapist.
  - Palpable tumors may be initially treated with neoadjuvant chemotherapy to downsize them if they are too large to result in a good cosmetic outcome.
  - Nonpalpable tumors will require preoperative ultrasound-guided, stereotactically placed, or on rare occasions, MRI-directed needle localization.
  - Size and extent of lesion relative to breast size will dictate the ability to perform breast-conserving surgery and the cosmetic outcome.
  - Centrally located tumors may require resection of the nipple-areolar complex.
  - Multifocality is the presence of satellite tumors within the index quadrant. If they are close enough together to permit resection through a single incision, breast conservation remains an option.
  - Multicentricity, the presence of tumors in different quadrants of the breast, is usually taken as a contraindication to breast conservation.
  - Calcifications that are associated with a malignancy may be treated with breast conservation unless they involve too extensive an area for a good cosmetic outcome or if they involve the entire breast.

- Breast conservation may not be an option:
  - When extensive resection would lead to poor cosmesis
    - Large tumor size relative to breast size
    - Diffuse suspicious calcifications
    - Multicentric disease
    - Inflammatory carcinoma
    - Locally advanced disease
  - When medical contraindications are present
    - Previous chest wall irradiation
    - Active collagen vascular disease
    - Presence of a pacemaker
    - Significant cardiac disease
    - Significant pulmonary disease
  - When the patient is pregnant
    - Radiotherapy is contraindicated in pregnancy but may be delayed until after delivery if other treatment is ongoing.

STEP 3: OPERATIVE STEPS

1. ANESTHESIA

- Monitored anesthesia care with local anesthetic is usually sufficient for a small lumpectomy.

- Larger resection or resection in the vicinity of the nipple-areolar complex may require a general anesthetic.

- General anesthesia is usually preferable for lumpectomy combined with sentinel node biopsy and axillary dissection.

2. INCISION

◆ The curvilinear incision is placed along Langer's lines over a palpable mass in the upper hemisphere **(Figures 9-1 and 9-2)**. Some surgeons prefer a radial incision in the inferior hemisphere, particularly if skin must be removed. Shortening the distance between the nipple and inframammary crease gives much poorer cosmesis than medial/lateral narrowing of the breast.

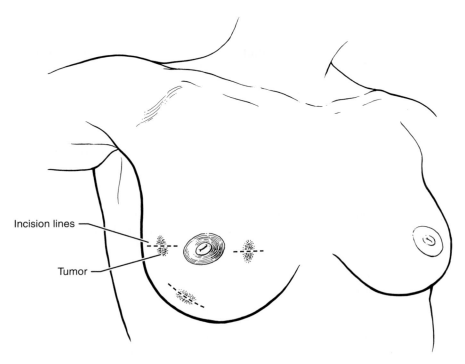

FIGURE 9–1

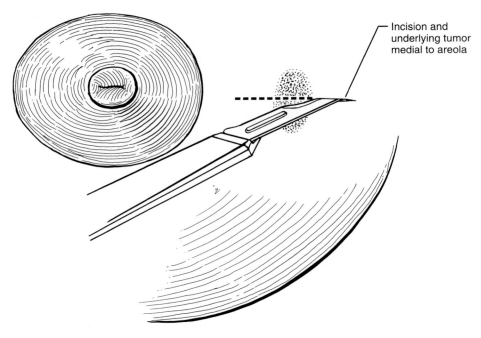

FIGURE 9–2

- When a nonpalpable lesion is localized with a wire, review of the mammogram with attention to the lesion and the wire tip dictates the placement of the incision. The entrance point of the wire may be far removed from the lesion, and an incision placed at the entry point of the wire may lead to extensive unnecessary dissection of normal breast tissue. Multiple bracketing wires may be used for extensive calcifications.

- Some radiologists inject a small amount of methylene blue at the tip of the wire to aid the surgeon.

- Skin excision is usually unnecessary unless the tumor is too close to achieve a clear margin.

3. DISSECTION

- Dissection of the area of interest may be performed with sharp dissection **(Figure 9-3)** or electrocautery.

- If electrocautery is used, the skin edges are at risk from thermal injury, and there may be significant cautery artifact of the specimen, making histopathologic evaluation of the margins difficult for the pathologist.

- Sharp dissection is an alternative and requires meticulous hemostasis once the lesion is removed.

- When the tumor is located, a 1-cm margin of normal tissue may be grasped with Allis forceps **(Figure 9-4)**. If the glandular tissue is almost completely replaced with adipose tissue, traction with instruments on the friable fatty tissue can damage the surrounding normal margin and preclude accurate margin assessment. In these cases, gentle pressure should be applied to separate the area of interest from the remaining breast. The incision may need to be larger for better visibility.

- The pectoralis fascia is removed in cases in which the tumor approaches the chest wall.

- When the specimen is resected, it is oriented for the pathologist with marking sutures so that the medial, lateral, superior, inferior, posterior, and anterior margins can be evaluated for proximity of the tumor cells.

- The presence of the lesion is placed on a grid, and the location of the lesion is confirmed by specimen mammogram. The radiologist can place marking needles in the specimen for the pathologist to identify the lesion.

- The submission of separate shaved margins from the cavity is a technique that provides additional information about margins.

- The cavity is demarcated with metal clips for the radiation oncologist, unless partial breast irradiation with a MammoSite balloon catheter is anticipated. The balloon is susceptible to rupture from the sharp metallic clips.

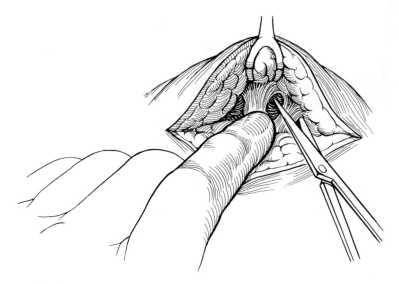

FIGURE 9–3

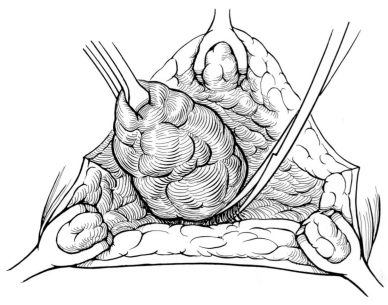

FIGURE 9–4

4. CLOSING

- Surgeons vary in their recommendation for closure of the partial mastectomy defect. In most cases, the defect in the breast can be closed by approximating the fascia of the superficial subcutaneous adipose tissue and the skin **(Figure 9-5)**. The cavity is allowed to accumulate a fibrinous seroma, which helps maintain the natural shape of the breast.

- Some surgeons are concerned that lack of cavity closure will leave a dimple in the contour and therefore elect to close the parenchyma. The goal in breast conservation is to remove the tumor with a healthy margin to reduce risk of recurrence, minimize deformity, and preserve the location of the nipple.

- Oncoplastic advancement flaps may be helpful when a large cavity remains but should be applied only by individuals experienced in the techniques. When applying oncoplastic procedures that shift tissues around, the surgeon must be reasonably certain that the margins are free of tumor.

- Reapproximation of the subcutaneous fat with an absorbable suture leads to better skin closure (see Figure 9-5).

- Skin closure may be performed with absorbable or nonabsorbable sutures or Dermabond, according to individual preference.

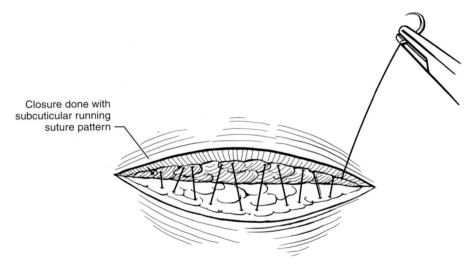

Closure done with subcuticular running suture pattern

FIGURE 9–5

5. PROCESSING OF RESECTED SPECIMEN

- Orientation of the specimen is the responsibility of the surgeon, and any concerns should be communicated to the pathologist.

- The specimen may not be a perfect sphere or rectangle but rather an irregular specimen that requires detailed orientation.

- Specimen mammography aids the surgeon who can perform additional resections at the time of lumpectomy.

- Specimen mammography aids the pathologist who can process the areas of interest in greater depth.

- Pathologic processing is most helpful when multicolor inking of the specimen margins is performed.

6. REEXCISION LUMPECTOMY

- If the margins demonstrate transected tumor, discussion for reexcision lumpectomy or mastectomy must be undertaken.

- If reoperation is desired by the patient, the same incision may be used.

- Multicolored inking of the initial lumpectomy specimen can identify a specific margin that is positive, and re-resection may be limited to the affected margin.

STEP 4: POSTOPERATIVE CARE

- A variety of dressings can be used, from Opsite alone to fluffs and a specialized postsurgical bra.

- Showers may be taken in 48 hours.

- Tub baths and swimming are avoided until the wound is completely healed.

- Strenuous exercise should be avoided in the first week to prevent bleeding.

- Silicone-based sheets, such as Biodermis, may be applied to reduce scarring by direct pressure.

- A sports bra worn 24 hours a day may be comfortable for some, whereas others find any form of bra uncomfortable.

STEP 5: PEARLS AND PITFALLS

- Discussion with the interdisciplinary team will sequence treatment in the most appropriate manner.

- Surgical planning preoperatively with the radiologist is critical to achieve negative margins the first time.

- Complex resections may require input from a plastic surgeon, especially when contralateral symmetry may be an issue.

- Large excisions may require oncoplastic techniques to rearrange the remaining breast parenchyma.

- Maintenance of the nipple-areolar complex in the native position results in the best cosmetic outcome.

- Specimen orientation by the surgeon and communication with the radiologist and pathologist is critical.

- Specimen mammography and communication of the findings to the surgeon and pathologist are essential to take additional margins at the first operation.

- Specimen multicolor inking aids in determining the location of a close margin, so re-resection is limited to the area of residual tumor and not on the negative margins.

SELECTED REFERENCES

1. Anderson BO, Masetti R, Silverstein MJ: Oncoplastic approaches to partial mastectomy: An overview of volume-displacement techniques. Lancet Oncol 2005;6:145-157.
2. Fisher B, Anderson S, Bryant J, et al: Twenty-year follow-up of a randomized trial comparing total mastectomy, lumpectomy, and lumpectomy plus irradiation for the treatment of invasive breast cancer. N Engl J Med 2002;347:1233-1241.
3. Schwartz GF, Veronesi U, Clough KB, et al: Consensus conference on breast conservation. J Am Coll Surg 2006;203:198-207.
4. Veronesi U, Cascinelli N, Mariani L, et al: Twenty-year follow-up of a randomized study comparing breast-conserving surgery with radical mastectomy for early breast cancer. N Engl J Med 2002;347:1227-1232.
5. Iglehart JD, Kaelin CM: Diseases of the breast. In Townsend C Jr, Beauchamp R, Evers B, Mattox K (eds): Sabiston Textbook of Surgery. Philadelphia, Elsevier Saunders, 2004, pp 867-927.

CHAPTER 10

MODIFIED RADICAL MASTECTOMY

Baiba J. Grube

STEP 1: SURGICAL ANATOMY

- A comprehensive understanding of the location of the mammary gland in relation to the chest wall musculature, the fascial boundaries, the lymphatic drainage pathways, the vascular supply to the breast and the associated supporting structures, and the innervation of the breast and surrounding tissues is essential for appropriate surgical management.

- **Figure 10-1** demonstrates the breast gland and the rich intraparenchymal lymph channels coursing toward the deeper major nodal reservoirs.

- **Figure 10-2** illustrates the relationship of the nodal basins to the chest wall musculature. The lymph nodes lateral to the pectoralis minor constitute level I nodes, those immediately beneath the pectoralis minor level II nodes, and those medial to it level III. The interpectoral nodes (Rotter's nodes) are located between the pectoralis major and minor muscles and are part of level III nodes. Internal mammary nodes are located medially along internal mammary vessels beneath the sternum. Unnamed intramammary lymph nodes can be present in all quadrants of the breast.

DEFINITION

- Modified radical mastectomy constitutes the removal of the breast parenchyma, the nipple-areolar complex, and levels I and II axillary lymph nodes.

- Other types of mastectomy procedures include the following:
  - Total mastectomy (removal of the breast only) may be combined with sentinel node biopsy.
  - Patey's modified radical mastectomy includes dissection of level III nodes reached by division or resection of the pectoralis minor muscle.
  - Radical mastectomy further removes the pectoralis major and minor muscles.
  - Extended radical mastectomy also eradicates the internal mammary lymph nodes.
  - Nipple-sparing mastectomy preserves the nipple and areola.
  - Areola-sparing mastectomy preserves the areola, usually with resection of the nipple.

STEP 2: PREOPERATIVE CONSIDERATIONS

- Selection of a surgical option for local control of breast cancer is a complex decision that is based on tumor features, body habitus, and individual patient choice. Interdisciplinary discussion with radiation oncologists, medical oncologists, and plastic surgeons in addition to the oncologic surgeon provides a comprehensive understanding of the options available to the patient.

- Modified radical mastectomy may be an option for a diagnosis of the following:
  - Invasive breast cancer
  - Multicentric invasive breast cancer
  - Invasive breast cancer after previous chest irradiation
  - Invasive breast cancer when postoperative radiotherapy maybe contraindicated (e.g., connective tissue disease, presence of a pacemaker)
  - Invasive breast cancer in a pregnant patient
  - Palliative resection in stage IV breast cancer for local control

- Lumpectomy with axillary lymph node dissection may be an alternative procedure to modified radical mastectomy for many women, especially in the current era of mammographic screening and identification of early stage disease, or with the use of induction chemotherapy to reduce the size of a larger primary tumor.

- Discussion of the planned procedure with the anesthesiologist is critical.
  - Long-acting paralytic agents should be avoided when an axillary dissection is planned so that intact motor nerve function can be detected.
  - Inhalation agents may be varied if immediate reconstruction is planned with autologous tissue.

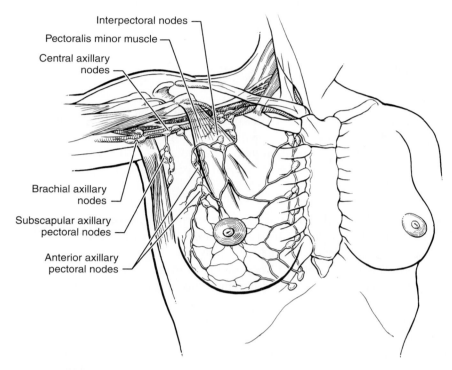

Interpectoral nodes
Pectoralis minor muscle
Central axillary nodes
Brachial axillary nodes
Subscapular axillary pectoral nodes
Anterior axillary pectoral nodes

FIGURE 10–1

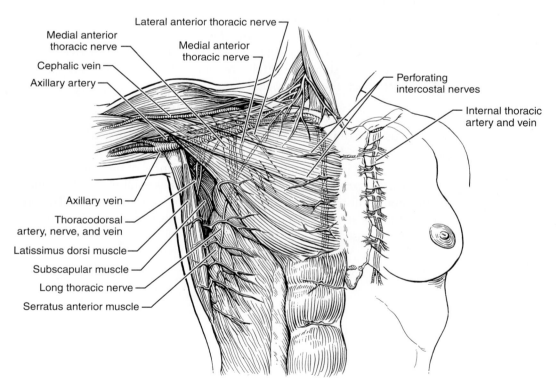

Lateral anterior thoracic nerve
Medial anterior thoracic nerve
Medial anterior thoracic nerve
Cephalic vein
Axillary artery
Perforating intercostal nerves
Internal thoracic artery and vein
Axillary vein
Thoracodorsal artery, nerve, and vein
Latissimus dorsi muscle
Subscapular muscle
Long thoracic nerve
Serratus anterior muscle

FIGURE 10–2

STEP 3: OPERATIVE STEPS

1. INCISION

♦ The patient is placed supine, close to the edge of the operating table with the arm extended on a padded arm board, with or without a wedge. The arm may be prepped separately and covered in a sterile stockinette to allow free rotation of the arm medially, to relax the pectoralis major and minor muscles, and to permit better exposure of the axilla.

♦ The type of incision depends on whether immediate reconstruction is planned or a delayed procedure is anticipated. If no reconstruction or a delayed procedure is planned, an elliptical incision is made to include a previous surgical biopsy site if present **(Figure 10-3)**. The incision is usually placed horizontally to include the nipple-areolar complex, but in some cases may be oriented at different angles to include a previous surgical biopsy site. If delayed reconstruction is anticipated, the medial extent of the incision may be angled slightly caudad to permit sufficient skin for reconstruction of the medial cleavage and to avoid a scar that may be visible with low décolletage. The width of skin resection should permit a tension-free closure but avoid redundant skin folds. A good way to judge the amount of skin to be resected is to draw a transverse or angled line through the nipple and move the inferior flap upward with gentle tension and draw a mark on the skin where it intersects the transverse line. A similar action should be performed for the superior flap.

♦ If immediate reconstruction is planned, discussion with the plastic surgeon for placement of incisions is important. The most natural appearance to the native breast is a skin-sparing mastectomy that is accomplished by resecting the nipple-areolar complex and leaving most of the skin envelope behind. If the nipple areolar-complex is small relative to the breast, a transverse incision can be extended laterally, resembling a tennis racquet, for a short distance sufficient to reach the axillary nodes.

♦ A marking pen is used to draw the planned incision. The skin is incised with a no. 15 scalpel and extended through the dermis into the subcutaneous adipose tissue to expose the superficial investing fascia of the breast **(Figure 10-4)**. The thickness of the flaps will vary according to body mass index. In very lean individuals this can be just millimeters thick and may require subcutaneous infusion of tumescence solution for easier dissection. The breast parenchyma lies closest to the skin at the nipple-areolar complex and increases in thickness toward the periphery of the breast.

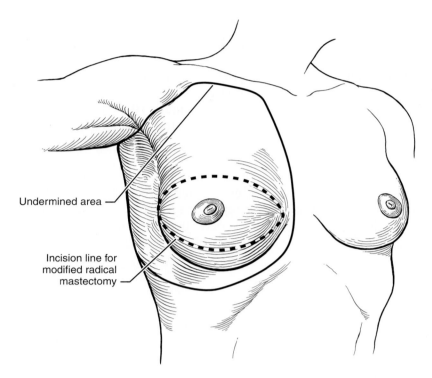

Undermined area

Incision line for
modified radical
mastectomy

FIGURE 10–3

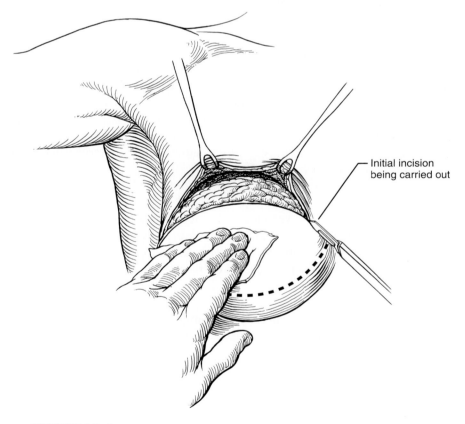

Initial incision
being carried out

FIGURE 10–4

2. DISSECTION

- Dissection is initiated by elevating the skin edges with skin hooks or Freeman rake retractors and may be performed with electrocautery as illustrated or by sharp dissection with a no. 10 scalpel or curved Gorney scissors **(Figure 10-5)**. If sharp dissection is undertaken, subcutaneous injection of a dilute saline solution with epinephrine may reduce bleeding.

- As the flaps are elevated, the assistant holds upward tension on the skin flaps while the surgeon uses countertraction on the breast parenchyma. These counter forces help expose the fine avascular areolar fascial plane separating the subcutaneous fat from breast parenchyma. Excessive bleeding indicates that the dissection is not in the correct anatomic plane that separates the glandular tissue from the subcutaneous adipose tissue.

- Dissection is continued circumferentially following the superficial fascia to its fusion with the muscular fascia around the anatomic borders of the breast. These are defined by the pectoralis major muscle below the clavicle superiorly, the margin of the sternum medially, the inframammary fold overlying the rectus abdominis muscle inferiorly, and the serratus anterior muscle to the latissimus dorsi muscle laterally. Dissection along the latissimus dorsi muscle continues to the level of its tendinous insertion just inferior to the axillary vein.

- The resection of the breast off the chest wall posteriorly includes the retromammary fascia with the investing fascia of the pectoralis major muscle.

- The mammary gland with the superficial fascia and the posterior investing fascia of the pectoralis major muscle is resected from superomedial to inferolateral, exposing the axillary fat pad containing the draining lymph nodes and the lateral aspect of the pectoralis major muscle **(Figure 10-6)**. Care should be taken to dissect the fascia in the avascular plane parallel to the muscle fibers to avoid transection of muscle fibers, especially along the sternal insertion medially and along the rectus sheath inferiorly. The fascia of the serratus anterior muscle should be left intact if immediate implant reconstruction is planned, unless contraindicated by disease.

- Perforating muscular blood vessels and intercostal vessels should be ligated with 3-0 silk ligatures or be cauterized. Care should be taken to avoid traction on these vessels, which have a tendency to retract and be an occasional source of postoperative bleeding. Blind dissection for these vessels may lead to entry into the chest cavity and pneumothorax.

- The breast remains attached laterally exposing the axilla, the pectoralis major muscle medially, and the latissimus dorsi muscle laterally.

- The boundaries of the axilla are defined by the pectoral muscles medially, the latissimus dorsi muscle laterally, the axillary vein superiorly, and the subscapularis and teres major muscles posteriorly.

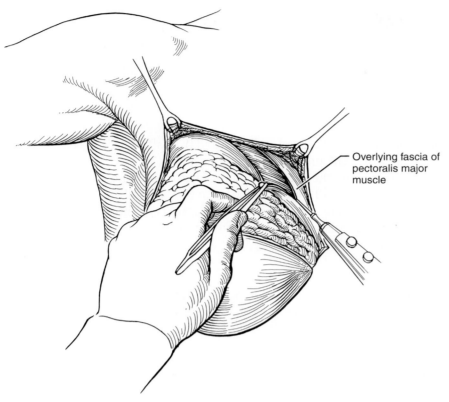

Overlying fascia of
pectoralis major
muscle

FIGURE 10–5

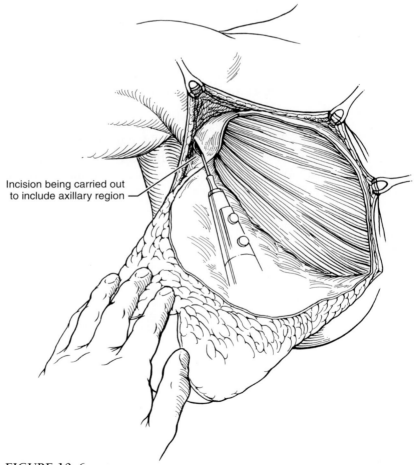

Incision being carried out
to include axillary region

FIGURE 10–6

◆ Dissection of the axilla is undertaken by incising the fascia of the pectoralis major muscle from inferior to superior **(Figure 10-7)**. Care must be exercised to avoid injury to the medial anterior thoracic nerve (medial pectoral nerve), which may penetrate both pectoral muscles and emerge medially or may course along the lateral aspect of the pectoralis minor muscle. Injury to this nerve may lead to atrophy of part of the pectoralis major muscle.

◆ The fascia along the pectoralis major muscle is incised and retracted medially with a small or medium Richardson retractor, exposing the underlying pectoralis minor muscle **(Figure 10-8)**. The clavipectoral fascia along the pectoralis minor muscle is then incised, and the retractor is replaced exposing the level II nodes posterior to the pectoralis minor muscle. The arm may now be rotated medially to take tension off the pectoral muscles and expose the axillary contents. Care must be taken to avoid traction of the extremity and the brachial plexus in the anesthetized patient.

◆ The intercostal brachial cutaneous nerve may be identified coursing transversely below the axillary vein and should be preserved if free of matted tumor-laden nodes to avoid bothersome sensory dysesthesias along the medial aspect of the upper arm.

◆ Dissection medially should be cautious, with attention to the long thoracic nerve, which lies on the serratus anterior muscle beneath the fascia. Retraction of the fascia off the chest wall will pull the long thoracic nerve off the chest wall and place it at risk of injury. The nerve can be identified deep to the intercostal brachial nerve or higher, inferior to the axillary vein on the chest wall, where it is less likely to have been pulled away from the serratus anterior muscle into the axillary fat. The nerve should be protected and preserved. The function can be confirmed by very gentle compression and demonstration of contraction of the serratus muscle in the unparalyzed individual. Injury to the long thoracic nerve causes a winged scapula.

◆ Lateral dissection of the axilla is along the latissimus dorsi muscle to the tendinous insertion. The axillary vein overlies the tendinous insertion, and care should be taken to proceed cautiously from lateral to medial and from superficial to deep, with careful visualization of underlying structures.

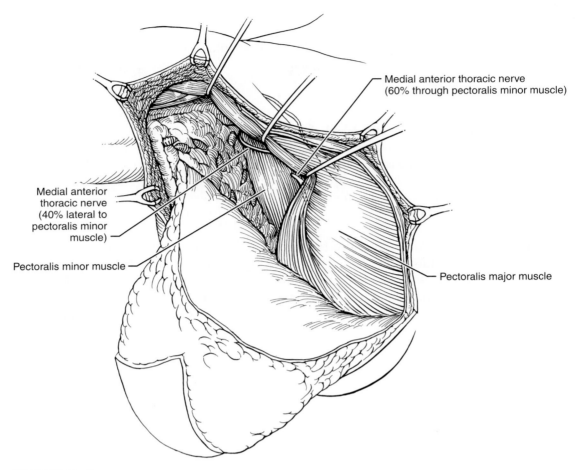

Medial anterior thoracic nerve
(60% through pectoralis minor muscle)

Medial anterior
thoracic nerve
(40% lateral to
pectoralis minor
muscle)

Pectoralis minor muscle

Pectoralis major muscle

FIGURE 10–7

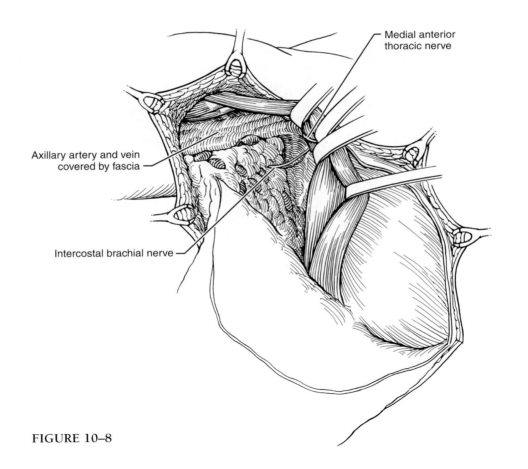

Medial anterior
thoracic nerve

Axillary artery and vein
covered by fascia

Intercostal brachial nerve

FIGURE 10–8

- The superior extent of the axillary dissection should begin approximately 5 mm below the axillary vein to preserve the lymphatics of the arm and reduce the likelihood of upper extremity lymphedema (**Figure 10-9**).

- **Figures 10-9, 10-10, and 10-11** show dissection with exposure of the brachial plexus above the axillary vein for anatomic orientation, but the dissection should stop just below the vein. This tissue is rich in lymphatics and blood vessels, which should be ligated with fine silk ties or Weck Hemoclips. Preservation of the lymphatics surrounding the axillary vein reduces the risk of lymphedema.

- The thoracodorsal artery and vein with the thoracodorsal nerve medially will be identified in the lateral third of the axillary artery (see Figure 10-10). The thoracodorsal trunk courses on the medial aspect of the latissimus dorsi muscle. Transection of the thoracodorsal nerve leads to weakened shoulder adduction. Once the thoracodorsal trunk is identified, lateral dissection is safe as long as the intercostal brachial cutaneous nerve is visualized as it emerges from the axillary fat pad, approximately halfway up the latissimus dorsi muscle coursing toward the arm.

- Dissection of the axilla is carried out from superior to inferior, maintaining visualization of the nerves at risk. As the fatty tissue is swept inferiorly, lymphatics and blood vessels are transected.

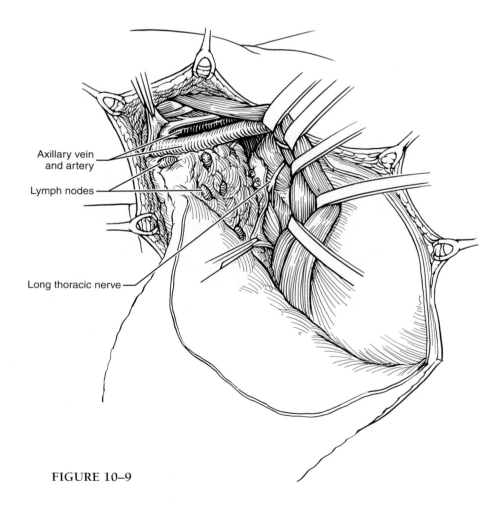

Axillary vein
and artery

Lymph nodes

Long thoracic nerve

FIGURE 10–9

◆ The axilla and breast are removed and identified with sutures that distinguish the apex of the axilla and the orientation of the breast. The axilla and the chest wall are visualized (see Figure 10-11). The cavity is irrigated with warm saline. Any residual bleeding vessels are cauterized or ligated.

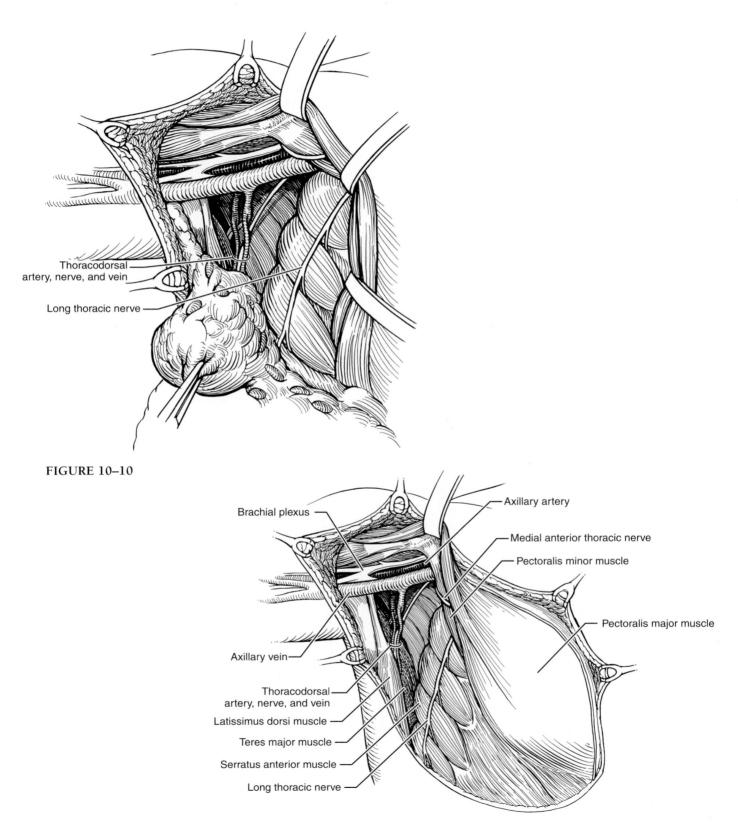

Thoracodorsal artery, nerve, and vein

Long thoracic nerve

FIGURE 10–10

Brachial plexus

Axillary artery

Medial anterior thoracic nerve

Pectoralis minor muscle

Pectoralis major muscle

Axillary vein

Thoracodorsal artery, nerve, and vein

Latissimus dorsi muscle

Teres major muscle

Serratus anterior muscle

Long thoracic nerve

FIGURE 10–11

3. CLOSING

◆ Two closed suction drains, such as #10 Jackson-Pratt drains, are inserted through separate small stab incisions inferior and lateral to the skin incision, one oriented toward the axilla and the second anteriorly beneath the skin flaps. The drains are secured in place with 2-0 silk sutures.

◆ The skin is closed in two layers with absorbable sutures, a deep layer of 3-0 Vicryl sutures, and a subcuticular closure with 4-0 Monocryl sutures **(Figure 10-12)**. Steri-Strips or Dermabond may be used for skin approximation. A light dressing or special mastectomy bra is applied with loose fluff gauze dressings.

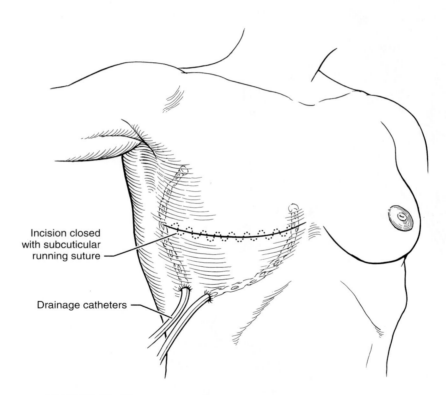

Incision closed
with subcuticular
running suture

Drainage catheters

FIGURE 10–12

STEP 4: POSTOPERATIVE CARE

- Drains are emptied 2 to 3 times per day and drain output is recorded on a log.
  - Drainage may be sanguinous immediately postoperatively, but should be dilute.
  - Continued postoperative frank bloody output indicates ongoing bleeding and warrants return to the operating room.
  - Drainage clears to serosanguinous, then clear and straw-colored.
  - Cloudy fluid may indicate bacterial infection and should be cultured.

- Drains are removed when the output is less than 30 mL for 2 consecutive days.
  - Drains usually remain for 7 to 10 days.
  - Seroma may form after drain removal.
    - Aspirate in clinic if large, suspicious for infection, or uncomfortable.
    - Multiple aspirations may be required.
    - Compression dressing may reduce likelihood of seroma reaccumulation.
    - Some seromas reabsorb without aspiration if they are small.

- Dressings are removed after 48 hours.
  - Pain out of proportion to the procedure may indicate a significant hematoma, for which dressings should be removed earlier.
  - Other indications include fever and excessive drainage.

- Shower may be acceptable after 48 hours when dressings are removed.
  - The surgical site is bathed with mild soap and water, patted dry, and redressed around the drain site.
  - The incision may be left open according to individual preference.

- Tub baths are usually not advised while drains are in place.

- Antibiotics are usually not needed but may be considered on an individual basis for the following:
  - Previous surgical biopsy
  - Immunocompromised individuals
  - Local wound conditions

- Limited exercises are initiated on postoperative day 1 and increased to range-of-motion and strengthening exercises after the drains are removed.
  - Consultation with American Cancer Society for Reach to Recovery is helpful.
  - Consultation with occupational therapy for rehabilitation is useful.

- Individuals are monitored for lymphedema.

- Patient education about long-term precautions for protection of the affected extremity include the following:
  - Avoidance of blood pressure measurements and phlebotomy sticks on the affected extremity
  - No intravenous infusion lines
  - No constrictive clothing
  - Electric razors for shaving
  - Protective gloves for tasks that may lacerate the skin and lead to infection
  - Early intervention with antibiotics for a hand or arm infection, often requiring hospitalization for parenteral antibiotics

- Compression sleeve and glove may be indicated for cases of extensive nodal disease, combination surgery and radiotherapy, and evidence of lymphedema, as well as for prophylaxis for air travel.

- Postoperative radiotherapy or chemotherapy is not initiated for 2 to 3 weeks.

- Skin flap loss may require local care with wet to dry dressings or silver sulfadiazine (Silvadene) cream if limited or surgical revision if skin loss is extensive.

- A bra and prosthesis are measured and fitted for long-term symmetry or for a short interval while the patient is awaiting autologous or implant reconstruction.

- Scarring maybe reduced with application of a silicone sheet, such as Biodermis.

STEP 5: PEARLS AND PITFALLS

- Discussion with the interdisciplinary team will sequence treatment in the most appropriate manner.

- Surgical planning in conjunction with the plastic surgeon will result in optimal cosmetic outcome.

- Skin-sparing mastectomy leads to the best cosmetic appearance of the reconstructed breast.

- Gentle handling of the skin flaps reduces the risk of flap loss.

- Preservation of the fascia of the serratus anterior muscle on the chest wall and identification of the long thoracic nerve underlying it on the chest wall will reduce the risk of transection and the winged scapula deformity.

- Dissection along the lateral aspect of the latissimus dorsi muscle reduces the likelihood of injury to the thoracodorsal trunk and weakened shoulder adduction.

- Preservation of the medial pectoral nerve prevents atrophy of the pectoralis major muscle and chest wall contour.

- Preservation of the intercostal brachial cutaneous nerves maintains sensation to the medial aspect of the upper extremity and prevents bothersome dysesthesias.
    - Preservation of fatty tissue and lymphatic channels from the arm around the axillary vein reduces the risk of lymphedema.
    - In obese patients, anatomic boundaries may be more difficult to identify and require wider exposure, increased operative time, and patience during the procedure.
    - The pulse in the axillary artery is a landmark that can help orient the surgeon to stay inferior.

SELECTED REFERENCES

1. Fisher B, Anderson S, Bryant J, et al: Twenty-year follow-up of a randomized trial comparing total mastectomy, lumpectomy, and lumpectomy plus irradiation for the treatment of invasive breast cancer. N Engl J Med 2002;347:1233-1241.
2. Iglehart JD, Kaelin CM: Diseases of the breast. In Townsend C Jr , Beauchamp R, Evers B, Mattox K (eds): Sabiston Textbook of Surgery. Philadelphia, Elsevier Saunders, 2004, pp 867-927.
3. Staradub VL, Morrow M: Modified radical mastectomy with knife technique. Arch Surg 2002;137: 105-110.
4. Stolier AJ, Grube BJ: Areola-sparing mastectomy: Defining the risks. J Am Coll Surg 2005;201:118-124.
5. Veronesi U, Cascinelli N, Mariani L, et al: Twenty-year follow-up of a randomized study comparing breast-conserving surgery with radical mastectomy for early breast cancer. N Engl J Med 2002;347: 1227-1232.

CHAPTER 11

SENTINEL LYMPH NODE BIOPSY

Celia Chao

INTRODUCTION

Regional lymph node status is the most powerful predictor of recurrence and survival in patients with breast cancer and melanoma. Nodal staging remains an essential component in the decision-making process to offer adjuvant therapy for both breast cancer and melanoma. Over the last century, experience with surgical clearance of a nodal basin has shown that this procedure can result in significant morbidity: pain, paresthesias, seroma, infection, limitation of limb motion, lymphedema, and lymphangitis. Sentinel lymph node (SLN) biopsy has proven to be a highly accurate technique with minimal morbidity. The development and adaptation of SLN biopsy has revolutionized the staging of melanoma and breast cancer.

STEP 1: SURGICAL ANATOMY

- SLN biopsy is most commonly performed for breast cancer. Although the same principles and techniques apply to SLN biopsy for primary malignant melanoma, this chapter describes in detail SLN biopsy for breast cancer. **Figure 11-1** demonstrates the lymphatic drainage of a breast cancer to the axillary lymph nodes.

STEP 2: PREOPERATIVE CONSIDERATIONS

- The SLN is defined as the first draining lymph node in the axilla to receive lymphatic drainage from a primary breast tumor. Should regional metastatic disease exist, the SLN is the node most likely to contain metastases. Conveniently, if the SLN is negative for metastasis, then the remainder of the nodal basin should also be negative. Therefore, the SLN should reflect the histopathologic status of the entire axilla. In 1992, Morton's group performed SLN biopsy in more than 500 patients with melanoma, removing the SLN, as well as the remaining regional lymph nodes. The pathology of the SLN predicted the remaining regional nodal status with 99% accuracy. His pioneering work was validated by studies at other institutions with completion lymphadenectomy, histopathologic nodal examination, and long-term follow-up to identify potential recurrences in undissected nodal basins following a negative SLN biopsy. Similarly, Giuliano reported initial experience with SLN biopsy for breast cancer using vital blue dye injection, including validation with histopathologic examination of the non-SLN.

◆ Definitions: Successful SLN biopsy is judged by two critical parameters: the SLN identification rate and the false-negative rate. The SLN *identification rate* is the frequency of finding and removing an SLN. When the SLN cannot be identified, a standard level I/II axillary dissection must be performed. The *false-negative rate* is the proportion of patients with positive lymph nodes who are incorrectly staged by the SLN biopsy procedure. Understanding that no staging procedure is 100% accurate, we accept a small false-negative rate (5% or less) to spare most true-negative patients the morbidity of a full level I and II axillary dissection.

◆ Pathologic examination of the SLN: By examining serial sections, a more thorough evaluation of the nodal specimen is possible. The SLN biopsy identifies the node(s) that should be more closely scrutinized. Such a focused examination would be prohibitively costly and time-consuming if performed on the entire contents of an axillary dissection.

◆ A team approach: Implementation of SLN biopsy requires the cooperative efforts of multiple disciplines: surgeons and the operating room staff and colleagues from the departments of radiology, nuclear medicine, pathology, and anesthesiology. The "team" must agree on a protocol: how to perform injections, how to dispose of radioactive waste, what type of radionuclide to use, and which adaptation of a SLN pathology protocol should be used.

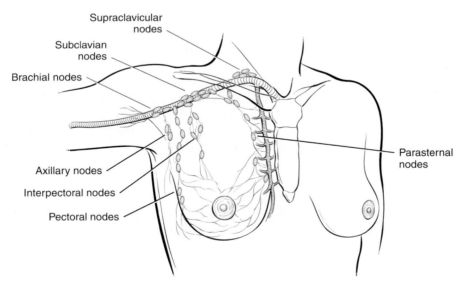

FIGURE 11–1

STEP 3: OPERATIVE STEPS

- Patient eligibility: SLN biopsy is appropriate for patients with T1-T3 breast cancers without palpable nodal metastases (clinical N0). SLN biopsy is applicable for patients undergoing either a breast-conserving operation or mastectomy and is equally accurate after open excisional breast biopsy or needle biopsy that has been performed for diagnosis. The procedure is most appropriate for biopsy-proven invasive cancer, including multifocal/multicentric disease. SLN biopsy can be considered for ductal carcinoma in situ, in which there is a high likelihood of an invasive component, or if mastectomy is considered. Contraindications include pregnancy, palpable axillary nodal metastases, hypersensitivity to either blue dye or technetium sulfur colloid, and prior major breast or axillary operations that could interfere with lymphatic drainage.

- Dual-agent injection technique: Intraoperative lymphatic mapping using vital blue dye, radioactive colloid, or a combination of both is performed to identify the SLN. I advocate the use of dual-agent injection to facilitate SLN localization. The combination of the two techniques—visualization of the blue dye and intraoperative gamma probe detection—provides overlapping and complementary ability to discriminate the SLN. Some SLNs may be blue-stained but not radioactive ("blue, not hot"), and others may be radioactive but not blue ("hot, not blue"); but most SLNs will be both blue and hot. Use of dual agents provides more accurate nodal staging than the use of either agent alone.

- I recommend preoperative dermal radioactive colloid injection using 0.5 mCi of 0.2 μm technetium-99 sulfur colloid in a volume of 0.2 to 0.5 mL at least 30 minutes before operation. The use of filtered or unfiltered colloid has been shown to be equivalent in terms of identification rates and false-negative rates. Equal injections into the dermis (intradermally) are accomplished using a tuberculin syringe with a 25- to 30-gauge needle (raising a wheal) immediately anterior (superficial) to the tumor site, using four to five separate injections **(Figure 11-2)**. The use of routine lymphoscintigraphy has been shown to be neither necessary nor helpful in SLN biopsy for breast cancer. However, because of less predictable drainage patterns, such as bilateral drainage basins, or the possibility of interval node involvement, a lymphoscintigram is recommended routinely for melanoma.

- Injection in the areolar border has been shown to be accurate for breast cancers located in any quadrant or centrally. Embryologically, all the lymphatic drainage of the breast converges in the periareolar or subareolar plexus of lymphatics. Therefore injection of the areola will accurately reflect the drainage of tumors in any part of the breast. This technique has been advocated for patients with multicentric or multifocal breast cancer.

- Following radioactive colloid injection, the patient is taken to the operating room. For patient comfort, I perform almost all SLN biopsies with the patient under general anesthesia, without muscle relaxant, although it is possible to use local anesthesia. Patients should be counseled preoperatively that the blue dye injection will impart a change to the color of their urine and that there is a small chance of allergic reaction to the dye (approximately 1 in 10,000). Adverse reactions, including anaphylactic reactions, to vital blue dye are rare but have been documented. Allergic reaction to the blue dye may manifest as blue-colored hives.

◆ Patients will occasionally have a noticeably blue tattoo on the skin after the procedure. They should be told that this color will fade and disappear with time. The anesthesiologist should be aware that pseudohypoxia is often seen intraoperatively as a result of the blue dye, which interferes with pulse oximetry, falsely lowering oxygen saturation readings. The use of radioactive colloid is safe, and numerous reports have documented the relatively low amount of radiation exposure associated with its use.

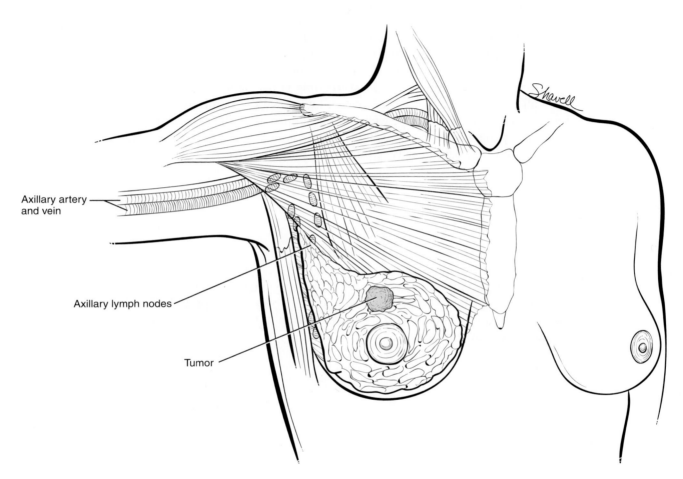

Axillary artery and vein

Axillary lymph nodes

Tumor

FIGURE 11–2

◆ For beginners, I recommend that the entire arm (limb) be prepped and draped into the operative field. This allows for mobility of the arm and offers potentially easier access to the SLN(s). After the patient is prepped and draped, 5 mL of Lymphazurin (1% isosulfan blue) dye can be injected peritumorally, in a subareolar location, or subdermally (deeper than intradermal, no wheal), taking care to disperse the dye around the tumor **(Figure 11-3)**. For melanoma, 1 mL of blue dye intradermally (raising a wheal) is sufficient. A 5-minute massage of the area following blue dye injection helps stimulate lymphatic uptake toward the axilla or nodal basin of interest. Peritumoral injection of isosulfan blue dye is performed by injecting 1 mL in each of four corners intraparenchymally around the tumor, with the final 1 mL injected superficial to the tumor (between the tumor and the skin). For palpable tumors, the injection is easily accomplished. For nonpalpable tumors, the injection is guided by ultrasound or by judging the depth and direction of the imbedded wire following standard needle localization. It is helpful for the radiologist to mark on the skin anterior to the tumor with an indelible marker at the time of needle localization. It is not advisable to inject all of the blue dye or radioactive colloid down the localization needle, because this does not disperse the blue dye well and may concentrate the dye deep within the breast tissue. For patients who previously have undergone excisional biopsy, injection should be made around the biopsy cavity, avoiding the seroma cavity.

1. INCISION

◆ The hand-held gamma counter is used to locate the SLN transcutaneously, and a 3-cm incision is made in line with the usual axillary dissection incision, usually just lateral to the pectoralis muscle edge and just below the hairline **(Figure 11-4)**. The localization of the "hot spot" allows for planning of a small incision over the suspected site of the SLN. If a hot spot is not identified, a curved transverse incision in the lower axilla just below the hairline provides excellent exposure.

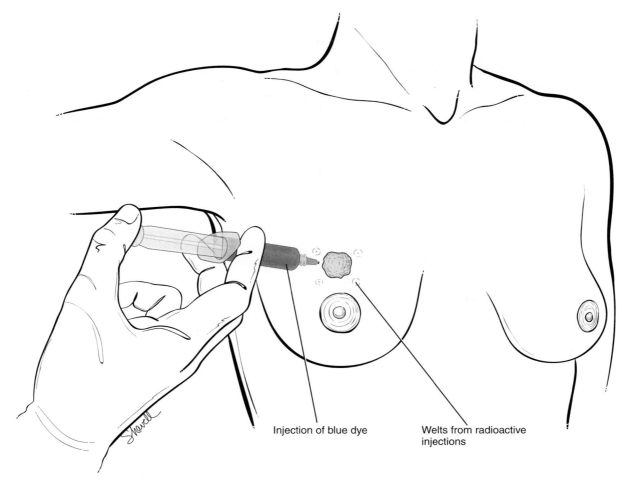

FIGURE 11–3

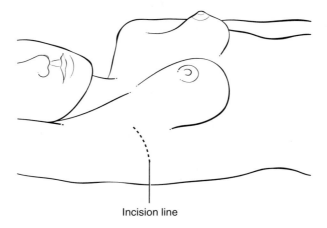

FIGURE 11–4

2. DISSECTION

◆ After dissecting through the subcutaneous tissue, the surgeon divides the clavipectoral fascia to gain exposure to the axillary contents. The gamma counter is used to help locate the SLN. As the dissection continues, the signal from the probe should increase in intensity **(Figure 11-5).** If there is difficulty in identifying an SLN, the clavipectoral fascia along the lateral border of the pectoralis major and minor muscles should be divided to easily access the entire axilla. This is accomplished by elevating and rotating the arm (which has been incorporated in the sterile field) medially.

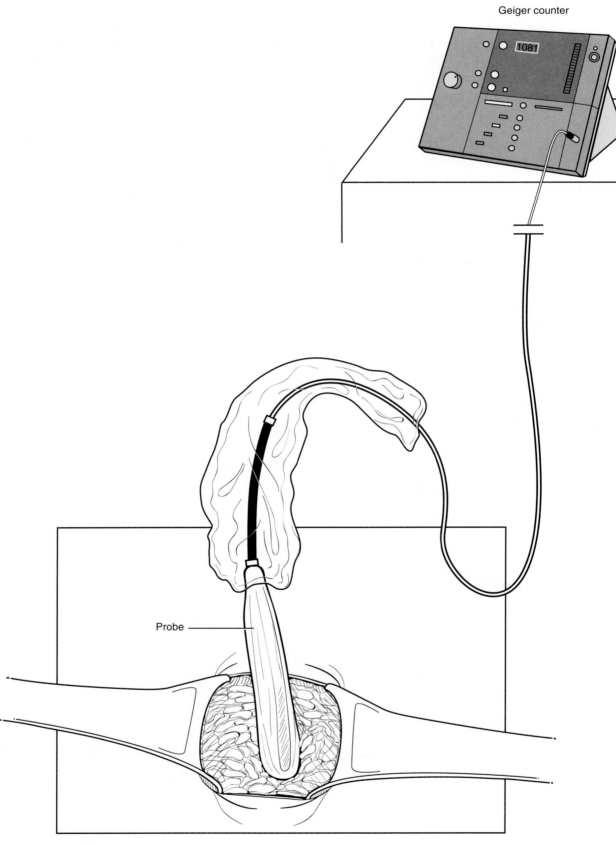

Geiger counter

Probe

FIGURE 11–5

◆ Using a combination of the visualization of blue dye in the afferent lymphatics and lymph nodes themselves, as well as the hand-held gamma probe, the location of the SLN is pinpointed **(Figure 11-6).** Care should be taken not to disrupt the capsule of the lymph node. Hemoclips are used for hemostasis and to clip the afferent lymphatic channels. Meticulous clipping of the lymphatics will prevent postoperative lymphocele formation. This is important because a closed suction drain is not placed for SLN biopsy.

◆ After the SLN is removed, ex vivo radioactive counts are obtained, and the node may be sent to pathology for frozen section analysis if it was harvested for breast cancer (see "Pearls and Pitfalls"). The background radioactivity in the axilla is then surveyed. False-negative rates are lowest if all blue nodes, blue-stained afferent lymphatic channels leading to an SLN, and nodes greater than 10% of the ex vivo count of the hottest SLN are harvested (the 10% rule). That is, if there is focal activity of 10% or greater of the ex vivo counts of the hottest SLN, a diligent search should be made for another SLN. The node is placed on the gamma probe (pointing away from the breast and up toward the ceiling) to obtain an ex vivo radioactive count. If the highest reading ("hottest node") recorded is 7099 counts per second, then any additional lymph node remaining in the axilla with counts greater than 710 (10% of the hottest node) should be removed as another SLN.

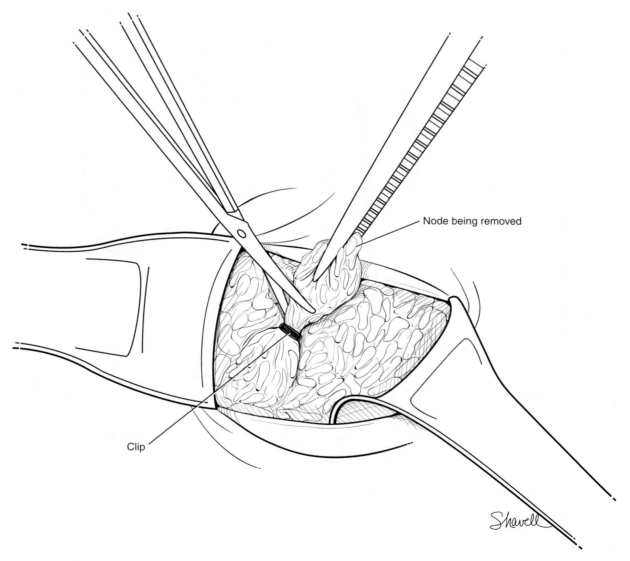

Node being removed

Clip

FIGURE 11–6

- After removal of blue and/or hot nodes, palpation of the surgical bed for enlarged, firm, or otherwise suspicious lymph nodes should be performed. A pathologic lymph node may not be hot or blue for two reasons: (1) the lymph node is completely replaced with tumor and the lymphatics are "blocked" from uptake of any tracer, and (2) unexplainable false-negative results do occur. A tumor-positive, nonradioactive or nonblue node should still be considered a "sentinel" node when removed because it accurately staged the axilla of that patient. If no SLN can be identified, then a default level I/II axillary dissection must be performed. On average, two to three SLNs are removed per case for breast cancer, and one to two for melanoma.

- SLN biopsy is followed by either breast-conserving therapy or mastectomy. If mastectomy is planned, it is helpful to perform the SLN biopsy first by opening a small portion of the axillary portion of the mastectomy incision before raising the flaps. Depending on the tumor location, raising the entire superior flap may result in blue dye spillage into the axilla, which can make identification of the SLN difficult.

3. CLOSING

- The axilla is irrigated and hemostasis is achieved. The wound is closed in two layers: an interrupted watertight layer with absorbable sutures that reapproximates the clavipectoral fascial layer and a subcuticular layer to close the skin edges.

STEP 4: POSTOPERATIVE CARE

- Should the patient require a completion axillary lymph node dissection, the previous SLN biopsy scar should be removed en bloc with the specimen.

STEP 5: PEARLS AND PITFALLS

- Unless formally trained during residency or fellowship, all surgeons must climb the learning curve and begin to learn this procedure by offering SLN biopsy with planned backup axillary dissection. This will allow the individual surgeon to calculate his or her own identification and false-negative rates. Surgeons who wish to adopt this technology must ensure that in their own hands, a false-negative rate of 5% or lower and an identification rate of 95% or higher are achieved. The false-negative rate significantly decreased from 9% for surgeons who performed 20 or fewer procedures to a rate of 1.9% for those who performed more than 20 procedures. It must be emphasized, however, that false-negative results and non-identification of the SLN can occur even after appropriate surgical training. Patients must be told of the small risk of a false-negative result and balance this against the benefits of a less invasive procedure. If staged to be SLN negative, the patient may have a small lifetime risk of axillary recurrence due to the potential of a false-negative result.

- Although limited data suggest that SLN biopsy may be feasible following previous SLN biopsy, previous neoadjuvant chemotherapy, or radiotherapy, if successful mapping is not achieved by the technical criteria defined previously, the standard levels I and II axillary dissection should be performed. Many studies demonstrate adequate identification rates, but few report false-negative rates in these clinical circumstances.

- The role for SLN biopsy in inflammatory breast cancer has not been defined.

- Some surgeons advocate frozen section analysis of the SLN, whereas others never use frozen section analysis because of the issue of sampling error in this setting. The decision to incorporate frozen section evaluation into one's program depends on the comfort level of the pathologist and surgeon. Patients are informed preoperatively that frozen section analysis may miss some positive SLNs, which subsequently will be found on final patho-logic sections. The sensitivity of frozen section analysis decreases with micrometastatic deposits, defined as tumor 2 mm or smaller in the SLN. If there is a positive SLN found on frozen section examination, this is an indication for completion axillary dissection under the same anesthetic setting. If frozen section evaluation is not used, the patient can return to the operating room (1 or 2 weeks later) for completion level I/II node dissection after final sections have been confirmed to be tumor-positive.

- For melanoma, frozen section analysis is never recommended. Because both serial section-ing and immunohistochemistry for tumor markers (e.g., S-100, MART-1) are required, per-manent sections are necessary for accurate histopathologic diagnosis.

- Injection technique: Many centers perform peritumoral injection of both blue dye and radioactive colloid. However, peritumoral injection of radioactive colloid results in a large zone of diffusion that can obscure the objective of locating the axillary SLN, especially for upper outer quadrant tumors. To minimize this "shine-through" effect, some centers use a sterile lead shield to block the radioactive interference from the upper outer quadrant of the breast. Furthermore, peritumoral injection results in relatively little uptake of the tracer from the breast tissue compared with dermal injection. Studies have shown that dermal in-jection of radioactive colloid significantly improves SLN identification rate and minimizes the false-negative rate. For instance, dermal injection of radioactive colloid is associated with SLNs that are fivefold to sevenfold more radioactive, or hot, than with the peritumoral injection method. When the dermal injection is used, the skin overlying the tumor can be retracted medially, away from the axilla, to facilitate accurate gamma probe localization.

STEP 6. CONCLUSION

- Implementation of SLN biopsy requires multidisciplinary cooperation and high standards of quality control. Ongoing studies, such as the American College of Surgeons Oncology Group Trials Z0010 and Z0011 and the NSABP trial B-32, should provide answers to many of the remaining clinically relevant questions.

SELECTED REFERENCES

1. Morton DL, Wen DR, Wong JH, et al: Technical details of intraoperative lymphatic mapping for early stage melanoma. Arch Surg 1992;127:392-399.
2. Giuliano AE, Kirgan DM, Guenther JM, Morton DL: Lymphatic mapping and sentinel lymphadenectomy for breast cancer. Ann Surg 1994;220:391-401.
3. McMasters KM, Giuliano AE, Ross MI, et al: Sentinel lymph node biopsy for breast cancer: Not yet the standard of care. N Engl J Med 1998;339:990-995.
4. McMasters KM, Chao C, Wong SL, et al: Sentinel lymph node biopsy in patients with ductal carcinoma-in-situ: A proposal. Cancer 2002;95:15-50.
5. McMasters KM, Wong SL, Chao C, et al: Defining the optimal surgeon experience for breast cancer sentinel lymph node biopsy: A model for implementation of new surgical techniques. Ann Surg 2001;234:292-300.

CHAPTER 12

EXCISION OF BENIGN BREAST LESION

Courtney M. Townsend, Jr.

STEP 1: SURGICAL ANATOMY

- ◆ Knowledge of breast anatomy is important. Benign lesions are usually fibroadenomas, papillomas, or fibrocystic condition.

- ◆ Fibroadenomas usually occur in younger women, often in their 20s, and often are characterized by a round, smooth, "slippable" mass. Indication for operation is patient concern, because fibroadenoma is not a premalignant lesion.

STEP 2: PREOPERATIVE CONSIDERATIONS

- ◆ I favor the patient having general anesthesia for all of these resections for the following reasons:
  - ◆ In young women with dense breast tissue, local anesthetic diffuses poorly. Resecting a lesion at any depth or size often is much more uncomfortable than one would think.
  - ◆ With fibrocystic condition in premenopausal or postmenopausal women, the fibrous nature of the reaction sometimes is such that local anesthetic does not diffuse well throughout the breast. If local anesthetic is chosen, however, I always avoid the use of epinephrine because bleeding, which occurs some time later, may not be detected at the time of operation.
  - ◆ Many lesions can be reached through an areolar margin incision, even though they appear initially to be some distance from the areolar margin. However, if a lesion is too far from the areolar margin, then an incision directly over the lesion in Langer's lines paralleling the areolar margin should be used. Radial incisions are to be avoided **(Figures 12-1 and 12-2).**
  - ◆ A preoperative mammogram is required for all patients who are to have a breast operation.
  - ◆ Prophylactic antibiotics are given.

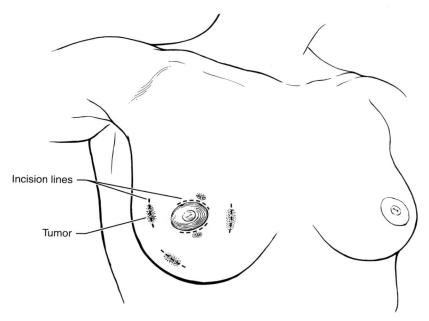

Incision lines

Tumor

FIGURE 12–1

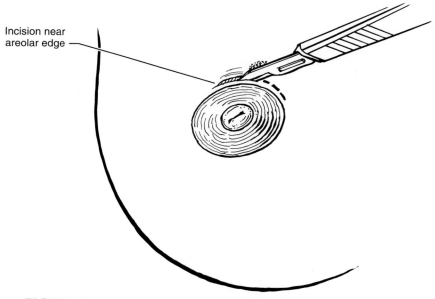

Incision near
areolar edge

FIGURE 12–2

STEP 3: OPERATIVE STEPS

1. INCISION

◆ Regardless of the size of the incision, flaps are raised after the skin incision has been carried down through the intramammary fat.

2. DISSECTION

◆ The lesion is then approached directly or, if it is not a palpable lesion, the area of breast tissue into which the localizing wire disappears is resected **(Figures 12-3 and 12-4)**.

◆ The portion of tissue into which the wire disappears is excised blindly and the specimen mammography is required to determine that the lesion has been removed.

◆ For a solid lesion, the margin is easily determined. I use a traction suture placed in a figure-of-eight fashion rather than clamps.

◆ Before final removal of the lesion, the borders are marked. I use a short suture on the superior margin, a long suture for the lateral margin, and a traction suture of intermediate length marks the superficial margin.

◆ Hemostasis is achieved with coagulating cautery, and the wound is irrigated with hydrogen peroxide to aid in detection of bleeders.

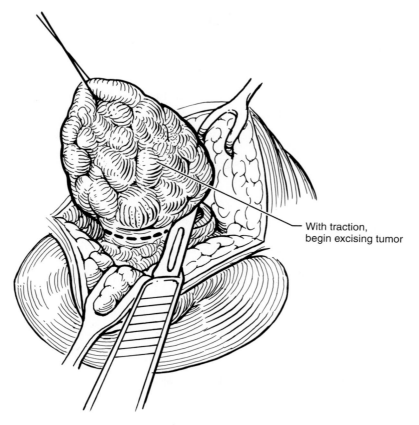

With traction, begin excising tumor

FIGURE 12–3

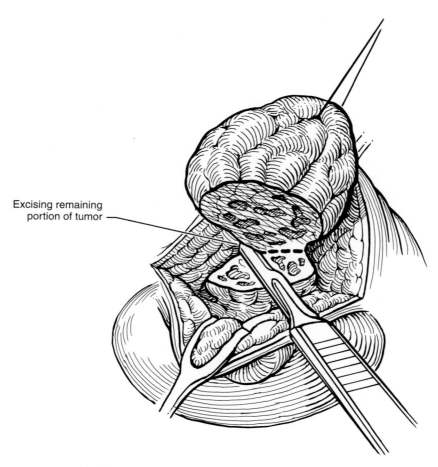

Excising remaining portion of tumor

FIGURE 12–4

3. CLOSURE

- The breast tissue is not closed and the wound is closed with subcuticular absorbable sutures **(Figures 12-5 and 12-6)**.

- The wound is covered with a plastic dressing.

STEP 4: POSTOPERATIVE CARE

- I prefer nonopioid analgesics.

- An ice pack is used for the first 12 to 24 hours.

- I recommend that the patient wear a new sports bra for support and wear it until the discomfort has disappeared.

STEP 5: PEARLS AND PITFALLS

- Avoid local anesthetic in dense breasts.

- Avoid epinephrine if local anesthetic is to be used.

- Traction sutures prevent destruction of the specimen to be excised by multiple applications of forceps or clamps. I use coagulating cautery for dissection and therefore take a more generous margin because there may be coagulation artifact produced in the specimen.

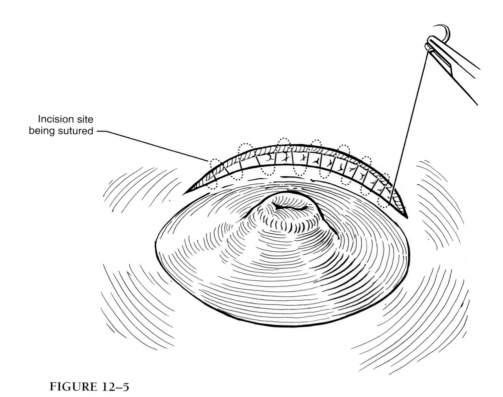

Incision site being sutured

FIGURE 12–5

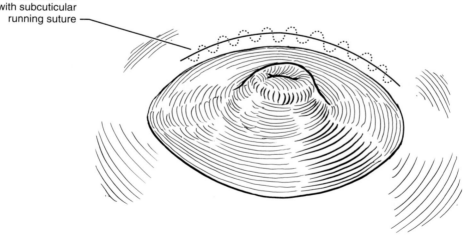

Incision closed with subcuticular running suture

FIGURE 12–6

CHAPTER 13

MAJOR DUCT EXCISION

Courtney M. Townsend, Jr.

STEP 1: SURGICAL ANATOMY

- ◆ A comprehensive understanding of the location of the mammary gland in relation to the chest wall musculature, the fascial boundaries, the lymphatic drainage pathways, the vascular supply to the breast and the associated supporting structures, and the innervation of the breast and surrounding tissues is essential for appropriate surgical management.

STEP 2: PREOPERATIVE CONSIDERATIONS

- ◆ Bilateral nipple discharge, which is usually seen in postmenopausal patients, is sometimes sufficiently voluminous to cause problems with soiling.

- ◆ Bilateral nipple discharge is rarely due to neoplastic lesions and almost always due to duct ectasia. As noted, the lobes of the breast are drained by ducts that coalesce in the subareolar area into 5 to 10 lactiferous ducts, each of which opens independently in the nipple.

- ◆ Diagnosis of duct ectasia is made when single-digit compression is carried out and discharge from multiple ducts in the nipple is noted, usually bilaterally.

- ◆ Preoperative mammography is required for all patients.

- ◆ General anesthesia is used.

STEP 3: OPERATIVE STEPS

1. INCISION

- ◆ When resection is required, it is performed through an areolar margin incision. The areola is elevated from the intramammary fat and all of the ducts together can be identified and dissected free from the undersurface of the nipple (**Figures 13-1 and 13-2**).

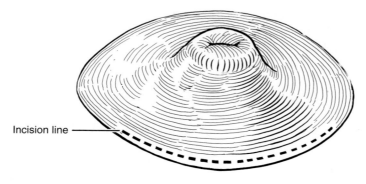

Incision line ————

FIGURE 13–1

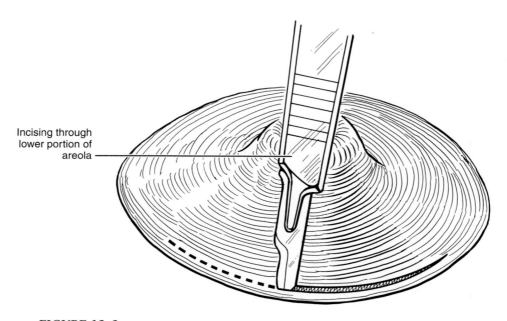

Incising through
lower portion of
areola ————

FIGURE 13–2

2. DISSECTION

- The ducts are ligated and divided, as a group, in the subareolar area, and an inverted cone excision removing the lactiferous ducts is carried out in a circumferential fashion **(Figures 13-3 and 13-4).**

- Dissection and hemostasis are carried out with cautery.

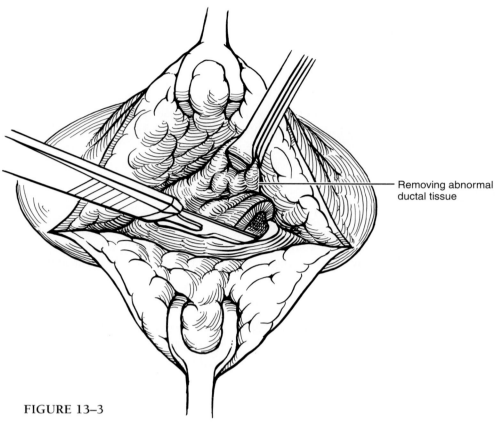

Removing abnormal ductal tissue

FIGURE 13–3

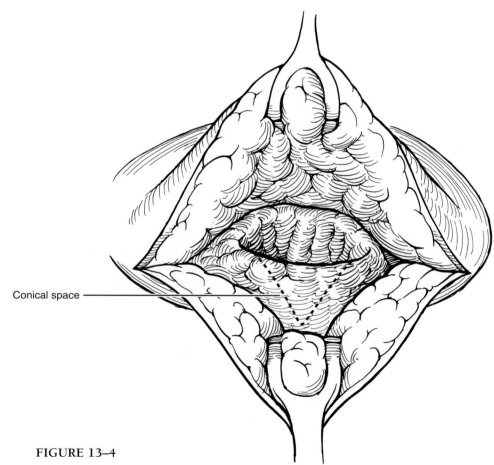

Conical space

FIGURE 13–4

3. CLOSURE

◆ The breast tissue is not closed.

◆ The wound is irrigated with hydrogen peroxide and, after hemostasis is secured, the wound is closed with running subcuticular absorbable sutures **(Figure 13-5)**.

STEP 4: POSTOPERATIVE CARE

◆ I recommend that all patients who are going to have partial mastectomy for benign or malignant conditions wear a new sport or jogging bra after the procedure, because it gives good nonrigid support to the breast.

◆ An ice pack is often helpful to relieve localized pain, and one or two doses of nonopioid analgesic is usually all that is required. The dressing can be removed in the bath 24 to 36 hours after the operation and no further dressing needs to be used.

STEP 5: PEARLS AND PITFALLS

◆ I do not close the breast tissue because of the distortion that would occur.

◆ The extent of breast tissue excised is different from when resecting an area of pathologic nipple discharge. This is a method to ablate the ducts; therefore, less extensive breast tissue resection is required.

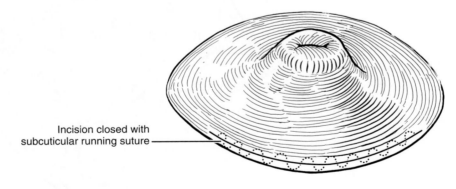

Incision closed with
subcuticular running suture

FIGURE 13–5

CHAPTER 14

INTRADUCTAL PAPILLOMA

Courtney M. Townsend, Jr.

STEP 1: SURGICAL ANATOMY

◆ The ducts draining the 15 to 20 lobes of the breast tissue coalesce into 5 to 10 lactiferous ducts, each of which opens separately in the nipple.

◆ Understanding that the subareolar ducts represent components from multiple glands, excision extends from the immediate area under the nipple in which the involved duct is identified to encompass the tissue drained. It is excised en bloc so that the specimen is much larger than simply a duct as shown in **Figure 14-1.**

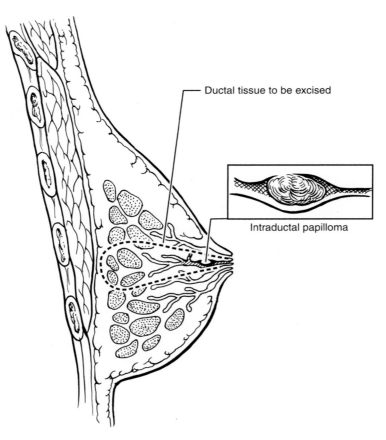

Ductal tissue to be excised

Intraductal papilloma

FIGURE 14–1

STEP 2: PREOPERATIVE CONSIDERATIONS

- Pathologic nipple discharge is spontaneous, persistent, nonlactational, and unilateral. A single-duct opening in the nipple can be identified as the source of the discharge.

- The color and consistency of the discharge play no role in determination for resection once the criteria for pathologic nipple discharge are met.

- Everyone with a breast complaint, including nipple discharge, should have a bilateral mammogram. The object of the mammogram is not to determine whether operation for pathologic nipple discharge will be performed but to search for occult cancer in both breasts.

- Ductography is not required to identify the segment of breast to be resected.

- Cytologic examination of nipple discharge is not required.

- Pathologic nipple discharge requires resection and pathologic examination of the tissue. The danger is that intraductal papillary cancer could be overlooked.

STEP 3: OPERATIVE STEPS

- I prefer that the patient has general anesthesia, although local anesthesia may be used.

1. INCISION

- The area of breast in which the lesion is located can be identified by single-digit compression from periphery toward the areola **(Figure 14-2)**.

2. DISSECTION

- The duct opening through which discharge flows can be identified; that identifies the area for the excision. An areolar margin incision is used, and the areola is elevated from underlying intramammary fat. The involved duct can usually be identified as distended and often containing a dark substance visible through the wall of the duct **(Figure 14-3)**.

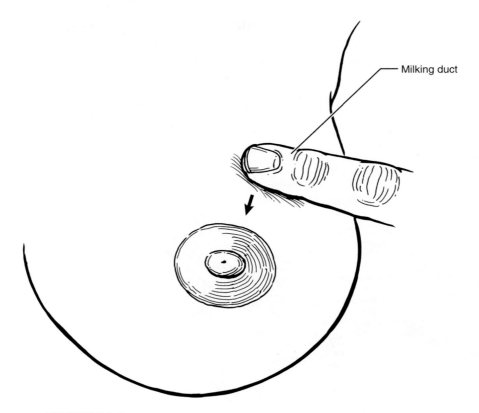

Milking duct

FIGURE 14–2

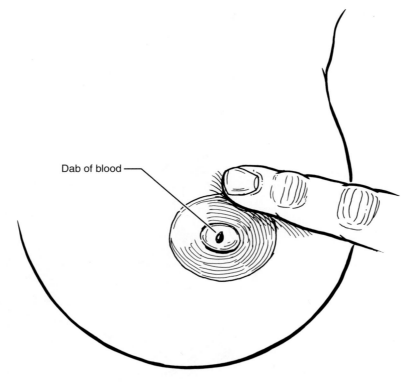

Dab of blood

FIGURE 14–3

◆ If the involved duct cannot be identified, single-digit compression in the area after the areola is raised can be carried out to elicit discharge from the nipple, which is noted so that the area of resection can be identified **(Figure 14-4)**.

◆ Once the duct is isolated below the nipple, it is dissected free from the surrounding tissue, ligated, and divided just below the nipple **(Figures 14-5 and 14-6)**.

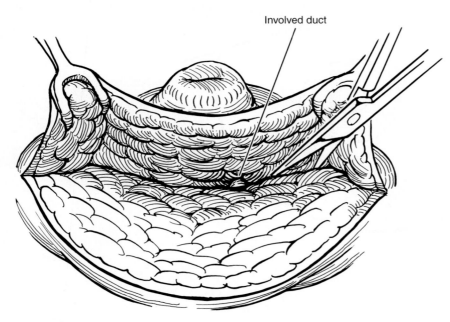

Involved duct

FIGURE 14–4

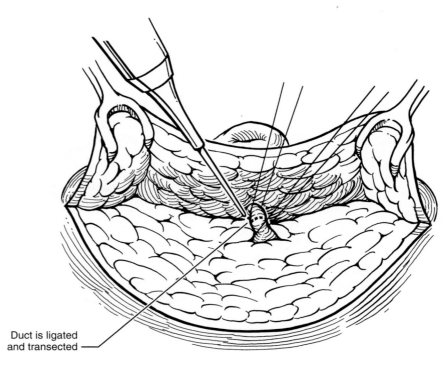

Duct is ligated
and transected —

FIGURE 14–5

◆ The segment drained by the duct is then excised by sharp dissection **(Figure 14-7)**. (I prefer cautery. Although the illustration shows specimen grasped with forceps, I have come to prefer use of a traction suture placed in a figure-of-eight fashion to avoid clamp dislodgment with tearing breast tissue).

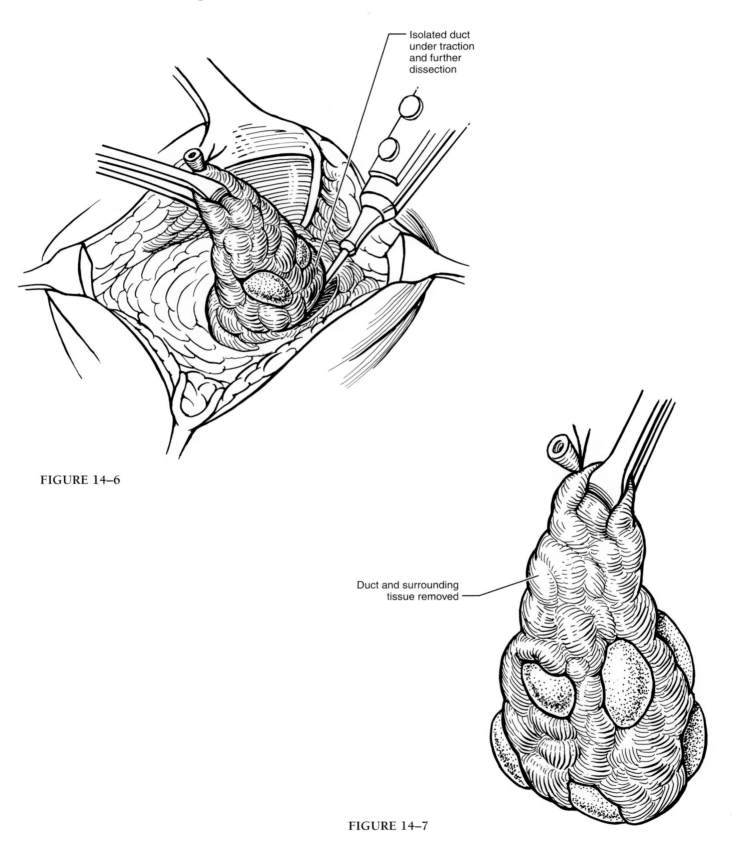

Isolated duct
under traction
and further
dissection

FIGURE 14–6

Duct and surrounding
tissue removed

FIGURE 14–7

◆ After the specimen is excised, the wound is irrigated. I use hydrogen peroxide because it helps localize any bleeding. Direct cautery through the foam of the peroxide can be carried out.

3. CLOSURE

◆ The breast tissue is not closed. After hemostasis is secured, the incision is closed with running subcuticular absorbable sutures and a clear plastic dressing is applied.

STEP 4: POSTOPERATIVE CARE

◆ I recommend that all patients who are going to have partial mastectomy for benign or malignant conditions wear a new sport or jogging bra after the procedure, because it gives good, nonrigid support to the breast.

◆ An ice pack is often helpful to relieve localized pain, and one or two doses of nonopioid analgesic is usually all that is required. The dressing can be removed in the bath 24 to 36 hours after the operation, and no further dressing needs to be used.

STEP 5: PEARLS AND PITFALLS

◆ The most important determination to be made is that pathologic nipple discharge is present and that resection will be required. Every patient must have a preoperative mammography, but there is no need for ductography or for cannulation of the ductal opening at the time of operation.

◆ The duct can be identified with digital compression after the incision is made, or often the duct can be visualized and seen to be dilated, containing the dark fluid.

THE ESOPHAGUS

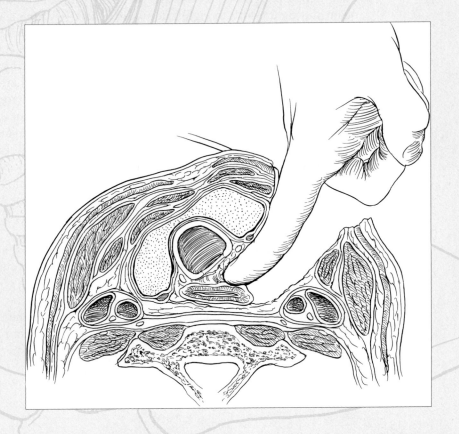

CHAPTER 15

ZENKER'S DIVERTICULA

David B. Loran and Joseph B. Zwischenberger

STEP 1: SURGICAL ANATOMY

- A comprehensive understanding of the anatomy of the esophagus is critical before undertaking surgical procedures on the esophagus.

- **Figure 15-1** demonstrates key anatomic structures that must be considered in surgical correction of Zenker's diverticula.

STEP 2: PREOPERATIVE CONSIDERATIONS

- Pharyngoesophageal (Zenker's) diverticula, the most common diverticula of the esophagus, occur during the fifth to eighth decades of life. They are classified as pulsion diverticula and consist of mucosal and submucosal esophageal layers. Zenker's diverticula are believed to result from either an uncoordinated relaxation or incomplete relaxation of the upper esophageal sphincter (cricopharyngeal muscle) during swallowing, resulting in higher than normal bolus pressures in the lower pharynx. This leads to herniation of the esophageal mucosa between the oblique fibers of the inferior constrictor muscle (superiorly) and the transverse fibers of the cricopharyngeal muscle (inferiorly) (see Figure 15-1). Small diverticula rarely produce symptoms. However, progressive enlargement of the diverticula leads to pronounced symptoms. Upper esophageal dysphagia, foul breath, and spontaneous regurgitation of undigested food material are characteristically seen. Rarely is a palpable mass encountered. Late manifestations include weight loss, hoarseness, and pulmonary abscess. Any symptomatic Zenker's diverticulum should be corrected.

- Barium esophagram is obtained to confirm the presence of a pharyngoesophageal diverticulum and localize it to the left or right side to assist in planning the surgical approach.

- Anesthetic approach is dictated by the comorbidities of the patient and by surgeon preference. The procedure can be performed satisfactorily under a regional cervical block or a general anesthetic.

◆ The patient is placed supine on the operating room table, with the head slightly extended and turned away from the side of the incision. Some surgeons prefer to have the patient semirecumbent or seated.

◆ Betadine preparation of the skin should be applied to cover the entire neck and upper chest. This should include the area from the mastoid process to the spinous processes posteriorly, along the angle of the mandible anteriorly, and to the level of the nipples inferiorly.

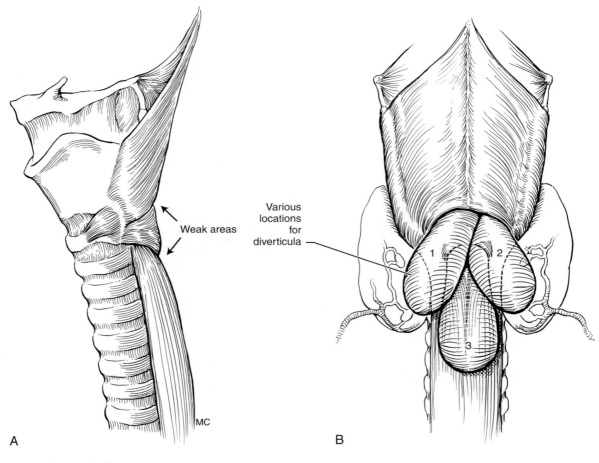

A

B

FIGURE 15–1

STEP 3: OPERATIVE STEPS

1. INCISION

♦ Almost all diverticula are best approached through the left side of the neck. Various incisions can be used based on surgeon preference and patient anatomy. Most surgeons use an incision along the anterior border of the sternocleidomastoid muscle, from the level of the hyoid bone to 1 cm above the clavicle. Alternatively, a transverse cervical incision can be used within a prominent cervical fold centered over the middle third of the sternocleidomastoid muscle (**Figure 15-2**).

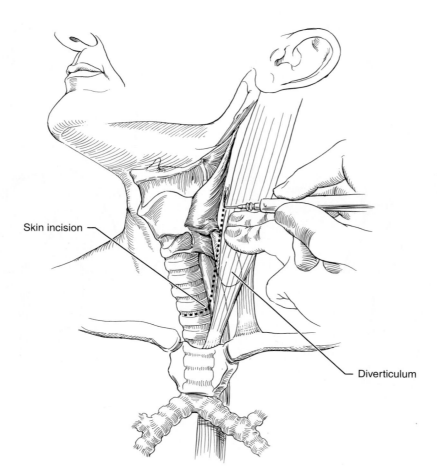

FIGURE 15–2

2. DISSECTION

◆ The incision is carried through the platysma to expose the deep cervical fascia. The sterno-cleidomastoid muscle and carotid sheath are retracted laterally to expose the retroesopha-geal space. Sometimes ligation of the middle thyroid vein is needed to adequately retract the thyroid gland and larynx medially. Care should be taken to avoid excessive retraction on the thyroid so that the recurrent laryngeal nerve, which courses superiorly in the tra-cheoesophageal groove, is not injured.

◆ The omohyoid muscle, which can be divided, is retracted superiorly to complete exposure of the area and should bring into view the diverticulum as it emerges superior to the crico-pharyngeal muscle **(Figure 15-3)**.

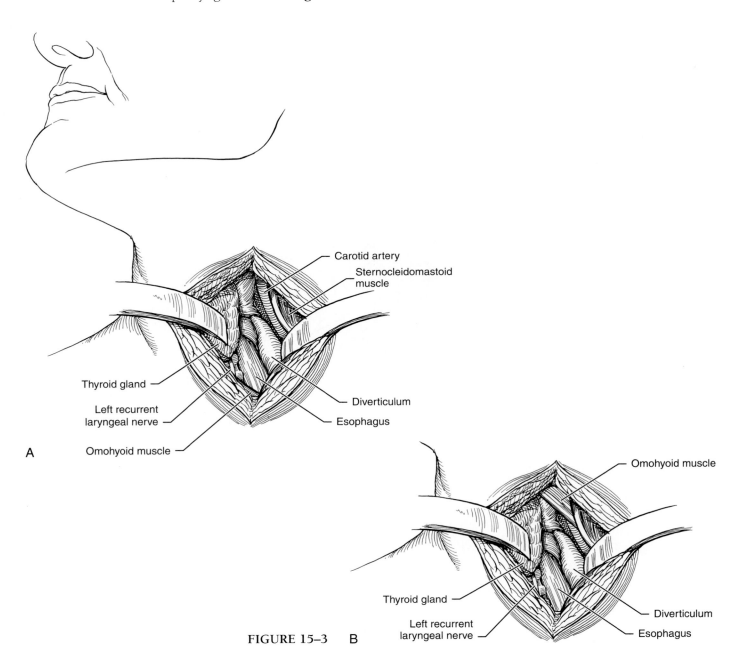

FIGURE 15–3   B

◆ The diverticulum is grasped with an Allis or Babcock clamp and dissected free from the surrounding fibroadipose tissue to adequately expose the neck. A 36F to 40F bougie is placed into the pharynx by the anesthesiologist to help prevent narrowing of the esophagus with diverticulectomy and to facilitate dissection. A myotomy is performed with a no. 15 blade scalpel or Bovie electrocautery unit on low settings between a dissecting hemostat from the base of the diverticula through the entire length of the transverse cricopharyngeal muscle fibers and extended onto the longitudinal muscle fibers of the upper esophagus over a total length of 8 to 10 cm **(Figure 15-4)**.

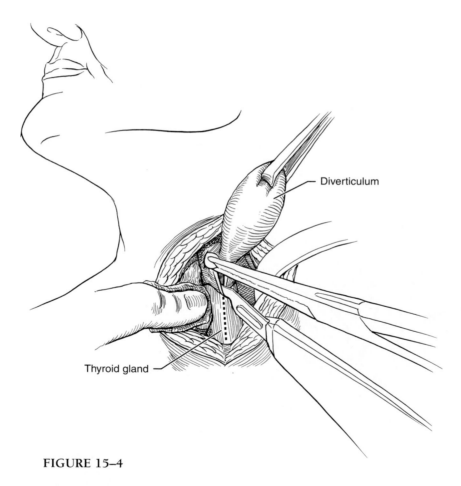

FIGURE 15–4

◆ The base of the diverticulum is now easily seen. Diverticula that measure less than 2 cm long usually do not require resection, and the mucosa will retract once the myotomy is performed. Those diverticula larger than 2 cm will require resection or "pex." Many surgeons prefer to tack, or pex, the pouch cephalad on the pharynx **(Figure 15-5).**

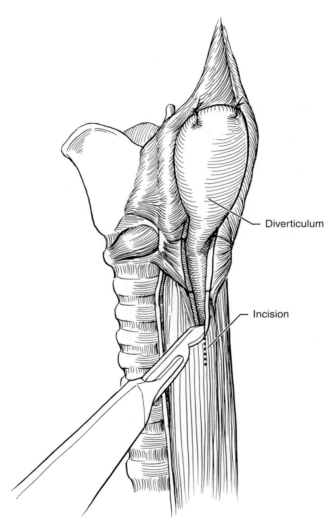

— Diverticulum

— Incision

FIGURE 15–5

◆ A stapling device with 4.8-mm staples is oriented along the longitudinal esophageal axis with the bougie in place and is fired to resect the diverticulum (**Figures 15-6 and 15-7**).

◆ Alternatively, the diverticula can be resected with a no. 15 blade scalpel and the mucosal defect closed with a running 4-0 absorbable suture.

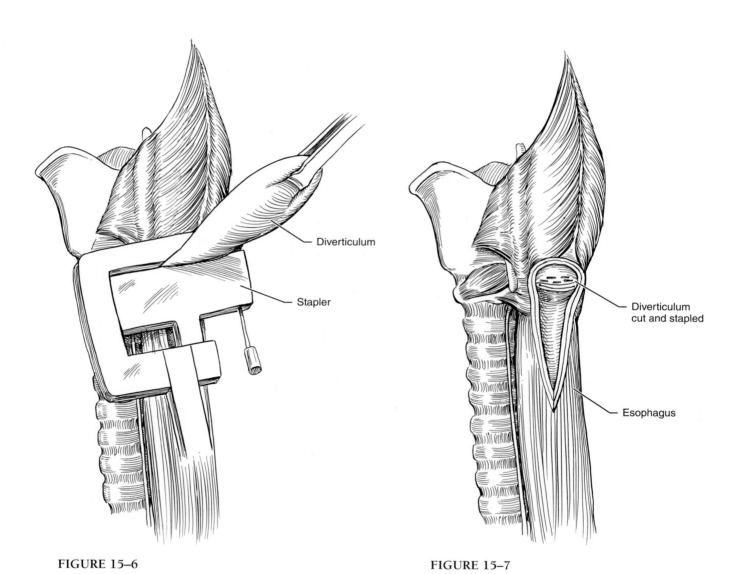

FIGURE 15–6   FIGURE 15–7

◆ The bougie is removed and the surgeon guides placement of a nasogastric (NG) tube into the lower pharynx to check for mucosal leaks. The surgical bed is filled with water to cover the suture/staple line while the anesthesiologist gently injects air through the NG tube. If no air bubbles are seen, mucosal integrity is intact. The staple line is left uncovered and a small Jackson-Pratt drain is placed in the surgical bed and exited through a separate stab incision in the neck laterally **(Figure 15-8)**. A leak can be closed primarily with fine interrupted sutures and reinforced with muscle coverage.

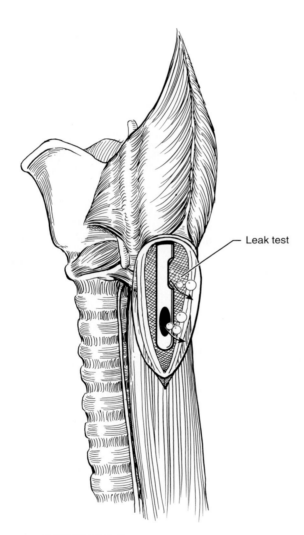

FIGURE 15–8

3. CLOSING

◆ Alternatively, if the muscular layers are intact they can be reapproximated. Retractors are removed and the platysma is closed with interrupted stitches using 4-0 absorbable suture. The drain is secured to the skin with a 4-0 silk stitch (**Figures 15-9 and 15-10**).

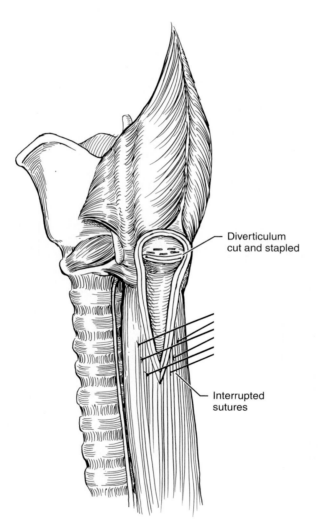

Diverticulum cut and stapled

Interrupted sutures

FIGURE 15–9

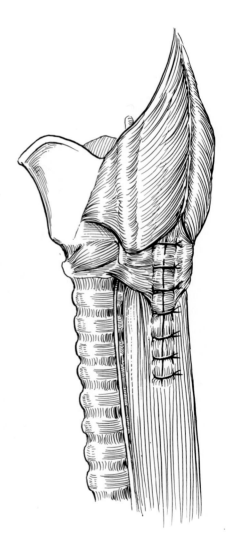

FIGURE 15–10

STEP 4: POSTOPERATIVE CARE

◆ After recovery from anesthesia, the patient is returned to a floor bed, with no food allowed overnight. On the second postoperative day, a contrast esophageal swallow study is performed and a diet started if no leak is present.

◆ The following day, the drain can be removed if no increase in output is observed after initiation of a diet. The patient can be discharged to home by the third or fourth postoperative day.

STEP 5: PEARLS AND PITFALLS

◆ Recognize that Zenker's diverticula are the sequelae of cricopharyngeal/esophageal dysmotility. Many patients will present with cricopharyngeal dysfunction (choking or aspiration or both) without a Zenker's diverticulum. The goal of the operation is to address the dysmotility in a two-step process: myotomy followed by management of the diverticulum.

◆ Recent retrospective reports with endoscopic stapler-assisted diverticulotomy and carbon dioxide laser endoscopic diverticulotomy present alternative therapies for Zenker's diverticula. Advocates note shorter operative time, shorter hospital stay, and quicker return to diet. The techniques have not been shown to be superior to an open procedure, with a recurrence rate of approximately 10%. Carbon dioxide laser endoscopic diverticulotomy is also an alternative to open surgery, but likewise results in a higher failure rate.

SELECTED REFERENCES

1. Wirth D, Kern B, Guenin MO, et al: Outcome and quality of life after open surgery versus endoscopic stapler-assisted esophagodiverticulostomy for Zenker's diverticulum. Dis Esophagus 2006;19:294-298.
2. Chang CY, Payyapilli RJ, Scher RL: Endoscopic staple diverticulostomy for Zenker's diverticulum: Review of literature and experience in 159 consecutive cases. Laryngoscope 2003;113:957-965.
3. Chang CW, Burkey BB, Netterville JL, et al: Carbon dioxide laser endoscopic diverticulotomy versus open diverticulectomy for Zenker's diverticulum. Laryngoscope 2004;114:519-527.

CHAPTER 16

ESOPHAGECTOMY—TRANSHIATAL

David B. Loran and Joseph B. Zwischenberger

STEP 1: SURGICAL ANATOMY

- A comprehensive understanding of the anatomy of the esophagus is critical before undertaking surgical procedures on the esophagus.

- **Figure 16-1** demonstrates key anatomic structures that must be considered before performing a transhiatal esophagectomy.

STEP 2: PREOPERATIVE CONSIDERATIONS

- Indications for transthoracic esophagectomy include carcinoma, caustic injury with stricture or dysplastic mucosal changes, and other benign diseases. Most surgeons agree benign disease is best treated with transhiatal esophagectomy, which eliminates the risk of intrathoracic anastomotic leak and spares the patient the discomfort of thoracotomy without compromising outcomes. Carcinoma at any level of the esophagus can be safely resected by transhiatal approach. In performing a transhiatal esophagectomy, the surgeon removes accessible cervical, intrathoracic, and intra-abdominal lymph nodes for staging, but a complete en bloc resection of adjacent lymph node–bearing tissue is not accomplished.

- Transhiatal esophagectomy results in a lower incidence of pulmonary complications compared with a transthoracic approach. Anastomotic leak rates range from 12% to 15% but have been shown to be approximately 3% with a stapled technique. When a leak does occur, the associated morbidity and mortality are less than that seen for leaks from an intrathoracic esophagogastrostomy.

- Informed consent is obtained and the patient is made nothing-by-mouth status at least 8 hours before the procedure. A bowel preparation can be given to the patient the day before the procedure, in case the colon is needed as a reconstruction conduit. In the operating room, a radial artery catheter should be used for continuous blood pressure monitoring, because retrocardiac dissection can cause periods of hypotension. Central venous access is not routinely necessary; however, if needed, the right neck veins should be used to allow the surgeon complete access to the left side of the neck during operation. A standard endotracheal tube is used for intubation.

◆ General endotracheal anesthesia is mandatory for this procedure. Close cooperation and communication between anesthesiologist and surgeon must be maintained, especially during the transhiatal dissection when transient hypotension is expected. During this time, inhalation anesthetics that can contribute to hypotension should be discontinued, and the inspired oxygen concentration should be increased.

◆ The patient is placed supine on the operating table with the head slightly extended and turned to the right. Arms are tucked and protected close to the patient's body to allow the surgeon unimpeded access to the neck, chest, and abdomen.

◆ The skin over the entire neck, chest, and abdomen should be prepped with povidone-iodine (Betadine).

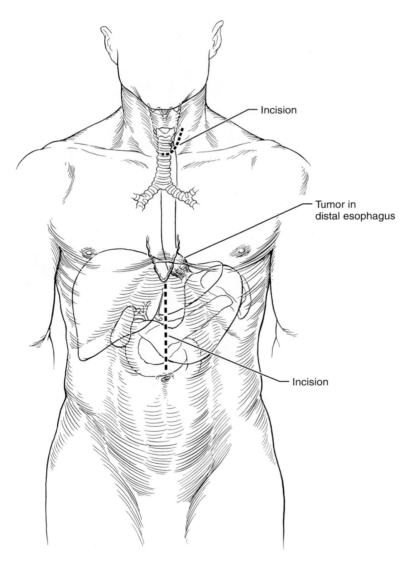

FIGURE 16–1

STEP 3: OPERATIVE STEPS

1. INCISION

◆ An upper midline supraumbilical incision from the xiphoid process to the umbilicus is used to begin the abdominal portion of the procedure. The exposure should be extended cephalad to excise the xiphoid process to gain maximum access to the esophageal hiatus. A self-retaining retractor can facilitate exposure of the upper abdomen (**Figures 16-1 and 16-2**).

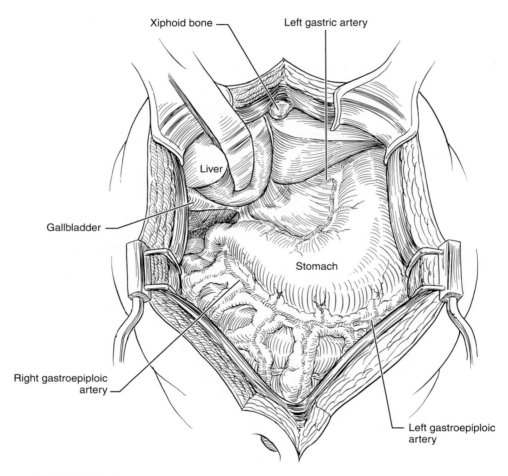

FIGURE 16–2

2. DISSECTION

◆ Upon entering the abdomen, the surgeon should perform careful inspection to search for metastatic disease and to ensure the stomach is free from scarring, shortening, or disease that will preclude its use as a suitable conduit for reconstruction.

◆ The surgeon must be intimately familiar with the arterial anatomy of the upper abdomen and early in the course of the dissection must identify the left gastroepiploic artery and protect this artery throughout the operation **(Figure 16-3)**.

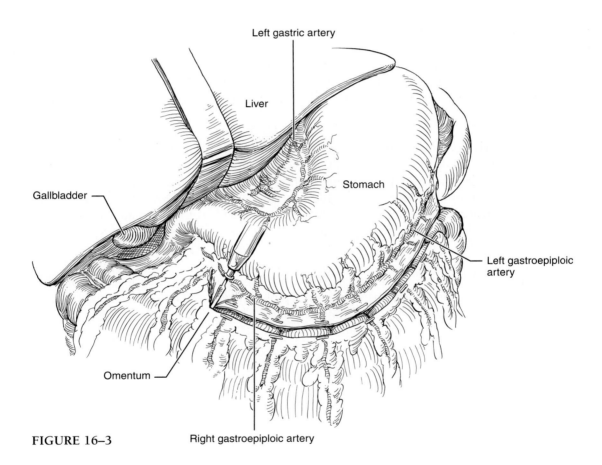

FIGURE 16–3

◆ To begin mobilization of the stomach, the left triangular ligament is taken down and the left liver lobe is retracted to the right. The greater omentum is separated from the greater curve of the stomach, beginning at an avascular plane approximately at the greater curve's midpoint. Dissection is then carried superiorly to the esophageal hiatus, carefully ligating the left gastroepiploic artery and all short gastric vessels. Care must be taken to avoid pinching a portion of the stomach wall within ligature ties of the short gastric vessels, which can later lead to necrosis and perforation of the gastric wall. Once the surgeon has reached the esophageal hiatus, the peritoneum is incised and the distal esophagus encircled with a Penrose drain to aid in esophageal retraction and dissection. The lesser omentum is dissected from the lesser curve of the stomach, and the left gastric artery is ligated because its branches supply the lesser curve. All lymph nodes in the area should be included with the specimen. Identification and preservation of the right gastric artery along this dissection plane is attempted **(Figure 16-4)**.

◆ Next a pyloromyotomy is performed from 1 to 2 cm on the anterior gastric wall through the pylorus extending approximately 0.5 to 1.0 cm onto the duodenum. We prefer to use a fine-tipped hemostat and needle-tipped Bovie for careful dissection of the stomach and duodenum muscular wall away from the underlying mucosa. The surgeon must ensure the mucosa has not been violated. If the lumen of the bowel has been entered, the mucosal defect is closed primarily and Heineke-Mikulicz pyloroplasty is performed **(Figure 16-5)**.

◆ The hiatus is enlarged by small radial incisions of the crura to allow much of the esophageal dissection under direct vision through the hiatal keyhole. To complete the abdominal portion of the procedure, the Penrose drain is retracted downward, and the distal 10 to 15 cm of esophagus is mobilized through the hiatus by blunt and sharp dissection. At this point the surgeon must determine that the distal esophagus is free from adhesions or tumor or both to proceed with the operation.

◆ To complete gastric mobilization, the remaining greater omentum is freed from the greater curve again, preserving the right gastroepiploic artery, and a Kocher maneuver is performed to ensure maximum gastric mobility.

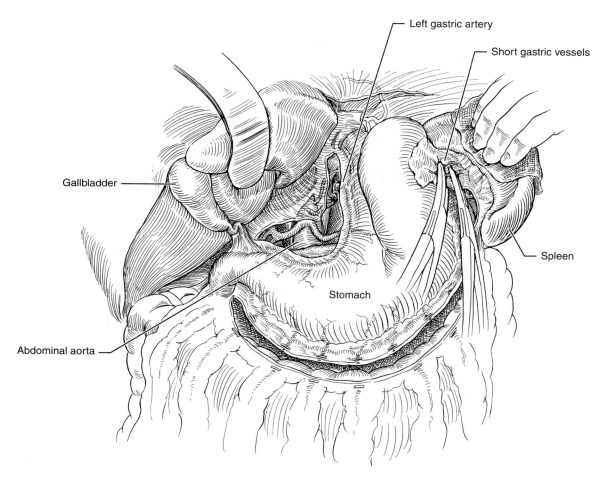

FIGURE 16–4

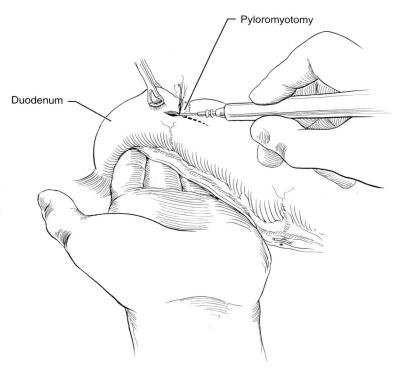

FIGURE 16–5

◆ The cervical dissection begins by placing an incision along the anterior border of the left sternocleidomastoid muscle from the hyoid bone to 1 cm above the clavicle. The incision is carried through the platysma to expose the deep cervical fascia (**Figure 16-6**).

◆ The sternocleidomastoid muscle and carotid sheath are retracted laterally while the thyroid gland and trachea are retracted medially to expose the proximal esophagus. Occasionally the middle thyroid vein and inferior thyroid artery need to be divided for adequate exposure. Care should be taken to avoid excessive retraction or placing instruments in the tracheo-esophageal groove, where the recurrent laryngeal nerve can be injured (**Figure 16-7**).

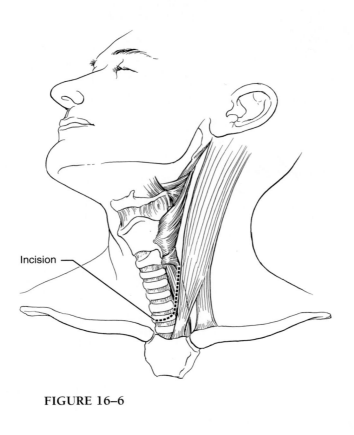

Incision

FIGURE 16–6

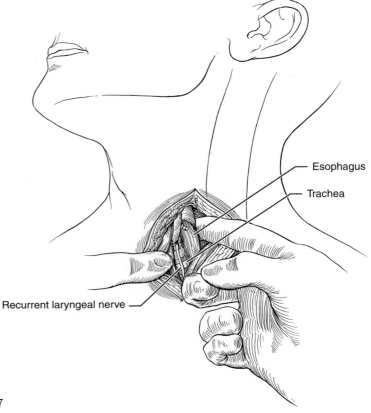

Esophagus

Trachea

Recurrent laryngeal nerve

FIGURE 16–7

◆ The cervical esophagus is mobilized by blunt dissection, beginning in the prevertebral space and working medially. The tracheoesophageal groove is opened with blunt dissection that is continued medially to connect with the prevertebral dissection (**Figures 16-8 and 16-9**).

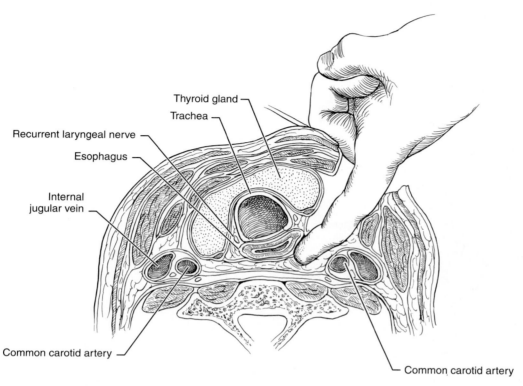

Thyroid gland

Trachea

Recurrent laryngeal nerve

Esophagus

Internal jugular vein

Common carotid artery

Common carotid artery

FIGURE 16–8

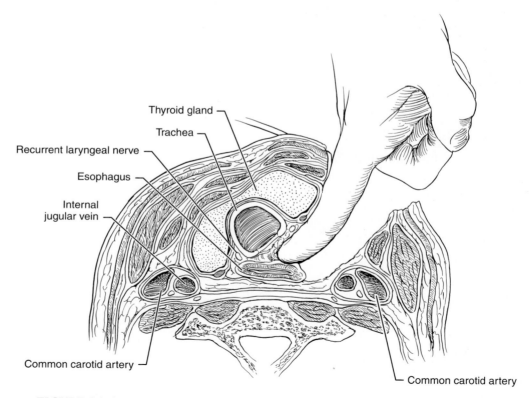

Thyroid gland

Trachea

Recurrent laryngeal nerve

Esophagus

Internal jugular vein

Common carotid artery

Common carotid artery

FIGURE 16–9

◆ Now that the proximal and distal esophagus is mobilized, the transhiatal dissection is begun to fully mobilize the remaining esophagus is continued. Continuous traction is placed on each of the Penrose drains encircling the ends of the esophagus while the surgeon bluntly develops the prevertebral plane with his or her right hand through the hiatus and left hand through the cervical incision (**Figure 16-10**).

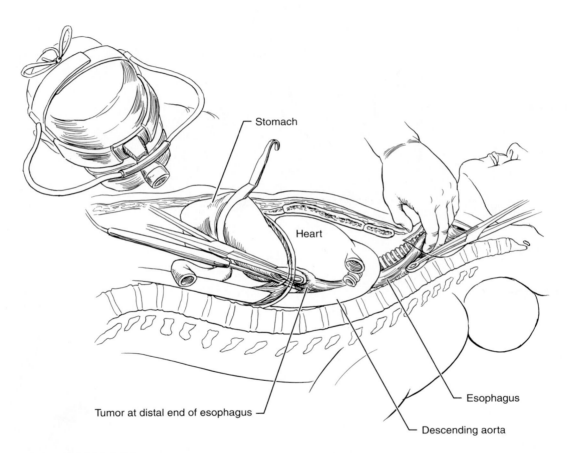

FIGURE 16–10

◆ A Penrose drain is looped around the esophagus and retracted superiorly while blunt dissection of the esophagus is continued to the level of the carina. Dissection can be performed under direct vision through the enlarged hiatus, by blunt finger dissection, or using a thoracoscope **(Figure 16-11)**.

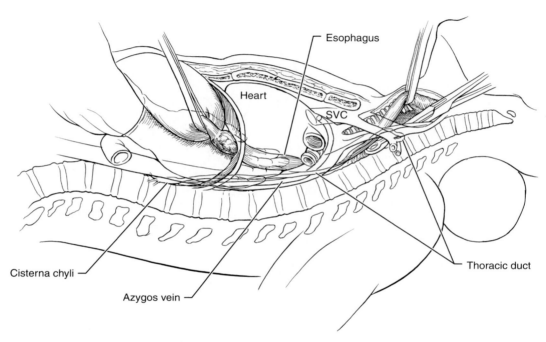

FIGURE 16–11

◆ A sponge on a stick can help facilitate this dissection from the cervical incision. Once the entire posterior esophagus is mobilized, the anterior section is mobilized in similar fashion. During the anterior dissection, the surgeon must be careful not to injure the membranous portion of the trachea. The lateral esophageal attachments can be freed under direct vision from the hiatus with superior retraction of the chest wall. Lymph nodes in the subcarinal area should be dissected free and removed with the specimen. If the lateral attachments cannot be viewed, an alternative method is to insert the surgeon's right hand through the hiatus and pin the esophagus against the spine between the index and middle fingers. The lateral tissue is then stripped from the esophagus by blunt dissection **(Figures 16-12 to 16-14)**.

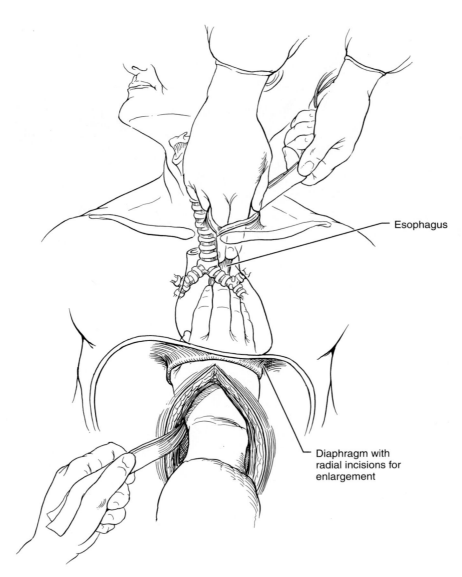

Esophagus

Diaphragm with radial incisions for enlargement

FIGURE 16–12

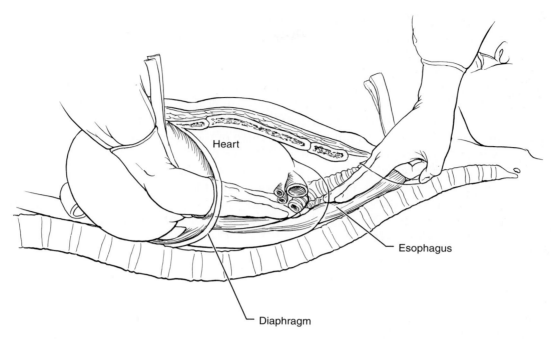

Heart

Esophagus

Diaphragm

FIGURE 16–13

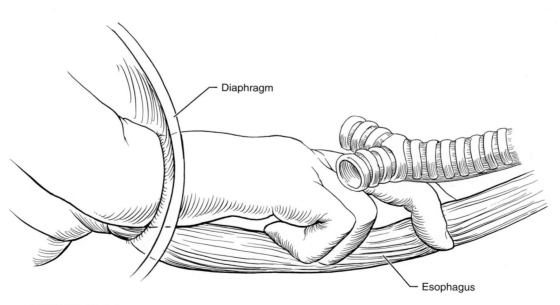

Diaphragm

Esophagus

FIGURE 16–14

- Once the esophagus is fully mobilized, the cervical esophagus is divided obliquely with a gastrointestinal anastomosis (GIA) stapling device **(Figure 16-15)**.

- The esophagus is pulled from the posterior mediastinum and delivered into the abdomen. At this point the surgeon should inspect the surgical bed for bleeding and insert a gauze pack into the posterior mediastinum to tamponade any minor oozing while the stomach is prepared. The fundus and distal greater curve of the stomach are grasped and held on tension while the esophagus is pulled at a 90-degree angle. A GIA stapling device can be used to resect a portion of the lesser curve and gastric cardia to gain a 4- to 6-cm margin from a distal esophageal tumor. For benign disease, only the cardia is resected to maximize collateral flow through the stomach. This process also "tubularizes" the stomach in preparation for use as a conduit. The staple line can be oversewn with 3-0 silk interrupted Lembert stitches **(Figure 16-16)**.

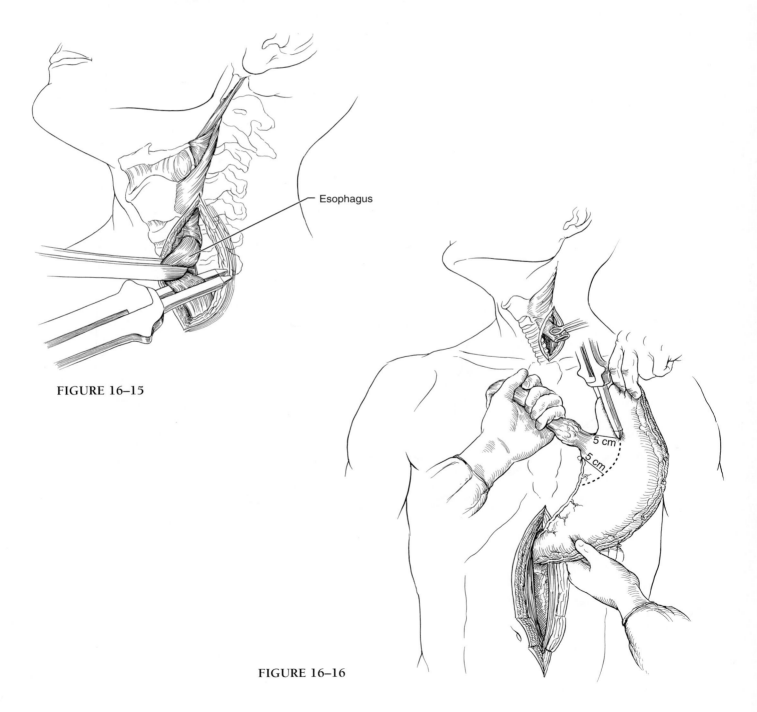

Esophagus

FIGURE 16–15

5 cm

5 cm

FIGURE 16–16

◆ The stomach is then manipulated through the enlarged hiatus to the cervical incision. A Babcock clamp can be inserted from the cervical incision into the posterior mediastinum to help grasp and deliver the fundus of the stomach into the neck **(Figure 16-17)**.

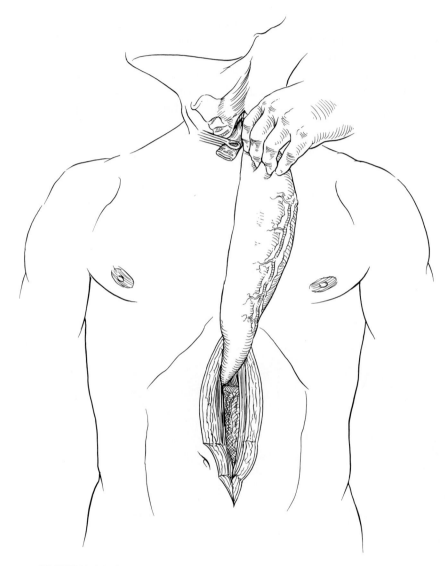

FIGURE 16–17

- Alternatively, a Penrose drain can be sutured to the apex of the stomach and delivered into the cervical incision to help provide traction. Both techniques use more pushing from the diaphragm side rather than pulling from the neck side. The surgeon must be careful to avoid twisting the stomach, which will compromise gastric blood flow and can lead to conduit necrosis with anastomotic breakdown **(Figures 16-18 to 16-20).**

- The abdominal portion of the procedure is completed before the cervical anastomosis is performed. This allows time to assess the viability of the gastric conduit. In the abdomen, the hiatus is closed by approximating the crura with 2-0 Vicryl figure-of-eight stitches to easily allow 2 fingerbreadths between the stomach and hiatus. The stomach is also tacked to the diaphragm with interrupted 3-0 silk stitches to prevent subsequent gastric herniation into the chest. At this point a jejunostomy feeding tube can be placed according to surgeon preference.

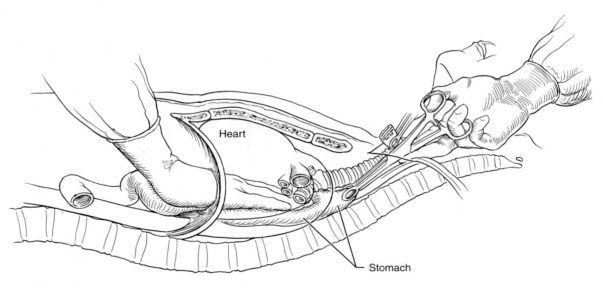

FIGURE 16–18

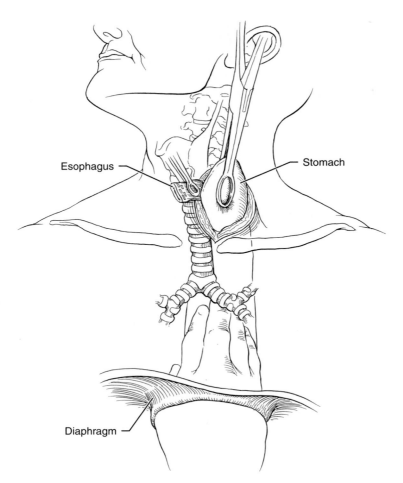

Esophagus

Stomach

Diaphragm

FIGURE 16–19

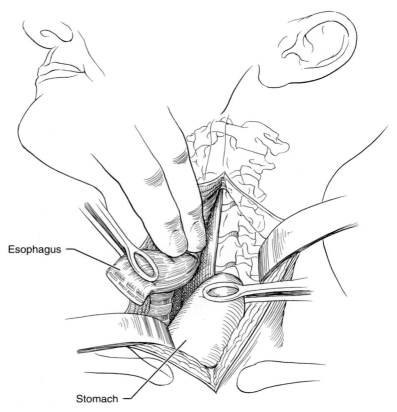

Esophagus

Stomach

FIGURE 16–20

◆ Many techniques have been described to complete the cervical esophagogastric anastomosis. Stapled anastomoses have shown a lower incidence of anastomotic leak over hand-sewn anastomoses. Once an adequate length of stomach (4 to 5 cm) has been mobilized above the clavicles, the suture line from the lesser curve is oriented toward the patient's right, and a traction suture is placed on the anterior wall of the stomach at the lower aspect of the neck wound (**Figures 16-21 and 16-22**).

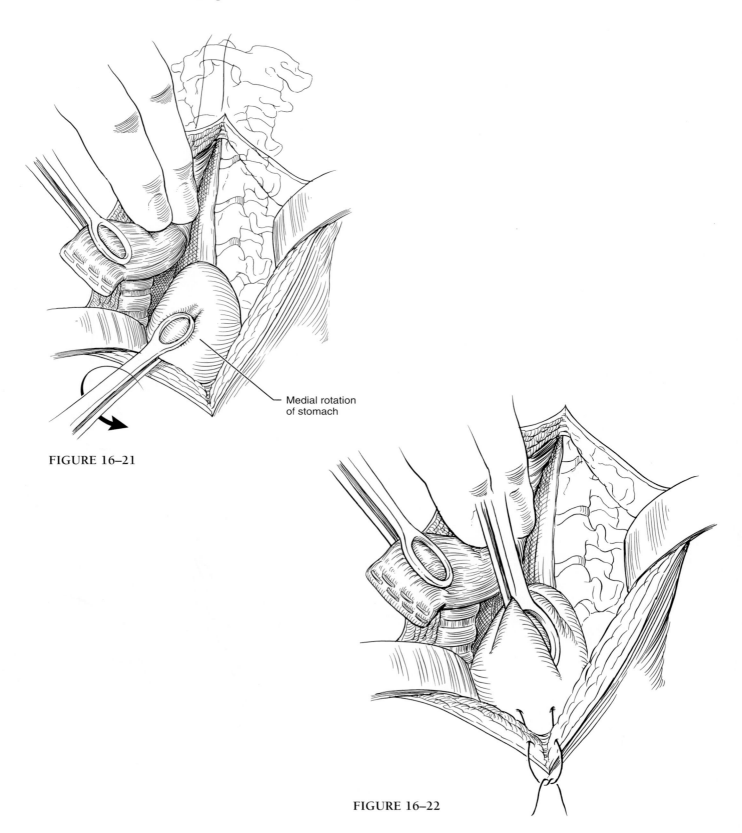

Medial rotation
of stomach

FIGURE 16–21

FIGURE 16–22

◆ A 1.0- to 1.5-cm gastrotomy is performed on the anterior gastric wall, 3 to 4 cm distal to the tip of the fundus lying high in the neck (**Figures 16-23 and 16-24**).

◆ An atraumatic clamp is placed parallel to the esophageal staple line, keeping the oblique orientation to ensure the anterior portion of the esophagus is longer than the posterior portion to facilitate the anastomosis.

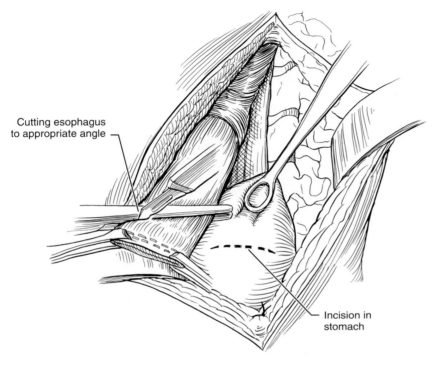

Cutting esophagus to appropriate angle

Incision in stomach

FIGURE 16–23

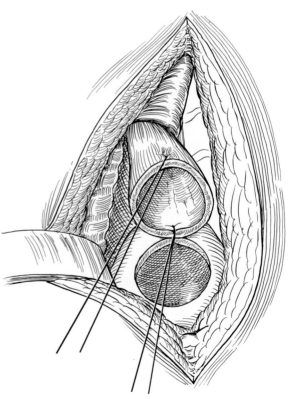

FIGURE 16–24

◆ A traction stitch is placed on the anterior corner of the cervical esophagus and pulled caudad while one arm of the endoscopic gastrointestinal anastomosis (EndoGIA) stapling device is placed through the gastrotomy toward the fundus and the other arm placed into the esophagus along its posterior wall. The stapling device is fired and individual 4-0 absorbable sutures are then placed at the corners of the stapled anastomosis. At this point the anesthesiologist inserts a nasogastric (NG) tube while the surgeon guides the tube through the partially completed anastomosis and into the distal stomach (**Figure 16-25**).

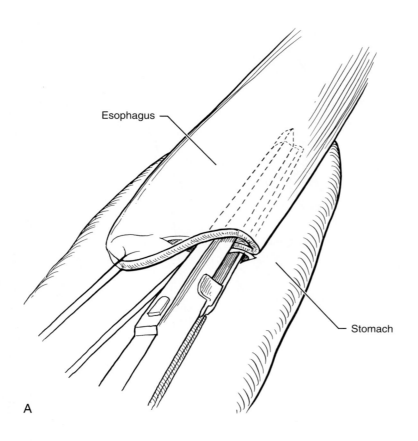

A

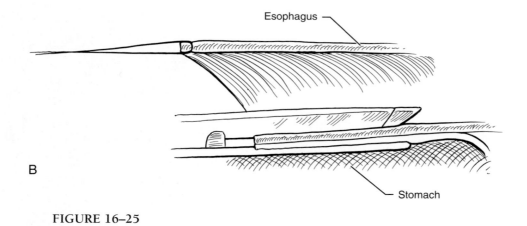

B

FIGURE 16–25

◆ The remaining small opening between the esophagus and gastrotomy is closed in two layers. A running 4-0 absorbable suture is used for the first layer followed by interrupted 4-0 Lembert stitches to complete the anastomosis **(Figure 16-26)**.

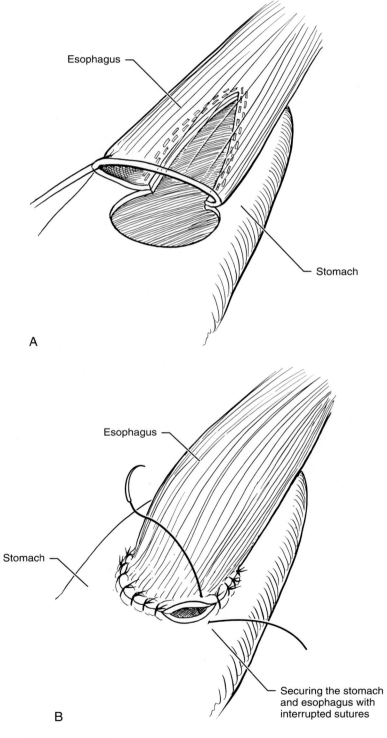

FIGURE 16–26

♦ The neck wound is filled with saline and the anesthesiologist gently introduces 50 mL of air into the NG tube while the surgeon occludes the distal stomach and observes for air bubbles at the anastomosis in the neck. The completed anastomosis should lie high in the neck without tension **(Figure 16-27)**.

3. CLOSING

♦ Before closure, the entire stomach should be inspected for areas of necrosis. The abdominal fascia is closed with an 0-looped running polydioxanone suture (PDS) or according to surgeon preference, then the skin closed with staples. In the neck, a small Jackson-Pratt drain is placed in the surgical bed and exited through a separate stab incision in the lateral neck. The platysma is approximated with a running 4-0 absorbable suture, then the skin closed with a second 4-0 to 5-0 absorbable stitch. A chest radiograph should be obtained in the operating room to ensure no pneumothorax or hemothorax is present. If pneumothorax or hemothorax is present, appropriate chest tubes should be inserted.

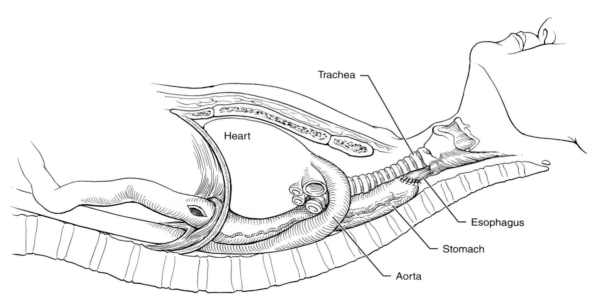

FIGURE 16–27

STEP 4: POSTOPERATIVE CARE

- The need for extensive postoperative monitoring in the intensive care unit (ICU) is based on surgeon preference, patient comorbidities, blood loss, and length of procedure. However, routine ICU care is not required postoperatively.

- Hallmarks to a rapid recovery lie in adequate pain control, physical therapy, and pulmonary toilet.

- The esophagogastrostomy should be evaluated on postoperative day 4 or 5 with a contrast swallow study. If no leak is present, a diet is initiated and the drain is removed as long as the output does not increase with feeding.

- If an anastomotic leak occurs, the neck incision should be opened and packed with moist gauze 2 to 3 times daily. The wound is allowed to granulate and close secondarily.

STEP 5: PEARLS AND PITFALLS

- Identify and preserve the right gastroepiploic and right gastric arteries during mobilization of the stomach.

- Vagal fibers around the midesophagus can be difficult to dissect bluntly. Using the vertebral bodies posteriorly as an anvil against which to compress tissues can facilitate blunt dissection.

- Communicate with the anesthesiologist, especially during transthoracic dissection when periods of hypotension are common.

- Keep dissection close to the proximal esophagus to minimize potential injury to the recurrent laryngeal nerves.

SELECTED REFERENCES

1. Orringer MB, Marshall B, Iannettoni MD: Eliminating the cervical esophagogastric anastomotic leak with a side-to-side stapled anastomosis. J Thorac Cardiovasc Surg 2000;119:277-288.
2. Orringer MB, Marshall B, Stirling MC: Transhiatal esophagectomy for benign and malignant disease. J Thorac Cardiovasc Surg 1993;105:265-276.

CHAPTER 17

ESOPHAGECTOMY—TRANSTHORACIC (IVOR LEWIS)

David B. Loran and Joseph B. Zwischenberger

STEP 1: SURGICAL ANATOMY

- ◆ A comprehensive understanding of the anatomy of the esophagus is critical before undertaking surgical procedures on the esophagus.

- ◆ **Figure 17-1** demonstrates key anatomic features that should be considered before performing a transthoracic esophagectomy.

STEP 2: PREOPERATIVE CONSIDERATIONS

- ◆ Indications for transthoracic esophagectomy include carcinoma, caustic injury with stricture or dysplastic mucosal changes, and other benign diseases. Most surgeons agree that benign disease is best treated with transhiatal esophagectomy, which eliminates the risk of intrathoracic anastomotic leak and spares the patient the discomfort of thoracotomy without compromising outcomes. If dense adhesions are expected, a transthoracic approach can afford a safer dissection of the intrathoracic esophagus under direct vision and eliminate the blind dissection and potential for massive hemorrhage, which is rarely associated with transhiatal esophagectomy. For tumors of the proximal esophagus and mid-esophagus, a right thoracotomy is preferred, whereas a left thoracotomy is preferred for distal esophageal tumors.

- ◆ Advocates of the transthoracic approach for cancer resection point out that a more complete lymph node dissection can be accomplished by direct visualization of the operative field. Advocates of the transhiatal approach point to a perceived overall lower morbidity rate. Despite multiple studies over the years with trends in both directions, the aggregate experience has shown no difference in morbidity, mortality, or outcome between the transthoracic and transhiatal approaches. The most important determining criteria are experience of the surgeon, need for exposure, and patient selection.

- ◆ Informed consent is obtained and the patient is made nothing-by-mouth status at least 8 hours before the procedure. A bowel preparation can be given to the patient the day before the procedure in case the colon is needed as a reconstruction conduit. In the operating room, a radial artery catheter should be used for continuous blood pressure monitoring.

Central venous access is not routinely necessary. However, if access is needed, the contralateral neck veins should be used to allow the surgeon complete access to the neck during operation. A double-lumen endotracheal tube is used to deflate and retract the lung to facilitate dissection.

◆ General endotracheal anesthesia is mandatory for this procedure.

◆ The patient is placed supine on the operating table with the head slightly extended. A roll is placed under the patient to slightly elevate the side of the patient in anticipation of a thoracotomy. The patient's arm is either elevated and draped out of the field or prepped into the field to allow its mobility during the procedures. Alternatively, the patient can be placed supine during the abdominal portion of the procedure, then re-prepped and draped in the lateral position for the thoracic portion.

◆ The skin over the entire neck, chest, and abdomen should be prepped with povidone-iodine (Betadine).

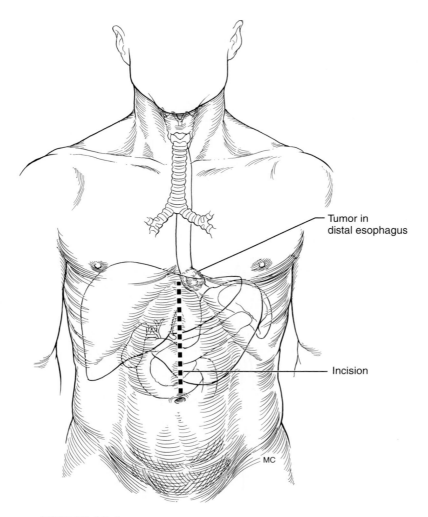

Tumor in distal esophagus

Incision

MC

FIGURE 17–1

STEP 3: OPERATIVE STEPS

1. INCISION

- ◆ Transthoracic esophagectomy uses two incisions: a midline abdominal incision and a thoracotomy. An upper midline supraumbilical incision from the xiphoid process to the umbilicus is used to begin the abdominal portion of the procedure. The incision should be extended cephalad to the left of the xiphoid process to adequately expose the esophageal hiatus. A self-retaining retractor can facilitate exposure of the upper abdomen.

- ◆ A right thoracotomy is recommended for a mid-thoracic or upper thoracic cancer. A left thoracotomy is recommended for a cancer in the lower one third of the thorax or in the esophagus **(Figure 17-2)**.

2. DISSECTION

- ◆ The stomach is completely mobilized as previously described for transhiatal esophagectomy (Chapter 16). A lateral thoracotomy is performed in the sixth to seventh intercostal space and the lung is retracted cephalad. If a right thoracotomy is used, the azygous vein should be identified and suture ligated to better reduce the risk of postoperative hemorrhage **(Figure 17-3)**.

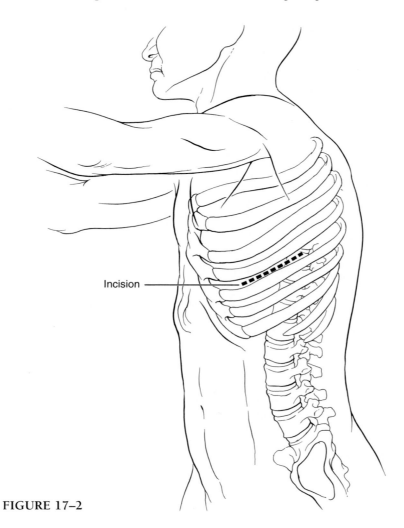

Incision

FIGURE 17–2

◆ The pleura overlying the esophagus is incised and the esophagus is dissected free from its bed. A Penrose drain is used to encircle the esophagus and provide retraction during the dissection. The surgeon should be able to include the lymph nodes surrounding the esophagus in the dissection **(Figure 17-4).** Care must be taken not to injure the posterior membranous trachea during mobilization of the esophagus or tumor or both. Once the esophagus is mobilized it is transected at a point at least 4 cm proximal to the tumor.

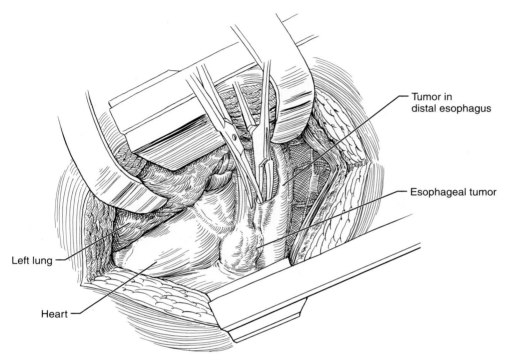

Tumor in distal esophagus

Esophageal tumor

Left lung

Heart

FIGURE 17–3

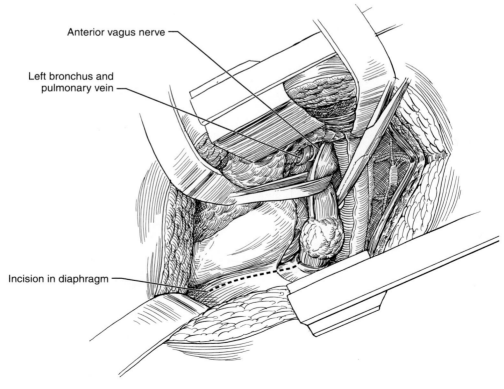

Anterior vagus nerve

Left bronchus and pulmonary vein

Incision in diaphragm

FIGURE 17–4

◆ The stomach, which has been previously mobilized, should be gently elevated into the chest **(Figure 17-5)**.

◆ An endoscopic gastrointestinal anastomosis (GIA) stapling device is used to resect the cardia and proximal fundus along the lesser curve with at least a 5-cm margin. This staple line can be oversewn with interrupted 3-0 silk Lembert stitches **(Figure 17-6)**.

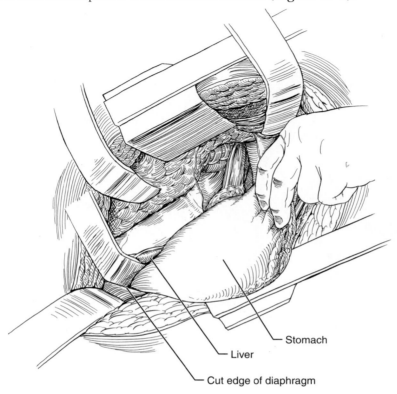

Stomach

Liver

Cut edge of diaphragm

FIGURE 17–5

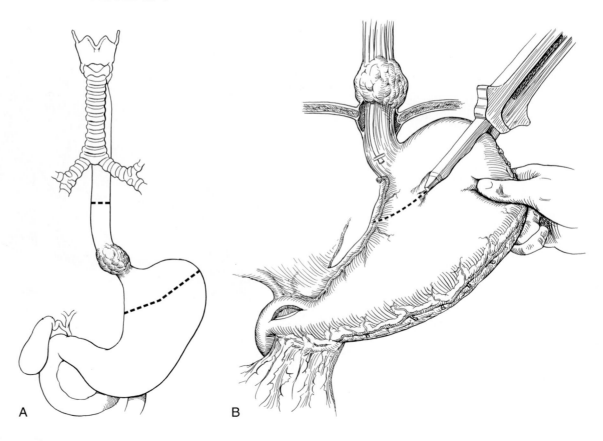

FIGURE 17–6   A   B

◆ The stomach is placed as high in the chest cavity as possible to avoid undue tension at the anastomotic site. A stapled anastomosis using an end-to-end anastomosis (EEA) stapling device can be used via a 1.0- to 1.5-cm gastrotomy or, alternatively, a hand-sewn anastomosis can be performed. The hand-sewn anastomosis is performed in two layers. First, the posterior row of interrupted 3-0 silk stitches is placed between the posterior wall of the esophagus, approximately 0.5 to 1.0 cm proximal to the cut end of the esophagus and the fundus of the stomach (**Figures 17-7 and 17-8**).

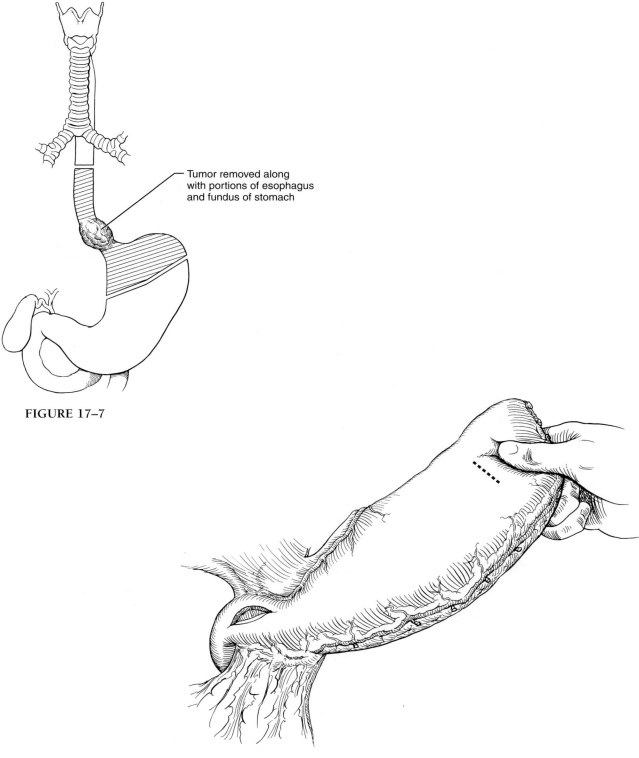

Tumor removed along
with portions of esophagus
and fundus of stomach

FIGURE 17–7

FIGURE 17–8

◆ At this point, the anesthesiologist places a nasogastric tube as the surgeon guides it from the esophagus, through the gastrotomy, and into the stomach. A running 4-0 absorbable suture is used to perform the mucosa-mucosa anastomosis. An anterior row of interrupted 3-0 silk Lembert stitches completes the anastomosis **(Figure 17-9)**.

◆ The stomach should be tacked to the prevertebral fascia and esophageal hiatus with interrupted 3-0 silk stitches once the anastomosis is complete. A 36F chest tube is placed into the right side of the chest and exited through a separate stab incision below the thoracotomy.

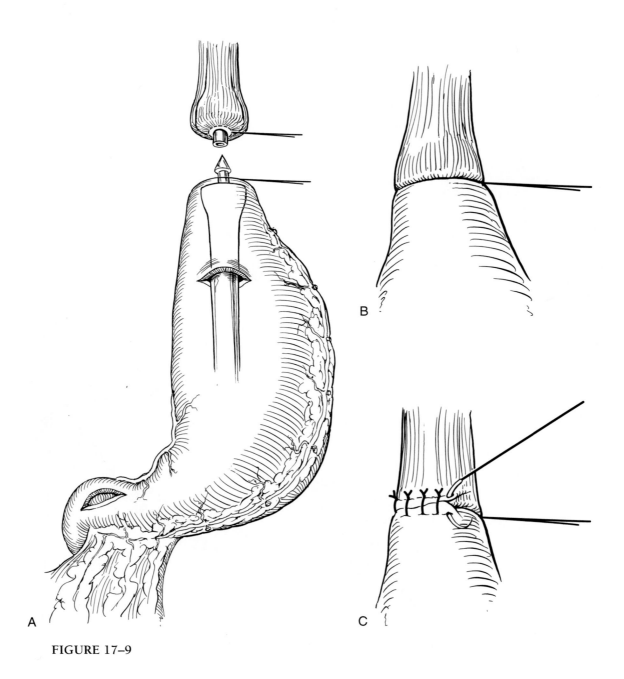

FIGURE 17–9

3. CLOSING

◆ The abdominal incision is closed according to surgeon preference. The fascia is usually closed with a no. 0 or no. 1 interrupted or running absorbable monofilament suture, and skin is closed with staples. The thoracotomy is closed with interrupted no. 1 or no. 2 Vicryl figure-of-eight stitches. Muscle layers are individually reapproximated with running 2-0 Vicryl suture, and the skin is closed with staples or running 4-0 absorbable suture. Sterile dressings are applied (**Figure 17-10**).

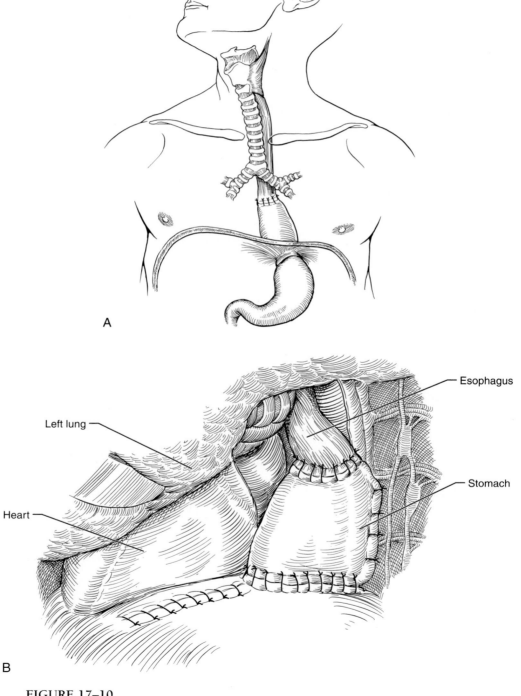

FIGURE 17–10

STEP 4: POSTOPERATIVE CARE

◆ Routine intensive care unit monitoring is not mandatory following transthoracic esophagec-tomy, but the decision is made for each individual based on length of operation, surgeon preference, patient comorbidities, and blood loss. On postoperative day 4 or 5, a contrast esophageal swallow study is performed to evaluate the anastomosis for leak. If no leak is present, a diet is initiated and output from the chest tube is monitored. Assuming no increase in output with feeding and a fully expanded lung and drained right hemithorax, the chest tube can be removed. Ambulation and chest physiotherapy should be initiated on postoperative day 1 and continued until discharge.

STEP 5: PEARLS AND PITFALLS

◆ Identify and preserve the right gastric and right gastroepiploic arteries when mobilizing the stomach.

◆ Test the esophagogastric anastomosis under water before closing to ensure no gross anasto-motic dehiscence is present.

◆ Avoid injury to the posterior membranous trachea during esophageal mobilization.

◆ Act quickly to ensure adequate drainage of the thorax and mediastinum if signs of anasto-motic leak occur in the postoperative period.

SELECTED REFERENCES

1. Junginger T, Gockel I, Heckhoff S: A comparison of transhiatal and transthoracic resections on the prog-nosis in patients with squamous cell carcinoma of the esophagus. Eur J Surg Oncol 2006;32:749-755.
2. Hulscher JB, van Sandick JW, de Boer AG, et al: Extended transthoracic resection compared with limited transhiatal resection for adenocarcinoma of the esophagus. N Engl J Med 2002;347:1662-1669.

CHAPTER 18

ESOPHAGOGASTRECTOMY

Joseph B. Zwischenberger and Edward Y. H. Chan

STEP 1: SURGICAL ANATOMY

- A comprehensive understanding of the anatomy of the thorax, esophagus, stomach, and abdomen is critical before undertaking surgical procedures on the esophagus and stomach.

STEP 2: PREOPERATIVE CONSIDERATIONS

- Indications: Indications for esophagogastrectomy include malignant tumor of the lower esophagus or esophagogastric junction, which precludes a clear tumor margin to allow use of the stomach for esophageal reconstruction. Malignancies of the esophagogastric junction are most commonly adenocarcinomas of gastric origin (**Figure 18-1**).

- A left thoracoabdominal approach is indicated if the tumor location necessitates resection of the distal esophagus and proximal stomach and when a Roux-en-Y anastomosis is to be used to reconstruct the resected stomach. If removal of the proximal stomach only is required to obtain adequate surgical margins, an anastomosis may be made between the distal stomach and the esophagus in the chest. However, this reconstructive approach may be associated with reflux esophagitis and dysphagia. Some surgeons prefer the alternative of a total resection of the stomach and distal esophagus with a Roux-en-Y jejunal interposition with an end-to-end anastomosis with the remaining esophagus. For a total esophagogastrectomy, a colon interposition is required. A double-contrast barium enema and colonoscopy will aid selection of the right (preferred), transverse, or left colon. During the procedure, length and blood supply also influence colon selection.

- Preoperative planning: Informed consent is obtained and the patient is made nothing-by-mouth status at least 8 hours before the procedure. A bowel preparation is necessary the day before the procedure in case the colon is needed as a reconstruction conduit. In the operating room, a radial artery catheter should be used for continuous blood pressure monitoring. Central venous access is not routinely necessary; however, if access is needed, the right neck veins should be used to allow the surgeon complete access to the left side of the neck during operation. A double-lumen endotracheal tube is used to deflate and retract either lung to facilitate dissection. If a colonic interposition is planned, mesenteric angiography should be performed on patients with risk factors for atherosclerotic disease.

◆ Anesthesia: General endotracheal anesthesia is mandatory for this procedure.

◆ Position: The patient is placed in the right lateral (left thoracoabdominal) position.

◆ Operative preparation: The skin over the entire neck, chest, and abdomen should be prepped with povidone-iodine (Betadine).

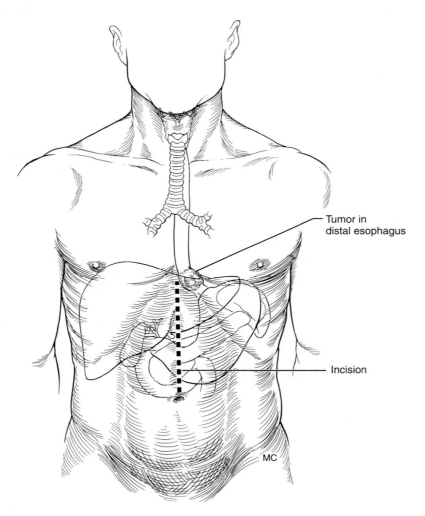

FIGURE 18–1

STEP 3: OPERATIVE STEPS

1. INCISION

◆ Incision and exposure: A left thoracotomy is performed between the sixth and seventh ribs. The serratus anterior muscle is separated to expose the intercostal muscles, which are removed from the superior aspect of the seventh rib to enter the chest **(Figure 18-2)**.

◆ A thoracoabdominal incision may provide greater exposure. However, this approach leads to longer operative time and may result in an unstable costal arch, chondritis, or persistent pain. A separate midline abdominal incision is often better tolerated (see Figure 18-1).

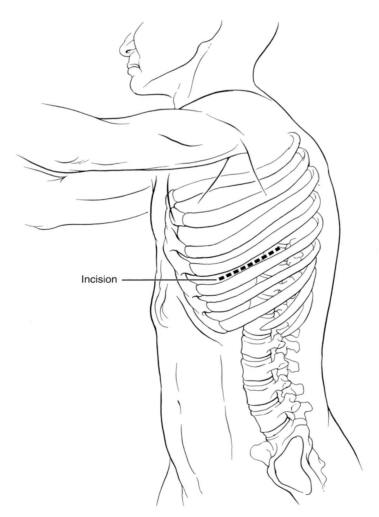

Incision

FIGURE 18–2

2. DISSECTION

◆ Diaphragm incision: The left thorax is entered and a semilunar incision is made in the diaphragm near the costal arch, 2 cm from the costal margin. Retraction of the cut edge of the diaphragm exposes the left lobe of the liver and the left upper abdomen. Radial incisions may be made to expose and resect the adjacent diaphragm to achieve tumor-free margins when the tumor invades the crus. Crural resection has a greater risk of diaphragmatic paralysis postoperatively **(Figures 18-3 and 18-4)**.

◆ The abdomen should be carefully examined for peritoneal or hepatic metastases. The cardia of the stomach should be palpated through the lesser sac, and the mobility of the tumor should be assessed. If there are metastases or the tumor is fixed to the aorta or spine, the tumor is not resectable.

◆ Esophageal mobilization: The pleura of the mediastinum is opened with visualization of the esophagus and the esophageal tumor. Mobilization of the esophagus from the aorta is achieved and the esophagus proximal to the tumor is encircled by a Penrose drain. The surgeon must identify the anterior vagus nerve and the left bronchus and pulmonary vein. The esophageal vessels should be dissected, ligated, and divided. To provide local clearance of the tumor, the surgeon should take 1 cm of the crura in continuity with the tumor (see Figure 18-4).

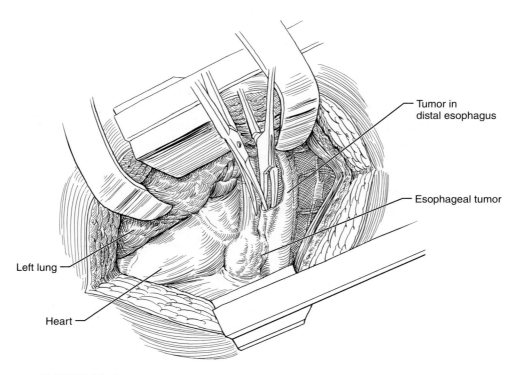

Tumor in distal esophagus

Esophageal tumor

Left lung

Heart

FIGURE 18–3

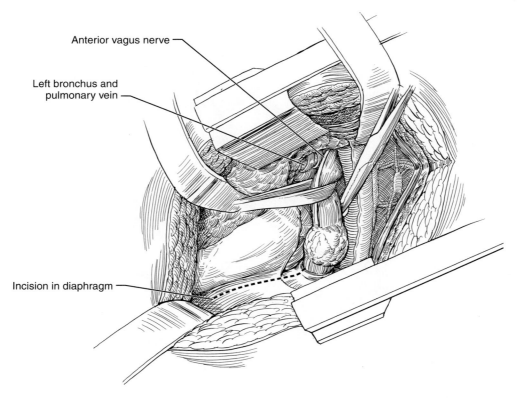

Anterior vagus nerve

Left bronchus and pulmonary vein

Incision in diaphragm

FIGURE 18–4

◆ Mobilization of the stomach: The mobilization of the stomach proceeds along the greater curvature in the direction of the pylorus, with division of the omentum maintaining a 1-cm margin from the right gastroepiploic artery and vein. Attention should be paid to avoiding excessive traction on the omental artery arcade. The right gastroepiploic vessels should be preserved until the extent of dissection is determined. The stomach is retracted to the right to provide tension on the short gastric vessels. Dissection proceeds cephalad along the greater curvature until the proximal stomach and distal esophagus are freed **(Figure 18-5)**.

◆ The freed stomach is reflected to visualize the celiac axis on the posterior aspect. The posterior gastric artery and recurrent branch of the left inferior phrenic artery should be identified, ligated, and divided. Node-bearing tissue is removed from the superior aspect of the pancreas, around the celiac axis, and along the left gastric artery for en bloc removal with the specimen. The left gastric artery and vein are ligated.

◆ The lesser sac is examined to determine whether the pancreas or spleen is involved with the tumor. The lesser omentum is divided and removed from the right side of the esophagus to the pylorus, with care taken to preserve the right gastric artery and vein.

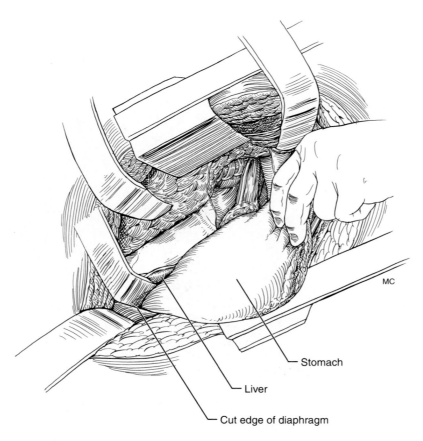

MC

Stomach

Liver

Cut edge of diaphragm

FIGURE 18–5

3. SELECTION OF PARTIAL OR TOTAL GASTRECTOMY

◆ Proximal esophagogastrectomy with esophagogastrostomy should be undertaken if the tumor can be adequately resected with a 5-cm margin by removal of the proximal stomach. The stomach has a blood supply that is less likely to be affected by atherosclerotic disease and requires only a single anastomosis, as opposed to using an intestinal conduit.

◆ Gastric remnant reconstruction: The margin of resection should be 4 to 6 cm from the esophagogastric junction, from halfway on the lesser curvature to a medial point on the fundus. A gastrointestinal anastomosis (GIA) stapler is placed at a right angle and transects the proximal stomach from the lesser curvature toward the fundus. The staple line is oversewn with inverting 3-0 suture. Care should be taken to maintain tension along the stomach to prevent shortening of the lesser curvature. A pyloromyotomy may be necessary to prevent gastric stasis secondary to division of the vagus nerves (**Figure 18-6**).

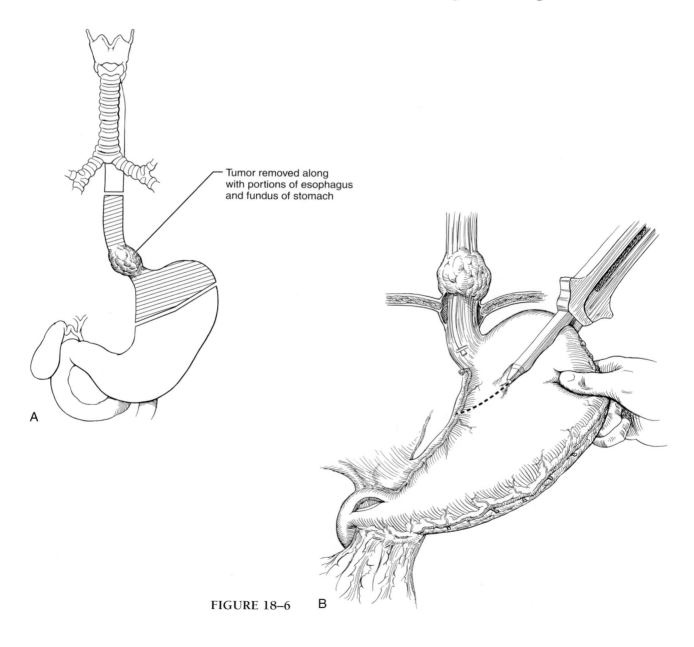

Tumor removed along with portions of esophagus and fundus of stomach

FIGURE 18–6   B

A

◆ The gastric remnant is brought into the thorax through the hiatus and behind the proximal esophagus. The margin should be at least 10 cm. If the margin is adequate, the posterior wall of the esophagus is anastomosed to the end of the gastric tube. If the margin is inadequate, the gastric tube length should be determined. If the length of stomach is inadequate to achieve a clear proximal remnant, the left side of the colon can be used as an alternative between the gastric remnant and the cervical esophagus **(Figure 18-7).**

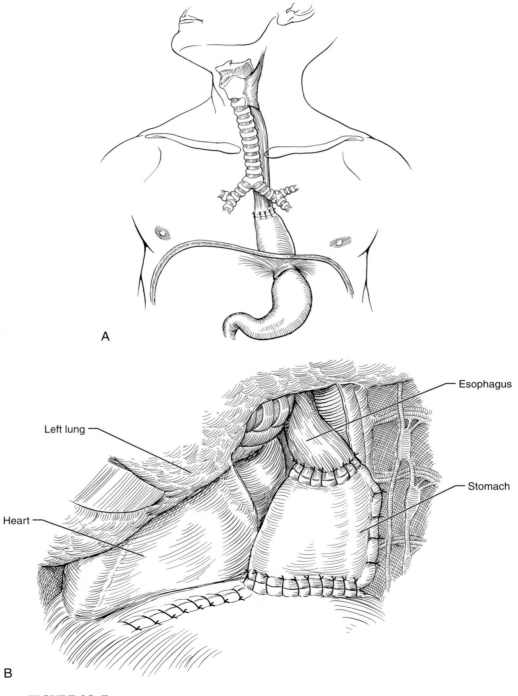

FIGURE 18–7

◆ Esophagogastric anastomosis: The esophagus is cut at a 45-degree angle with the anterior wall longer than the posterior wall. Stay sutures should be placed with 4-0 Vicryl at the midpoint of the anterior wall, as well as the posterior wall. A 2-cm gastrotomy is made between the stapled end of the lesser curvature and the greater curvature. The stay suture from the posterior esophageal wall is passed through the full thickness of the cephalad portion of the gastrotomy. A 45-mm endoscopic GIA stapler is placed with the thick part in the stomach and the narrow part in the esophagus. Two suspension sutures are tied on each side of the anastomosis, one at the tip and one at the base. The stapler is fired to complete the posterior section of the anastomosis (**Figure 18-8, A-B**).

◆ Care should be paid to ensure that the staple line is adequately clear of the previous staple line along the lesser curvature. Overlap of the staple lines could result in ischemia and a subsequent leak.

◆ The anterior portion of the anastomosis is made in two layers: the inner layer with continuous full-thickness 4-0 inverting polydioxanone structure (PDS) and the outer layer with interrupted sutures. Particular attention should be given to where the hand-sewn portion intersects with the stapled portion at the corners. Start the inner layer at the corner and incorporate at least 5 mm of the staple line (**Figure 18-8, C**).

◆ Total gastrectomy with Roux-en-Y esophagojejunostomy is undertaken if a proximal gastrectomy does not allow the tumor to be resected with adequate 5-cm margins on the stomach.

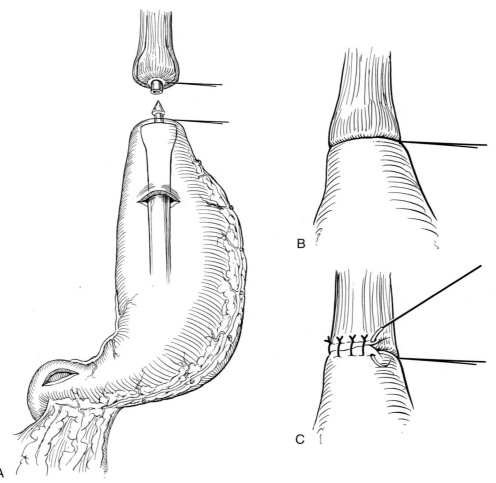

FIGURE 18–8

◆ The right gastroepiploic and right gastric vessels are suture-ligated and divided distal to the pylorus. The duodenum is divided distal to the pylorus with a linear stapler. The staple line should be inverted with interrupted 3-0 nonabsorbable sutures and covered with omentum to prevent duodenal stump blowout (**Figures 18-9 and 18-10**).

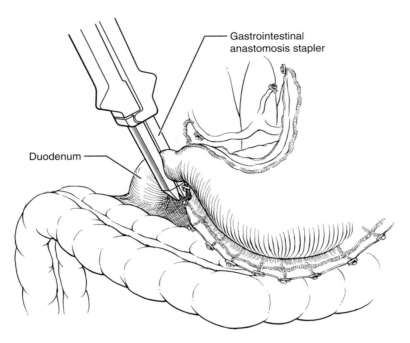

FIGURE 18–9

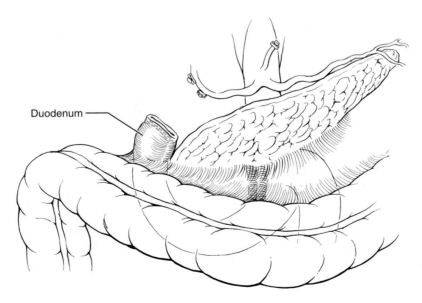

FIGURE 18–10

◆ The esophagus is mobilized to the level of the inferior pulmonary vein. A monofilament nylon purse-string suture is placed around the circumference of the proximal esophagus. The esophageal lumen should be distended with a no. 24 Foley catheter and a 20-mL balloon, which is advanced into the esophagus and gently inflated **(Figure 18-11)**.

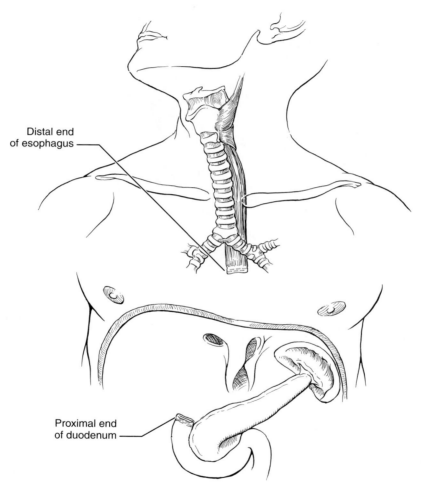

FIGURE 18–11

◆ A jejunal interposition is created using the Roux-en-Y technique **(Figures 18-12 and 18-13)**. The jejunum should be mobilized sufficiently to permit anastomosis with the thoracic esophagus, necessitating division of several jejunal arteriovenous arcades.

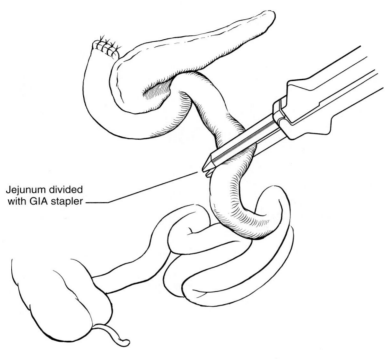

Jejunum divided with GIA stapler

FIGURE 18–12

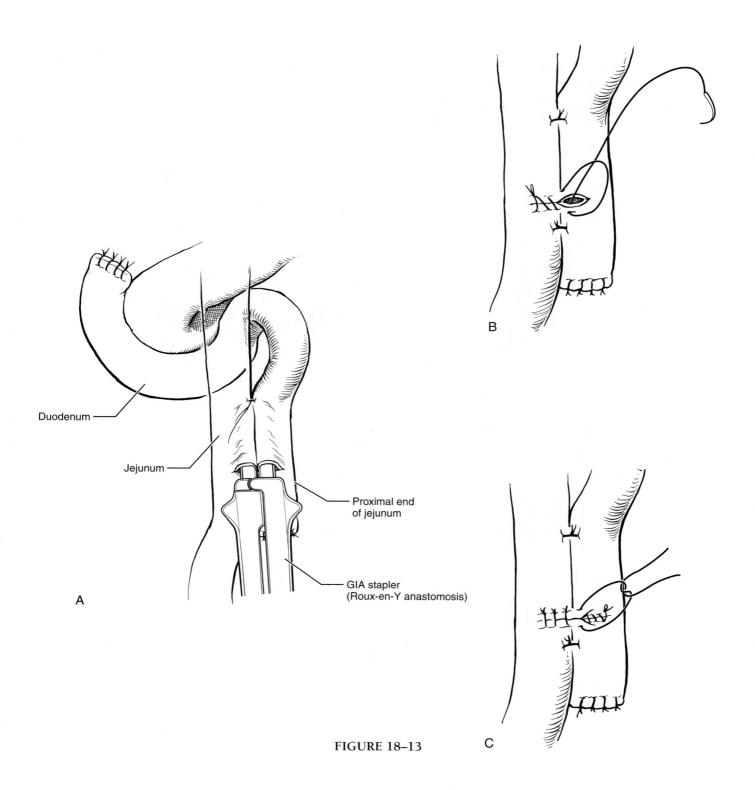

Duodenum

Jejunum

Proximal end
of jejunum

GIA stapler
(Roux-en-Y anastomosis)

A

B

C

FIGURE 18–13

◆ Loading: An end-to-end anastomosis (EEA) stapler is passed through the jejunum into the esophagus and fired. The jejunum is anchored to the proximal esophagus. To minimize bile reflux, the surgeon should anastomose the duodenal loop to the jejunum at least 50 cm distal to the esophagojejunal anastomosis. The blind end of the jejunal loop is stapled closed (**Figures 18-14 and 18-15**).

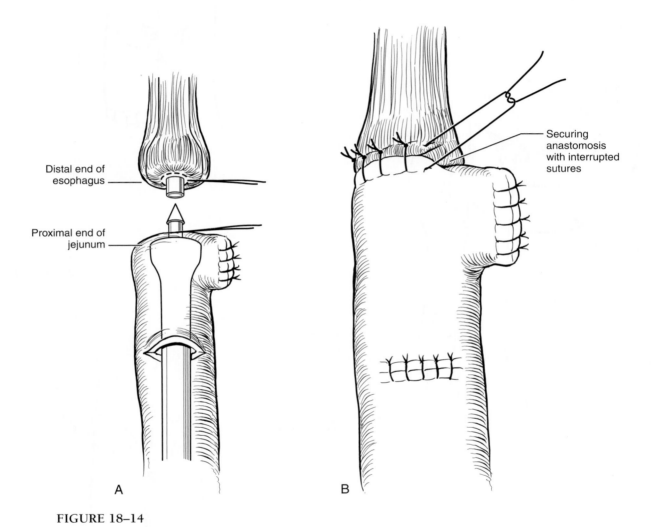

Distal end of esophagus

Proximal end of jejunum

Securing anastomosis with interrupted sutures

A

B

FIGURE 18–14

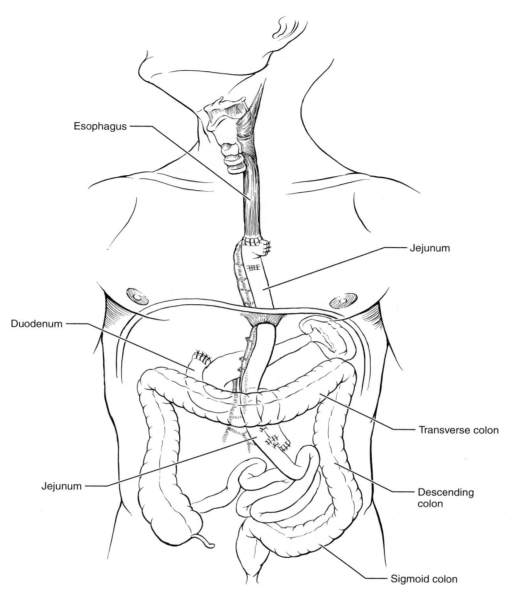

FIGURE 18–15

4. CLOSING

◆ In repairing the diaphragm, the gastric or jejunal interposition is secured to the crura with interrupted sutures. The remainder of the diaphragm is closed with interrupted mattress sutures. A chest tube should be placed into the pleural space near the anastomosis to ensure adequate fluid drainage. The left lung is reexpanded and the costal cartilages are left to float free. Tissue and skin are closed according to surgeon preference.

◆ Total gastrectomy with descending colon graft: Whereas the stomach is better than the colon as an esophageal substitute, the colon may be used if the stomach is not a viable option because of prior surgery or tumor extension. The descending colon is preferred to the ascending colon, because the smaller lumen is more similar in diameter to the esophagus. However, the inferior mesenteric artery that supplies the descending colon is more likely to have atherosclerotic disease than other mesenteric vessels **(Figure 18-16)**.

◆ After the surgeon thoroughly explores the abdomen for metastases, the length of the required graft should be measured. The middle colic artery should be clamped with a bulldog clamp to evaluate the adequacy of collateral circulation.

◆ The descending colon is prepared by mobilizing the splenic flexure and separating the attached omentum. The remaining colon is reanastomosed and the mesentery is reapproximated **(Figures 18-17 and 18-18)**.

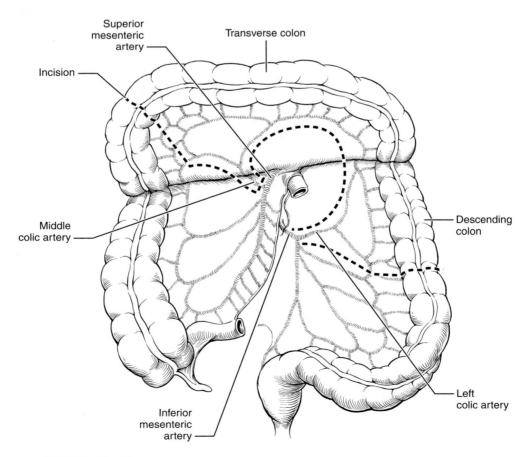

FIGURE 18–16

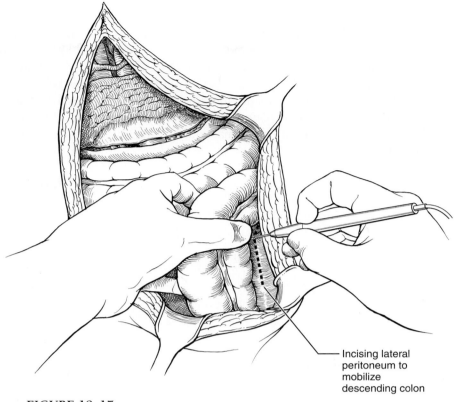

Incising lateral
peritoneum to
mobilize
descending colon

FIGURE 18–17

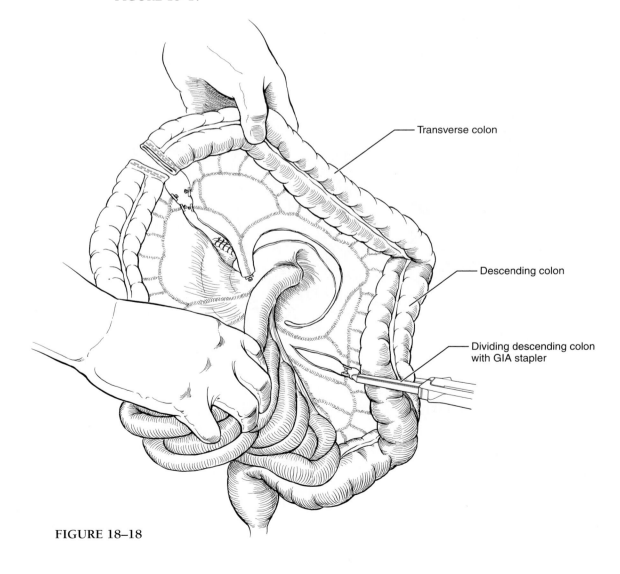

Transverse colon

Descending colon

Dividing descending colon
with GIA stapler

FIGURE 18–18

◆ The proximal end of the anastomosis may be performed first to measure the length of the graft more accurately **(Figure 18-19)**. The colon is passed along the posterior mediastinum, which is the shortest route between the stomach and the esophagus **(Figure 18-20)**. The substernal and transpleural routes are also secondary possibilities but may result in greater kinking of the graft and subsequent emptying problems **(Figures 18-21 and 18-22)**. The proximal anastomosis may be hand-sewn in two layers or stapled **(Figure 18-23)**. The distal anastomosis between the proximal jejunum and colon is closed with an EEA stapler **(Figure 18-24)**.

Text continued on p. 225

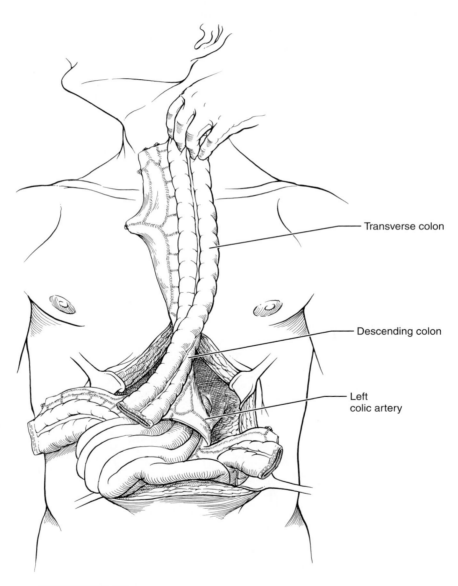

Transverse colon

Descending colon

Left
colic artery

FIGURE 18–19

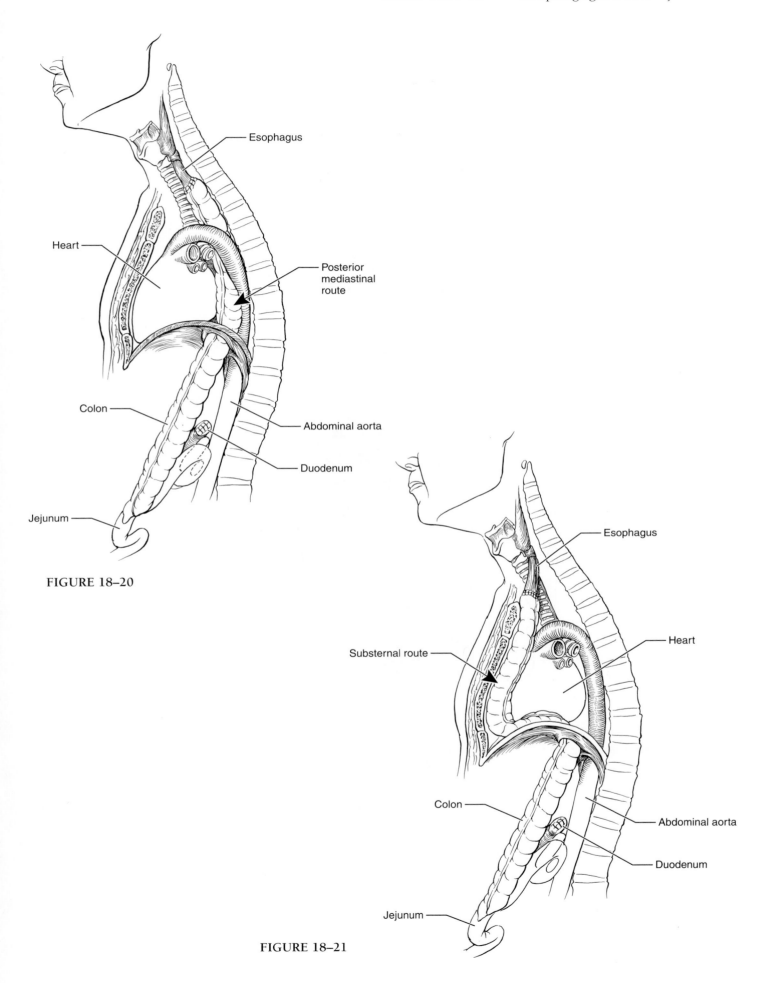

Esophagus

Heart

Posterior
mediastinal
route

Colon

Abdominal aorta

Duodenum

Jejunum

FIGURE 18–20

Esophagus

Substernal route

Heart

Colon

Abdominal aorta

Duodenum

Jejunum

FIGURE 18–21

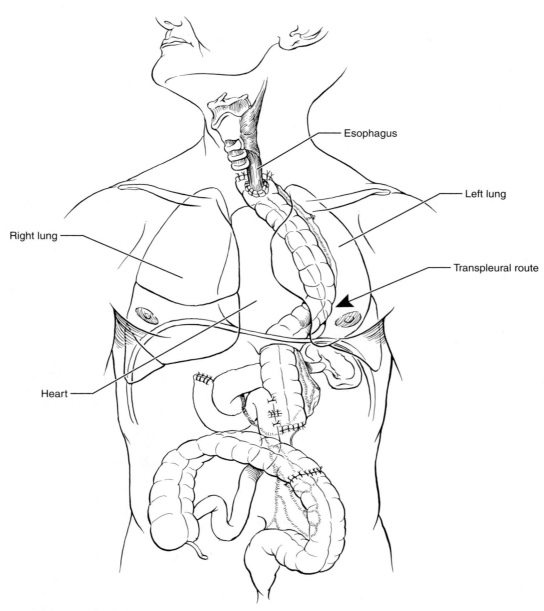

FIGURE 18–22

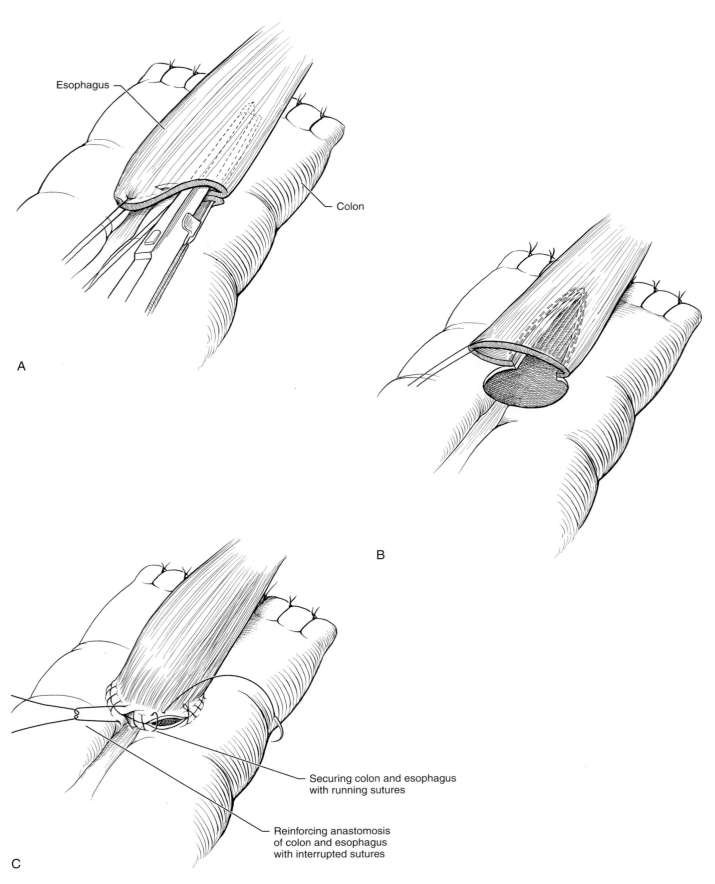

A

Esophagus

Colon

B

C

Securing colon and esophagus
with running sutures

Reinforcing anastomosis
of colon and esophagus
with interrupted sutures

FIGURE 18–23

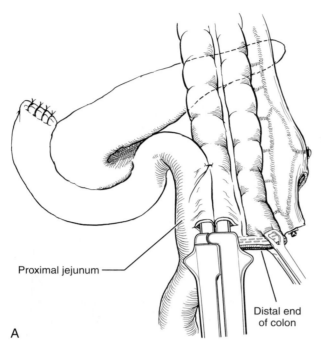

Proximal jejunum

Distal end
of colon

A

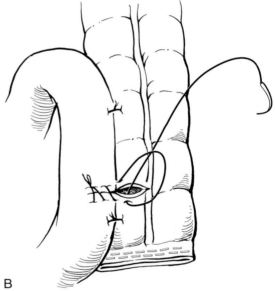

B

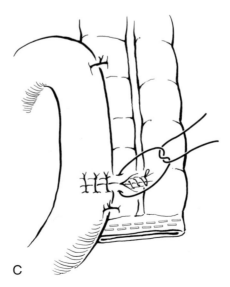

C

FIGURE 18–24

◆ The graft should be sutured to the crus of the diaphragm to avoid migration of the colon into the thoracic cavity. The remainder of the closure is carried out as described previously **(Figure 18-25).**

◆ Total gastrectomy with ascending colon graft: The ascending colon may be used if the descending colon has been affected by severe diverticular disease, atherosclerotic disease of the inferior mesenteric artery, or splenic vein thrombosis that extends to the inferior mesenteric vein.

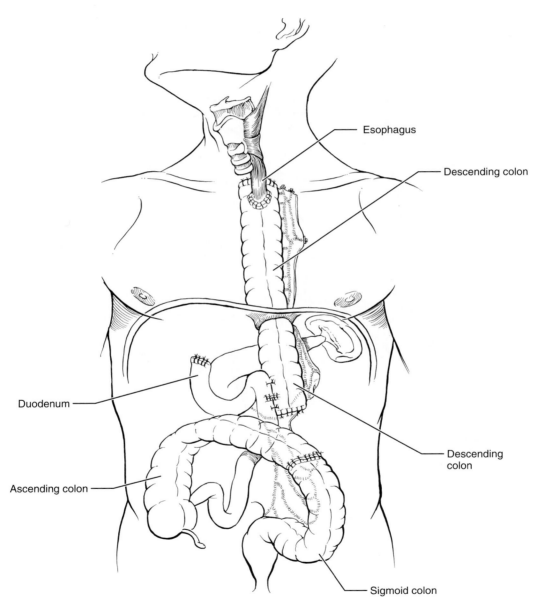

FIGURE 18–25

◆ The blood supply of the right colon from the marginal artery should be inspected by clamping the ileocolic and right colic arteries. The ascending colon is harvested, leaving the marginal artery intact **(Figure 18-26)**.

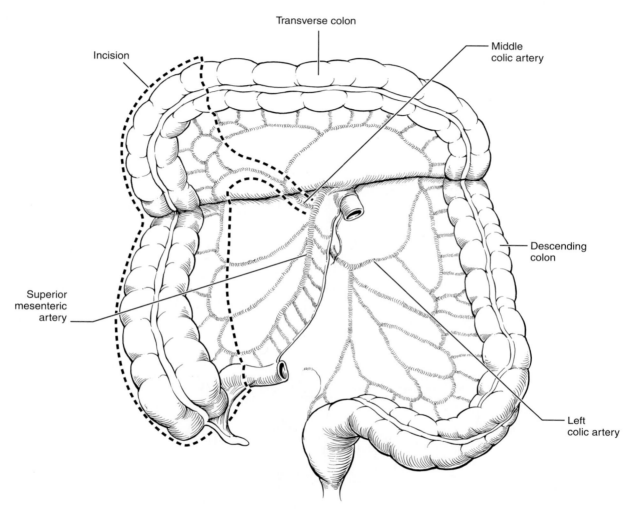

FIGURE 18–26

◆ A section of ileum and the ileocecal valve may be included as part of the graft, because the size of the ileum matches well with that of the esophagus and because the valve may provide some protection against reflux. However, reflux esophagitis is unusually high in the neck and the valve may result in mild obstruction.

◆ After measuring out the length of colon needed, the surgeon divides the ascending colon with a GIA stapler and reanastomoses the remaining colon. The graft is rotated and the proximal end is brought into the neck for the anastomosis. The distal anastomosis can be performed with an EEA stapler or a side-to-side stapled technique. The closure is performed as described previously **(Figure 18-27).**

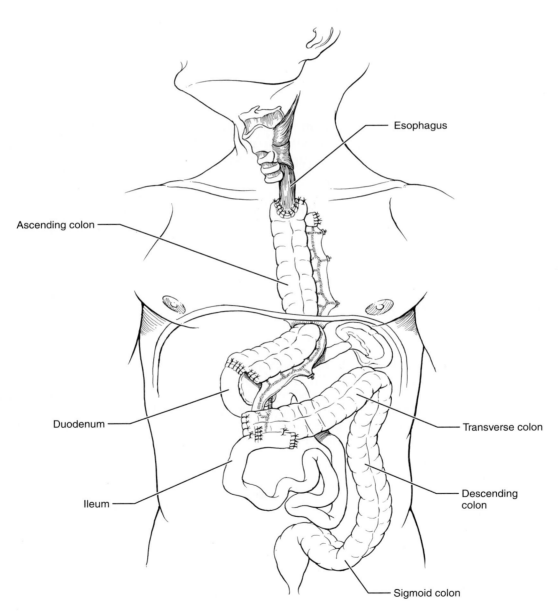

FIGURE 18–27

STEP 4: POSTOPERATIVE CARE

♦ After recovery from anesthesia, the patient can be taken to a floor bed.

♦ The patient should be encouraged to ambulate as early as postoperative day 1. Incentive spirometry and good pulmonary physiotherapy are essential.

♦ The nasogastric tube may be removed on the second postoperative day, and jejunostomy tube feedings are started. Sips of clear liquids may be allowed when bowel function normalizes. Between postoperative days 5 and 7, a barium swallow should be performed to evaluate the anastomosis. If the anastomosis is intact, a soft diet is started. As diet is advanced, bulky food and carbonated beverages should be avoided.

STEP 5: PEARLS AND PITFALLS

♦ When using a jejunal graft, one should be prepared to substitute a colonic graft if the jejunum is inadequate, either because the length is insufficient to replace the full length of the esophagus or because the blood supply is damaged during harvesting.

♦ Studies comparing the quality of life of patients after esophagectomy with age-matched controls demonstrated no significant differences in outcomes between the populations.

SELECTED REFERENCES

1. Meneshian A, Heitmiller RF: Surgical management of esophageal cancer. In Yuh D (ed): Johns Hopkins Manual of Cardiothoracic Surgery. New York, McGraw-Hill, 2007, pp 273-294.
2. Deschamps C, Nichols FC III, Cassivi SD, et al: Long-term function and quality of life after esophageal resection for cancer and Barrett's. Surg Clin North Am 2005;85:649-656.
3. Linden PA, Swanson SJ: Esophageal resection and replacement. In Sellke F (ed): Sabiston & Spencer: Surgery of the Chest. Philadelphia, Elsevier, 2005, pp 627-651.

CHAPTER 19

OPEN HELLER MYOTOMY

David B. Loran and Joseph B. Zwischenberger

STEP 1: SURGICAL ANATOMY

- ◆ A comprehensive understanding of the anatomy of the thorax and esophagus is critical before undertaking surgical procedures on the esophagus.

- ◆ **Figure 19-1, A,** demonstrates key anatomic structures that must be considered in an open Heller myotomy.

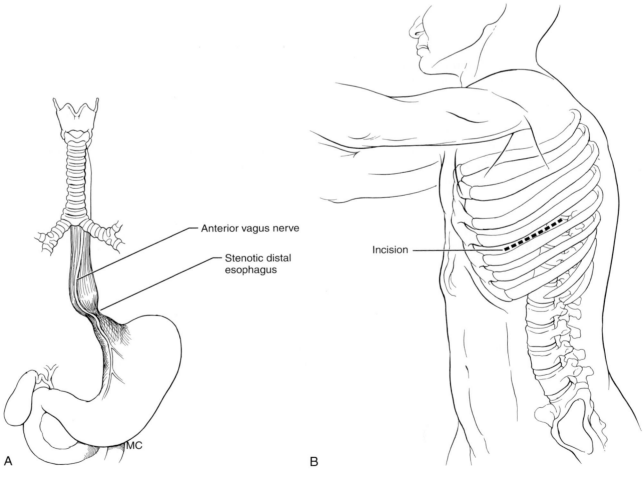

Anterior vagus nerve

Stenotic distal esophagus

Incision

A

B

FIGURE 19–1

STEP 2: PREOPERATIVE CONSIDERATIONS

- The word achalasia means "failure to relax," which characterizes the pathophysiologic dysfunction of the lower esophageal sphincter in this disease. The sustained high-pressure zone is believed to be due to denervation or dysfunction of the nerves in Auerbach's plexus, which leads to the loss of inhibitory effects of these ganglia on the muscles of the lower esophageal sphincter. Initiation of swallowing is normal; however, the esophagus cannot empty properly, which leads to varying degrees of dysphagia. Typical symptoms include odynophagia, foul breath, regurgitation of undigested food, and the patient describing a sensation of food "getting stuck" in his or her lower chest. Late symptoms result from the sequelae of continued aspiration and include hoarseness, pneumonitis, pneumonia, and lung abscess.

- Diagnosis is based on patient symptoms and objective testing. Barium esophagram will show a mild to severely dilated esophageal body with a characteristically smooth "bird-beak" tapering at the distal esophagus. Manometry is the gold standard for diagnosis of achalasia and will show a loss of propulsive contractions in the esophageal body. Resting pressures at the lower esophageal sphincter can be normal to elevated with incomplete or completely absent relaxation upon swallowing. Esophagoscopy with biopsy is sometimes needed to rule out distal esophageal stricture due to esophagitis or carcinoma, which can mimic achalasia.

- Once the diagnosis of achalasia is made, treatment usually begins with nonsurgical therapies. Botulinum toxin injected via an endoscope into the area of the lower esophageal sphincter can relieve symptoms in 50% to 65% of patients for as long as 18 months. Most have recurrence of symptoms beyond this time. Pneumatic or forceful bougie dilation of the lower esophageal sphincter has a long-term success rate approaching 70%. The gold standard for treatment of achalasia is surgical myotomy, with long-term success rates of 90% to 95%. Patients are usually treated with one or two attempts of nonsurgical therapies before being referred to a surgeon for myotomy. Those who are poor surgical candidates can be treated nonsurgically indefinitely.

- Informed consent is obtained from the patient who is given nothing by mouth 8 hours before the procedure.

- General endotracheal anesthesia is administered for this procedure.

- The patient is placed in the lateral decubitus position with the right side down and secured to the operating table. The bed can be bent at the seventh to eighth intercostal space to facilitate exposure.

- The skin is prepped with povidone-iodine (Betadine), from the top of the shoulder superiorly to the iliac crest inferiorly, then between the midline anteriorly and spinous processes posteriorly.

STEP 3: OPERATIVE STEPS

1. INCISION

- A muscle-sparing minithoracotomy incision measuring 8 to 10 cm is placed in the seventh intercostal space **(Figure 19-1, B)**. The serratus anterior muscle is separated to expose the intercostal muscles, which are removed from the superior aspect of the eighth rib to enter the chest. A rib retractor is placed.

2. DISSECTION

- A size 40F to 44F bougie or Maloney dilator is placed by the anesthesiologist to facilitate dissection. The inferior pulmonary ligament is divided and the lung is retracted cephalad. The mediastinal pleura overlying the esophagus is incised from the gastroesophageal junction to the inferior pulmonary vein to expose the esophagus. This segment of esophagus is mobilized anteriorly if only a myotomy is planned or is completely mobilized and encircled with a Penrose drain if an antireflux procedure is added to the myotomy **(Figure 19-2)**.

- Care should be taken during this dissection not to injure either vagus nerve located at the lateral margins of the distal esophagus. Usually the vagus nerves are adherent and should not be mobilized (see Figure 19-2, B-C).

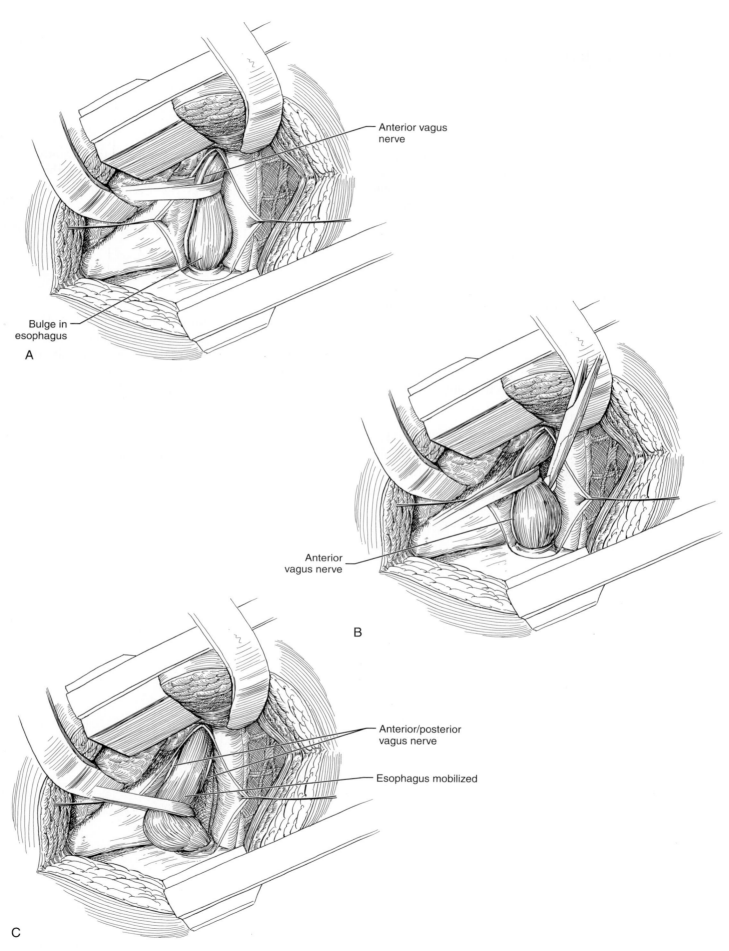

Anterior vagus
nerve

Bulge in
esophagus

A

Anterior
vagus nerve

B

Anterior/posterior
vagus nerve

Esophagus mobilized

C

FIGURE 19–2

◆ The esophageal musculature is incised from the inferior pulmonary vein to the esophageal hiatus and extended onto the cardia of the stomach for approximately 1 to 2 cm **(Figure 19-3)**.

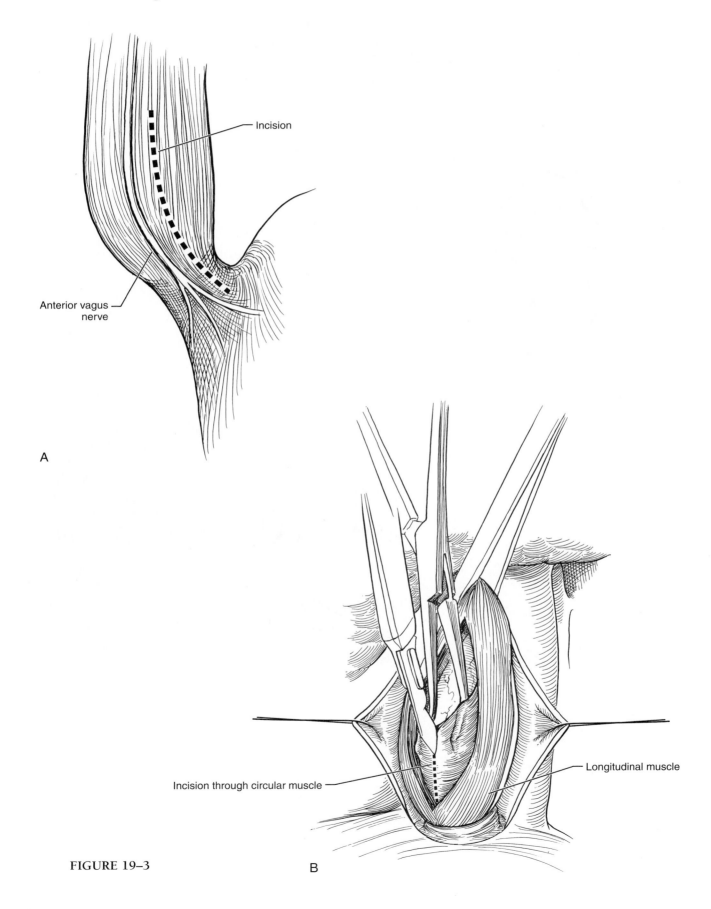

FIGURE 19–3

◆ The esophageal muscle is gently divided longitudinally until the mucosa is seen to bulge from underneath **(Figure 19-4).**

◆ A right-angle clamp or peanut dissector is used to raise the muscular wall from the mucosa over approximately 50% of the esophageal circumference. Care must be taken not to enter the esophageal lumen through the mucosa.

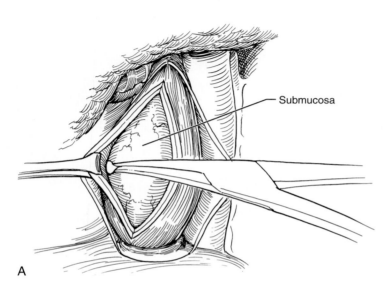

Submucosa

A

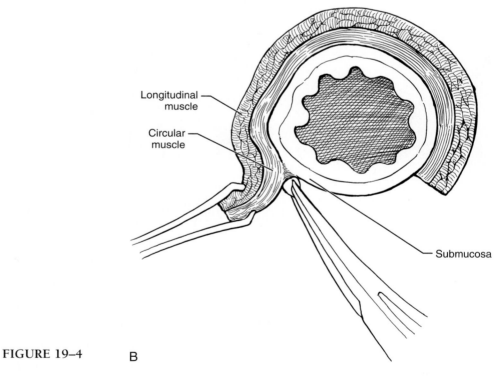

Longitudinal muscle

Circular muscle

Submucosa

FIGURE 19–4   B

◆ For the surgeon to inspect mucosal integrity, the bougie can be removed from the esophagus upon completion of the myotomy and replaced by a nasogastric (NG) tube. The chest cavity is filled with saline irrigation while the anesthesiologist gently injects air through the NG tube and the surgeon looks for air bubbles. If no air bubbles are seen, the Penrose drain is removed and the esophagus returns to its normal position **(Figure 19-5)**. If the mucosa has been violated, the defect should be closed primarily with absorbable suture reapproximating the muscle fibers. An opposite site is then used for the myotomy.

◆ Following completion of the myotomy, a chest tube is placed in the pleural space and exited through a separate incision in the lateral chest wall.

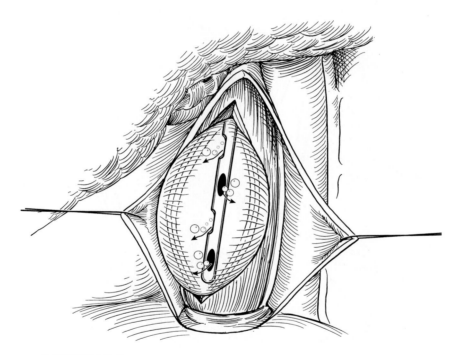

FIGURE 19–5

◆ Antireflux procedure, if added, is either a Belsey Mark IV (270 degree), Nissen (360 degree), or Dor (180 degree). Most surgeons add an antireflux procedure but no individual technique has proven superior **(Figure 19-6)**.

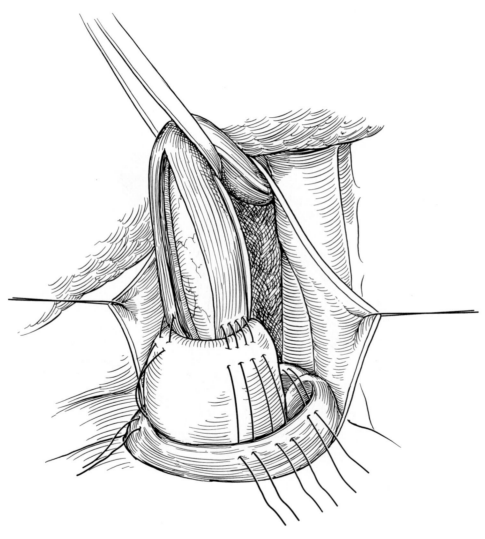

FIGURE 19–6

3. CLOSING

◆ The rib retractor is removed, and interrupted 0 Vicryl sutures are placed around the seventh and eighth ribs for closure of the chest cavity. Muscle layers are reapproximated with running 2-0 absorbable suture. The skin is closed with staples or a running 4-0 absorbable stitch. The chest tube is secured with a 2-0 silk drain stitch (**Figure 19-7**).

STEP 4: POSTOPERATIVE CARE

◆ After recovery from anesthesia, the patient can be taken to a floor bed.

◆ The chest tube should initially be placed to 15 to 20 cm H_2O wall suction and the patient kept NPO.

◆ On the second postoperative day, a contrast esophagram is obtained to ensure there is no leak from the myotomy site. With no leak present, a diet is initiated. If no esophageal leak is found, the lung is fully expanded. If there is no air leak present in the chest tube, the tube is removed. Patients are usually ambulatory by the second postoperative day and discharged to home by the third postoperative day.

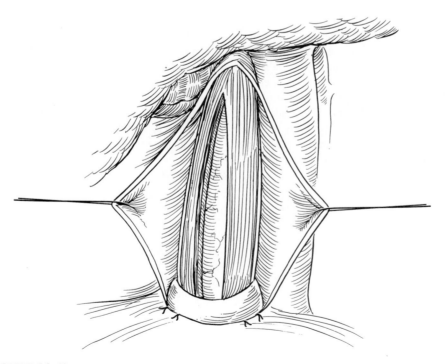

FIGURE 19–7

STEP 5: PEARLS AND PITFALLS

◆ Without fundoplication, approximately 60% of patients report symptoms of reflux, most of which can be managed medically. Most surgeons therefore add an antireflux procedure to the myotomy. No technique has proven superior, but most avoid a 360-degree fundoplication because of its higher rate of dysphagia.

◆ In prospective studies, laparoscopic Heller myotomy has been shown to achieve comparable outcomes with open surgery, with longer operative time and shorter hospital stay. Long-term follow-up has demonstrated satisfactory outcomes in 80% to 90% of cases.

◆ Patients with esophageal dilation of up to 6 cm have had patient satisfaction of greater than 90% from laparoscopic Heller myotomy.

◆ Patients with a sigmoid esophagus should be considered for myotomy first, then esophagectomy if symptoms do not resolve. Studies have demonstrated good to excellent patient satisfaction in 54% to 71% of patients at 7 to 11 years follow-up with myotomy of the sigmoid esophagus.

SELECTED REFERENCES

1. Tsiaoussis J, Athanasakis E, Pechlivanides G, et al: Long-term functional results after laparoscopic surgery for esophageal achalasia. Am J Surg 2007;193:26-31.
2. Constantini M, Zaninotto G, Guirroli E, et al: The laparoscopic Heller-Dor operation remains an effective treatment for esophageal achalasia at a minimum 6-year follow-up. Surg Endosc 2005;19:345-351.
3. Bonatti H, Hinder RA, Klocker J, et al: Long-term results of laparoscopic Heller myotomy with partial fundoplication for the treatment of achalasia. Am J Surg 2005;190:874-878.
4. Douard R, Gaudric M, Chaussade S, et al: Functional results after laparoscopic Heller myotomy for achalasia: A comparative study to open surgery. Surgery 2004;136:16-24.
5. Gaissert HA, Lin N, Wain JC: Transthoracic Heller myotomy for esophageal achalasia: Analysis of long-term results. Ann Thorac Surg 2006;81:2044-2049.

THE ABDOMEN

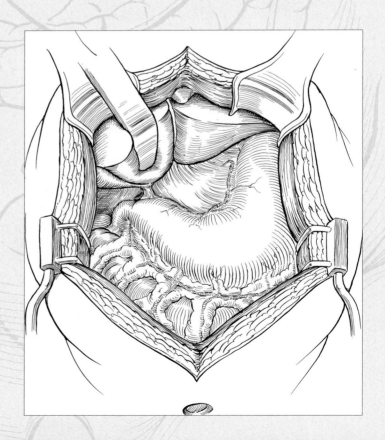

CHAPTER 20

STAMM GASTROSTOMY

Dennis C. Gore

STEP 1: SURGICAL ANATOMY

- Allows gastric decompression

- Access for enteral feeding **(Figure 20-1)**

STEP 2: PREOPERATIVE CONSIDERATIONS

- Anesthesia: general

- Position: supine

STEP 3: OPERATIVE STEPS

1. INCISION

- Incision and exposure: upper midline

- Use scalpel to create stab wound through skin and anterior fascia just lateral to rectus abdominus muscle left of midline (see Figure 20-1).

2. DISSECTION

- With retraction and visualization, the surgeon should use forceps through the stab wound to enter through the peritoneum and into the abdomen.

- The surgeon should use the same forceps to grasp a mushroom catheter (12F) and retract the external end of the catheter through the stab wound **(Figure 20-2).**

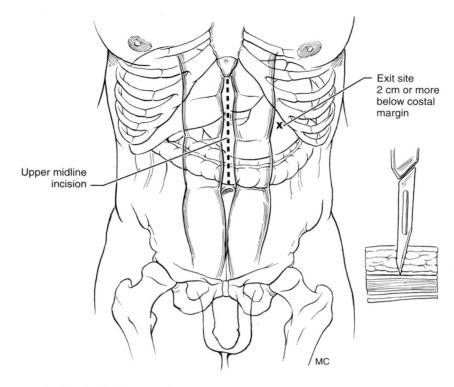

Exit site
2 cm or more
below costal
margin

Upper midline
incision

MC

FIGURE 20–1

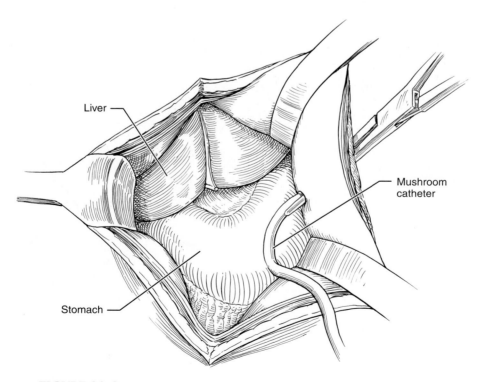

Liver

Mushroom
catheter

Stomach

FIGURE 20–2

◆ Place 2-0 silk purse-string suture to the anterior wall of the stomach **(Figure 20-3)**.

◆ Using two Babcock clamps for traction, the surgeon uses the cautery to create gastrotomy within the purse-string suture **(Figure 20-4)**.

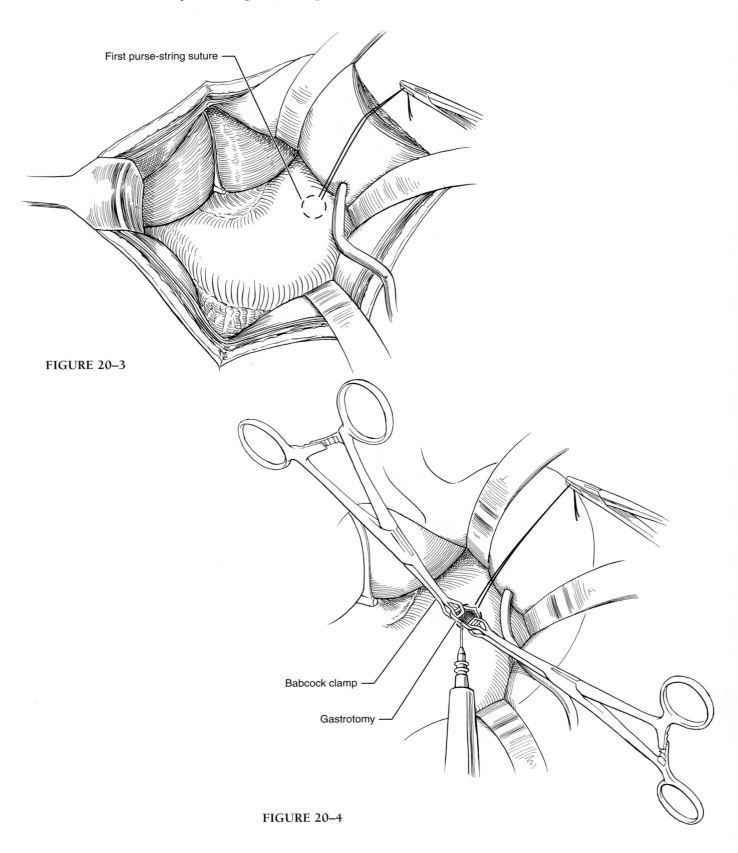

First purse-string suture

FIGURE 20–3

Babcock clamp

Gastrotomy

FIGURE 20–4

◆ Two Babcock clamps are used for traction and forceps are used to stent the mushroom catheter tip, which is placed through gastrotomy **(Figure 20-5, A)**.

◆ The first purse-string suture is secured around the catheter **(Figure 20-5, B)**.

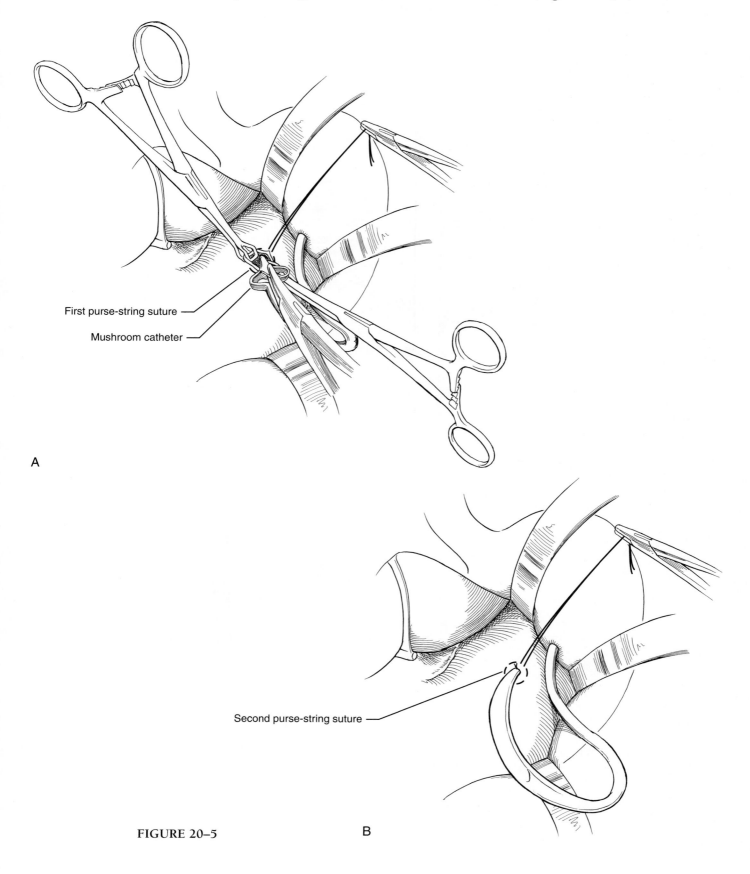

First purse-string suture —

Mushroom catheter —

A

Second purse-string suture —

FIGURE 20–5

B

- The second purse-string of 2-0 silk sutures is placed around the tube and secured **(Figure 20-6)**.

- 2-0 silk sutures are used to anchor the anterior wall of the stomach to the peritoneum in simple, interrupted fashion **(Figure 20-7)**.

- The mushroom catheter is retracted to approximate the anterior stomach wall with the peritoneum, then secured, and silk sutures are tied.

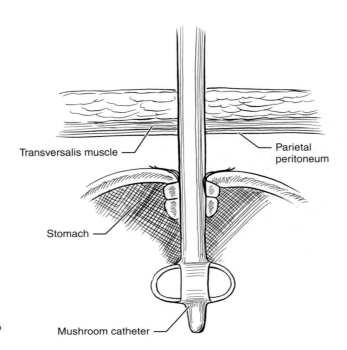

Transversalis muscle —

Stomach —

Parietal peritoneum

FIGURE 20–6

Mushroom catheter —

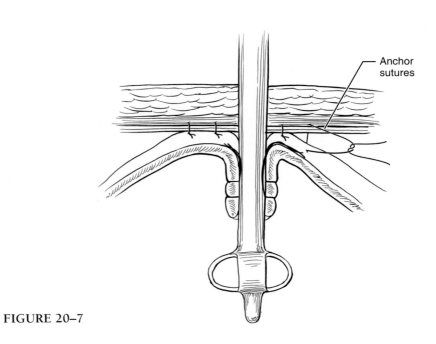

Anchor sutures

FIGURE 20–7

3. CLOSING

◆ Closure of fascia with suture

◆ Closure of skin

STEP 4: POSTOPERATIVE CARE

◆ Routine

STEP 5: PEARLS AND PITFALLS

◆ Two Babcock clamps grasping the edges of the gastrotomy along with a forceps inserted into the tip of the mushroom catheter and then held under tension provide an excellent means of retraction for placing the mushroom catheter within the stomach.

◆ The catheter should remain in place until the gastrostomy tract and the anterior stomach wall are securely healed to the peritoneal surface, which usually takes 10 days.

◆ First place all the sutures from the stomach to the peritoneum, then retract the catheter to approximate the anterior surface of the stomach to the peritoneum and secure ligatures. This sequence allows good visualization and room for placing sutures.

SELECTED REFERENCES

1. Zollinger RM Jr, Zollinger RM: Atlas of Surgical Operations. New York, MacMillan, 1983, p 30.

CHAPTER 21

WITZEL JEJUNOSTOMY

Dennis C. Gore

STEP 1: SURGICAL ANATOMY

 ◆ See Figure 21-1.

STEP 2: PREOPERATIVE CONSIDERATIONS

 ◆ Indication: access for enteral feeds

 ◆ Anesthesia: general

 ◆ Position: supine

STEP 3: OPERATIVE STEPS

 1. INCISION

 ◆ Periumbilical midline laparotomy **(Figure 21-1)**.

 2. DISSECTION

 ◆ After entering the peritoneal cavity, use scalpel to create stab wound through skin and anterior fascia, just lateral to rectus abdominus muscle, usually to the left (see Figure 21-1).

 ◆ With retraction and visualization, use forceps through stab wound to enter through peritoneum and into abdomen **(Figure 21-2)**.

 ◆ Use this same forceps to grasp mushroom catheter (20F) and retract external end of catheter through stab wound.

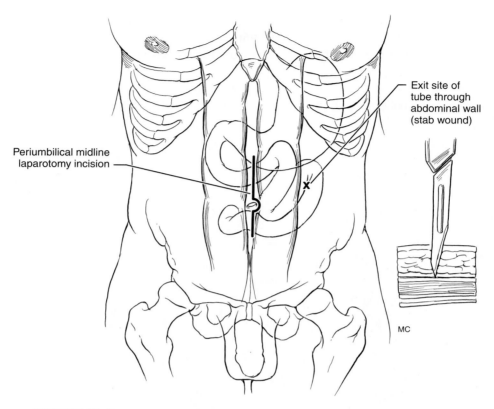

Periumbilical midline
laparotomy incision

Exit site of
tube through
abdominal wall
(stab wound)

MC

FIGURE 21-1

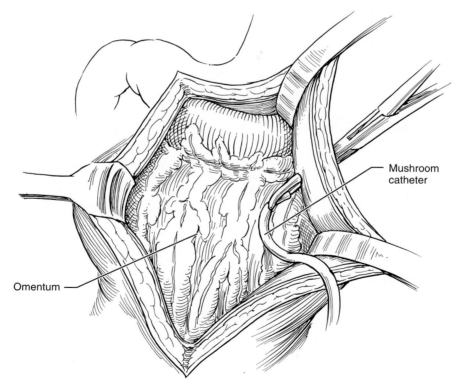

Mushroom
catheter

Omentum

FIGURE 21-2

◆ Place 3-0 silk suture as purse string into antimesenteric wall of selected jejunum, usually approximately 30 cm distal to ligament of Treitz yet with sufficient mobility to reach peritoneum at the site of the catheter exit (**Figure 21-3**).

◆ Using two Babcock clamps for traction, use cautery to create enterotomy within purse string (Figure 21-3).

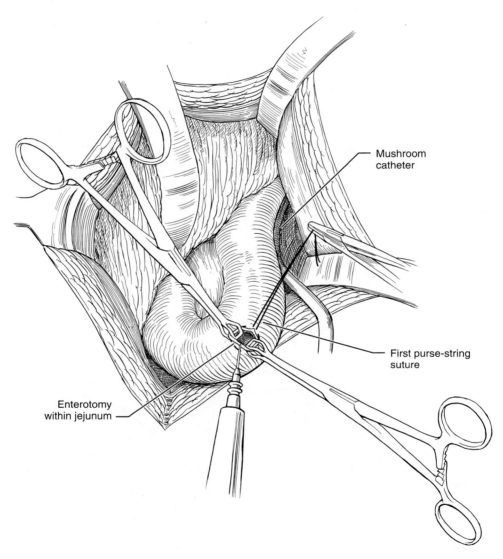

Mushroom catheter

First purse-string suture

Enterotomy within jejunum

FIGURE 21–3

◆ Using two Babcock clamps for traction, use forceps to stent mushroom catheter tip and place through enterotomy and advance tip 8 cm distally into intestine **(Figure 21-4)**.

◆ Secure purse string around catheter.

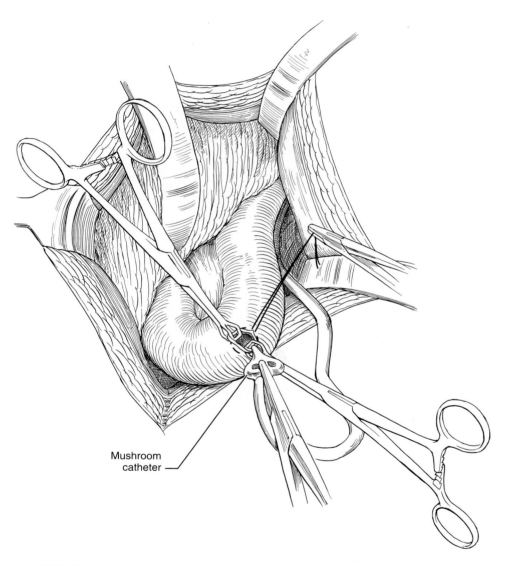

Mushroom
catheter —

FIGURE 21–4

◆ Place multiple 3-0 silk interrupted sutures at 1-cm intervals for 6 to 8 cm proximal to enterotomy and incorporate bowel wall on both sides of catheter **(Figure 21-5).**

◆ Tie sutures, thereby burying catheter within wall of intestine (see Figure 21-5, B).

◆ Place several additional 3-0 silk sutures at 1-cm intervals in a Lembert fashion, incorporating enterotomy and continuing distally for 3 to 5 cm (see Figure 21-5, C).

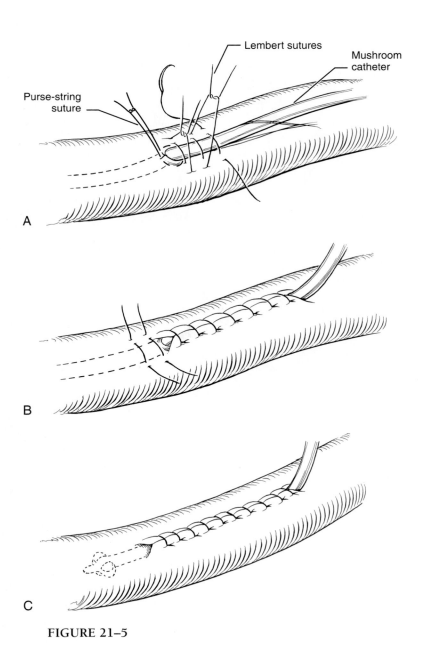

FIGURE 21–5

◆ Use several 3-0 silk sutures to anchor the antimesenteric wall of jejunum to peritoneum **(Figure 21-6).**

◆ Retract mushroom catheter to approximate antimesenteric jejunal wall with enterotomy to peritoneum, secure silk sutures.

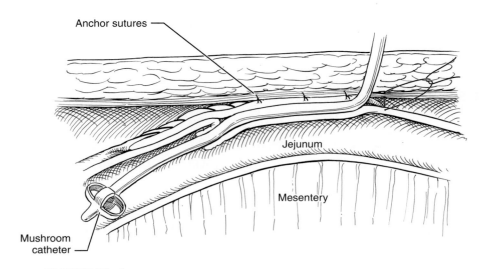

FIGURE 21–6

3. CLOSING

- Close fascia with suture.

- Close skin.

STEP 4: POSTOPERATIVE CARE

- Routine: start feeds

STEP 5: PEARLS AND PITFALLS

- Use of two Babcock clamps grasping edges of enterotomy in conjunction with forceps inserted into tip of mushroom catheter provides an excellent means for placing catheter through enterotomy.

- Catheter should remain in place for at least 2 weeks to allow enterotomy tract and jejunum to heal securely to peritoneum.

- Broad attachment of jejunal loop to peritoneum is advisable to minimize angulation of small intestine.

- First place all the sutures from the antimesenteric edge of jejunum to peritoneum, and then retract the catheter to approximate the jejunum to peritoneum and secure ligatures. This sequence allows good visualization and space for placing sutures.

SELECTED REFERENCES

1. Zollinger RM Jr, Zollinger RM: Atlas of Surgical Operations. New York, Macmillan, 1983, p 92.

CHAPTER 22

PERCUTANEOUS GASTROSTOMY FEEDING TUBE PLACEMENT (BY SURGEON OR GASTROENTEROLOGIST)

Dennis C. Gore

STEP 1: SURGICAL ANATOMY

◆ See **Figure 22-1.**

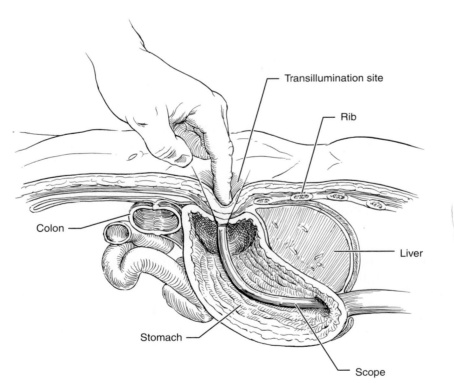

FIGURE 22–1

STEP 2: PREOPERATIVE CONSIDERATIONS

- Percutaneous endoscopic feeding tube placement is indicated for patients who have a functional gastrointestinal tract but are unable or unwilling to meet nutritional demands by mouth, in general for a period longer than 30 days (nasogastric or orogastric tubes are recommended for shorter-term use). In addition, the patient's potential survivability should be good if adequate nutrition is achieved. Potential candidates include those with neurologic deficits, psychomotor deficits, pseudodementia with starvation, facial trauma, facial tumors that will not immediately threaten the patient's life, and prolonged ventilation assistance, again with good survivability.

- Placement can be done at bedside, in the endoscopy suite, or in the operating room.

- Obtain informed consent. Often these patients cannot consent for themselves, so proper planning with family members is important.

- Visualize the patient's abdomen. Prior surgery may preclude proper placement. Adhesions may prevent transillumination (at which point the procedure should be stopped to avoid insertion into an overlying loop of bowel), or displacement of the stomach may cause placement too close to ribs or belt line.

- If the patient has an oral or upper airway tumor, he or she may not be a candidate for endoscopy or passage of the scope.

- Ensure there is no evidence of gastric outlet obstruction, in which case a jejunostomy feeding tube may be required.

- Patients with excessive reflux or nonfunctional esophageal sphincters may not be good candidates for gastrostomy feeding tubes, which can increase risk of aspiration.

- Some surgeons advocate one dose of preoperative antibiotic, such as a first-generation cephalosporin, but this is not universal practice.

- Blood pressure, pulse oximetry, and electrocardiogram should be monitored in all patients during the procedure.

- Place the video camera on the patient's right to facilitate viewing during the procedure.

◆ Two operators are required—one for endoscopy and one for feeding tube insertion.

◆ **Sedation/anesthesia considerations:** Often these patients can be comatose or altered in level of consciousness, so less sedation is required. Usually 1 to 2 mg of a benzodiazapine and a small dose of narcotic can relax the patient to allow passage of the endoscope, which may be eased if the patient can cooperate with swallowing. Topical spray to the oropharynx will facilitate endoscopy. The abdominal insertion site should receive local anesthetic.

◆ **Positioning/preparation:** Patients are placed supine, often with the head of the bed raised at 30 degrees to prevent aspiration. A bite block is used in the mouth to prevent the patient from biting the scope or the surgeon. Suction should be available for secretions and to prevent risk of aspiration. The abdominal site is prepped widely with povidone-iodine (Betadine) or sterile soap, and sterile drapes are applied. The endoscopist should be at the patient's head on the left and the assistant on the right by the patient's abdomen.

STEP 3: OPERATIVE STEPS

In both methods currently used, at least two persons are needed to perform the procedure—one to perform the endoscopic visualization and the other to perform insertion of the tube under sterile technique. Both are performed using a prepackaged kit available from several manufacturers.

1. INCISION

- **Sheath method (Russell technique) (rarely used):** After the patient is adequately sedated and the abdomen is prepped in sterile technique, the endoscope is passed via the mouth into the stomach. The stomach is insufflated and transilluminated (see Figure 22-1). The lack of transillumination precludes safe placement **(Figure 22-2).** Once the light source is visible through the skin, an area is marked for insertion (the site should be 2 cm away from the costal margin) and lidocaine is injected. A no. 11 blade is used to make a small incision (0.5 mm) in the skin. A 14- to 18-gauge needle is then passed through the incision with the tip identified on the video screen and endoscopy camera **(Figure 22-3).** The guidewire is then passed through the needle and identified inside the stomach and the needle is removed. The dilator and then the sheath are passed in turn over the guidewire. Once the sheath is confirmed within the stomach, the feeding tube is passed through the sheath into the stomach. Again after visualization of the tube, the balloon of the feeding tube is inflated inside the stomach.

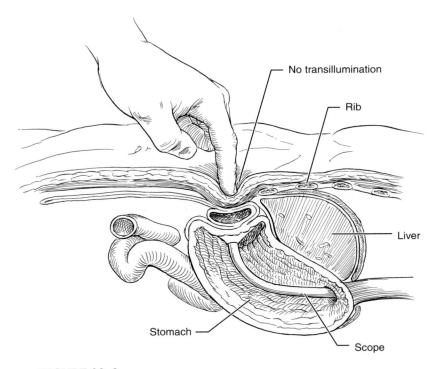

FIGURE 22–2

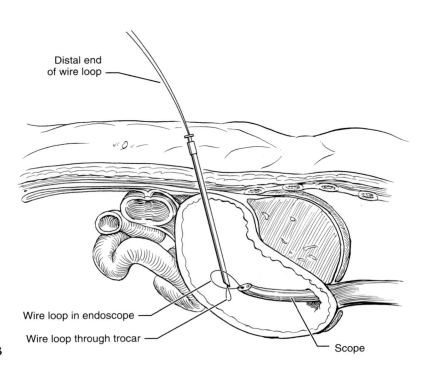

FIGURE 22–3

◆ **Pull method (Ponsky):** After the patient is adequately sedated and prepped using sterile technique, the endoscope is passed via the mouth into the stomach. Visualization and insufflation of the stomach is performed with transillumination (see Figure 22-1). After identification of an appropriate insertion site on the stomach (2 cm away from the costal margin), the area is marked and lidocaine is injected. A small incision is made (1 cm) with the no. 11 blade, and a 14- to 18-gauge needle is passed through the incision into the stomach with visualization via the endoscope (see Figure 22-3). A braided suture is passed through the needle and encircled by a snare passed through the endoscope. Once the "rope" is securely entrapped, the needle is removed and the entire endoscope with snare and attached rope is withdrawn through the mouth **(Figure 22-4).** The feeding tube is then attached to the rope and lubricated well. The assistant then withdraws the rope from the stomach wall, and the tube is carefully guided through the patient's mouth into the stomach and is pulled into position **(Figure 22-5).** Once the feeding tube has been drawn through the skin to approximately 4 cm, the endoscope is reinserted into the stomach to ensure proper seating of the feeding tube. A skin disc is placed to help hold the tube in position against the abdomen **(Figure 22-6).**

◆ **Push method (Sacks-Vine):** After the patient is adequately sedated and prepped using sterile technique, the endoscope is passed via the mouth into the stomach. Visualization and insufflation of the stomach is performed with transillumination (see Figure 22-1). After identification of an appropriate insertion site on the stomach (2 cm away from the costal margin), the area is marked and lidocaine is injected. A small incision is made (1 cm) with the no. 11 blade, and a 14- to 18-gauge needle is passed through the incision into the stomach with visualization via the endoscope (see Figure 22-3). A guidewire is passed through the needle and encircled by a snare passed through the endoscope. Once the guidewire is securely entrapped, the needle is removed and the entire endoscope with snare and attached guidewire is withdrawn through the mouth (see Figure 22-4). Once enough guidewire is visible through the mouth, the feeding tube is then fed over the guidewire and lubricated well. The feeding tube is then fed through the mouth and pushed over the wire. The assistant keeps tension on the guidewire and grabs the tapered end of the feeding tube as it emerges on the skin. Once the feeding tube as been drawn through the skin to approximately 4 cm, the guidewire is withdrawn and the endoscope is reinserted into the stomach to ensure proper seating of the feeding tube. A skin disc is then guided over the feeding tube to help secure its position against the skin (see Figure 22-6).

2. DISSECTION

◆ Not applicable

3. CLOSING

◆ Not applicable

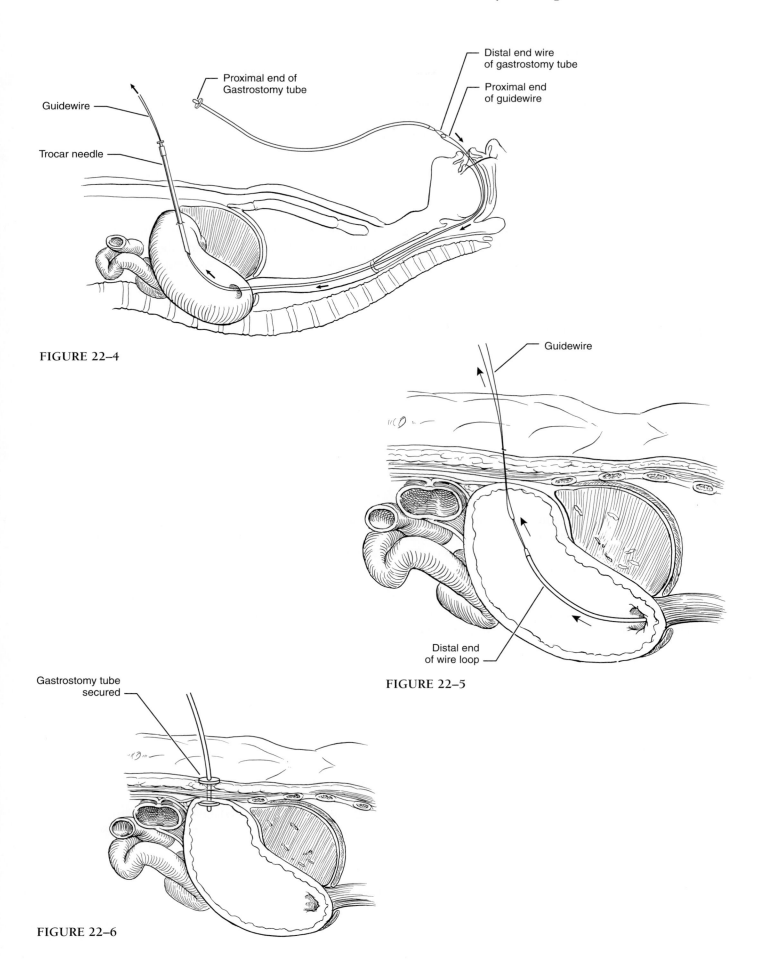

FIGURE 22–4

FIGURE 22–5

FIGURE 22–6

STEP 4: POSTOPERATIVE CARE

◆ The PEG tube is placed to gravity for the remainder of the procedure day with 30 to 60 mL of water or saline flush performed every 4 hours. If no signs of infection, abdominal sepsis, or ileus are seen the following morning, trickle feeds may be started and advanced as tolerated. The site should be kept clean and dry and the tube at approximately 3 to 5 cm depending on patient girth. Pills should not be inserted into the tube, and only liquid medications should be given.

◆ **Removal:** Most tubes are removed by gentle traction at the skin. If a balloon catheter type has been inserted, the balloon should be deflated first. If the tube breaks and the inner disc does not come out, endoscopic retrieval is necessary to avoid risk of bowel obstruction.

STEP 5: PEARLS AND PITFALLS

◆ Often patients are combative and accidentally dislodge tubes or break sterile fields. In addition, sedatives can disinhibit some patients. During the procedure, consider assistance or soft restraints.

◆ If transillumination cannot be performed, stop the procedure. This is a contraindication because adjacent viscera can be damaged.

◆ Early dislodgement may preclude replacement and require laparotomy. A Foley catheter can be used to maintain the tract once epithelialization has occurred, if the tube is displaced after that time. If a tube is reinserted, confirmation of placement should be made with a gastrograffin abdominal film.

◆ Excessive tension on the feeding tube can cause necrosis of the abdominal wall, site infection, and feed leakage. No gauze should be placed under the skin disc to help prevent this.

SELECTED REFERENCES

1. Eisen GM, Baron TH, Dominitz JA, et al: Role of endoscopy in enteral feeding. Gastrointest Endosc 2002;55:794-797.
2. Scott-Conner CEH (ed): The SAGES Manual: Fundamentals of Laparoscopy and GI Endoscopy. New York, Springer, 1999, pp 462-469.
3. Duh Q-Y, McQuaid K: Flexible endoscopy and enteral access. In Eubanks S, Swanström LL, Soper NJ, Leonard M (eds): Mastery of Endoscopic and Laparoscopic Surgery. Philadelphia, Lippincott Williams & Wilkins, 2000, pp 133-143.
4. Angus F: The percutaneous endoscopy gastrostomy tube, medical and ethical issues in placement. Am J Gastroenterol 2003;98:272-277.
5. Gopalan S: Enteral nutrition delivery technique. Curr Opin Clin Nutr Metab Care 2003;6:313-317.

CHAPTER 23

PYLOROPLASTY

Carlos A. Angel

STEP 1: SURGICAL ANATOMY

- The pylorus sits at the distal end of the stomach and is marked by thickening of the circular smooth muscle layer, thus forming the pyloric sphincter, which acts as a valve between the stomach and the duodenum and regulates gastric emptying. The pylorus does not have independent blood supply; rather, it gets its blood supply from the vessels that perfuse the distal stomach and proximal duodenum. Innervation of the pylorus is through the terminal branches of the right and the left vagus nerves. Any injury to these nerves or denervation of the pylorus will result in pylorospasm and delayed gastric emptying.

STEP 2: PREOPERATIVE CONSIDERATIONS

- Gastric drainage procedures such as pyloroplasties are indicated with truncal vagotomies in the management of peptic ulcer disease (pyloric, prepyloric, and duodenal ulcers), in selected patients who undergo transhiatal resection of the esophagus with gastric pull-ups, and in children undergoing fundoplication for gastroesophageal reflux disease with confirmed delay in gastric emptying. Three types of pyloroplasties have been classically described, namely, the Heineke-Mikulicz pyloroplasty, which is the easiest to perform and the most commonly used; the Finney pyloroplasty; and the Jaboulay pyloroplasty.

- Confirmation of the diagnosis of peptic ulcer disease or delay in gastric emptying should be documented before the procedure with endoscopy, contrast studies, or technetium-99 sulfur colloid meals.

- The Heineke-Mikulicz pyloroplasty is perhaps the most commonly performed because it is technically simple, carries low morbidity and mortality, and of all pyloroplasties it takes the least amount of time to complete.

STEP 3: OPERATIVE STEPS

1. INCISION

♦ After the antrum and duodenum are exposed, the pylorus is easily identified because it feels thicker that either the stomach or duodenum, and the pyloric vein, which runs across the pylorus transverse to the axis of the duodenum, serves as a clear landmark. A 3-cm full-thickness incision is made along the axis of the pylorus equidistant from both the stomach and the duodenum **(Figures 23-1 and 23-2)**. Holding stitches are placed at the midpoint of the incision on both the superior and inferior sides of the defect, and traction is used to align the tissue perpendicularly with respect to its original axis (see Figure 23-2). Closure is now performed in two layers. A running 3-0 absorbable suture layer is used to reapproximate the mucosa **(Figure 23-3)**, and interrupted 3-0 silk seromuscular stitches are used to complete the repair **(Figure 23-4)**. Care must be taken to avoid excessive invagination of the suture line. If tension is deemed to be excessive, mobilization of the duodenum with a Kocher maneuver may be required.

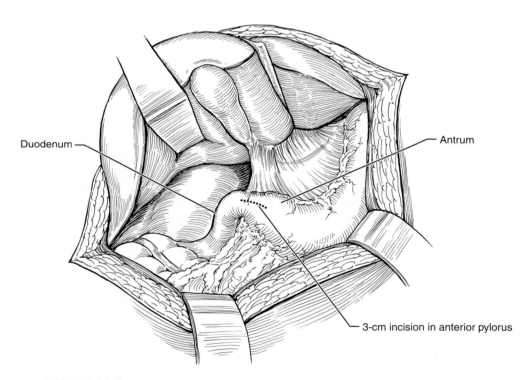

Duodenum

Antrum

3-cm incision in anterior pylorus

FIGURE 23–1

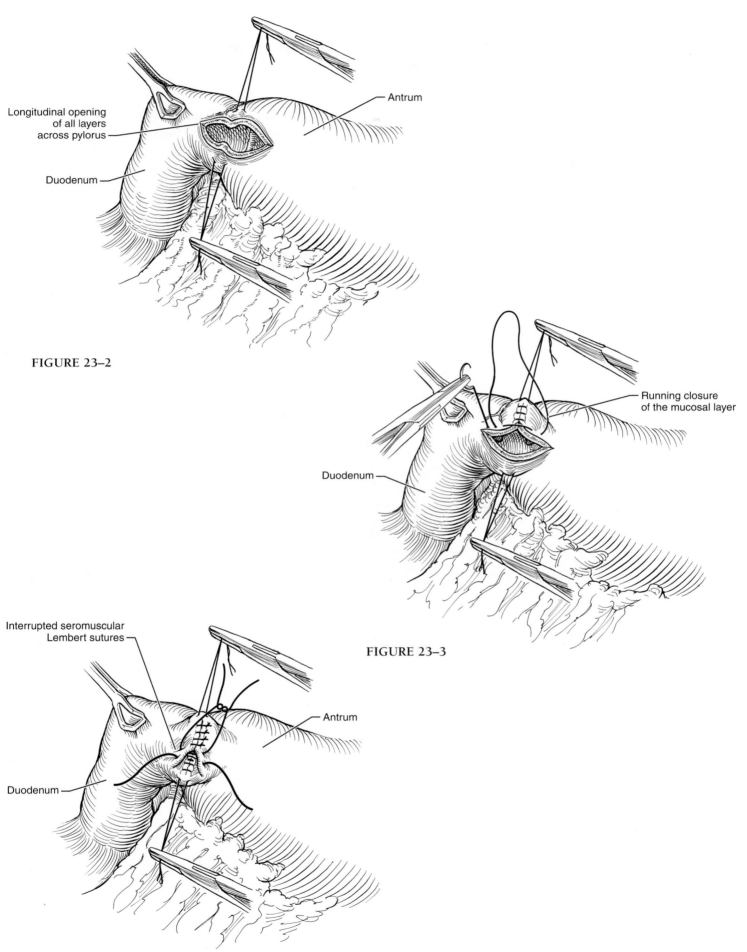

Longitudinal opening
of all layers
across pylorus

Antrum

Duodenum

FIGURE 23–2

Running closure
of the mucosal layer

Duodenum

FIGURE 23–3

Interrupted seromuscular
Lembert sutures

Antrum

Duodenum

FIGURE 23–4

2. DISSECTION, HEINEKE-MIKULICZ PYLOROPLASTY (STAPLED)

- A full-thickness 4- to 6-cm longitudinal incision is made along the axis of the pylorus, and two holding stitches are placed as described previously. An additional stitch is placed from the most proximal to the most distal point of the incision **(Figure 23-5)**. As these stitches are placed under traction, the longitudinal defect is converted into a transverse defect. A terminal anastomosis (TA)-55 linear stapling device is applied, making sure that all layers are involved and in such a manner that after its firing the result will be a transverse closure of the incision **(Figures 23-6 and 23-7)**. After the stapler is fired, excess pyloric tissue is removed with the scalpel, and subsequently the stapler is released (see Figures 23-6 and 23-7). Careful inspection of the staple line is mandatory. A stapled pyloroplasty such as the one described here requires a supple pylorus and should not be chosen when the pylorus is scarred and nonpliable.

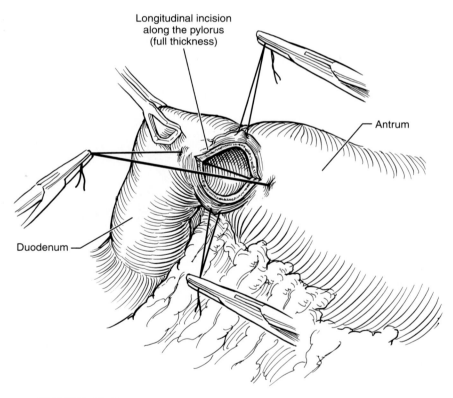

Longitudinal incision
along the pylorus
(full thickness)

Antrum

Duodenum

FIGURE 23–5

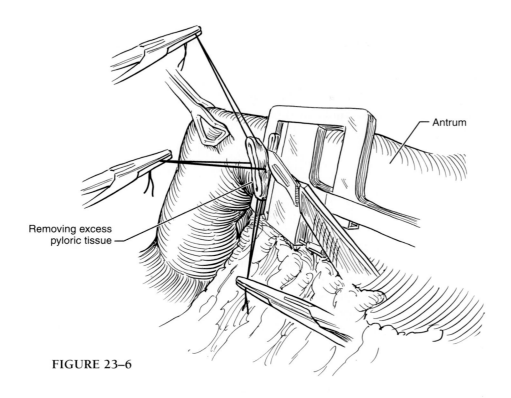

Antrum

Removing excess
pyloric tissue

FIGURE 23–6

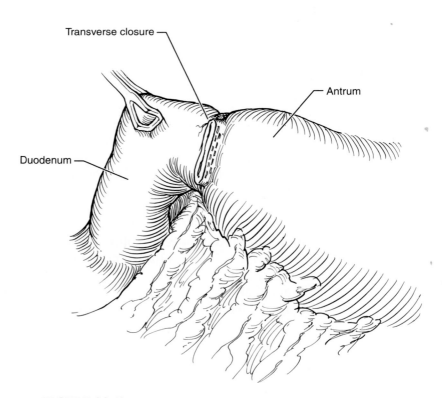

Transverse closure

Antrum

Duodenum

FIGURE 23–7

3. CLOSING

◆ The incision is closed in layers using 2-0 polyglactin in a running fashion. The subcutaneous tissue is reapproximated with a running 3-0 polyglactin suture. The skin can be stapled together or closed with a running subcuticular suture of 4-0 undyed absorbable monofilament and adhesive strips.

STEP 4: POSTOPERATIVE CARE

◆ The patient should have already received a preoperative dose of a prophylactic antibiotic such as cefazolin. Two additional doses are in order after the operation. Hydration will be maintained with an intravenous infusion of a balanced dextrose and electrolyte solution. Intravenous analgesics are used until the patient resumes enteral feeds. The decision to decompress the stomach with a nasogastric tube is up to the individual surgeon, and the current tendency is to use these tubes sparingly. Certainly, if the repair was deemed to be tenuous, a nasogastric tube could prove to be very helpful. After 2 to 3 days (on average), enteral feeds can be slowly and gradually resumed. The presence of bile in the gastric aspirate does not necessarily represent a persistent postoperative paralytic ileus, because it could be the result of the pyloroplasty itself and it should not be a reason for undue delays in resumption of enteral feeds. Pain, abdominal distention, tachycardia, and guarding should prompt the surgeon to order a contrast study to investigate for leaks in the suture line.

STEP 5: PEARLS AND PITFALLS

◆ Performance of this procedure in a scarred and nonpliable pylorus can potentially be plagued by complications. Poor selection of pyloroplasty technique will result in undue tension of the repair. On the other hand, excessive tension can also result in a supple pylorus from extending the initial incision too far proximally into the stomach and distally into the duodenum.

◆ **Complications:** Alkaline reflux, alkaline gastritis, and dumping syndrome can be seen after any pyloroplasty. Failure of the operation with delayed gastric emptying is the result of excessive invagination of one or both suture lines. Excessive tension of the suture line when performing this procedure in a pylorus that is acutely inflamed or ulcerated may result in disruption of the suture line, intestinal leaks, and intra-abdominal sepsis.

SELECTED REFERENCES

1. Economou SG, Economou TS: Atlas of Surgical Techniques. Philadelphia, Saunders, 1996, pp 224-227.
2. Mercer DM, Robinson EK: Stomach. In Townsend CM, Beauchamp RD, Evers MB, Mattox KL (eds): Sabiston Textbook of Surgery, 18th ed. Philadelphia, Saunders, 2008.

CHAPTER 24

FINNEY PYLOROPLASTY

Carlos A. Angel

INTRODUCTION

Finney, in 1902, described a gastric emptying procedure consisting of a horseshoe-shaped incision through the pylorus followed by a transverse repair in layers. In essence, Finney pyloroplasty is a side-to-side anastomosis of antrum and duodenum that, unlike the Jaboulay pyloroplasty, does not exclude the pyloric area. This procedure involves an extensive Kocher maneuver of the duodenum and can be performed with a classic handsewn two-layer technique as illustrated later, or using a gastrointestinal anastomosis (GIA) linear stapler to approximate antrum and duodenum with a single stab incision through the pylorus and closure of the defect with a terminal anastomosis (TA)-55 linear stapler.

STEP 1: SURGICAL ANATOMY

- The pylorus sits at the distal end of the stomach and is marked by thickening of the circular smooth muscle layer, thus forming the pyloric sphincter, which acts as a valve between the stomach and the duodenum and regulates gastric emptying. The pylorus does not have independent blood supply; rather, it gets its blood supply from the vessels that perfuse the distal stomach and proximal duodenum. Innervation of the pylorus is through the terminal branches of the right and left vagus nerves. Any injury to these nerves or denervation of the pylorus will result in pylorospasm and delayed gastric emptying.

STEP 2: PREOPERATIVE CONSIDERATIONS

- Confirmation of the diagnosis of peptic ulcer disease or delay in gastric emptying should be documented before the procedure with endoscopy, contrast studies, or technetium-99 sulfur colloid meals.

STEP 3: OPERATIVE STEPS

1. INCISION

◆ The operation can be performed through a limited midline supraumbilical laparotomy. The skin incision is made with the knife, and the rest of the layers are divided with electrocautery, taking care to stay in the midline and paying close attention to hemostasis. Once the peritoneum is opened, the surgeon's fingers or a malleable retractor is used to protect the intestines from enterotomies.

2. DISSECTION

◆ After mobilization of the duodenum, the midpoint of the pylorus is grasped and lifted with a Babcock forceps. A seromuscular suture line 5 cm long with interrupted 3-0 silk is placed to approximate the antrum and duodenum. These stitches should be placed as posteriorly as possible to diminish the tension on the anterior suture line **(Figure 24-1)**. A horseshoe-shaped incision involving all layers of the anterior wall of the antrum, pylorus, and duodenum is made. Hemostasis is achieved with electrocautery **(Figure 24-2)**. A continuous 3-0 absorbable stitch is used to reapproximate the mucosa, beginning posteriorly and finishing anteriorly **(Figures 24-3 and 24-4)**. The anastomosis is completed with 3-0 silk interrupted seromuscular stitches **(Figure 24-5)**.

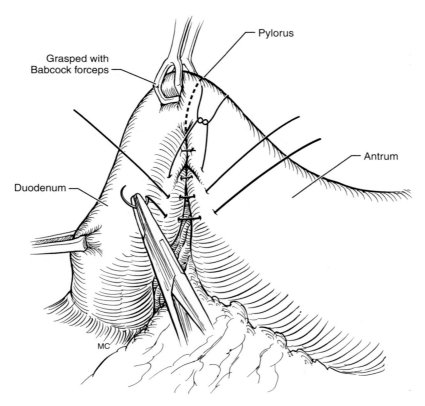

FIGURE 24–1

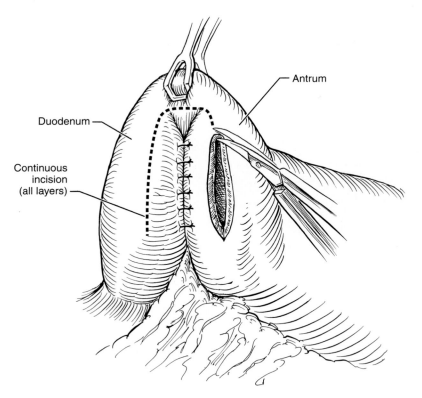

FIGURE 24–2

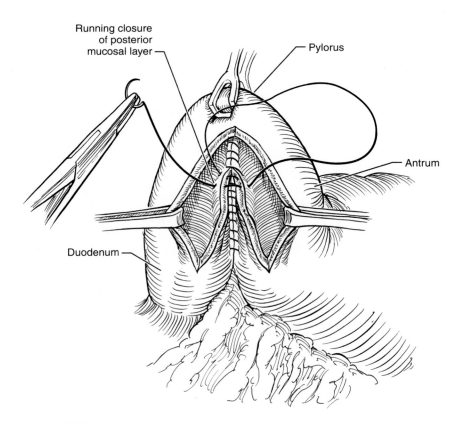

FIGURE 24–3

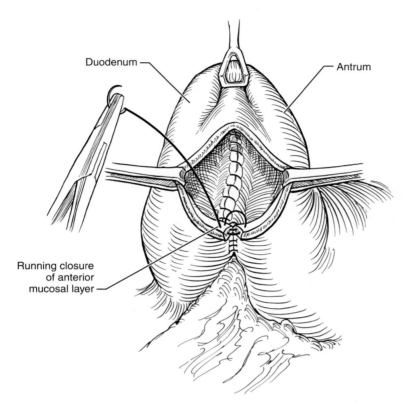

Duodenum

Antrum

Running closure
of anterior
mucosal layer

FIGURE 24–4

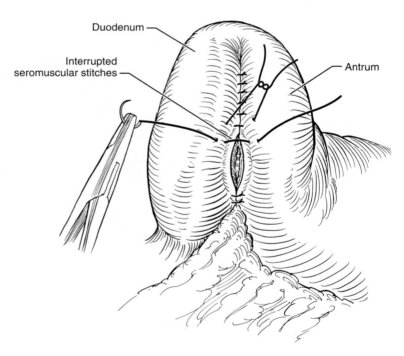

Duodenum

Interrupted
seromuscular stitches

Antrum

FIGURE 24–5

3. CLOSING

◆ The incision is closed in layers using 2-0 polyglactin in a running fashion. The subcutaneous tissue is reapproximated with a running 3-0 polyglactin suture. The skin can be stapled together or closed with a running subcuticular suture of 4-0 undyed absorbable monofilament and adhesive strips.

STEP 4: POSTOPERATIVE CARE

◆ The patient should have already received a preoperative dose of a prophylactic antibiotic such as cefazolin. Two additional doses should be given after the operation. Hydration will be maintained with an intravenous infusion of a balanced dextrose and electrolyte solution. Intravenous analgesics are used until the patient resumes enteral feeds. The decision to decompress the stomach with a nasogastric tube is up to the individual surgeon, and the current tendency is to use these tubes sparingly. Certainly, if the repair was deemed to be tenuous, a nasogastric tube could prove to be very helpful. After 2 to 3 days (on average), enteral feeds can be slowly and gradually resumed. The presence of bile in the gastric aspirate does not necessarily represent a persistent postoperative paralytic ileus, because it could be the result of the pyloroplasty itself, and it should not be a reason for undue delays in resumption of enteral feeds. Pain, abdominal distention, tachycardia, and guarding should prompt the surgeon to order a contrast study to investigate for leaks in the suture line.

STEP 5: PEARLS AND PITFALLS

◆ As mentioned previously, avoidance of tension on the suture line is essential. This is accomplished by a generous Kocher maneuver. Avoid approximating the antrum and duodenum in such a manner that both structures have to be excessively rolled inward to approximate the anterior layers. This can be achieved by placing the posterior seromuscular stitches as posterior as possible (taking care not to involve the ampulla of Vater in the suture line), giving ample room to perform the incisions in both the duodenum and antrum and complete the anastomosis with minimal tension.

◆ As with any pyloroplasty, alkaline reflux, alkaline gastritis, and dumping syndrome can be problematic. Suture line leaks can result from undue tension or the approximation of acutely inflamed or poorly perfused tissues.

SELECTED REFERENCES

1. Mercer DW: Stomach. In Townsend CM, Beauchamp RD, Evers MB, Mattox KL (eds): Sabiston Textbook of Surgery, 17th ed. Philadelphia, Saunders, 2004, pp 1265-1317.
2. Warner BW: Pediatric surgery. In Townsend CM, Beauchamp RD, Evers MB, Mattox KL (eds): Sabiston Textbook of Surgery, 17th ed. Philadelphia, Saunders, 2004, pp 2097-2132.

CHAPTER 25

JABOULAY SIDE-TO-SIDE GASTRODUODENOSTOMY

Carlos A. Angel

INTRODUCTION

This bypass operation is indicated in the presence of marked inflammation or scarring of the pylorus that precludes a Heineke-Mikulicz pyloroplasty. The procedure can be performed using a standard handsewn technique or a stapler. The handsewn technique described in this chapter is a two-layer anastomosis with a running inner layer of 3-0 absorbable sutures and a seromuscular outer layer of interrupted 3-0 silk sutures.

STEP 1: SURGICAL ANATOMY

◆ The pylorus sits at the distal end of the stomach and is marked by thickening of the circular smooth muscle layer, thus forming the pyloric sphincter, which acts as a valve between the stomach and the duodenum and regulates gastric emptying. The pylorus does not have independent blood supply; rather, it gets its blood supply from the vessels that perfuse the distal stomach and proximal duodenum. Innervation of the pylorus is through the terminal branches of the right and left vagus nerves. Any injury to these nerves or denervation of the pylorus will result in pylorospasm and delayed gastric emptying.

STEP 2: PREOPERATIVE CONSIDERATIONS

◆ Confirmation of the diagnosis of peptic ulcer disease or delay in gastric emptying should be documented before the procedure with endoscopy, contrast studies, or technetium-99 sulfur colloid meals.

STEP 3: OPERATIVE STEPS

1. INCISION

+ The operation can be performed through a limited midline supraumbilical laparotomy. The skin incision is made with the knife, and the rest of the layers are divided with electrocautery, taking care to stay in the midline and paying close attention to hemostasis. Once the peritoneum is opened, the surgeon's fingers or a malleable retractor can be used to protect the intestines from enterotomies.

2. DISSECTION

+ After wide mobilization of the duodenum with a generous Kocher maneuver, the pylorus is grasped with a Babcock forceps and a 3-0 silk stitch is placed approximately 7 cm distal from this point to approximate the antrum and duodenum (**Figures 25-1 and 25-2**). Approximately 6 to 8 cm of duodenum and antrum are approximated with 3-0 silk, interrupted seromuscular sutures (see Figure 25-2). The duodenum is incised down to the mucosa on both duodenal and antral sides. Bleeding points are cauterized (**Figure 25-3**). Antral and duodenal mucosas are sharply opened. Bleeding is controlled with cautery (**Figure 25-4**). The mucosa is approximated with a continuous, simple stitch of 3-0 absorbable suture, starting with the posterior portion and finishing anteriorly (**Figures 25-5 and 25-6**). The anastomosis is completed with interrupted 3-0 silk seromuscular stitches (**Figure 25-7**).

3. CLOSING

+ The incision is closed in layers using 2-0 polyglactin in a running fashion. The subcutaneous tissue is reapproximated with a running 3-0 polyglactin suture. The skin can be stapled together or closed with a running subcuticular suture of 4-0 undyed absorbable monofilament and adhesive strips.

STEP 4: POSTOPERATIVE CARE

+ The patient should have already received a preoperative dose of a prophylactic antibiotic such as cefazolin. Two additional doses are in order after the operation. Hydration will be maintained with an intravenous infusion of a balanced dextrose and electrolyte solution. Intravenous analgesics are used until the patient resumes enteral feeds. The decision to decompress the stomach with a nasogastric tube is up to the individual surgeon, and the current tendency is to use these tubes sparingly. Certainly, if the repair was deemed to be tenuous, a nasogastric tube could prove to be very helpful. After 2 to 3 days (on average), enteral feeds can be slowly and gradually resumed. The presence of bile in the gastric aspirate does not necessarily represent a persistent postoperative paralytic ileus, because it could be the result of the pyloroplasty itself and it should not be a reason for undue delays in resumption of enteral feeds. Pain, abdominal distention, tachycardia, and guarding should prompt the surgeon to order a contrast study to investigate for leaks in the suture line.

Text continued on p. 277

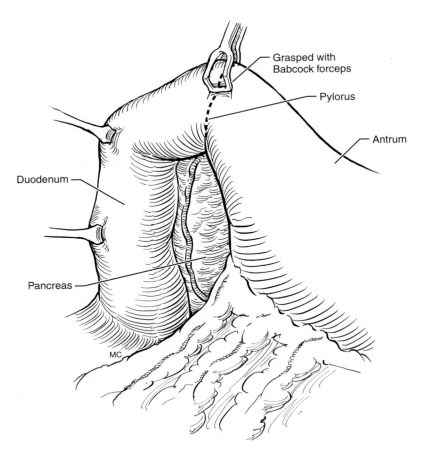

FIGURE 25–1

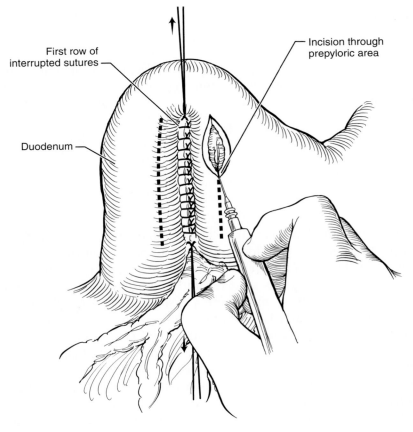

FIGURE 25–2

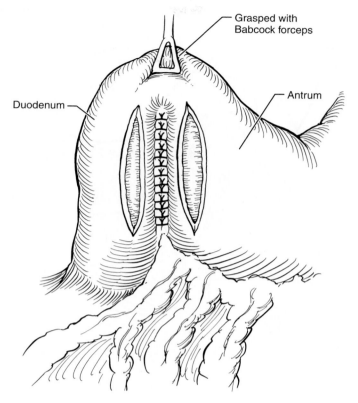

FIGURE 25–3

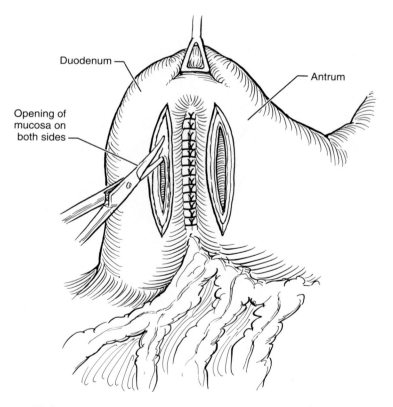

FIGURE 25–4

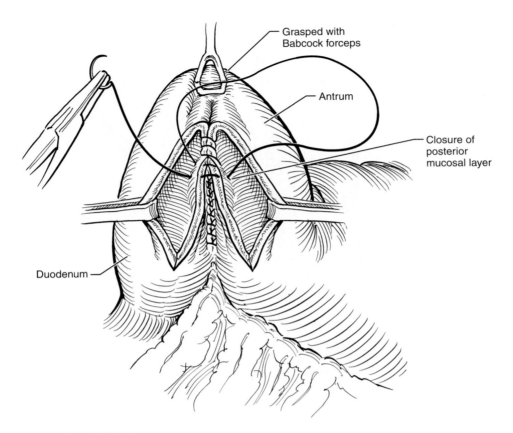

FIGURE 25–5

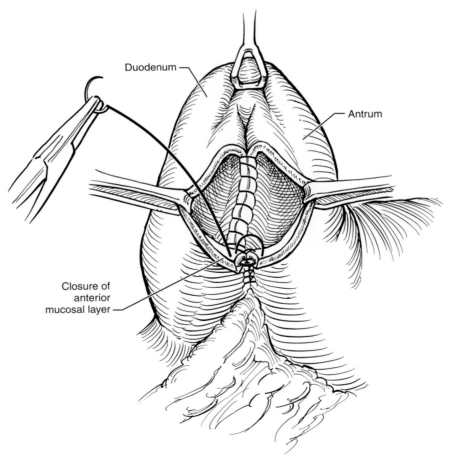

FIGURE 25–6

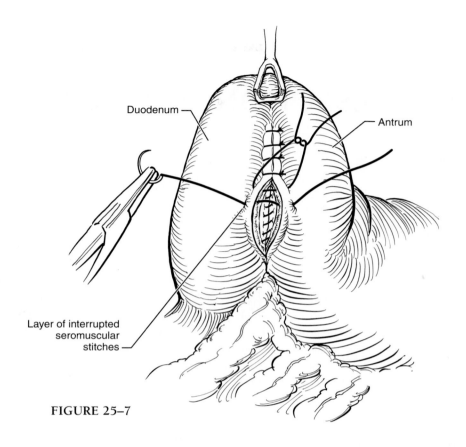

Duodenum

Antrum

Layer of interrupted
seromuscular
stitches

FIGURE 25–7

STEP 5: PEARLS AND PITFALLS

◆ As mentioned, avoidance of tension on the suture line is essential. This is accomplished by a generous Kocher maneuver. Avoid approximating the antrum and duodenum in such a manner that both structures have to be excessively rolled inward to approximate the anterior layers. This can be achieved by placing the posterior seromuscular stitches as posterior as possible (taking care not to involve the ampulla of Vater in the suture line), giving ample room to perform the incisions in both the duodenum and antrum and complete the anastomosis with minimal tension.

COMPLICATIONS

◆ As with any pyloroplasty, alkaline reflux, alkaline gastritis, and dumping syndrome can be problematic. Suture line leaks can result from undue tension or the approximation of acutely inflamed or poorly perfused tissues.

SELECTED REFERENCES

1. Mercer DW: Stomach. In Townsend CM, Beauchamp RD, Evers MB, Mattox KL (eds): Sabiston Textbook of Surgery, 17th ed. Philadelphia, Saunders, 2004, pp 1265-1317.
2. Warner BW: Pediatric surgery. In Townsend CM, Beauchamp RD, Evers MB, Mattox KL (eds): Sabiston Textbook of Surgery, 17th ed. Philadelphia, Saunders, 2004, pp 2097-2132.

CHAPTER 26

GASTRIC RESECTION: BILLROTH I

B. Mark Evers

STEP 1: SURGICAL ANATOMY

- The blood supply to the stomach is abundant. The right gastric artery, a branch from the hepatic artery, courses along the lesser curvature of the stomach to meet the left gastric artery, which is a branch of the celiac axis. The right gastroepiploic artery, a branch of the gastroduodenal artery, courses along the greater curvature of the stomach to meet the left gastroepiploic artery, which is a branch of the splenic artery. In addition, the stomach receives short gastric branches from the splenic artery. The venous drainage of the stomach is into the portal venous system (**Figure 26-1**).

STEP 2: PREOPERATIVE CONSIDERATIONS

- The Billroth I procedure for gastroduodenostomy is the most physiologic type of gastric resection, because it restores normal gastroduodenal continuity. It has been the preferred treatment of gastric ulcer or antral cancer by a number of surgeons; however, its use for duodenal ulcer has been less popular. The principal contraindications to a Billroth I operation include edema from acute or recurrent inflammation and scarring and deformation secondary to chronic disease.

STEP 3: OPERATIVE STEPS

1. INCISION

- An upper midline incision or subcostal incision is an acceptable option for performing this procedure. The line of division varies according to the extent of resection required. The dashed line indicates an approximate 50% gastric transection with a line from the lesser curvature slightly proximal to the incisura angularis (**Figure 26-2**).

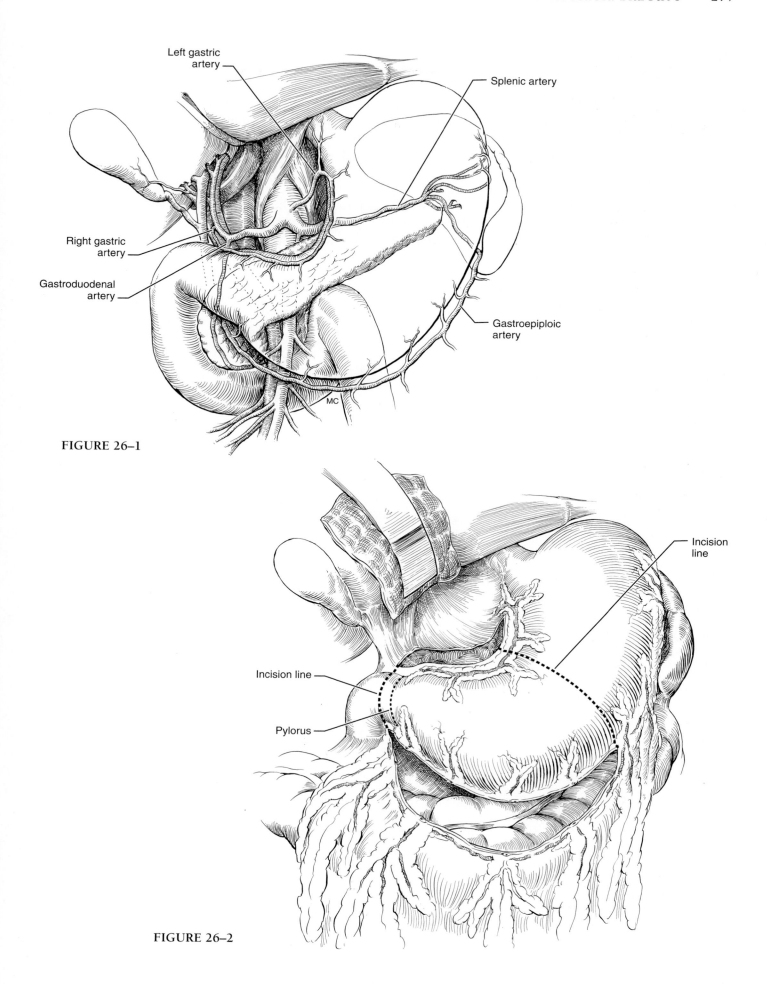

Left gastric artery

Splenic artery

Right gastric artery

Gastroduodenal artery

Gastroepiploic artery

MC

FIGURE 26–1

Incision line

Incision line

Pylorus

FIGURE 26–2

2. DISSECTION

- The greater curvature of the stomach is mobilized by serial division of the gastric branches of the gastroepiploic vessels. The lesser curvature is then mobilized by serially dividing the gastrohepatic ligament to the point of planned transection of the stomach. The left gastric vessels are then identified, clamped, and ligated **(Figure 26-3)**.

- After the lesser curvature has been mobilized, proximal to the left gastric artery and distal to the gastric duodenal artery, Kocher or Payr clamps are applied to the stomach and the stomach is divided with a scalpel **(Figure 26-4)**.

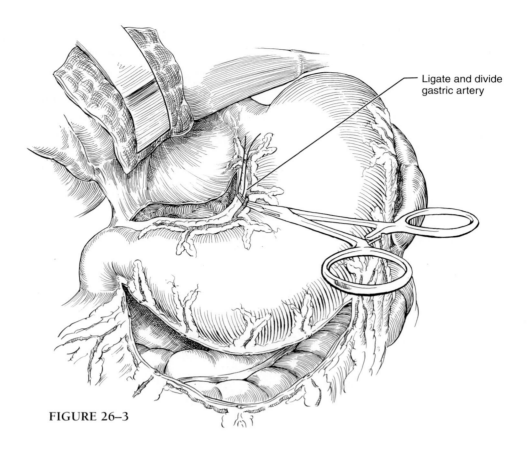

Ligate and divide gastric artery

FIGURE 26–3

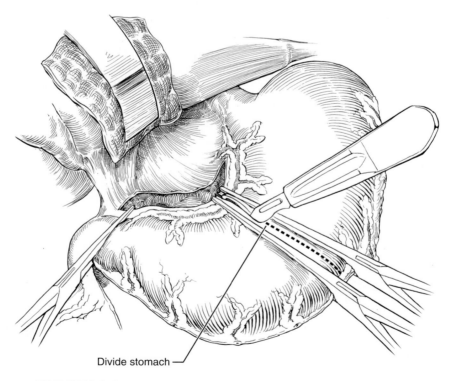

Divide stomach

FIGURE 26–4

◆ Excess gastric tissue is removed, which includes the crushed tissue from the placement of the clamp **(Figure 26-5)**.

◆ The lesser curvature side of the gastric division is then closed using a running nonabsorbable suture **(Figure 26-6)**, this is carried down to the point of the Kocher clamp, which is on the greater curvature side where the gastroduodenal anastomosis will be performed **(Figure 26-7)**.

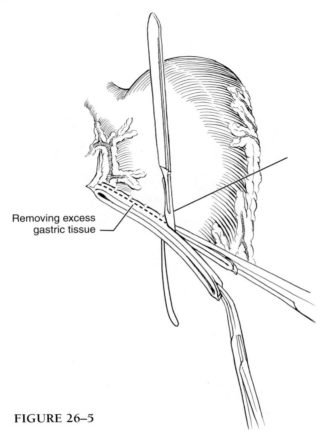

Removing excess
gastric tissue —

FIGURE 26–5

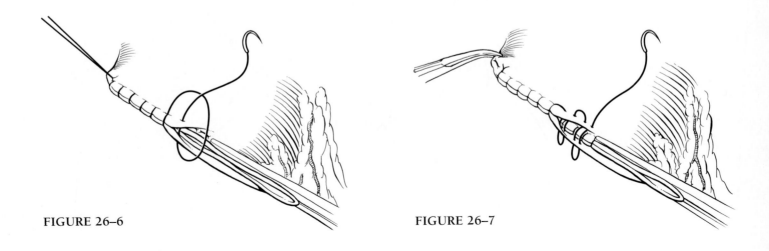

FIGURE 26–6

FIGURE 26–7

♦ After the distal stomach is fully mobilized, the proximal duodenum is divided between Kocher clamps just distal to the pylorus **(Figure 26-8)**.

♦ The gastroduodenal anastomosis is then performed by placing interrupted seromuscular sutures with 3-0 nonabsorbable sutures placed in Lembert fashion **(Figure 26-9)**.

♦ Excess duodenal tissue is removed using electrocautery **(Figure 26-10)**.

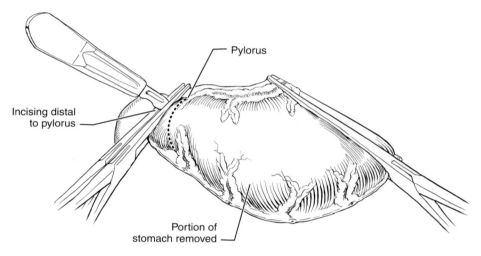

FIGURE 26–8

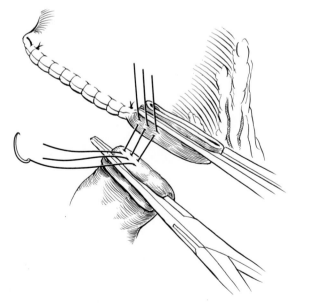

FIGURE 26–9

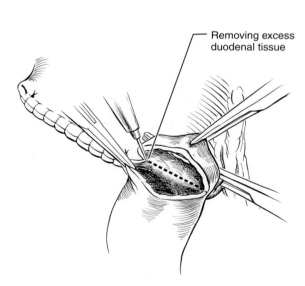

FIGURE 26–10

◆ The anastomosis is completed using a running full-thickness 3-0 absorbable suture such as chromic or Vicryl **(Figure 26-11).**

◆ At the end of the posterior row, the sutures are brought out and the corner is turned by converting to a running Connell suture. The continuous Connell suture is carried around anteriorly and tied together (see Figure 26-11).

◆ The anterior suture line is then reinforced with interrupted seromuscular 3-0 silk sutures **(Figure 26-12).**

◆ The completed gastroduodenal anastomosis is shown in **Figure 26-13.**

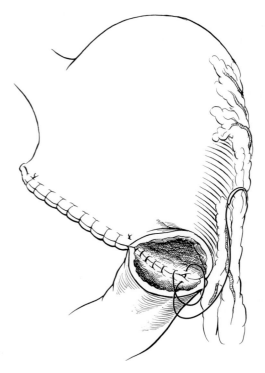

FIGURE 26–11

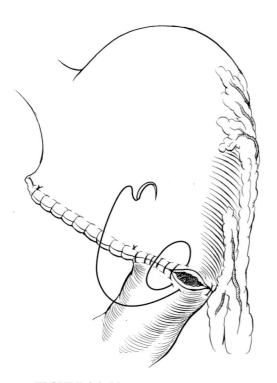

FIGURE 26–12

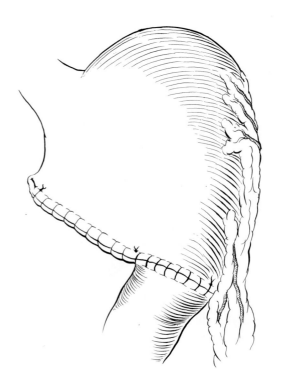

FIGURE 26–13

◆ **Figure 26-14** demonstrates transection of the duodenum using the stapler, usually a gastro-intestinal anastomosis (GIA) stapler. The lesser and greater curvatures have been dissected as noted previously, and the left gastric artery is divided between clamps.

◆ The proximal stomach is then stapled using the transanastomotic (TA) stapler device and transected staying right on the staple line using the scalpel **(Figure 26-15)**.

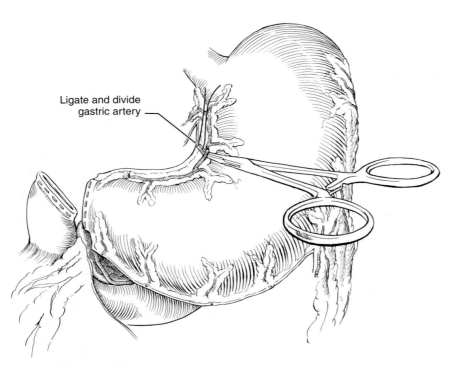

Ligate and divide
gastric artery

FIGURE 26–14

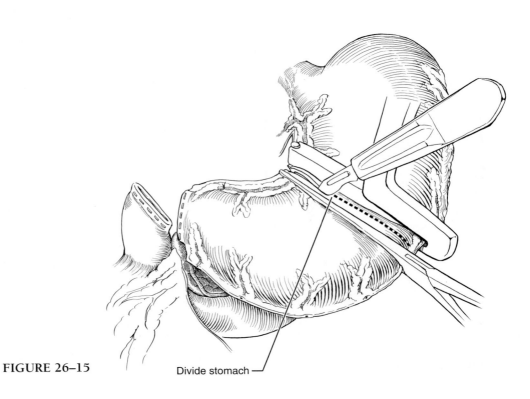

FIGURE 26–15   Divide stomach

◆ **Figure 26-16** shows the stapled end of the stomach and the duodenal stump.

◆ As shown in **Figure 26-17**, preparation for the gastroduodenal anastomosis is performed by trimming excess gastric tissue and opening the staple line on the greater curvature side of the stomach. This is accomplished with electrocautery. The staple line is also removed from the duodenal stump using electrocautery (see Figure 26-17).

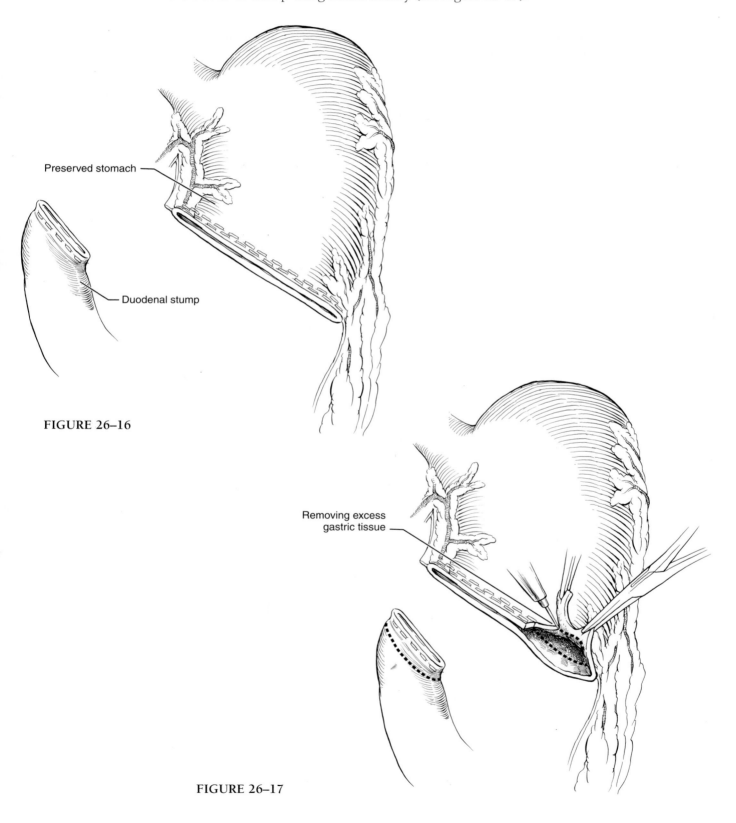

Preserved stomach

Duodenal stump

FIGURE 26–16

Removing excess gastric tissue

FIGURE 26–17

◆ The posterior gastroduodenal anastomosis is then performed by first placing interrupted 3-0 silk sutures in Lembert fashion **(Figure 26-18)**.

◆ The inner layer is performed using a running 3-0 nonabsorbable suture **(Figure 26-19)** and then carried anteriorly in a Connell fashion **(Figure 26-20)**.

◆ The anastomosis is completed with anterior interrupted 3-0 silk sutures placed in Lembert fashion **(Figure 26-21)**.

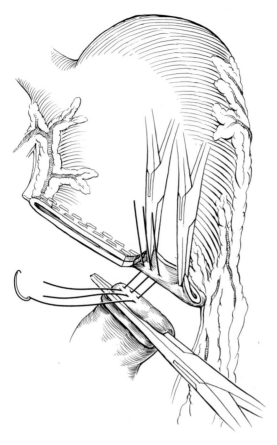

FIGURE 26–18

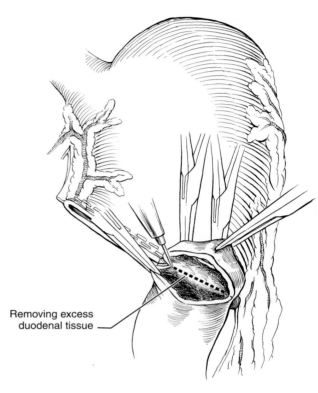

Removing excess
duodenal tissue

FIGURE 26–19

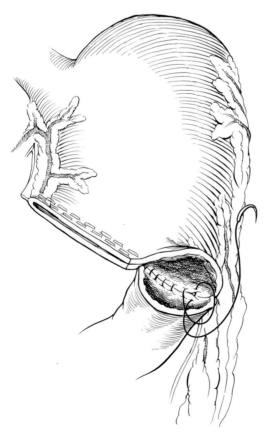

FIGURE 26–20

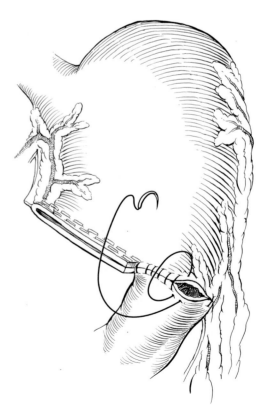

FIGURE 26–21

◆ The staple line is secured by running 3-0 silk sutures **(Figure 26-22)**.

◆ **Figure 26-23** shows the completed gastroduodenal anastomosis.

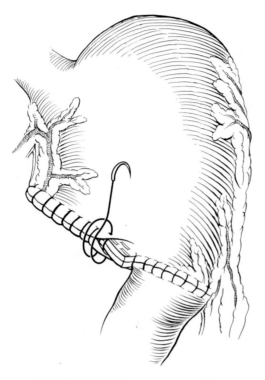

FIGURE 26–22

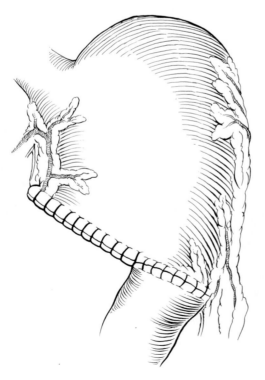

FIGURE 26–23

3. CLOSING

♦ The upper midline or subcostal incision is closed in usual fashion.

STEP 4: POSTOPERATIVE CARE

♦ Before closure, a nasogastric tube is positioned proximal to the suture line. When bowel activity has resumed, the nasogastric tube can be removed and clear liquids initiated. If there is no evidence of gastric retention, the feeding regimen can be progressed.

STEP 5: PEARLS AND PITFALLS

♦ The stomach and duodenum must be thoroughly mobilized for performance of the anastomosis.

♦ Duodenal edema, shortening, or deformity may prevent performance of a Billroth I anastomosis and require a Billroth II anastomosis for safe closure.

SELECTED REFERENCES

1. Mercer DW, Robinson EK: Stomach. In Townsend CM Jr (ed): Sabiston Textbook of Surgery: The Biological Basis of Modern Surgical Practice, 18th ed. Philadelphia, Saunders, 2008, pp 1223-1277.
2. Thompson JC: Subtotal gastrectomy with stapled Billroth I anastomosis (also resection for benign distal gastric ulcer). In Thompson JC (ed): Atlas of Surgery of the Stomach, Duodenum and Small Bowel. St Louis, Mosby-Year Book, 1992, pp 45-53.
3. Thompson JC: Subtotal gastrectomy with stapled Billroth I anastomosis. In Thompson JC (ed): Atlas of Surgery of the Stomach, Duodenum and Small Bowel. St Louis, Mosby-Year Book, 1992, pp 55-59.

CHAPTER 27

GASTRIC RESECTION: BILLROTH II

B. Mark Evers

STEP 1: SURGICAL ANATOMY

- The vascular supply to the stomach has been previously described (see Figure 26-1).

STEP 2: PREOPERATIVE CONSIDERATIONS

- The Billroth II gastric resection is one of the most commonly performed procedures for cancer of the stomach and is also used for operative treatment of duodenal ulcer disease if gastric resection is required.

STEP 3: OPERATIVE STEPS

1. INCISION

- The patient is placed supine on the table, and an upper midline incision or subcostal incision is used as described for the Billroth I anastomosis.

2. DISSECTION

- **Figure 27-1** demonstrates transection of the stomach, indicating a 50% distal gastric resection, starting at the incisura on the lesser curvature as noted by the dashed line. The duodenum is transected distal to the pylorus. The greater curvature is mobilized by dividing the gastroepiploic vessels and is ligated with 2-0 silk sutures.

- The lesser curvature is then likewise mobilized to the incisura (see Figure 27-1).

- The left gastric artery and vein are ligated in continuity with 2-0 silk sutures and divided **(Figure 27-2)**.

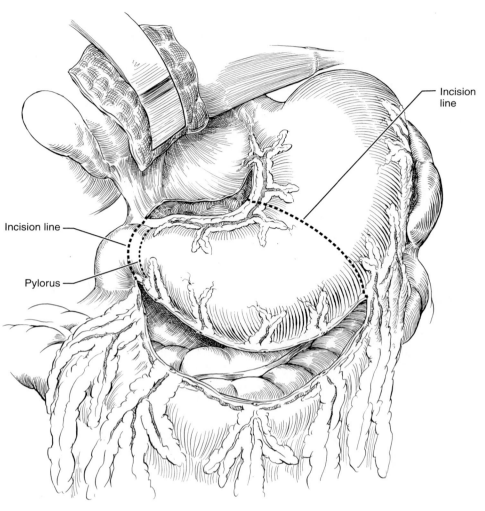

Incision
line

Incision line

Pylorus

FIGURE 27–1

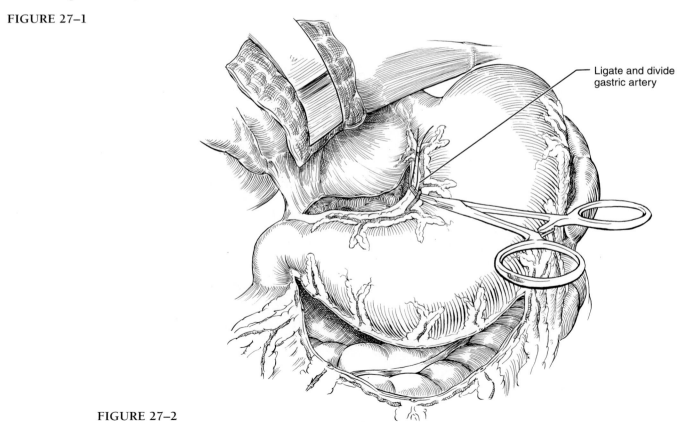

Ligate and divide
gastric artery

FIGURE 27–2

◆ The stomach is transected between Kocher or Payr clamps using the scalpel, and likewise, the first portion of the duodenum is transected between Kocher clamps **(Figure 27-3).**

◆ **Figure 27-4** demonstrates a stapled division of the stomach and duodenum with the duodenum stapled using a gastrointestinal anastomosis (GIA) stapler device and the stomach stapled using a transanastomotic (TA)-30 or TA-55 stapler. The stomach is then transected using the scalpel staying right on the staple line.

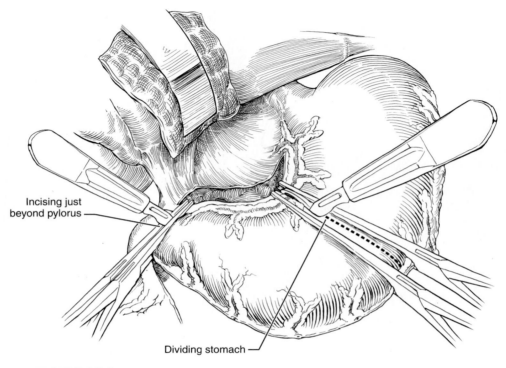

Incising just beyond pylorus

Dividing stomach

FIGURE 27–3

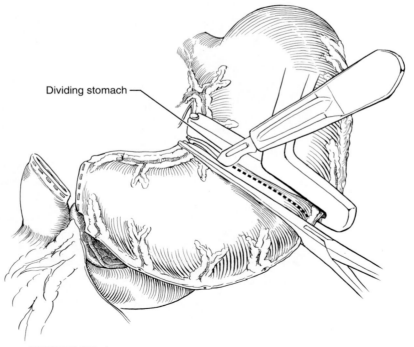

Dividing stomach

FIGURE 27–4

◆ **Figure 27-5, A** shows the duodenal stump closure performed using running nonabsorbable sutures. **Figure 27-5, B** shows a stapled closure of the duodenal stump. Interrupted seromuscular sutures are then placed over the first row of running sutures (**Figure 27-5, C**) or over the staple line (**Figure 27-5, D**). Some surgeons prefer to secure the duodenal stump to the pancreas as shown in **Figure 27-5, E.**

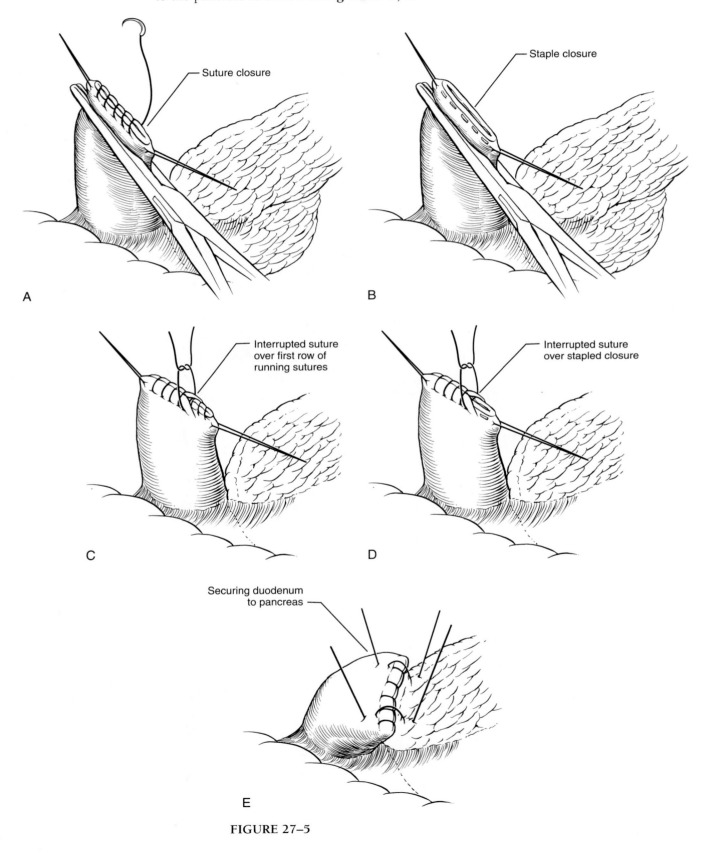

FIGURE 27–5

◆ Excess gastric tissue that had been crushed with the clamp is trimmed using the scalpel or electrocautery (**Figure 27-6, A**). Starting on the lesser curvature side, the stomach is closed with running nonabsorbable sutures (**Figure 27-6, B**). This is accomplished to the level of the Kocher clamp (**Figure 27-6, C**).

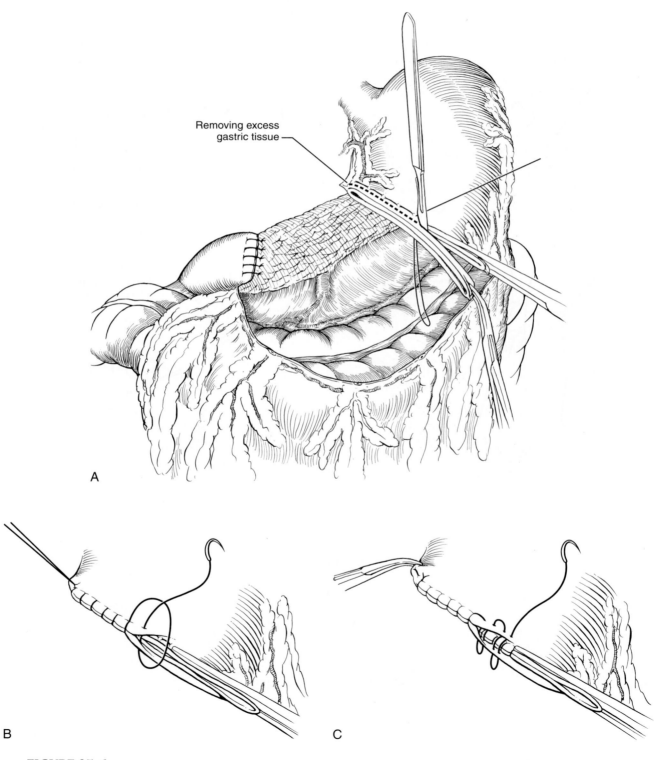

Removing excess
gastric tissue

A

B   C

FIGURE 27–6

◆ A loop of proximal jejunum is brought up in an antecolic fashion, and the anastomosis is performed in two layers. The outer layer is performed with interrupted 3-0 silk sutures placed in a Lembert fashion (**Figure 27-7**).

◆ The electrocautery is then used to open the jejunum at the dashed line as shown in **Figure 27-8**.

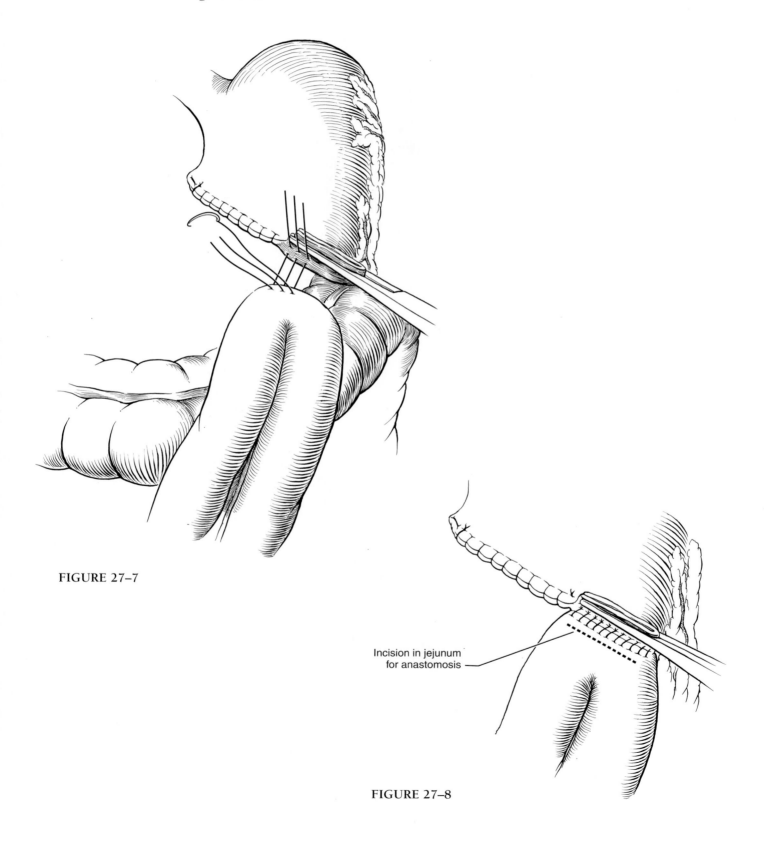

FIGURE 27–7

Incision in jejunum for anastomosis

FIGURE 27–8

◆ The inner row of the anastomosis is performed in a running fashion using a 3-0 nonabsorbable suture such as chromic or Vicryl. The suture is carried anteriorly in a Connell fashion **(Figures 27-9 and 27-10).**

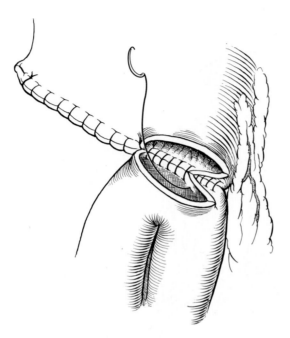

FIGURE 27–9

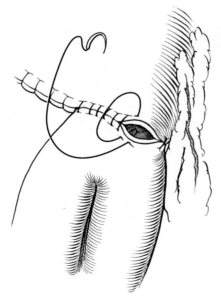

FIGURE 27–10

- The anastomosis is then completed anteriorly using interrupted 3-0 silk sutures placed in a Lembert fashion **(Figure 27-11)**.

- **Figure 27-12** demonstrates the completed Billroth II anastomosis (Hofmeister method).

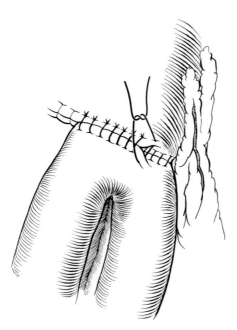

FIGURE 27–11

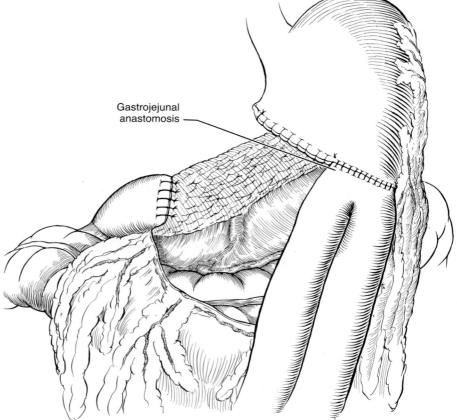

Gastrojejunal anastomosis —

FIGURE 27–12

◆ **Figure 27-13** shows the stapled end of the stomach, and in preparation for the gastrojejunal anastomosis, the end adjacent to the greater curvature is opened using electrocautery and excess gastric tissue is trimmed **(Figure 27-14)**.

◆ The gastrojejunal anastomosis is performed as previously described in two layers with an outer layer of 3-0 silk **(Figure 27-15)**, followed by opening the jejunum at the dashed line **(Figure 27-16)** and performing the inner layer of the anastomosis in a running fashion using a 3-0 nonabsorbable suture **(Figure 27-17)**, which is carried anteriorly in a Connell fashion **(Figure 27-18)**.

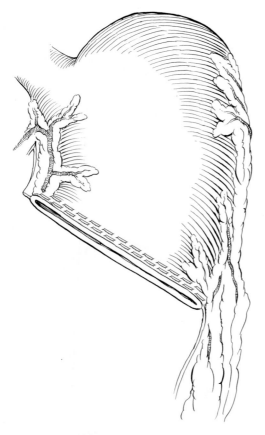

FIGURE 27–13

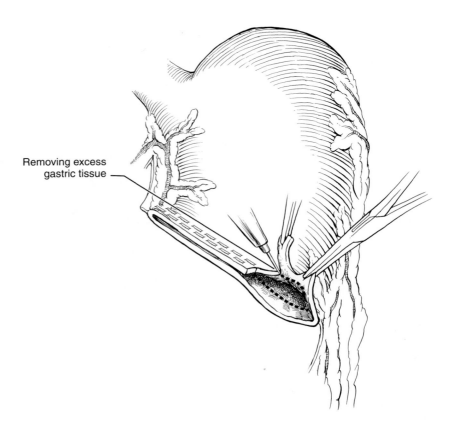

Removing excess gastric tissue

FIGURE 27–14

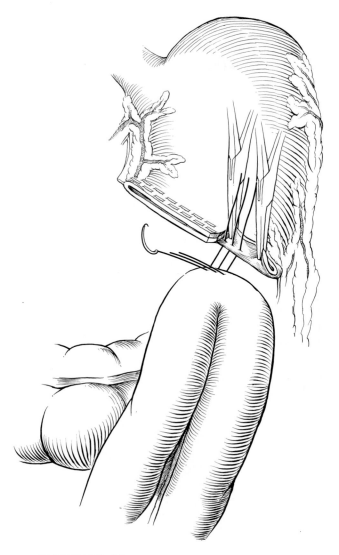

FIGURE 27–15

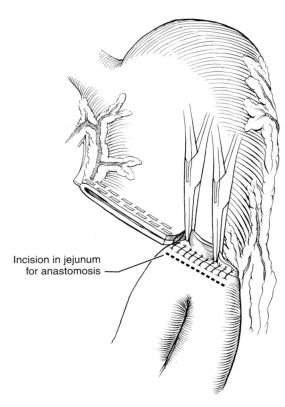

Incision in jejunum for anastomosis

FIGURE 27–16

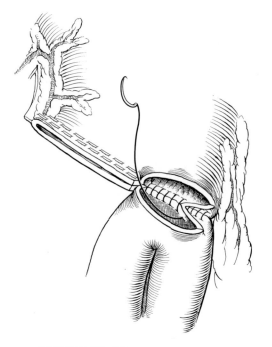

FIGURE 27–17

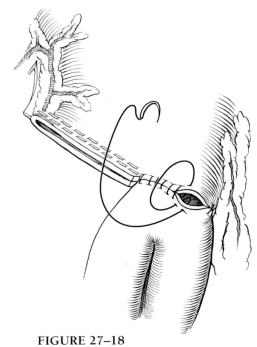

FIGURE 27–18

◆ The anterior suture line is then oversewn using 3-0 silk interrupted sutures, and likewise, the staple line is oversewn using running nonabsorbable sutures (**Figure 27-19**).

◆ **Figure 27-20** demonstrates the completed Billroth II anastomosis.

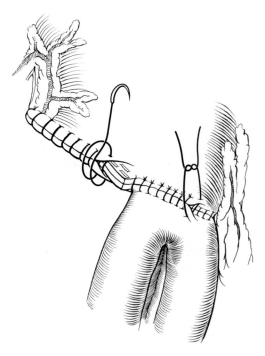

FIGURE 27–19

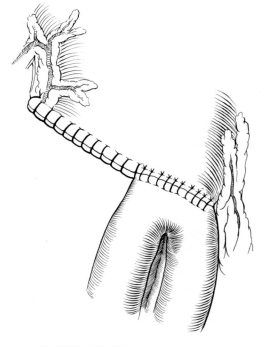

FIGURE 27–20

3. CLOSING

◆ The upper midline or subcostal incision is closed in the usual fashion.

STEP 4: POSTOPERATIVE CARE

◆ A nasogastric tube is positioned proximal to the suture line, and once bowel function has resumed the nasogastric tube can be removed and a liquid diet started. If there is no gastric retention, the diet can be rapidly advanced.

STEP 5: PEARLS AND PITFALLS

◆ In performing the Billroth II anastomosis, some surgeons prefer to use the Polya method, which uses the entire gastric opening for the gastrojejunal anastomosis. The choice between a Hofmeister or Polya method depends on the surgeon's preference.

◆ In operations for cancers of the stomach, most surgeons prefer the Billroth II anastomosis because local recurrence of the cancer would tend to cause earlier obstruction of a gastro-duodenostomy.

◆ In performing the Billroth II anastomosis, the choice of where the jejunal loop is brought anterior to the transverse colon or brought posterior to the transverse mesocolon is also a matter of the surgeon's preference.

SELECTED REFERENCES

1. Mercer DW, Robinson EK: Stomach. In Townsend CM Jr (ed): Sabiston Textbook of Surgery: The Biological Basis of Modern Surgical Practice, 18th ed. Philadelphia, Saunders, 2008, pp 1223-1277.
2. Thompson JC: Subtotal gastrectomy with stapled Billroth II anastomosis. In Thompson JC (ed): Atlas of Surgery of the Stomach, Duodenum and Small Bowel. St Louis, Mosby-Year Book, 1992, pp 61-65.

CHAPTER 28

TOTAL GASTRECTOMY

B. Mark Evers

STEP 1: SURGICAL ANATOMY

- A comprehensive understanding of the vascular anatomy of the stomach is required, and this is shown in Figure 26-1.

STEP 2: PREOPERATIVE CONSIDERATIONS

- Total gastrectomies are performed predominantly for gastric cancer. Total gastrectomy is now rarely performed for bleeding or Zollinger-Ellison syndrome, given the success with current medical regimens.

STEP 3: OPERATIVE STEPS

1. INCISION

- An upper midline incision carried inferior to the umbilicus, if needed, is commonly used for total gastrectomy (**Figure 28-1**). As an alternative incision, some surgeons prefer a bilateral subcostal incision, which affords excellent exposure to the stomach and distal esophagus.

2. DISSECTION

- Wide exposure is accomplished with various self-retaining retractors. A laparotomy pad is placed under the liver, and the liver is gently retracted cephalad (**Figure 28-2**).

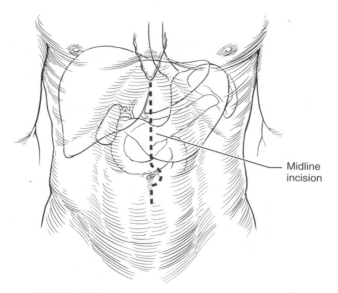

FIGURE 28–1

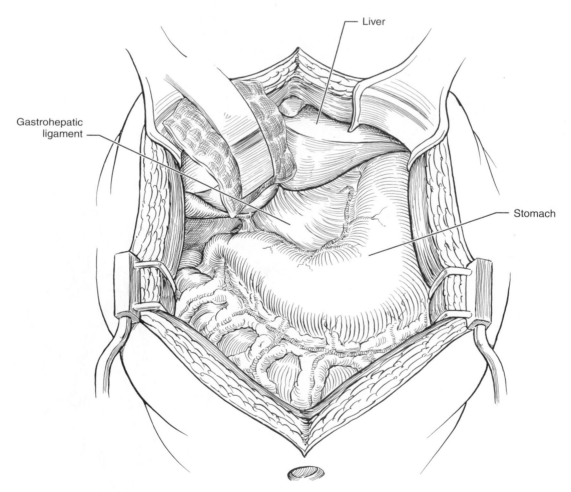

FIGURE 28–2

◆ The greater curvature of the stomach is mobilized by dividing the gastroepiploic vessels in the gastrocolic ligament and ligating with silk sutures. Likewise, the lesser curvature is mobilized by division of the gastrohepatic ligament (**Figure 28-3, A**).

◆ The short gastric vessels are divided between clamps and ligated with silk sutures. The spleen is gently retracted laterally to clearly identify the short gastric vessels (**Figure 28-3, B**).

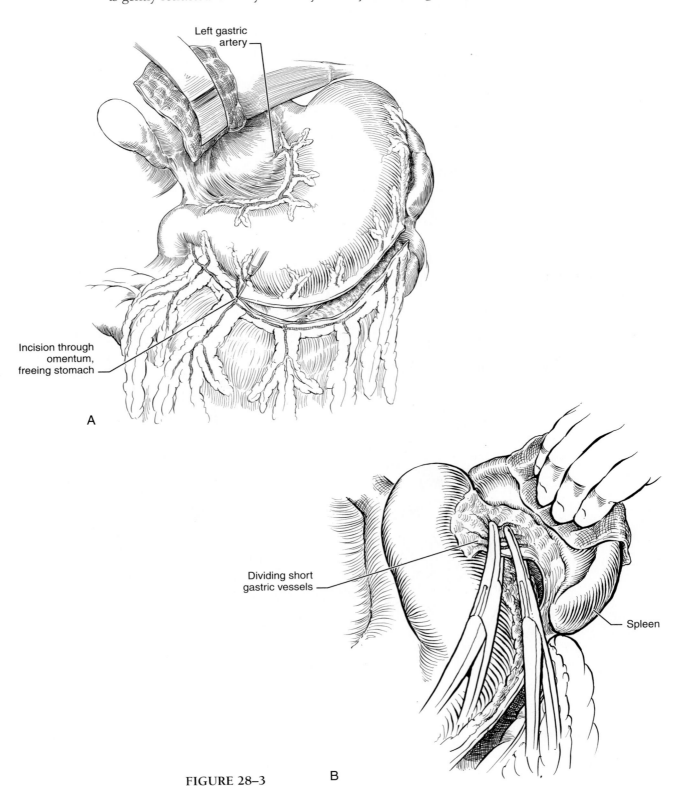

Left gastric artery

Incision through omentum, freeing stomach

A

Dividing short gastric vessels

Spleen

FIGURE 28–3   B

◆ As shown in **Figure 28-4,** the tumor is visualized in the distal and mid stomach.

◆ For an effective oncologic resection, the omentum is usually resected along with the stomach. The omentum is divided at its attachment to the transverse colon and then retracted cephalad. The stomach is likewise retracted cephalad to divide any remaining posterior attachments **(Figure 28-5).**

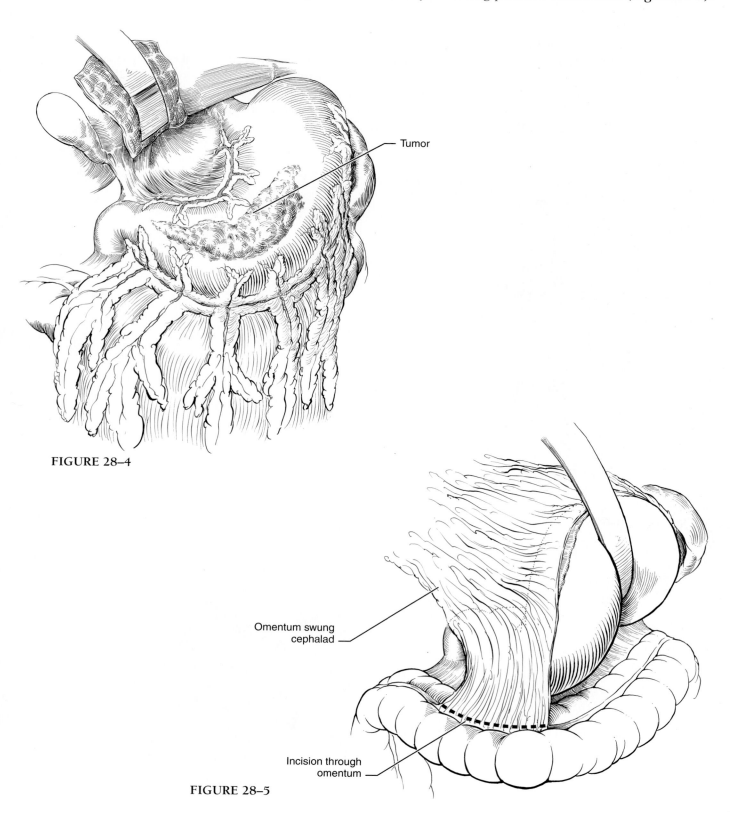

Tumor

FIGURE 28–4

Omentum swung cephalad

Incision through omentum

FIGURE 28–5

◆ **Figure 28-6** demonstrates dividing the right gastric artery to allow complete mobilization of the distal stomach and proximal duodenum.

◆ The division of the left gastric artery is accomplished for mobilization of the lesser curvature and access to the distal esophagus (**Figure 28-7**).

◆ As shown in **Figure 28-8, A,** the duodenum is transected distal to the pylorus using a gastrointestinal anastomosis (GIA) stapling device and, likewise, the distal esophagus is transected using the GIA device proximal to the gastroesophageal junction. **Figure 28-8, B** demonstrates suture closure of the duodenal stump, and **Figure 28-8, C** shows a stapled closure of the stump. Interrupted sutures are then placed over either the running suture (**Figure 28-8, D**) or the staple line (**Figure 28-8, E**).

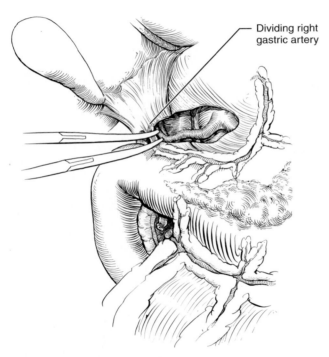

Dividing right gastric artery

FIGURE 28–6

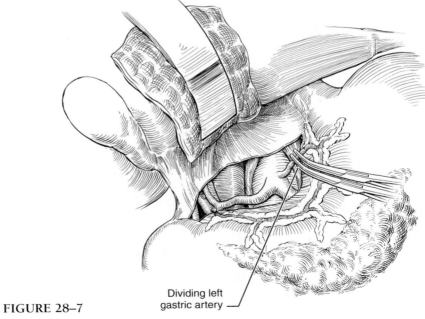

Dividing left gastric artery

FIGURE 28–7

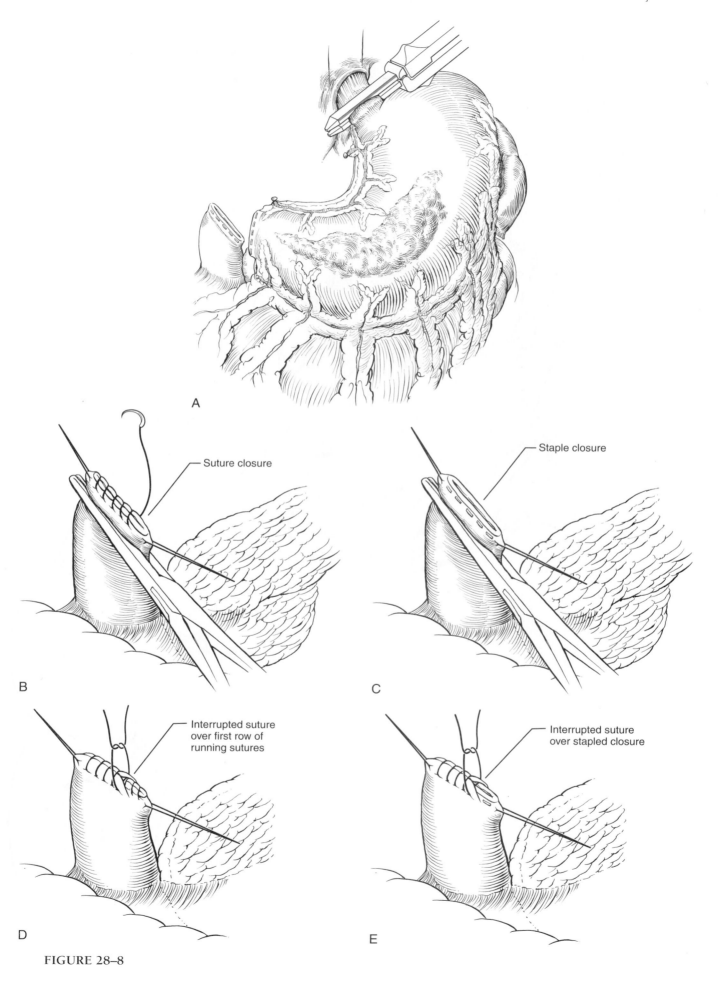

A

Suture closure

B

Staple closure

C

Interrupted suture
over first row of
running sutures

D

Interrupted suture
over stapled closure

E

FIGURE 28–8

◆ An opening is made in the mesocolon, taking care to not damage any vessels running in the mesocolon. The jejunum is then divided approximately 30 cm from the ligament of Treitz using the GIA device, and a Roux limb of approximately 40 to 50 cm is created (**Figure 28-9**).

◆ **Figure 28-10** demonstrates creation of the jejunojejunal anastomosis using the GIA device.

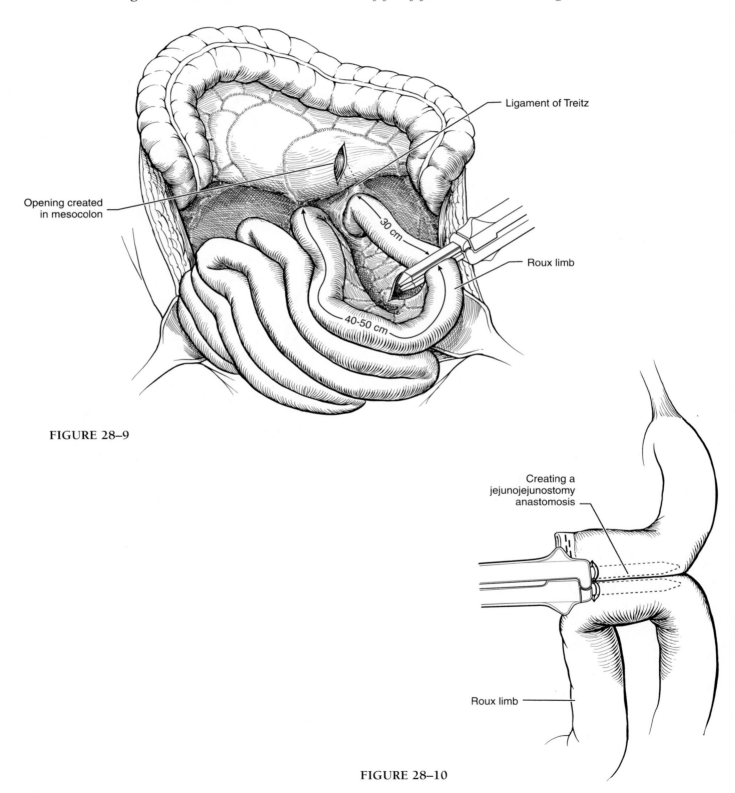

FIGURE 28–9

FIGURE 28–10

◆ The mesenteric rent that was created is now closed using a running (**Figure 28-11, A**) or interrupted suture (**Figure 28-11, B**).

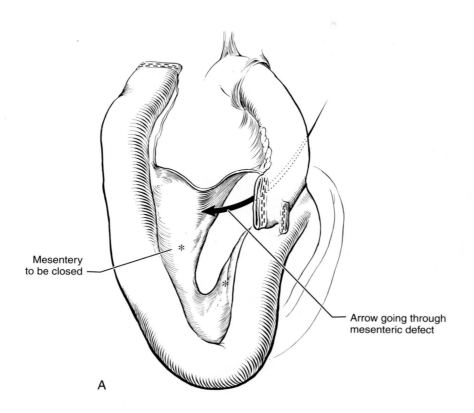

Mesentery
to be closed

Arrow going through
mesenteric defect

A

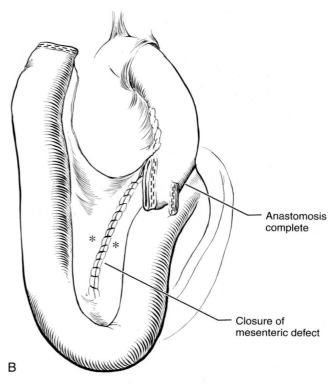

Anastomosis
complete

Closure of
mesenteric defect

B

FIGURE 28–11

◆ Stay sutures are placed on the free end of the jejunum and the jejunum is opened adjacent to the staple line. The end-to-end anastomosis (EEA) stapling device (without the anvil) is placed into the lumen of the free end of the jejunum. A point is selected approximately 4 to 5 cm from the free margin. The post on the EEA stapling device is extended and brought through the wall of the jejunum. Stay sutures are also placed on the distal esophagus, which is then opened and the anvil placed into the distal esophagus. A purse-string suture is then used to secure the anvil. The anvil is then placed into the post of the circular stapler and the tissue is approximated. Firing of the EEA stapler places a circular double ring of staples and extends a circular knife that excises the rings of the jejunum and esophagus inside the circle of staples **(Figure 28-12).**

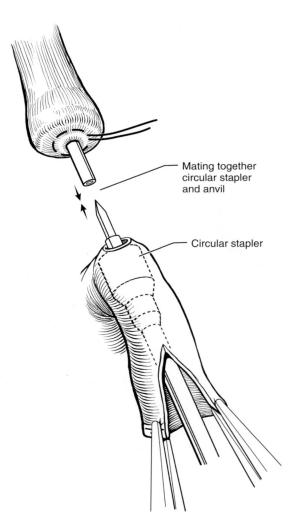

Mating together circular stapler and anvil

Circular stapler

FIGURE 28–12

◆ The redundant section of jejunum is then excised using a GIA stapling device. This converts the anastomosis functionally into an end-to-end esophagojejunostomy **(Figure 28-13)**.

◆ **Figure 28-14** demonstrates the completed esophagojejunal anastomosis with the Roux limb positioned in a retrocolic fashion.

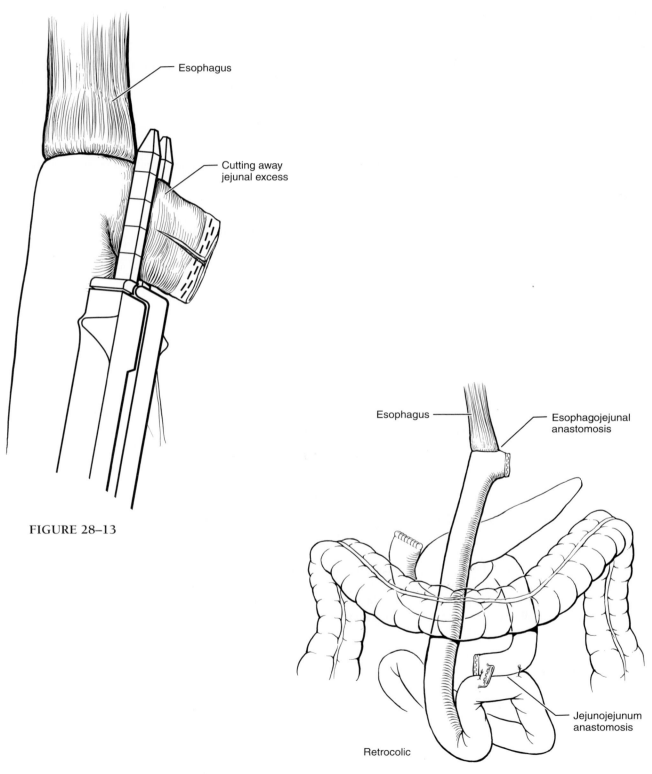

Esophagus

Cutting away jejunal excess

FIGURE 28–13

Esophagus

Esophagojejunal anastomosis

Jejunojejunum anastomosis

Retrocolic

FIGURE 28–14

3. CLOSING

- The midline or bilateral subcostal incisions are closed in the usual fashion.

STEP 4: POSTOPERATIVE CARE

- A nasogastric tube is positioned in the esophagus just proximal to the anastomosis. Once bowel function has resumed, oral feedings can be instituted when there is assurance that no anastomotic leak has occurred. Some surgeons prefer to perform a contrast study using water-soluble dye to ensure no leakage.

- Postgastrectomy patients require frequent small feedings. Adequate calorie intake may be problematic in the initial postoperative period.

- In addition, supplemental vitamin B_{12} is required at routine intervals.

STEP 5: PEARLS AND PITFALLS

- The use of the EEA stapling device has greatly simplified performing the esophagojejunal anastomosis.

- A Roux limb of 40 to 50 cm should be used to prevent complications of reflux into the Roux limb affecting the esophagojejunal anastomosis.

SELECTED REFERENCES

1. Mercer DW, Robinson EK: Stomach. In Townsend CM Jr (ed): Sabiston Textbook of Surgery: The Biological Basis of Modern Surgical Practice, 18th ed. Philadelphia, Saunders, 2008, pp 1223-1277.
2. Thompson JC: Total gastrectomy. In Thompson JC (ed): Atlas of Surgery of the Stomach, Duodenum and Small Bowel. St Louis, Mosby-Year Book, 1992, pp 153-165.

CHAPTER 29

OPEN AND LAPAROSCOPIC CLOSURE OF PERFORATED PEPTIC ULCER

B. Mark Evers

STEP 1: SURGICAL ANATOMY

- The usual site for a perforated peptic ulcer is anterior in the first portion of the duodenum just distal to the pylorus **(Figure 29-1)**.

- Patients with perforated peptic ulcers can be approached by either the standard open technique or laparoscopically.

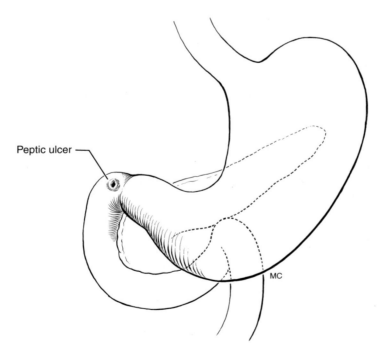

FIGURE 29–1

STEP 2: PREOPERATIVE CONSIDERATIONS

◆ The patient should be adequately hydrated before operation, and broad-spectrum antibiotics should be initiated in the preoperative period.

◆ Consideration should be given as to whether to perform simple closure of the perforation or to perform a more definitive operation if the patient has a history of chronic duodenal ulcer disease.

◆ However, with current medical regimens including drugs to eradicate *Helicobacter pylori,* the need to perform a more definitive ulcer operation at the time of closure of the perforation has greatly diminished.

STEP 3: OPERATIVE STEPS

1. INCISION

◆ If an open repair of a perforated ulcer is to be performed, this can be accomplished via an upper middle incision, which can be extended inferior to the umbilicus if necessary.

2. DISSECTION

Open:
◆ Upon entering the abdomen, the surgeon should locate the perforation. As stated previously, perforated peptic ulcers are routinely located anteriorly in the first portion of the duodenum **(Figure 29-2, A).**

◆ The abdomen should be copiously irrigated with warm saline, and, for a standard Graham closure, interrupted 3-0 silk sutures are placed in Lembert fashion across the ulcer **(Figure 29-2, B).**

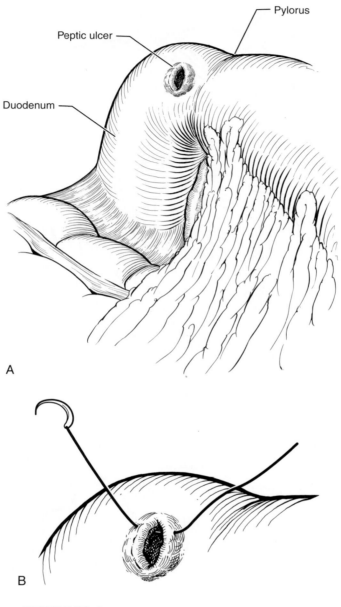

A

B

FIGURE 29–2

◆ Once the sutures are in place, a pedicle of omentum is placed across the base of the ulcer **(Figure 29-3)**. The sutures are then tied over the omental pedicle, thus sealing the perforation **(Figure 29-4)**.

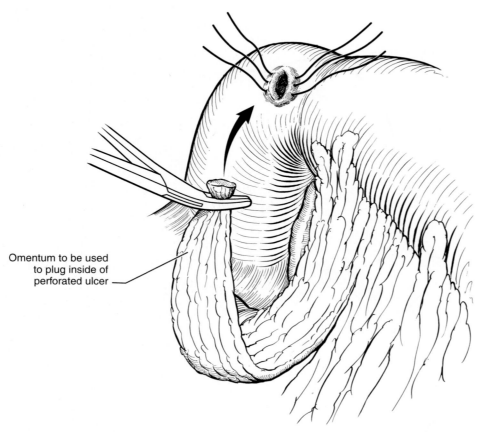

Omentum to be used
to plug inside of
perforated ulcer

FIGURE 29–3

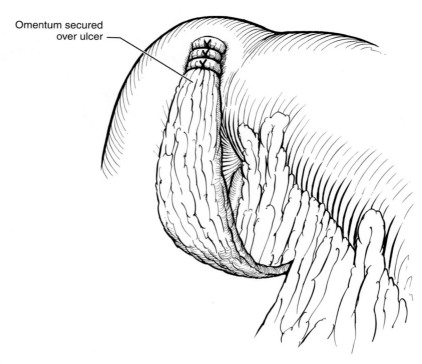

Omentum secured
over ulcer

FIGURE 29–4

◆ **Figure 29-5** illustrates a cross-section of the final repair showing the omental pedicle sealing the perforated ulcer.

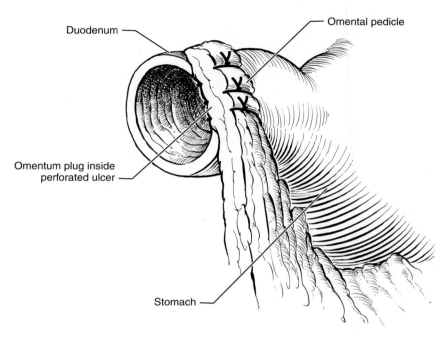

FIGURE 29–5

Laparoscopic:

◆ Depending on the preference of the surgeon and the patient's characteristics, a laparoscopic closure of the perforated ulcer can be accomplished.

◆ **Figure 29-6** illustrates port placement for performing the laparoscopic procedure. Trocars are placed subcostally and one below the xiphoid process. The camera port is placed superior to the umbilicus. Upon entering the abdomen, the surgeon achieves visualization of the perforated peptic ulcer (**Figure 29-7**).

Port Placement

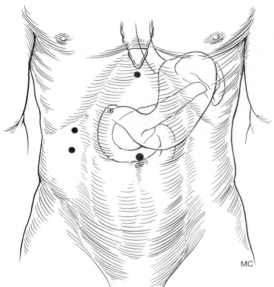

FIGURE 29–6

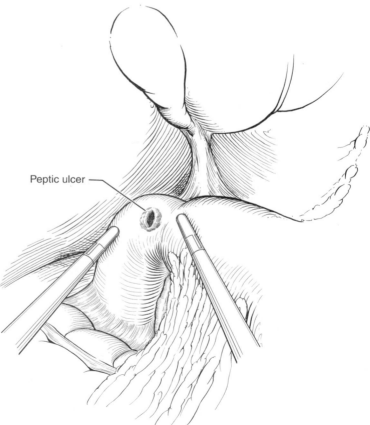

Peptic ulcer

FIGURE 29–7

◆ The closure of the perforation is achieved in a similar fashion as noted for the open procedure **(Figure 29-8, A)**. The stomach is grasped at the pylorus, and the duodenum is grasped distal to the perforation. Interrupted sutures are placed across the ulcer bed laparoscopically **(Figure 29-8, B)**.

◆ A pedicle of omentum is identified and grasped with the trocar and positioned over the ulcer bed **(Figure 29-9)**.

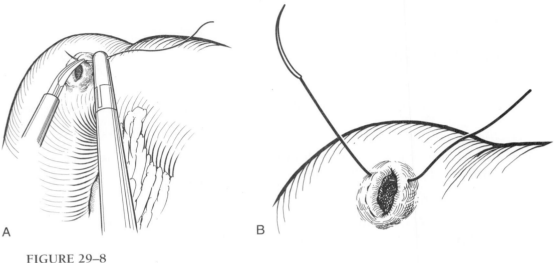

A

B

FIGURE 29–8

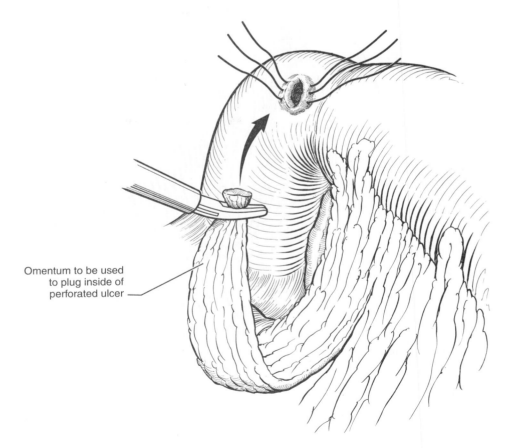

Omentum to be used
to plug inside of
perforated ulcer

FIGURE 29–9

◆ The interrupted sutures are tied over the omental pedicle **(Figure 29-10)**.

3. CLOSING

◆ If an open repair has been performed, the midline excision is closed in the usual fashion. If the operation is performed laparoscopically, the trocar sites are approximated using a subcuticular absorbable suture.

STEP 4: POSTOPERATIVE CARE

◆ Intravenous fluids and antibiotics should be continued over the postoperative period.

◆ Medical treatment for the ulcer disease should also be continued, as well as assessment of *H. pylori,* which should be treated if identified.

◆ With return of bowel function and absence of any signs of intra-abdominal sepsis, clear liquids can be instituted and the diet rapidly advanced as tolerated.

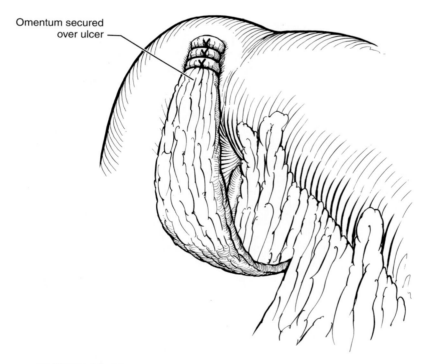

Omentum secured over ulcer

FIGURE 29–10

STEP 5: PEARLS AND PITFALLS

- The Graham closure of a perforated peptic ulcer is usually a highly effective and efficient way of controlling the perforation site.

- A well-vascularized pedicle of omentum must be selected and approximated under no tension.

- If the patient has a history of chronic ulcer disease that has been unsuccessfully treated with medical management, a more definitive ulcer operation, such as a truncal vagotomy and pyloroplasty, should be performed depending on the amount of contamination in the abdominal cavity and the duration of the perforation. However, as noted previously, the current medical regimens for ulcer treatment have greatly diminished the need for a definitive operation at the time of ulcer closure.

- The abdomen should be copiously irrigated with saline to decrease the chances of intra-abdominal abscess forming after the procedure.

SELECTED REFERENCES

1. Mercer DW, Robinson EK: Stomach. In Townsend CM Jr (ed): Sabiston Textbook of Surgery: The Biological Basis of Modern Surgical Practice, 18th ed. Philadelphia, Saunders, 2008, pp 1223-1277.
2. Thompson JC: Perforation of duodenal ulcer: Treatment by simple closure or by closure plus acid-reducing operation. In Thompson JC (ed): Atlas of Surgery of the Stomach, Duodenum and Small Bowel. St Louis, Mosby-Year Book, 1992, pp 113-119.

CHAPTER 30

BLEEDING DUODENAL ULCER

B. Mark Evers

STEP 1: SURGICAL ANATOMY

- Bleeding duodenal ulcers are normally located posteriorly in the first portion of the duodenum, with the bleeding due to penetration into the gastroduodenal artery **(Figure 30-1)**.

STEP 2: PREOPERATIVE CONSIDERATIONS

- Most patients with bleeding duodenal ulcers will stop bleeding and can be managed with nonoperative medical management or endoscopic treatment, which includes injection of the ulcer bed or actual ligation of the visible vessel. These techniques are usually highly effective; however, surgery is required if these measures are unsuccessful and the patient continues to bleed.

STEP 3: OPERATIVE STEPS

1. INCISION

- The abdomen is usually approached via an upper midline incision, which allows good exposure and can be performed quickly.

2. DISSECTION

- The first step is to perform a Kocher maneuver to mobilize the first and second portions of the duodenum, followed by a horizontal pyloroplasty, as noted by the dashed line in **Figure 30-2**.

- Traction sutures are placed in the mid-portion of the superior and inferior limbs of the pyloroplasty incision to afford exposure of the bleeding ulcer. Once the ulcer is identified, the ongoing bleeding can be controlled using a finger and placement of a 2-0 silk suture (U-stitch) to control the bleeding and occlude any collateral bleeding from the transverse pancreatic artery **(Figure 30-3)**.

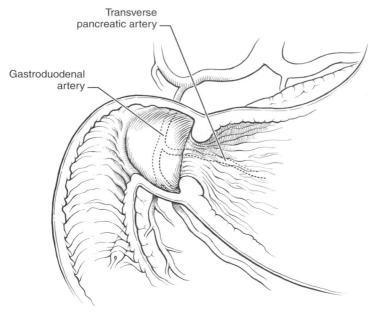

Transverse
pancreatic artery

Gastroduodenal
artery

FIGURE 30–1

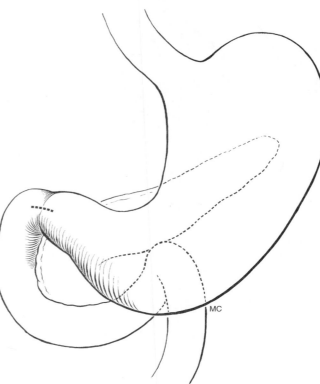

MC

FIGURE 30–2

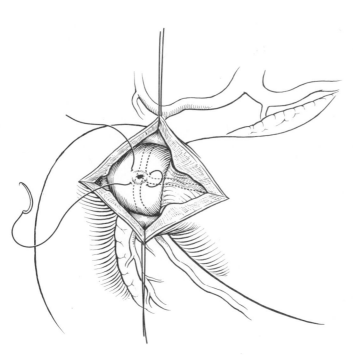

FIGURE 30–3

◆ After the U-stitch is tied, sutures are placed above and below the ulcer crater to ligate the gastroduodenal artery **(Figure 30-4)**.

◆ The horizontal pyloroplasty is then closed in a vertical fashion (Heineke-Mikulicz pyloroplasty), and a truncal vagotomy is performed **(Figure 30-5)**.

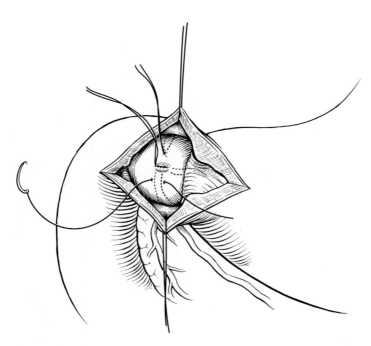

FIGURE 30–4

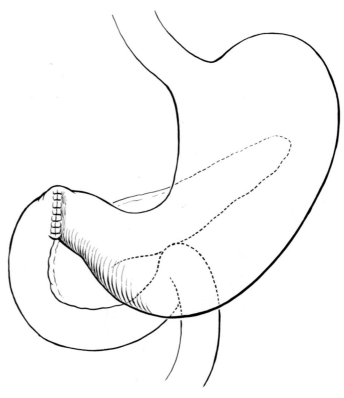

FIGURE 30–5

3. CLOSING

- The midline incision is closed in the usual fashion.

STEP 4: POSTOPERATIVE CARE

- Intravenous fluids are continued postoperatively.

- The patient is usually monitored in the intensive care unit for possible signs of rebleeding and to ensure adequate hemodynamics.

- Once bowel function resumes, the nasogastric tube can be discontinued and clear liquids initiated with rapid advancement of the diet as tolerated.

STEP 5: PEARLS AND PITFALLS

- In addition to the sutures placed above and below the ulcer crater, it is important to place the U-stitch to prevent rebleeding from a collateral anastomosis from the transverse pancreatic artery. The application of this technique has diminished the incidence of post–suture ligation rebleeding.

SELECTED REFERENCES

1. Mercer DW, Robinson EK: Stomach. In Townsend CM Jr (ed): Sabiston Textbook of Surgery: The Biological Basis of Modern Surgical Practice, 18th ed. Philadelphia, Saunders, 2008, pp 1223-1277.
2. Thompson JC: Pyloroplasty for bleeding duodenal ulcer using the U-stitch. In Thompson JC (ed): Atlas of Surgery of the Stomach, Duodenum and Small Bowel. St Louis, Mosby-Year Book, 1992, pp 109-111.

CHAPTER 31

TRUNCAL VAGOTOMY

B. Mark Evers

STEP 1: SURGICAL ANATOMY

- The vagus nerves are not always easily identified. Sometimes their location can be more quickly discovered by palpation. The left vagus nerve is usually located on the anterior surface of the esophagus, a little to the left of the midline, whereas the right vagus nerve is usually located a little to the right of the midline, posteriorly. The left vagus nerve is intimately associated with the anterior surface of the esophagus, whereas the right vagus nerve is located in the tissue adjacent to the posterior esophagus (**Figure 31-1**).

STEP 2: PREOPERATIVE CONSIDERATIONS

- Truncal vagotomy provides a safe and simple means for reducing acid secretion by the stomach. Because the vagus provides motor fibers to the circular muscle of the antrum, a truncal vagotomy must be accompanied by a procedure to facilitate gastric drainage, such as a pyloroplasty or gastroenterostomy. The advantages of truncal vagotomy are that it is safe and many of the serious late postgastrectomy sequelae can be avoided.

STEP 3: OPERATIVE STEPS

1. INCISION

- For an open truncal vagotomy procedure, a standard upper midline incision is performed.

- Retraction is obtained with self-retaining retractors, which allow excellent exposure of the distal esophagus and upper stomach.

2. DISSECTION

- The left lobe of the liver is retracted upward and toward the midline, so as to clearly expose the gastroesophageal junction. The peritoneal reflection at the diaphragm is incised to expose the esophagus as shown by the dashed line (**Figures 31-2 and 31-3**).

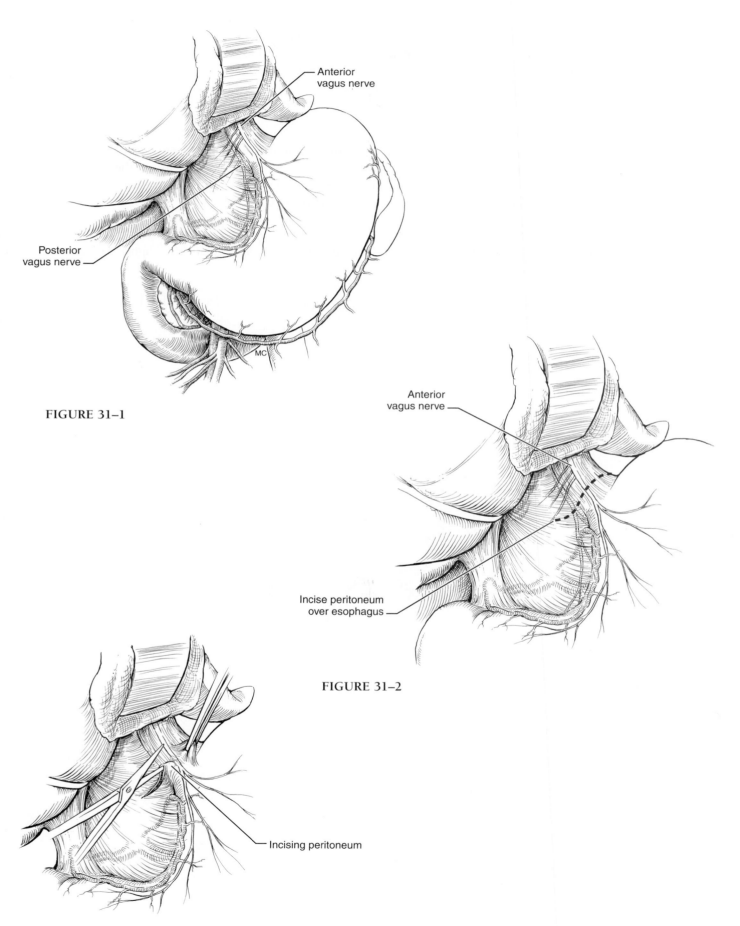

FIGURE 31–1

Anterior
vagus nerve

Posterior
vagus nerve

MC

Anterior
vagus nerve

Incise peritoneum
over esophagus

FIGURE 31–2

Incising peritoneum

FIGURE 31–3

◆ Once the peritoneum is incised, the index finger is placed around the esophagus to encircle it at the hiatus. Care should be taken to pass the finger around the esophagus above the diaphragm to ensure that the posterior vagus is included in this maneuver. A Penrose drain is then normally placed around the distal esophagus, and the anterior vagus nerve is identified lying in the substance of the anterior esophagus **(Figure 31-4)**.

◆ The anterior vagus nerve is then dissected and freed from the underlying esophagus **(Figure 31-5)**. In performing the truncal vagotomy, we place small metal clips on the vagus nerve and excise a 2-cm segment between the clips. Excised vagal segments are sent for pathologic examination of permanent sections **(Figure 31-6)**.

◆ Traction is placed on the Penrose drain and the posterior vagus nerve identified **(Figure 31-7)**.

◆ The procedure is repeated for the larger posterior nerve. Clips are placed and at least a 2-cm segment of the nerve is excised.

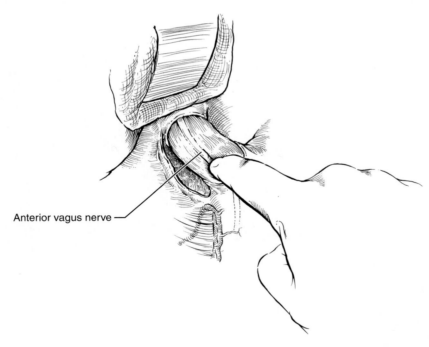

Anterior vagus nerve —

FIGURE 31–4

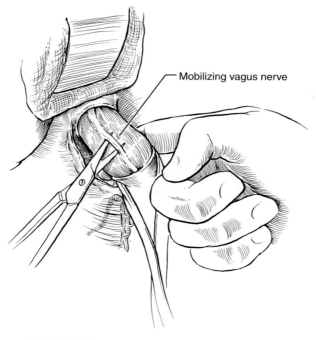

Mobilizing vagus nerve

FIGURE 31–5

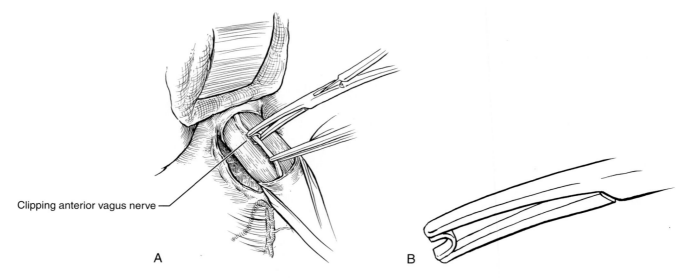

Clipping anterior vagus nerve

A

B

FIGURE 31–6

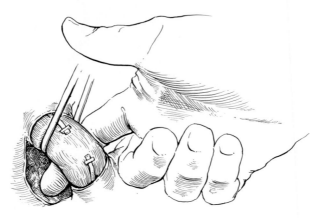

FIGURE 31–7

◆ Care should be taken to identify and divide any accessory vagal fibers. As many as five accessory vagal trunks have been reported, but most individuals have only two main trunks **(Figure 31-8).**

◆ A drainage procedure such as pyloroplasty or gastroenterostomy is then used to complete the procedure.

3. CLOSING

◆ The midline incision is closed in the standard fashion.

STEP 4: POSTOPERATIVE CARE

◆ A nasogastric tube is placed to suction, and when return of bowel function is noted, the nasogastric tube is removed and clear liquids started.

STEP 5: PEARLS AND PITFALLS

◆ Truncal vagotomy is usually a safe and effective method for definitive operative treatment of ulcer disease. The trunks should be clearly identified and at least a 2-cm segment excised and confirmed as nerve tissue by pathology.

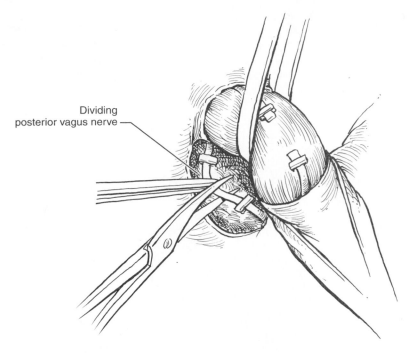

Dividing
posterior vagus nerve

FIGURE 31–8

◆ As noted, a careful assessment and identification of accessory vagal fibers should be undertaken to prevent ulcer recurrence.

◆ Truncal vagotomy must always be accompanied by a drainage procedure to prevent gastric stasis.

SELECTED REFERENCES

1. Mercer DW, Robinson EK: Stomach. In Townsend CM Jr (ed): Sabiston Textbook of Surgery: The Biological Basis of Modern Surgical Practice, 18th ed. Philadelphia, Saunders, 2008, pp 1223-1277.
2. Thompson JC: Truncal vagotomy. In Thompson JC (ed): Atlas of Surgery of the Stomach, Duodenum and Small Bowel. St Louis, Mosby-Year Book, 1992, pp 71-75.

CHAPTER 32

GASTROJEJUNOSTOMY

B. Mark Evers

STEP 1: SURGICAL ANATOMY

- Understanding the anatomy of the stomach and small bowel and determining whether an antecolic or retrocolic approach is more appropriate are key points in this procedure.

STEP 2: PREOPERATIVE CONSIDERATIONS

- Gastrojejunostomy can be performed in an antecolic fashion, which provides a quick and effective method of connecting the distal stomach to the jejunum. In some instances, the more direct path is a retrocolic anastomosis involving placement of the jejunal loop through the transverse colon mesentery.

- Gastrojejunostomy is usually performed to bypass an obstructed distal stomach or duodenum and provide relief. This is particularly useful in cancers that obstruct the duodenal lumen or the distal stomach and are not resectable. Gastrojejunostomy should also be considered in the patient who requires a drainage procedure in whom a pyloroplasty may not be safe because of chronic scarring of the duodenal bulb.

STEP 3: OPERATIVE STEPS

1. INCISION

- Using an open technique, an upper midline incision is usually performed. We are illustrating the open technique in this chapter; however, gastrojejunostomy may be also accomplished via laparoscopy.

2. DISSECTION

◆ To create an antecolic gastrojejunostomy, the surgeon identifies a convenient section of distal stomach and a loop of jejunum that is easily maneuverable to the stomach distal to the ligament of Treitz. A convenient location in the proximal jejunum is usually 15 to 20 cm distal to the ligament of Treitz.

◆ A posterior row of seromuscular 3-0 silk sutures are placed in Lembert fashion to connect the stomach and the jejunum. If a stapled anastomosis is to be performed, an enterotomy is created using electrocautery; likewise, a gastrotomy is also performed to facilitate placement of the stapler **(Figure 32-1)**.

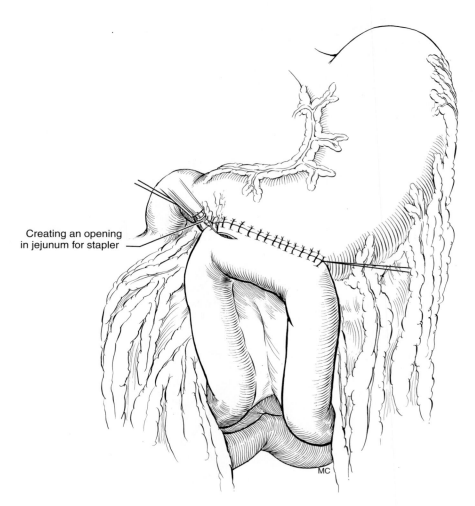

Creating an opening
in jejunum for stapler

FIGURE 32–1

- The gastrointestinal anastomosis (GIA) stapling device is placed through the holes created in the stomach and the jejunum, and the anastomosis is performed by firing the stapler (**Figure 32-2**).

- The enterotomy and gastroenterotomy are closed together using a transanastomotic (TA) stapling device (**Figure 32-3**).

- **Figure 32-4** demonstrates the complete antecolic gastrojejunostomy.

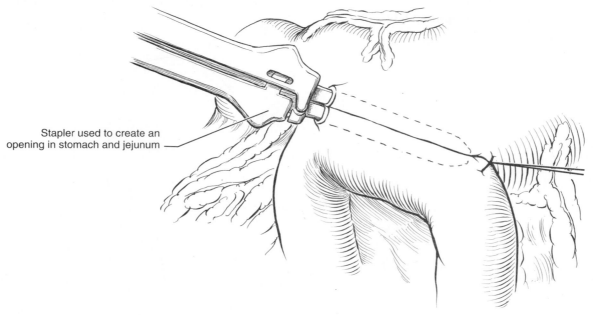

Stapler used to create an opening in stomach and jejunum

FIGURE 32–2

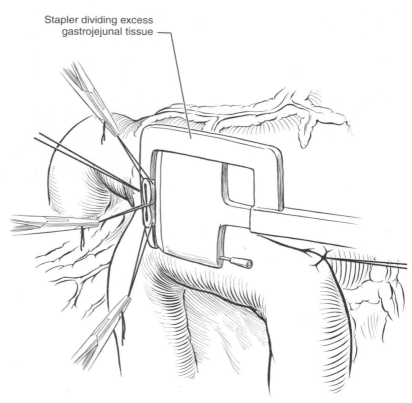

Stapler dividing excess gastrojejunal tissue

FIGURE 32–3

◆ **Figure 32-5** demonstrates the technique for a handsewn antecolic gastrojejunostomy. The posterior row of Lembert 3-0 silk sutures are placed as noted previously. Electrocautery is used to open the jejunum and the stomach, thereby creating the jejunal and gastric stomas (**Figure 32-6**).

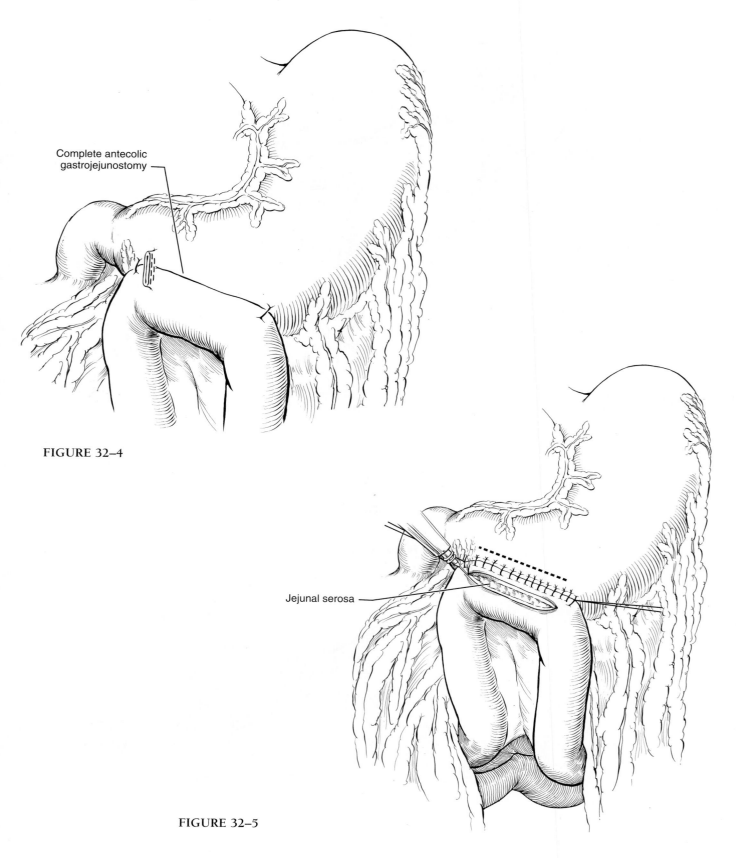

Complete antecolic
gastrojejunostomy

FIGURE 32–4

Jejunal serosa

FIGURE 32–5

◆ The inner layer of the anastomosis is performed using a running full-thickness absorbable suture, such as 3-0 chromic or Vicryl, which is then carried anteriorly in a Connell fashion **(Figure 32-7)**.

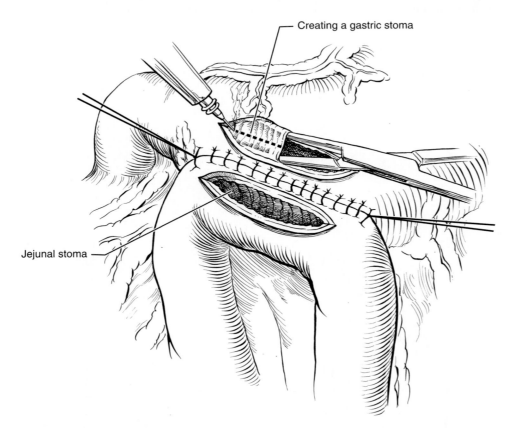

Creating a gastric stoma

Jejunal stoma

FIGURE 32–6

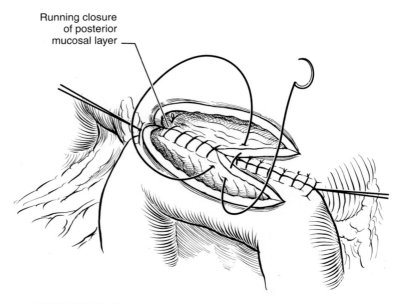

Running closure
of posterior
mucosal layer

FIGURE 32–7

◆ Interrupted 3-0 silk sutures, placed in Lembert fashion, complete the anterior portion of the two-layer gastrojejunostomy **(Figure 32-8)**.

◆ If a retrocolic gastrojejunostomy is thought to be necessary, sites for anastomosis to the stomach and jejunum are identified as shown in the dashed lines in **Figure 32-9**. The transverse colon is then lifted cephalad to visualize the mesentery and identify an avascular area in which to bring the jejunal loop, as noted by the dashed lines.

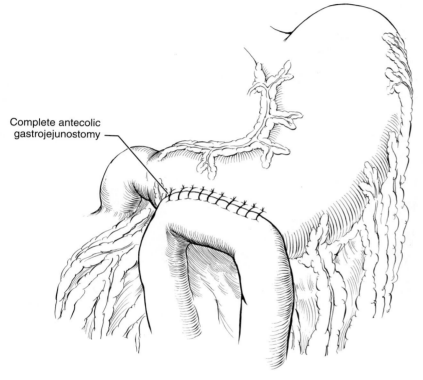

Complete antecolic gastrojejunostomy

FIGURE 32–8

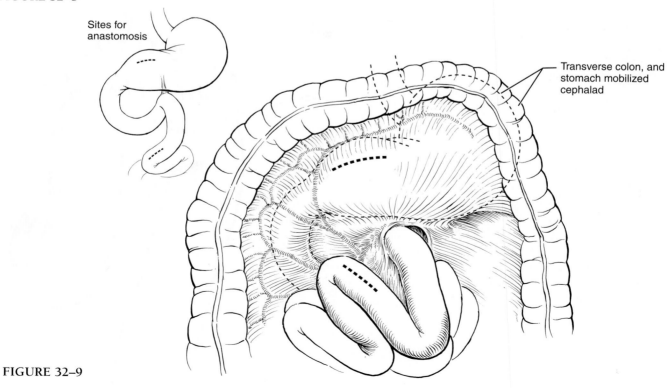

Sites for anastomosis

Transverse colon, and stomach mobilized cephalad

FIGURE 32–9

◆ A handsewn anastomosis is performed in the fashion already described using a two-layer anastomosis with a posterior row of 3-0 silk interrupted sutures. The jejunal and gastric stomas are then created using electrocautery **(Figure 32-10)**.

◆ The inner layer of the anastomosis is accomplished using a running full-thickness absorbable suture **(Figure 32-11)**.

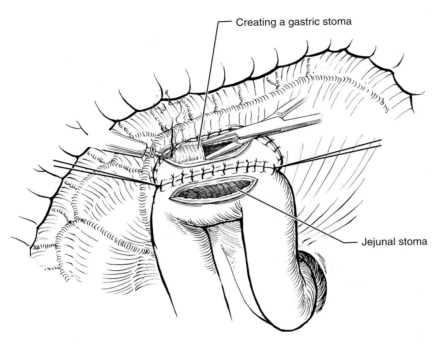

Creating a gastric stoma

Jejunal stoma

FIGURE 32–10

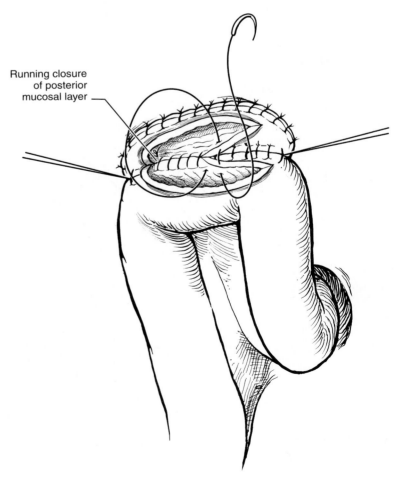

Running closure
of posterior
mucosal layer

FIGURE 32–11

◆ The retrocolic gastrojejunostomy is then completed using interrupted 3-0 silk seromuscular sutures placed anteriorly (**Figure 32-12**).

◆ Similar techniques are used to perform a stapled anastomosis (**Figure 32-13**).

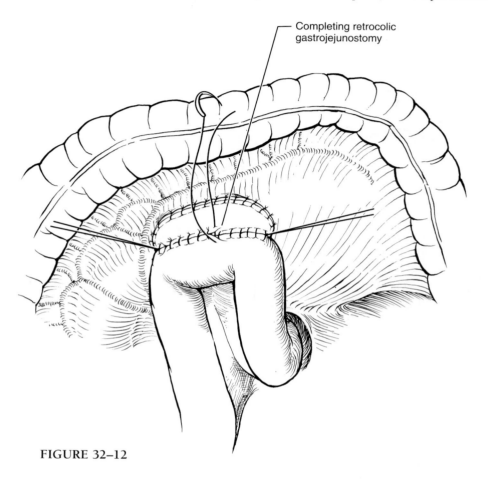

Completing retrocolic gastrojejunostomy

FIGURE 32–12

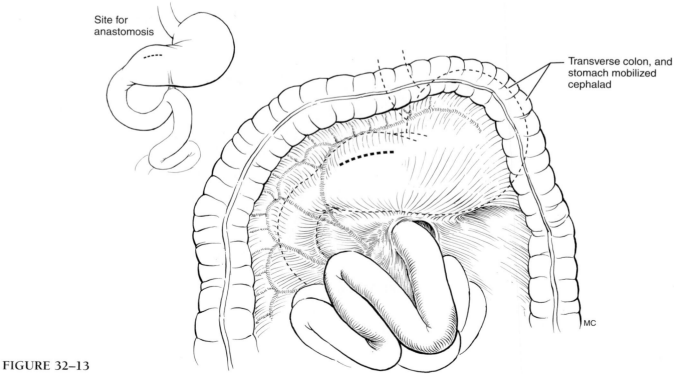

Site for anastomosis

Transverse colon, and stomach mobilized cephalad

MC

FIGURE 32–13

◆ The jejunal and gastric stomas are created using electrocautery. The opening should be large enough to allow entry of the stapling device **(Figure 32-14)**.

◆ The retrocolic gastrojejunostomy is then completed using the GIA stapler **(Figure 32-15)**.

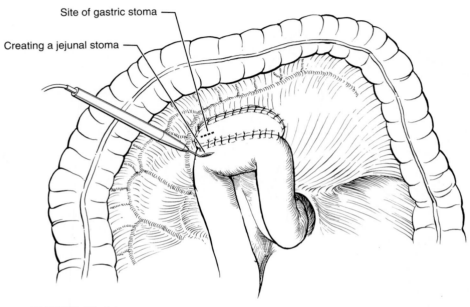

Site of gastric stoma

Creating a jejunal stoma

FIGURE 32–14

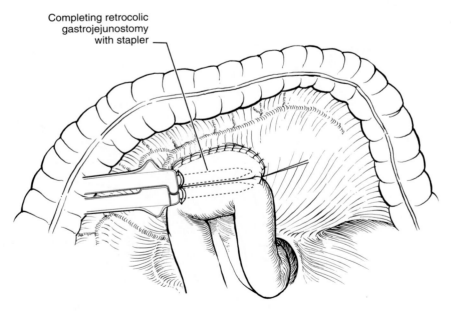

Completing retrocolic
gastrojejunostomy
with stapler

FIGURE 32–15

- The openings created in the stomach and jejunum are closed together using a GIA or a TA stapler (**Figure 32-16**).

- **Figure 32-17** demonstrates the completed retrocolic anastomosis.

3. CLOSING

- The midline incision is closed in the usual fashion.

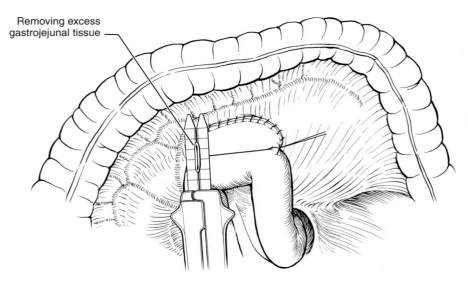

FIGURE 32–16

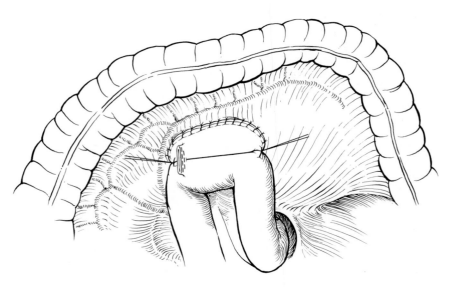

FIGURE 32–17

STEP 4: POSTOPERATIVE CARE

- ◆ Postoperative care is achieved as previously noted for other gastric procedures. A nasogastric tube is usually maintained postoperatively on suction, and once bowel function returns, the tube is removed and a diet initiated.

STEP 5: PEARLS AND PITFALLS

- ◆ If the retrocolic approach is used, most surgeons loosely suture the edges of the mesenteric rent to the jejunum, to minimize risk of herniation of a bowel loop.

- ◆ Care should be taken to clearly identify the proximal jejunum in which to make the gastrojejunostomy. A rare but tragic error is to mistakenly perform the anastomosis between the stomach and ileum.

SELECTED REFERENCES

1. Mercer DW, Robinson EK: Stomach. In Townsend CM Jr (ed): Sabiston Textbook of Surgery: The Biological Basis of Modern Surgical Practice, 18th ed. Philadelphia, Saunders, 2008, pp 1223-1277.
2. Thompson JC: Gastrojejunostomy. In Thompson JC (ed): Atlas of Surgery of the Stomach, Duodenum and Small Bowel. St Louis, Mosby-Year Book, 1992, pp 77-81.

CHAPTER 33

PYLOROMYOTOMY

Carlos A. Angel

STEP 1: SURGICAL ANATOMY

- The pylorus sits at the distal end of the stomach. It is marked by thickening of the circular smooth muscle layer, thus forming the pyloric sphincter, which acts as a valve between the stomach and the duodenum and regulates gastric emptying. The pylorus does not have independent blood supply; rather, it gets its blood supply from the vessels that perfuse the distal stomach and proximal duodenum. Innervation of the pylorus is through the terminal branches of the right and left vagus nerves. Any injury to these nerves or denervation of the pylorus will result in pylorospasm and delayed gastric emptying.

STEP 2: PREOPERATIVE CONSIDERATIONS

- The diagnosis is confirmed when, in an infant or child with a history of postprandial, non-bilious vomiting, the pyloric "olive" can be palpated. If this is not possible, hypertrophic pyloric stenosis can be confirmed by sonography when the pyloric muscle width is greater than 4 mm.

- These infants often present with hypochloremic metabolic alkalosis and dehydration. Intravenous hydration, correction of metabolic disturbances, and establishment of adequate urine output are imperative before pyloromyotomy.

- The operation is performed with the patient under general endotracheal anesthesia. Gastric contents are suctioned thoroughly. Rapid sequence induction is used to prevent aspiration of gastric contents.

- The patient is placed supine on the operating table. A folded towel under the thoracic vertebrae facilitates exposure to the pylorus. The abdomen is painted with iodine solution.

STEP 3: OPERATIVE STEPS

1. INCISION

◆ A transverse incision 2 to 3 cm long is made in the right upper quadrant. This incision can be made midway between the xiphoid and umbilicus, just off the midline to the right side. The anterior rectus fascia is opened in the direction of the incision, the rectus muscle is divided transversely using electrocautery, and the posterior rectus fascia and peritoneum are opened in the direction of the incision. If necessary, on the lateral side, the incision may be extended by division (for a short distance) of the internal oblique and transversus abdominis muscles to facilitate the delivery of the pyloric olive from the abdominal cavity **(Figure 33-1).** Alternatively, a transumbilical approach may be performed by making a semicircular incision superior to the umbilicus with a small cephalad extension (like a Mercedes Benz star). The skin is undermined, and the rectus fascia is opened in the midline for a distance of approximately 2.5 cm. The peritoneum is opened, and the pyloric tumor is delivered into the operating field by gentle traction on the antrum. After the pyloromyotomy, closure is performed with running 5-0 polyglactin sutures for the fascia, the most cephalad portion of the skin is reapproximated to the umbilicus, excess skin is trimmed on both the right and left sides, and skin closure is completed with 6-0 polyglactin sutures leaving a very well-hidden small semi-circular supraumbilical scar. Since there is more extensive dissection and undermining of the skin with this incision, I routinely administer a pre-operative dose and two post-operative doses of intravenous cefazolin to these patients.

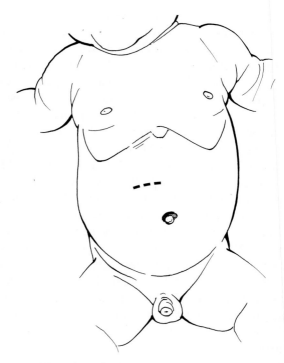

FIGURE 33–1

2. DISSECTION

◆ Upon entering the abdomen, the surgeon uses a small, malleable retractor over a moist gauze to retract the liver and the falciform ligament cephalad and to the right side of the patient. This maneuver usually exposes the greater curvature of the stomach. If the stomach is not exposed, gentle caudal traction on the transverse colon will expose the greater curvature of the stomach. Any attempts to grasp the pyloric tumor directly must be avoided because the tumor is friable and will easily tear and bleed. With the stomach firmly grasped (a sponge will help, because the stomach is slippery), the surgeon applies gentle to-and-fro rocking traction to deliver the pylorus out of the incision **(Figure 33-2)**. Palpation of the tumor will allow precise identification of the pyloroduodenal junction, because the tumor feels firm and the duodenum is very soft. There is a relative avascular plane on the anterior surface of the pylorus. A superficial serosal incision is made over this avascular plane, extending it distally just proximal to the pyloroduodenal junction and proximally to the junction of the antrum and pylorus; the length of this incision is 2 to 3 cm **(Figure 33-3)**. There is a critical zone of folded duodena mucosa in a very superficial position at the pyloroduodenal junction. This is the area where perforations more commonly occur. Using a knife handle or another blunt instrument, the surgeon splits the brittle pyloric muscle in the *middle* of the pyloromyotomy down to the submucosa by gently pushing over the incision while supporting the pylorus with the other hand. No attempts are made to split the muscle toward the duodenal side. Using a pyloric spreader or a hemostat (ensuring that the tips are well above the mucosa), the surgeon spreads the muscle beginning in the middle of the incision and then proceeding distally and proximally **(Figure 33-4)**. Hemostasis is performed with a fine-tipped cautery at low setting; touching the mucosa with the cautery must be avoided. Completeness of the pyloromyotomy is confirmed when the two halves of the muscle move independently from each other **(Figure 33-5)**. Now the pylorus is placed back in the abdomen and a clean gauze is placed on top of the pyloromyotomy for 2 minutes and subsequently inspected for the presence of bile, gastric juice, or excessive bleeding. Closure is performed in layers with running 5-0 or 6-0 polyglactin sutures. The skin is closed with a running 6-0 polyglactin subcuticular sutures after infiltration with 0.25% bupivacaine and is dressed with Steri-Strips.

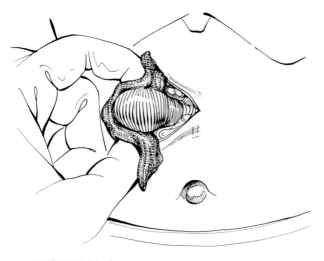

FIGURE 33–2

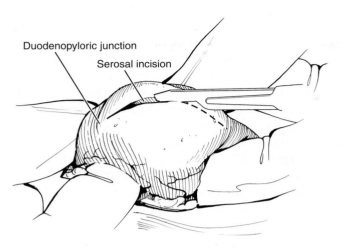

Duodenopyloric junction
Serosal incision

FIGURE 33–3

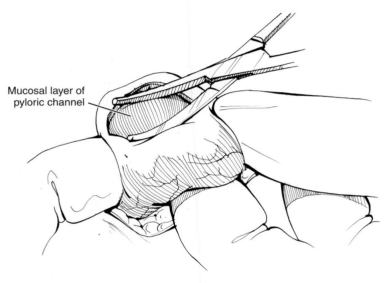

Mucosal layer of
pyloric channel

FIGURE 33–4

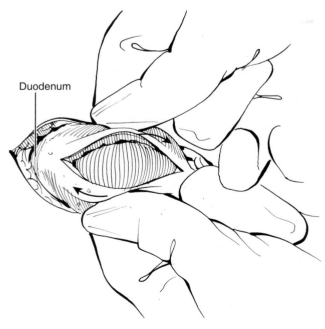

Duodenum

FIGURE 33–5

◆ **Laparoscopic pyloromyotomy:** The patient is placed across the operating table so that surgeon and patient are properly aligned. A 3-mm camera port is placed through the umbilicus with an open technique, and pneumoperitoneum is created to a maximum pressure of 8 mm Hg. A short (22 cm) 3-mm 30-degree telescope is introduced. Two additional 3-mm ports are placed in the upper quadrants lateral to the rectus muscles (alternatively, the 3-mm knife and grasper can be placed directly into the abdomen **(Figure 33-6)**. Atraumatic graspers are used to grasp the duodenum and rotate the pylorus to expose the avascular plane. An endoscopic pyloromyotomy knife (some surgeons prefer arthroscopy knives) is used to incise the pyloric serosa over the avascular plane **(Figure 33-7)**. One of the arms of the pyloric spreader is used to deepen this incision by pushing on the brittle muscle until it gives. This maneuver is performed in the *middle* of the incision and *never* close to the duodenum. The operation is complete by spreading the muscle until the mucosa prolapses and independent movement of both pyloric halves can be verified **(Figure 33-8)**. At this time a small amount of saline is instilled over the pylorus, and the anesthesiologist is asked to insufflate the stomach with air to check for leaks. All incisions are infiltrated with 0.25% bupivacaine and closed with 6-0 subcuticular, absorbable sutures or Steri-Strips.

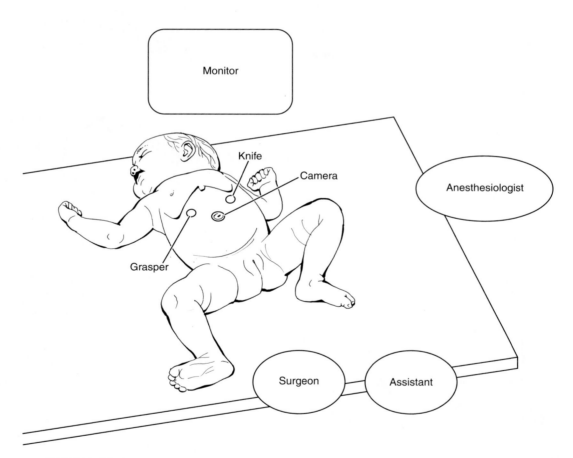

FIGURE 33–6

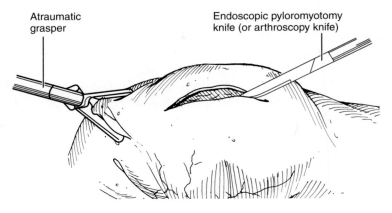

FIGURE 33–7

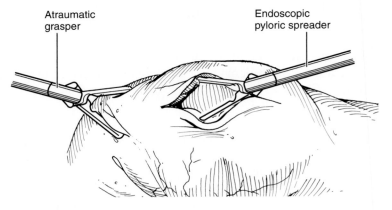

FIGURE 33–8

3. CLOSING

- The incision is closed in separate layers with running 5-0 or 6-0 polyglactin sutures. Posterior rectus fascia and peritoneum are closed together; no attempt is made to close the peritoneum by itself. The rectus muscle does not need to be reapproximated. After closure of the anterior rectus fascia, interrupted subcutaneous sutures of 6-0 polyglactin will obliterate any dead space. The skin is closed with subcuticular 6-0 undyed absorbable monofilament sutures and adhesive strips. Before closing, the skin is infiltrated with 0.25% bupivacaine without epinephrine at the appropriate dose.

STEP 4: POSTOPERATIVE CARE

- Maintenance intravenous fluids are continued until the patient is tolerating bottle feeds, which are started 4 to 6 hours after the operation and gradually advanced. It is a good practice to examine the patient's abdomen before proceeding with enteral feeds. Many surgeons use an electrolyte solution such as Pedialyte for the first feed. Some vomiting can be expected. Most patients are ready for discharge 24 to 48 hours after the procedure.

- **Complications:** The most dreaded complication of this procedure is duodenal perforation, which is reported in approximately 1% of open pyloromyotomies and between 1% and 2% of laparoscopic pyloromyotomies. Every effort must be made to identify this complication at operation, so that the entire pyloromyotomy can be closed with interrupted 4-0 silk sutures and a new pyloromyotomy performed. The patient is kept on intravenous fluids, antibiotics, and orogastric suction for 2 to 3 days. A contrast study to confirm patency of the pylorus and absence of leaks is performed before resuming enteral feeds. Failure to recognize a perforation results in life-threatening peritonitis and sepsis that mandates immediate resuscitation, and administration of broad-spectrum intravenous antibiotics, followed by laparotomy and washing of the abdominal cavity. The original pyloromyotomy is closed as described previously, and a new pyloromyotomy is performed.

- Postoperative care is done in a critical care setting, and the need for hemodynamic support is not unusual. These young patients have an increased incidence of wound infections and wound dehiscence.

- Up to one third of infants after an uncomplicated pyloromyotomy will experience vomiting, which is typically self-limited. Vomiting is usually managed by holding the next feed and resuming feeds 6 hours later. If vomiting persists, one must begin to consider the possibility of an incomplete pyloromyotomy. Although vomiting is not unusual after pyloromyotomy, abdominal distention is. Abdominal distention should prompt the surgeon to stop feeds and investigate for duodenal leaks. Wound infections after uncomplicated pyloromyotomy occur in approximately 2% of cases, and wound dehiscences are quite rare.

STEP 5: PEARLS AND PITFALLS

- ◆ Avoid incisions that extend into the duodenum. This will surely result in perforation, because the area of the distal pylorus and proximal duodenum is extremely thin. In fact, the scoring incision made over the pylorus should stop 2 to 3 mm short of the ring that is palpated at the distal pylorus. Spreading wide *proximal* to this area will result in disruption of the hypertrophic muscle fibers and release of the constrictive ring.

SELECTED REFERENCES

1. Lobe T, Kumar T: Pyloromyotomy. In Spitz L, Coran AG (eds): Operative Pediatric Surgery, 6th ed. London, Hodder Arnold, 2006, pp 367-375.
2. Ashcraft K: Atlas of Pediatric Surgery. Philadelphia, Saunders, 1994, pp 85-89.
3. Fujimoto T: Pyloromyotomy. In Najmaldin A, Rothenberg S, Crabbe D, Beasley S (eds): Operative Endoscopy and Endoscopic Surgery in Infants and Children. New York, Oxford University Press, 2005, pp 231-234.

CHAPTER 34

ROUX-EN-Y GASTRIC BYPASS (OPEN AND LAPAROSCOPIC)

Michael D. Trahan

STEP 1: SURGICAL ANATOMY

- Experience with the anatomy and surgical procedures of the esophagogastric junction are a prerequisite to a successful gastric bypass operation (**Figure 34-1**).

STEP 2: PREOPERATIVE CONSIDERATIONS

- The standard indications for a bariatric operation include either a body mass index of at least 40 kg/m^2 or a body mass index of at least 35 kg/m^2 with significant associated medical illness. Potential patients must also have tried multiple dietary, activity, and lifestyle modification programs. They should be free of substance abuse and psychologically stable so that they can make an intelligent decision regarding the risks of the operation and the need to dramatically alter their lifestyles.

- Bariatric operations should not be offered unless a dedicated team is in place for the thorough preoperative evaluation and close long-term follow-up that are required for every patient.

- Patients should receive prophylaxis against wound infection with an intravenous cephalosporin and against venous thrombosis with sequential compression devices and low-molecular-weight heparin before induction of anesthesia.

- General anesthesia is required for this operation. An anesthesia team specially trained and equipped for the morbidly obese patient is necessary.

- Obtaining a controlled airway can sometimes be quite challenging in the morbidly obese patient. A fiber-optic scope can be very helpful for an awake intubation. Elective tracheostomy is sometimes a good idea for the massively obese patient, especially one who already has some baseline respiratory dysfunction where airway control may continue to be a problem postoperatively.

- Each incision site is preemptively anesthetized with local anesthetic injection.

STEP 3: OPERATIVE STEPS

LAPAROSCOPIC

1. INCISIONS

- ◆ Six small incisions are used for the laparoscopic approach. The incision for the left-sided 12-mm trocar needs to be approximately 3 cm to later accommodate the circular stapler **(Figure 34-2)**.

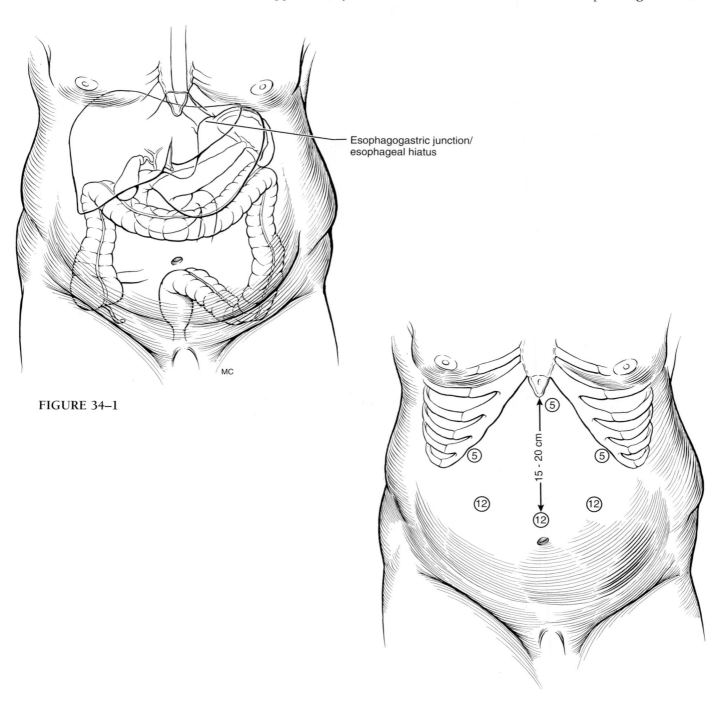

Esophagogastric junction/
esophageal hiatus

FIGURE 34–1

FIGURE 34–2

2. DISSECTION

♦ The 12-mm camera port is placed 15 to 17 cm from the xiphoid process in the midline. A port with internal visual capability is preferred. The umbilicus is not a useful landmark in the morbidly obese patient. The peritoneal cavity is inflated with carbon dioxide to 13 to 15 mm Hg.

♦ The remaining four ports (one 5 mm and one 12 mm in each of the upper abdominal quadrants as diagrammed) are then placed with internal visualization.

♦ A suture looped under the falciform ligament can often improve visualization and reduce interference with instrument introduction **(Figure 34-3)**.

♦ The omentum is divided in the midline all the way to and for a short distance along the transverse colon using the ultrasonic shears. This will allow placement of the Roux limb anterior to the colon and stomach with less tension. Adhesions to the abdominal wall may need to be divided first **(Figure 34-4)**.

♦ The omentum is placed above the transverse colon, which is then retracted superiorly by the assistant's grasping of the transverse mesocolon **(Figure 34-5)**.

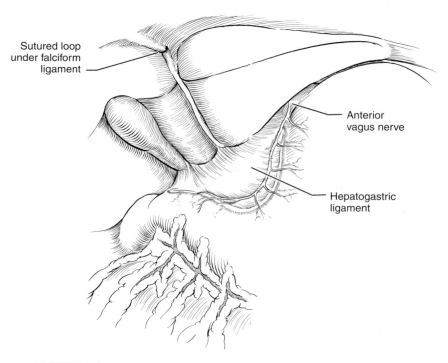

Sutured loop under falciform ligament

Anterior vagus nerve

Hepatogastric ligament

FIGURE 34–3

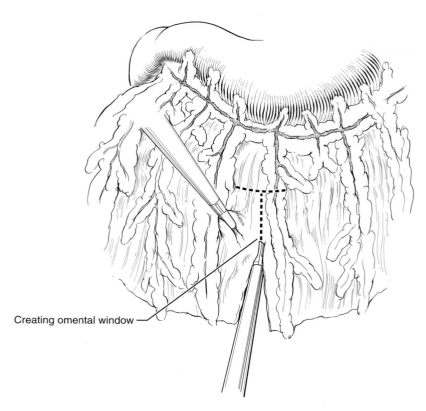

Creating omental window

FIGURE 34–4

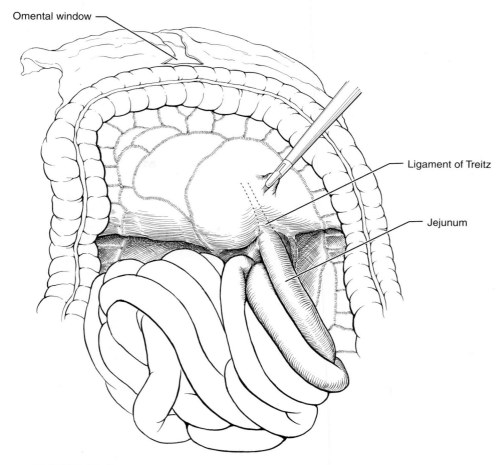

Omental window

Ligament of Treitz

Jejunum

FIGURE 34–5

◆ The ligament of Treitz is identified and followed until the mesentery lengthens (usually 30 to 40 cm). The jejunum is divided transversely with a linear cutting stapler loaded with 2.5-mm staples. A 45-mm stapler length is adequate (**Figure 34-6**).

◆ The mesentery of the distal aspect of the divided jejunum is incised next to the bowel wall to provide additional mobility of the Roux limb. Any ischemic area created by this maneuver will be trimmed during one of the final steps (**Figure 34-7**).

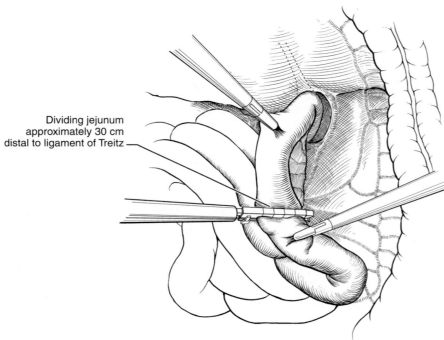

Dividing jejunum approximately 30 cm distal to ligament of Treitz

FIGURE 34–6

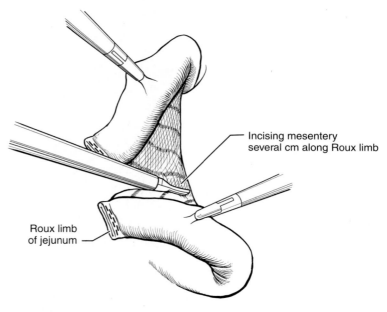

Incising mesentery several cm along Roux limb

Roux limb of jejunum

FIGURE 34–7

◆ The jejunum is followed for approximately 100 cm for a standard length gastric bypass. Here a small enterotomy is made on the antimesenteric border. Another small enterotomy is made at the antimesenteric corner of the proximal blind end of the jejunum. The enterotomies are only the length of the jaws of the ultrasonic shears **(Figure 34-8)**.

◆ With a jaw of the 2.5-mm stapler height linear cutter inserted though each of the enterotomies, the stapler is fired to create the anastomosis. Either one 60-mm stapler or two successive firings of the 45-mm stapler is used here **(Figure 34-9)**.

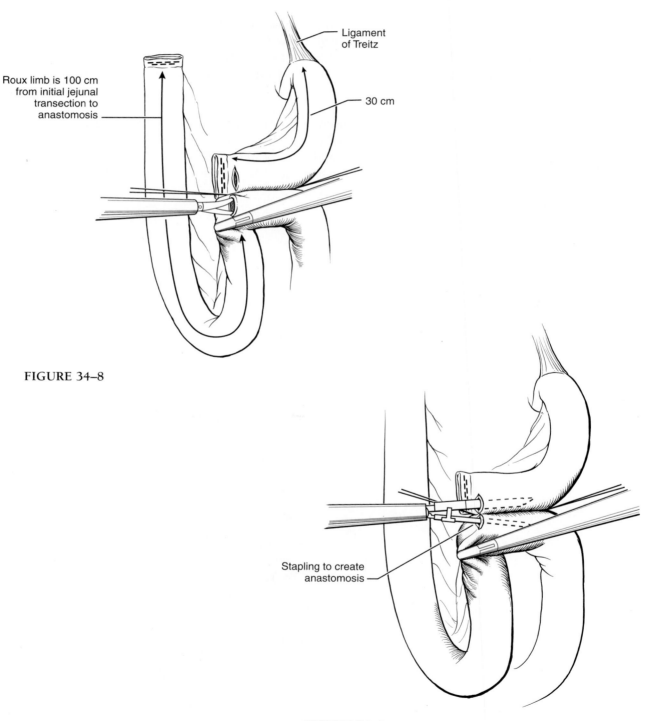

FIGURE 34–8

FIGURE 34–9

- The resulting enterotomy is closed with one 60-mm or two firings of the 45-mm linear stapler using the 2.5-mm stapler loads **(Figure 34-10)**.

- A seromuscular stitch of 2-0 silk is placed at the left side of the anastomosis, and the mesenteric defect is closed on the right side of the anastomosis with a running 2-0 silk suture, starting at the base of the defect and ending with a seromuscular bite of each portion of jejunum. This seromuscular bite is reported to decrease the risk of anastomotic obstruction **(Figure 34-11)**.

- The jejunojejunostomy is inspected for adequacy of the lumen and hemostasis of the suture and staple lines. The Roux limb is held in place as the omentum and colon are swept back downward. The patient is turned to the reverse Trendelenburg position. The telescope is exchanged for a 45-degree long scope. A table-mounted retractor is clamped to the bed.

- The 5- or 10-mm Fisher or Nathanson liver retractor is positioned to elevate the liver by direct insertion through the abdominal wall to the left of the midline in the epigastrium. This insertion site should be just at the caudal extent of the left lateral lobe. No attempt should be made to incise the lateral liver attachments. The retractor is secured to the table mount **(Figure 34-12)**.

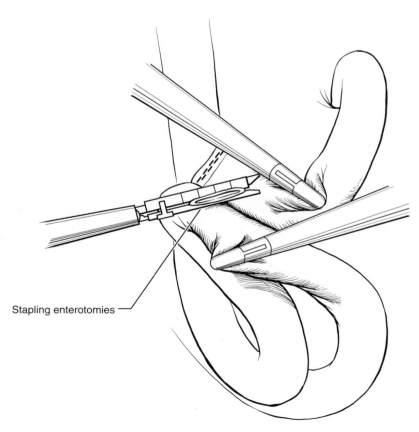

Stapling enterotomies

FIGURE 34–10

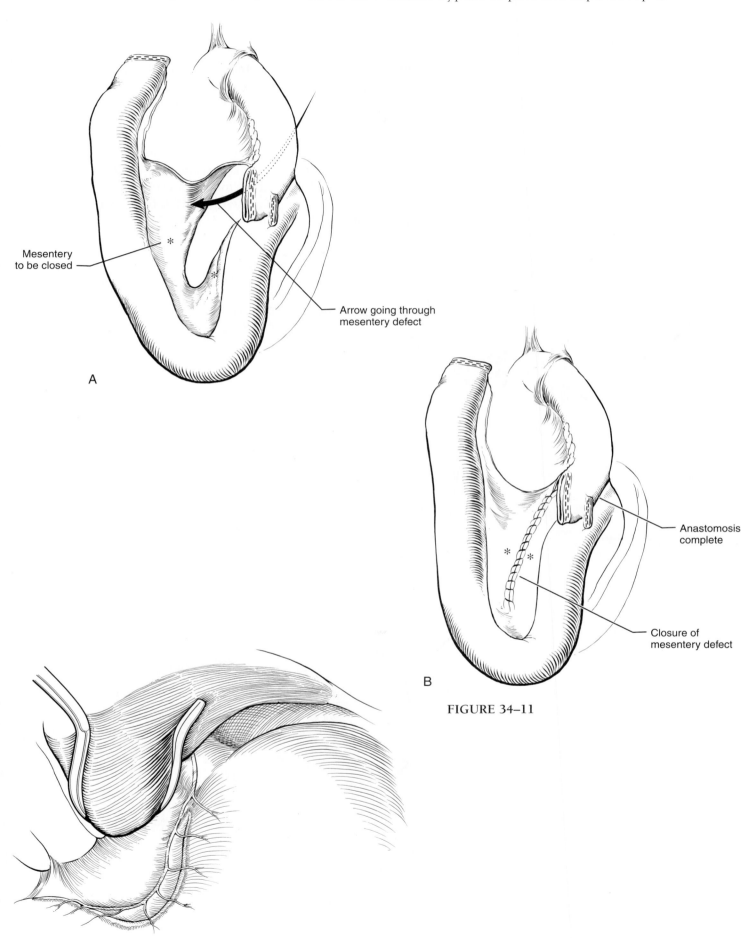

Mesentery to be closed

Arrow going through mesentery defect

A

Anastomosis complete

Closure of mesentery defect

B

FIGURE 34–11

FIGURE 34–12

◆ The peritoneum overlying the left crus of the diaphragm at the angle of His is disrupted bluntly and spread open to expose the diaphragmatic muscle. An articulating right-angled instrument is used to create a space by blunt dissection posterior to the stomach and along the crus. A thin veil of peritoneum is left between the stomach and spleen (**Figure 34-13**).

◆ A balloon-tipped orogastric tube is placed in the stomach to guide the pouch creation. The balloon is inflated to 20 mL and pulled back snuggly to the esophagogastric junction. Once the line of transection is identified, the balloon is deflated and the tube is pulled back into the esophagus. One must always be certain of the position of any esophageal tube, because stapling across the tubes can result in a difficult and lengthy revision (**Figure 34-14**).

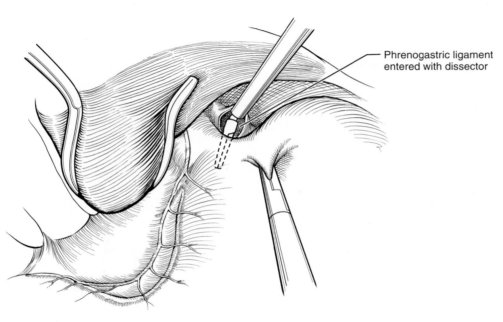

Phrenogastric ligament entered with dissector

FIGURE 34–13

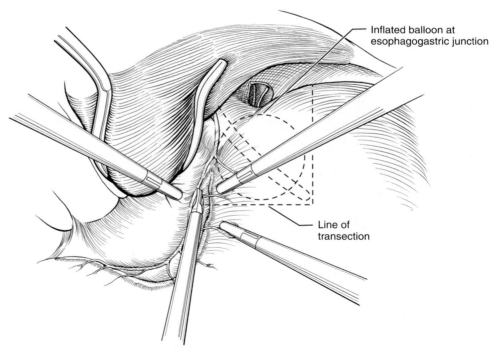

Inflated balloon at esophagogastric junction

Line of transection

FIGURE 34–14

◆ The assistant grasps the stomach in two places along the lesser curvature above and below the site of transection. The ultrasonic shears are used to carefully incise the peritoneum and underlying fat of the gastrohepatic ligament to enter the lesser sac without injuring the wall of the stomach, the vagus branches, or the vasculature of the pouch. There are a number of small veins that, when not entirely sealed with the shears, can cause troublesome bleeding. Therefore this dissection should be performed slowly and meticulously with a delicate combination of sweeping and sharp dissection with the ultrasonic device **(Figure 34-15)**.

◆ An articulating 45-mm linear cutting stapler loaded with 3.5-mm staples is angled, placed, and fired transversely across the lesser curvature approximately 3 to 4 cm distal to the esophagogastric junction at the site identified by the balloon to begin creation of the pouch (see Figure 34-15).

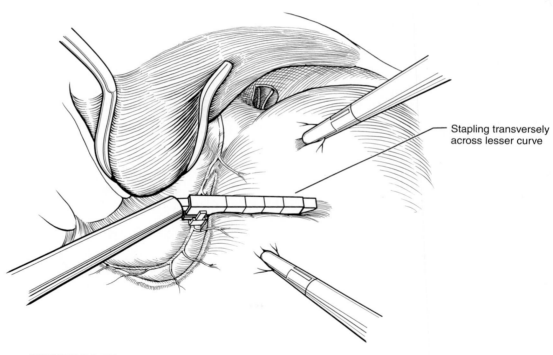

Stapling transversely across lesser curve

FIGURE 34–15

◆ A gastrotomy is made near the greater curvature of the stomach. The 12-mm port is removed from the left upper quadrant, and this incision is dilated sequentially up to 26 mm with Hegar dilators. The anvil of a 25-mm end-to-end stapler is loaded with the spike possessing a 2-0 polyester suture knotted through its eye. Using the 12-mm port facilitates insertion of the anvil into the peritoneal cavity **(Figure 34-16)**.

◆ The anvil is placed through the gastrotomy using an anvil grasper. The suture is threaded downward through the eye of a 5-mm articulating dissector **(Figure 34-17)**.

◆ The articulating dissector is placed through the gastrotomy and flexed so that its tip tents up the stomach at the staple line near the lesser curve. The ultrasonic dissector is activated while touching the tip of the articulating dissector to create a gastrotomy only big enough to pass the articulating dissector through it. The suture is then grasped, and once it is pulled through the tiny gastrotomy, the articulating dissector is straightened and removed (see Figure 34-17).

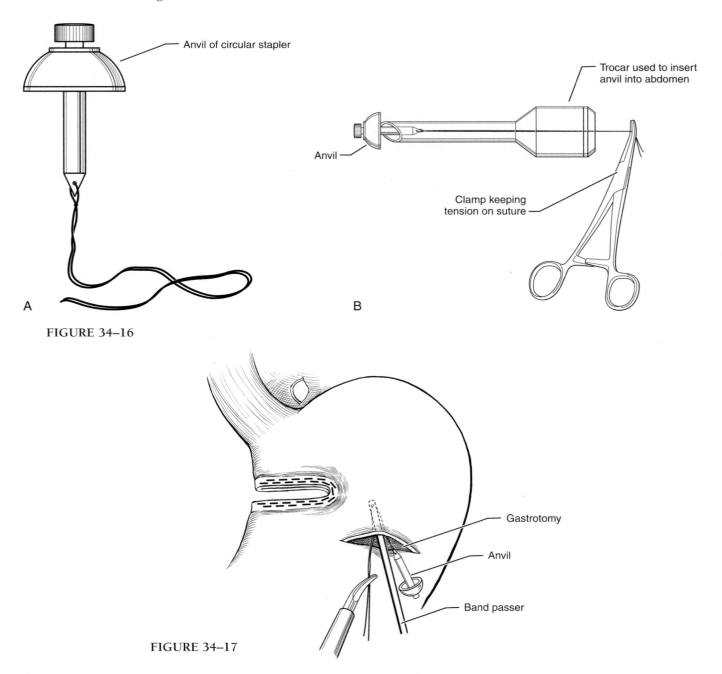

Anvil of circular stapler

Trocar used to insert anvil into abdomen

Anvil

Clamp keeping tension on suture

A

B

FIGURE 34–16

Gastrotomy

Anvil

Band passer

FIGURE 34–17

◆ The surgeon pulls the suture across the field to the patient's right while holding the stomach at the crotch of the staple line until the anvil trocar passes through the gastrotomy. Once the anvil is in position, the original gastrotomy is closed with the linear stapler containing 3.5-mm staples. Either one firing of the 60-mm or two firings of the 45-mm stapler is usually required **(Figure 34-18).**

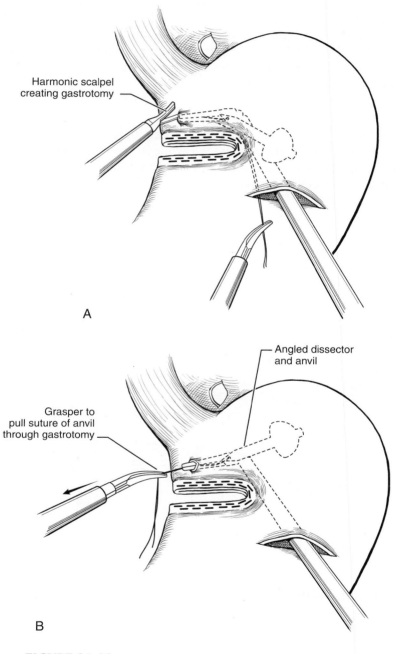

Harmonic scalpel
creating gastrotomy

A

Angled dissector
and anvil

Grasper to
pull suture of anvil
through gastrotomy

B

FIGURE 34–18

♦ The 60-mm linear stapler with 3.5-mm staple height is applied to the stomach paralleling the lesser curve through the 12-mm port on the left side. Downward pulling of the suture von the anvil facilitates proper placement. Before firing, the surgeon advances the orogastric tube until he or she can be certain that the tube is visible within the pouch and not within the main body of the stomach or caught by the stapler **(Figure 34-19)**.

♦ The 10-mm articulating dissector is placed through port two. Its tip is passed behind the stomach and flexed into the space created at the angle of His. Gentle side-to-side manipulation enlarges this opening. The assistant holds this instrument while the articulating 45-mm linear stapler loaded with 3.5-mm staples completes the division of the stomach, again confirming placement of the stapler by manipulation of the orogastric tube **(Figures 34-20 and 34-21)**.

♦ The anvil trocar can now be removed. It is helpful to note that a 90-degree rotation of the blue spike with a right-angled dissector while the anvil is held steady with an anvil grasper or other grasping instrument simplifies the detachment. The anvil grasper is applied to the anvil above the springs **(Figure 34-22)**.

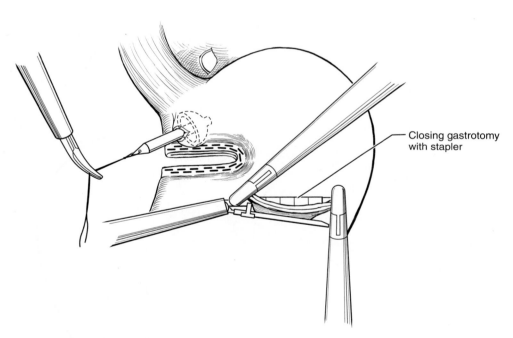

Closing gastrotomy with stapler

FIGURE 34–19

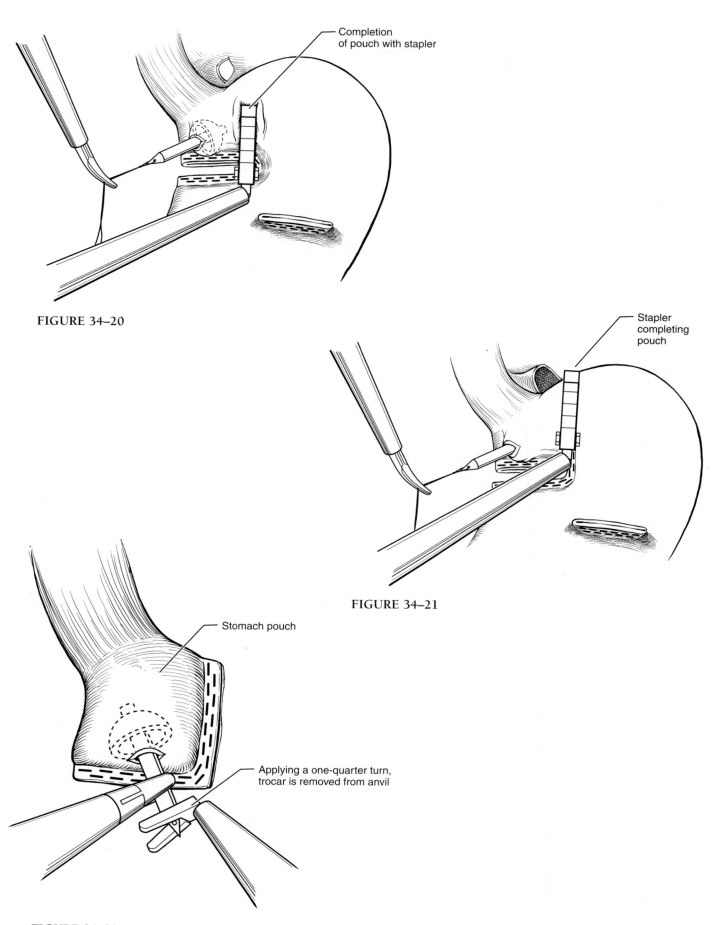

FIGURE 34–20

Completion of pouch with stapler

FIGURE 34–21

Stapler completing pouch

FIGURE 34–22

Stomach pouch

Applying a one-quarter turn, trocar is removed from anvil

◆ The jejunal Roux limb is opened longitudinally on its end **(Figure 34-23)**. The 12-mm port is removed again, and the circular stapler is placed through the dilated port site and into the lumen of the Roux limb. Once past the demarcated segment, the stapler is opened to pierce the antimesenteric border. Traction must be maintained on the bowel proximal and distal to the end of the stapler to keep the bowel from slipping off of the stapler trocar **(Figures 34-24 and 34-25)**.

◆ The stapler and anvil are mated together, and the instrument is closed and fired. The stapler is partially opened and removed. The redundant open segment of jejunum is trimmed and sealed by first incising the mesentery and then applying the linear stapler with 2.5-mm staples. Before firing the stapler, the orogastric tube should be passed through the gastroje-junostomy for the subsequent leak check. A seromuscular stitch of 2-0 Vicryl is placed at the right side of the gastrojejunostomy **(Figures 34-26, 34-27, and 34-28)**.

◆ A test for leaks and placement of a closed suction drain completes the procedure.

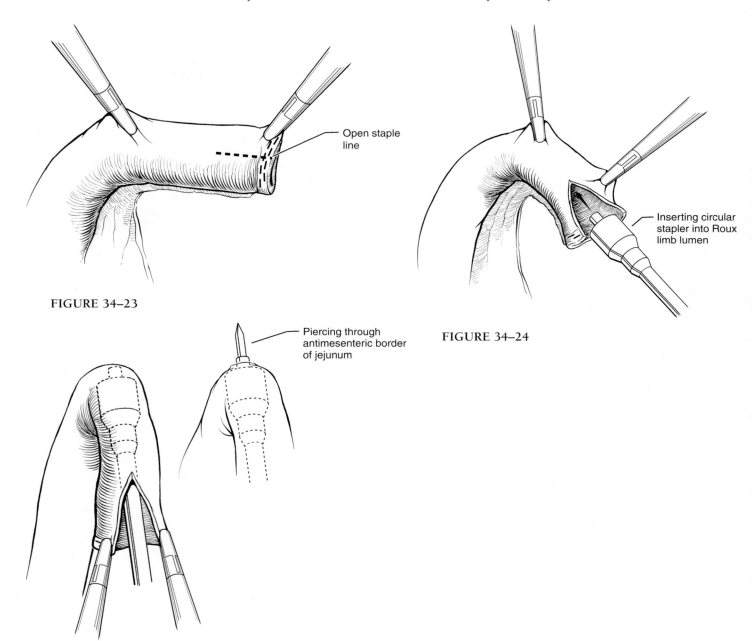

Open staple line

FIGURE 34–23

Inserting circular stapler into Roux limb lumen

FIGURE 34–24

Piercing through antimesenteric border of jejunum

FIGURE 34–25

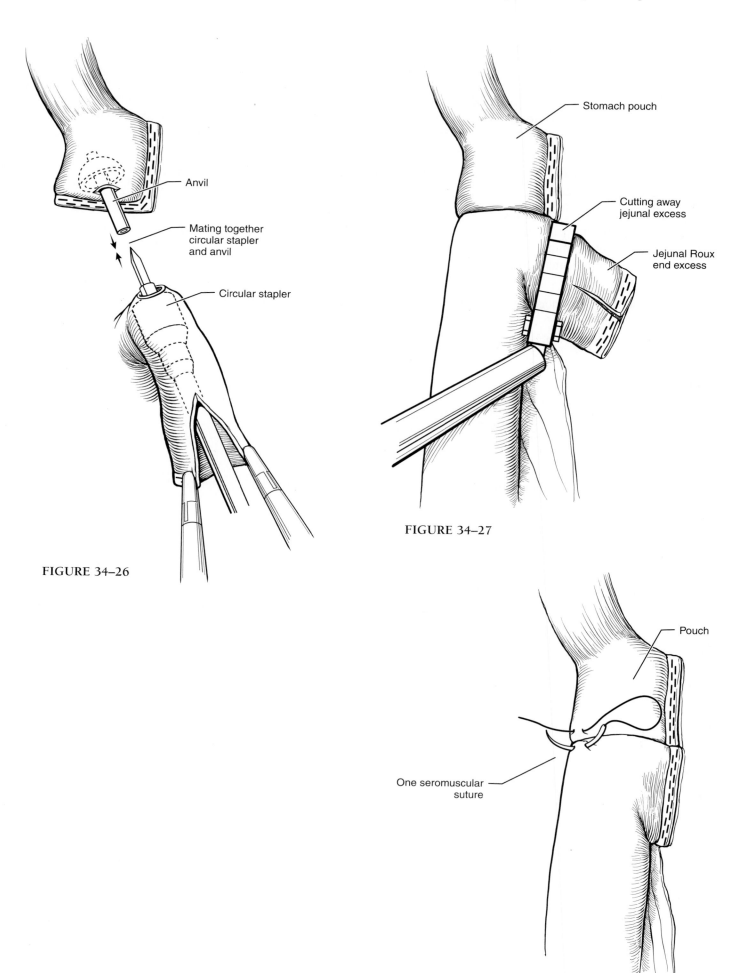

Anvil

Mating together
circular stapler
and anvil

Circular stapler

FIGURE 34–26

Stomach pouch

Cutting away
jejunal excess

Jejunal Roux
end excess

FIGURE 34–27

Pouch

One seromuscular
suture

FIGURE 34–28

3. CLOSURE

◆ The port site that had been dilated to 26 mm can be closed with two successive sutures of 0 Vicryl placed using the laparoscopic suture passer or fascial sutures through the open wound. There is no need to close the 5- and 12-mm port sites when using bladeless trocars.

◆ The instruments and ports are removed under direct visualization as the pneumoperitoneum escapes.

◆ The circular stapler site should be copiously irrigated before closure, because this site has been contaminated by the circular stapler and removal of the trimmed tissue from the stomach and small bowel.

◆ The skin incisions are closed with subcuticular sutures and either tissue adhesive or sterile tapes.

OPEN

1. INCISION

◆ A midline laparotomy from the xiphoid to near the umbilicus is preferred (**Figures 34-29 and 34-30**).

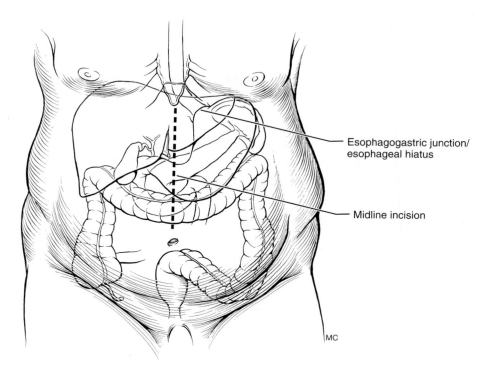

Esophagogastric junction/
esophageal hiatus

Midline incision

FIGURE 34–29

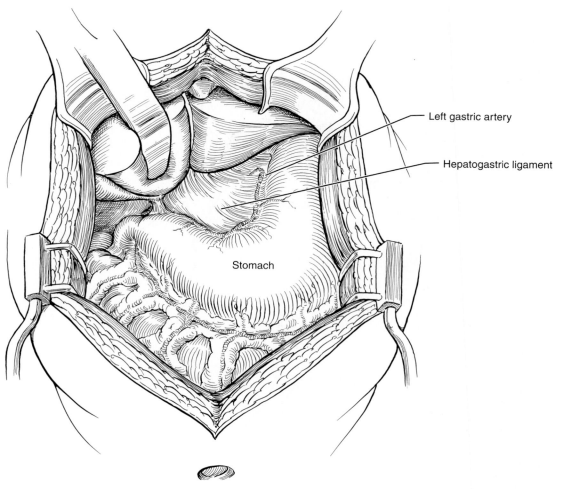

Left gastric artery

Hepatogastric ligament

Stomach

FIGURE 34–30

2. DISSECTION

- A table-mounted body wall retractor such as the Bookwalter model facilitates exposure.

- The omentum is divided in the midline all the way to and for a short distance along the transverse colon using the ultrasonic shears. This will allow placement of the Roux limb anterior to the colon and stomach with less tension. Adhesions to the abdominal wall may need to be divided first **(Figure 34-31).**

- The ligament of Treitz is identified, and the jejunum is divided approximately 40 cm distal to it. An opening is made in the transverse mesocolon if a retrocolic approach is favored **(Figure 34-32).**

- The mesentery of the distal aspect of the divided jejunum is incised next to the bowel wall to provide additional mobility of the Roux limb. Any ischemia area created by this maneuver will be trimmed during one of the final steps.

- The jejunum is followed for approximately 100 cm for a standard-length gastric bypass. Here a small enterotomy is made on the antimesenteric border. Another small enterotomy is made at the antimesenteric corner of the proximal blind end of the jejunum. The enterotomies are only large enough to accommodate the end of the stapler **(Figure 34-33).**

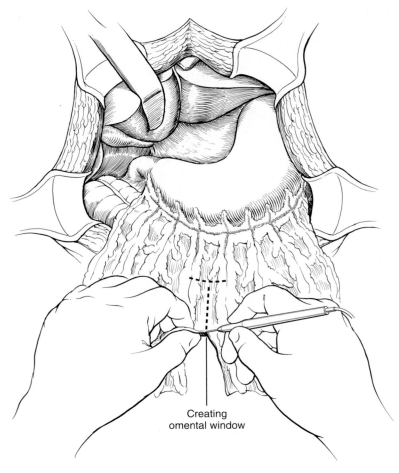

Creating
omental window

FIGURE 34–31

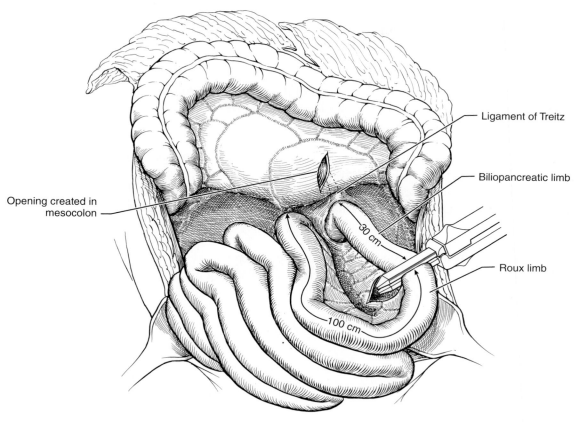

Ligament of Treitz

Biliopancreatic limb

Opening created in mesocolon

30 cm

Roux limb

100 cm

FIGURE 34–32

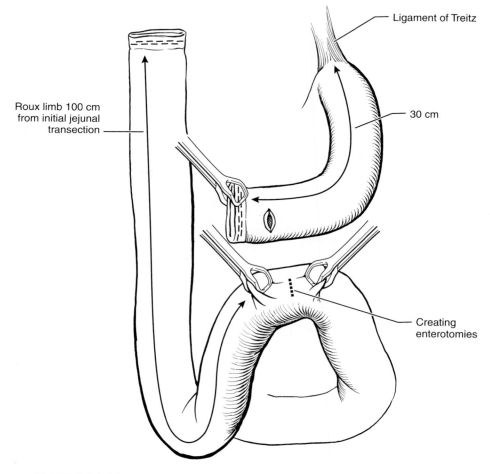

Ligament of Treitz

Roux limb 100 cm from initial jejunal transection

30 cm

Creating enterotomies

FIGURE 34–33

◆ With a jaw of the 2.5-mm stapler height linear cutter inserted though each of the enterotomies, the stapler is fired to create the anastomosis. Either one firing of the 60-mm stapler or two successive firings of the 45-mm stapler is used here **(Figure 34-34)**.

◆ The resulting enterotomy is closed with one firing of the 60-mm or two firings of the 45-mm linear stapler using the 2.5-mm stapler loads **(Figure 34-35)**.

◆ A seromuscular stitch of 2-0 silk is placed at the left side of the anastomosis. The mesenteric defect is closed from the right side with a running 2-0 silk suture, starting at the base of the defect and ending with a seromuscular bite of each portion of jejunum. This seromuscular bite is reported to decrease the risk of anastomotic obstruction **(Figure 34-36)**.

◆ The jejunojejunostomy is inspected for adequacy of the lumen and hemostasis of the suture and staple lines. The patient is turned to the reverse Trendelenburg position.

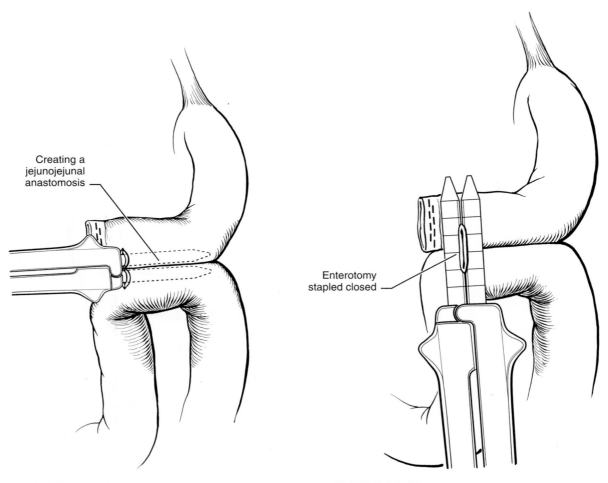

Creating a
jejunojejunal
anastomosis

Enterotomy
stapled closed

FIGURE 34–34   **FIGURE 34–35**

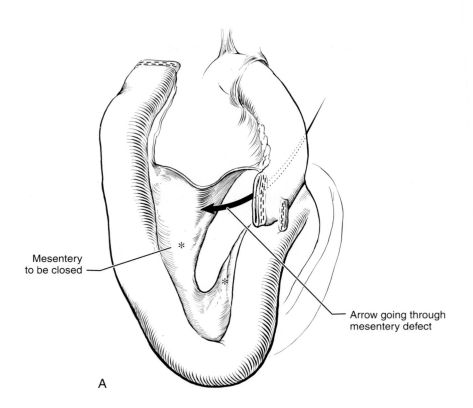

Mesentery
to be closed

Arrow going through
mesentery defect

A

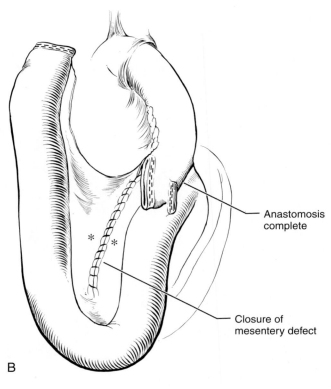

Anastomosis
complete

Closure of
mesentery defect

B

FIGURE 34–36

◆ The peritoneum overlying the left crus of the diaphragm at the angle of His is disrupted and spread open to expose the diaphragmatic muscle. Blunt dissection with a finger is used to enlarge this space posterior to the stomach and along the crus. A thin veil of peritoneum is left between the stomach and spleen **(Figure 34-37)**.

◆ A balloon-tipped orogastric tube is placed in the stomach to size the pouch. The balloon is inflated to 20 mL and pulled back snuggly to the esophagogastric junction. Once the line of transection is identified, the balloon is deflated and pulled back into the esophagus. One must be continuously aware of the position of all tubes in the esophagus, because stapling across the tubes requires a difficult and lengthy revision **(Figure 34-38)**.

◆ The cautery or ultrasonic shears is used to carefully incise the peritoneum and underlying fat of the gastrohepatic ligament to enter the lesser sac without injuring the wall of the stomach, the vagus branches, or the vasculature of the pouch. There are a number of small veins that, when not entirely sealed, can cause troublesome bleeding. Therefore this dissection should be performed slowly and meticulously, with a delicate combination of sweeping and judicious use of energy sources **(Figure 34-39)**.

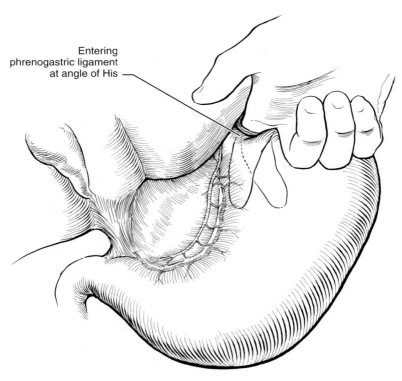

Entering phrenogastric ligament at angle of His

FIGURE 34–37

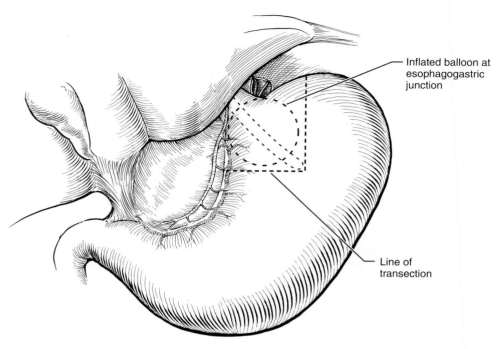

Inflated balloon at
esophagogastric
junction

Line of
transection

FIGURE 34–38

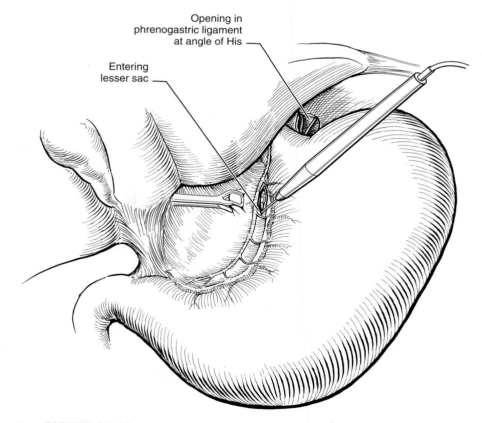

Opening in
phrenogastric ligament
at angle of His

Entering
lesser sac

FIGURE 34–39

◆ An articulating 45-mm linear cutting stapler loaded with 3.5-mm staples is angled, placed, and fired transversely across the lesser curvature approximately 4 cm distal to the esophagogastric junction at the site identified by the balloon to begin creation of the pouch (**Figure 34-40**).

◆ A gastrotomy is made near the greater curvature of the stomach. The anvil of a 25-mm end-to-end stapler is loaded with the spike that has a 2-0 polyester suture knotted through its eye. The anvil is placed through the gastrotomy. The suture is threaded downward through the eye of the 5-mm articulating dissector (**Figure 34-41**).

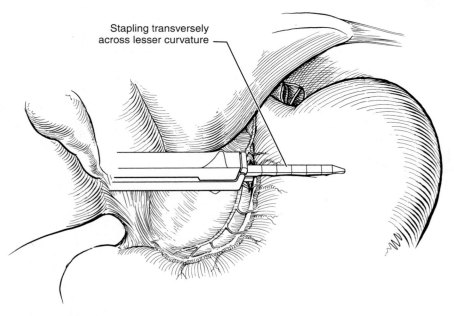

Stapling transversely across lesser curvature

FIGURE 34–40

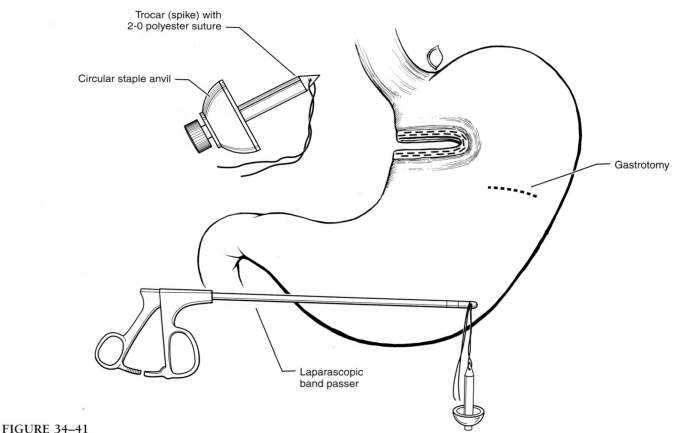

Trocar (spike) with 2-0 polyester suture

Circular staple anvil

Gastrotomy

Laparascopic band passer

FIGURE 34–41

◆ The articulating dissector is placed through the gastrotomy and flexed so that its tip tents up the stomach at the staple line near the lesser curve. The cautery or ultrasonic dissector is activated while touching the tip of the articulating dissector to create a gastrotomy only big enough to pass the articulating dissector through it. The suture is then grasped, and once it is pulled through the tiny gastrotomy, the articulating dissector is straightened and removed **(Figures 34-42 and 34-43).**

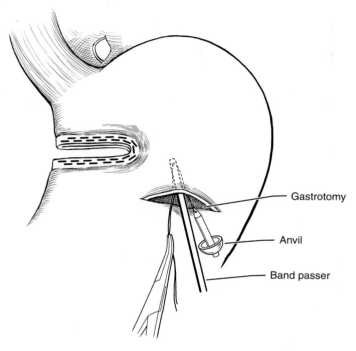

Gastrotomy

Anvil

Band passer

FIGURE 34–42

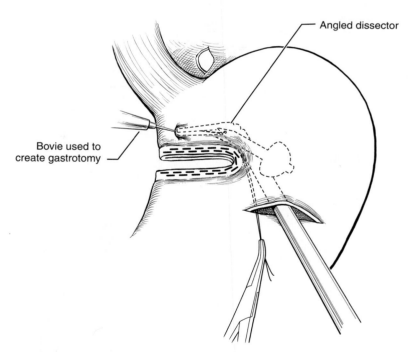

Angled dissector

Bovie used to create gastrotomy

FIGURE 34–43

◆ Once the anvil is in position, the original gastrotomy is closed with the linear stapler containing 3.5-mm staples **(Figure 34-44)**.

◆ The 60-mm linear stapler with 3.5-mm staple height is applied to the stomach paralleling the lesser curve. Downward traction on the suture on the anvil facilitates proper placement. Before firing the stapler, the orogastric tube is advanced until it can be certain that it is visible within the pouch and not within the main body of the stomach or caught by the stapler. This is repeated until the surgeon is certain the pouch has been completely separated from the main body of the stomach **(Figure 34-45)**.

◆ The spike is removed and discarded **(Figure 34-46)**.

◆ The jejunal Roux limb is opened longitudinally on its end **(Figure 34-47)**.

◆ The circular stapler is placed into the lumen of the Roux limb **(Figure 34-48)**.

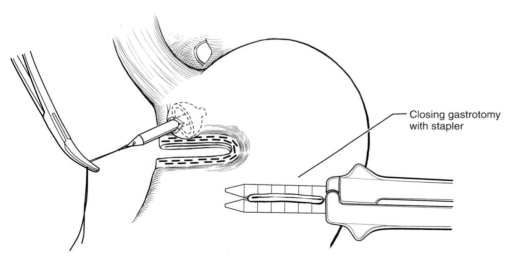

Closing gastrotomy with stapler

FIGURE 34–44

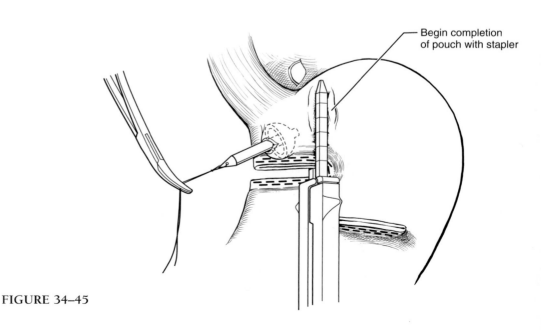

Begin completion of pouch with stapler

FIGURE 34–45

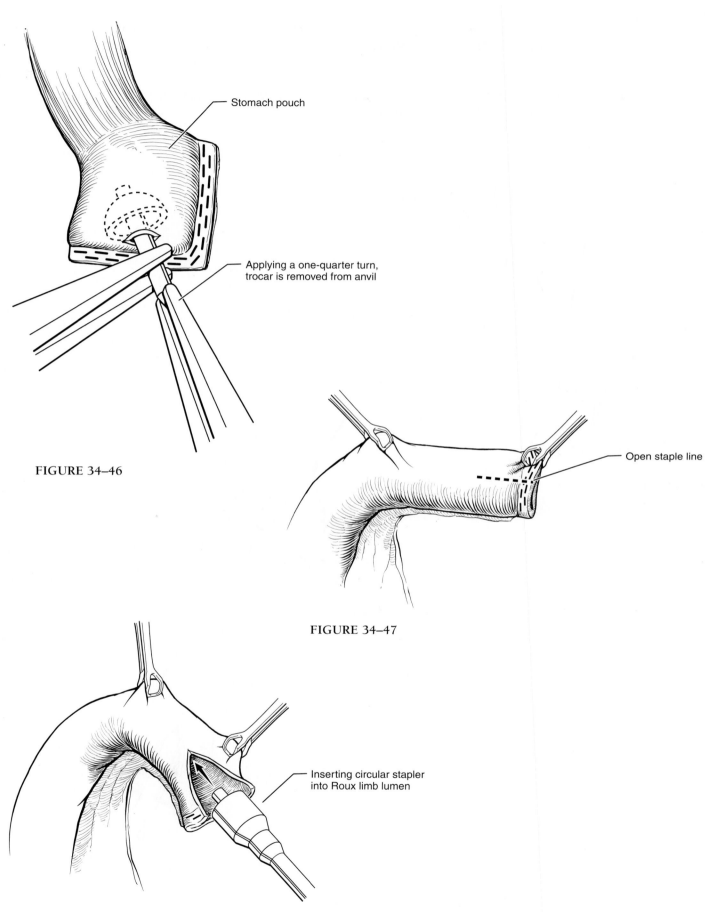

Stomach pouch

Applying a one-quarter turn, trocar is removed from anvil

FIGURE 34–46

Open staple line

FIGURE 34–47

Inserting circular stapler into Roux limb lumen

FIGURE 34–48

◆ Once past the demarcated segment, the stapler is opened to pierce the antimesenteric border **(Figure 34-49)**.

◆ The stapler and anvil are mated together, and the instrument is closed and fired. The stapler is partially opened and removed **(Figure 34-50)**.

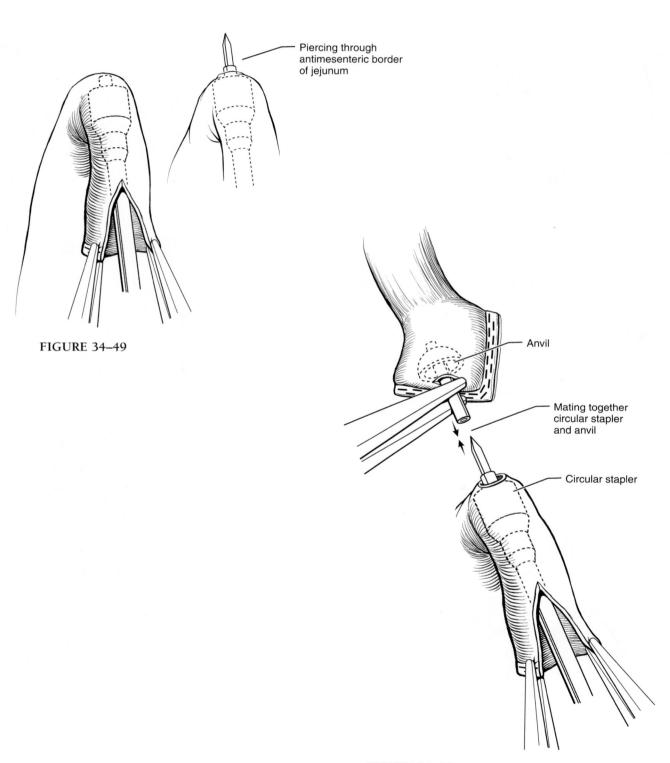

Piercing through antimesenteric border of jejunum

FIGURE 34–49

Anvil

Mating together circular stapler and anvil

Circular stapler

FIGURE 34–50

- The redundant open segment of jejunum is trimmed and sealed by first incising the mesentery and then applying the linear stapler with 2.5-mm staples. Before firing the stapler, the orogastric tube should be passed through the gastrojejunostomy for the subsequent leak check (**Figure 34-51**).

- A seromuscular stitch of 2-0 Vicryl is placed at the right side of the gastrojejunostomy (**Figure 34-52**).

- The leak check and placement of the closed suction drain complete the operation.

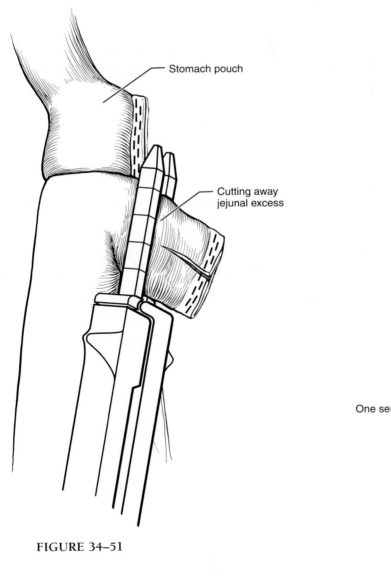

FIGURE 34–51

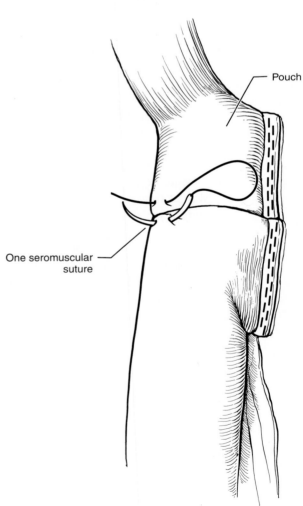

FIGURE 34–52

3. CLOSURE

- Interrupted #2 Vicryl sutures are used to close the abdominal fascia, and the skin is closed with staples after thorough irrigation.

STEP 4: POSTOPERATIVE CONSIDERATIONS

- Telemetry and pulse oximetry monitoring should be strongly considered for several hours postoperatively in these high-risk patients.

- Ambulation within the first 2 hours of emergence from anesthesia should help prevent venous thrombosis. Patients appropriately educated preoperatively will be anxious to get up out of bed.

STEP 5: PEARLS AND PITFALLS

- A thorough preoperative educational program is the best way to achieve the lowest risk of perioperative complications and highest patient compliance.

- Venous thrombosis and gastrointestinal leaks are among the most lethal perioperative complications, and surveillance for them is important.

- Despite prophylaxis with ambulation, sequential compression devices, and low-molecular-weight heparin, the risks of deep venous thrombosis and pulmonary embolism are still significant.

- Intraoperatively, a simple and quick way to test the integrity of the gastrojejunostomy is to occlude the Roux limb with an atraumatic instrument, flood the upper abdomen with saline, and inject boluses of air through the orogastric tube. Bubbles of air when present should be traced to their source to reinforce the staple line with Vicryl sutures. This procedure can also be performed with methylene blue injection through the orogastric tube.

◆ Another way to detect leaks in the early postoperative period is to place a closed suction drain at the gastrojejunostomy under the left lateral segment of the liver. This also helps protect against the progression of gastrojejunal leaks to peritonitis and abscess.

◆ Finally, consideration should be given to a contrast swallow with fluoroscopy before allowing any oral intake to screen for early postoperative leaks.

SELECTED REFERENCE

1. Brolin RE: The antiobstruction stitch in stapled Roux-en-Y enteroenterostomy. Am J Surg 1995;169: 355-357.

CHAPTER 35

Laparoscopic Placement of Adjustable Gastric Band (Pars Flaccida Approach)

Michael D. Trahan

STEP 1: SURGICAL ANATOMY

- Experience with the anatomy and a surgical procedure of the esophagogastric junction is a prerequisite to a successful gastric banding operation (see Figure 34-1).

STEP 2: PREOPERATIVE CONSIDERATIONS

- The standard indications for a bariatric operation include either a body mass index of at least 40 kg/m^2 or a body mass index of at least 35 kg/m^2 with significant associated medical illness. Potential patients must also have tried multiple dietary, activity, and lifestyle modification programs. They should be free of substance abuse and be psychologically stable so that they can make an intelligent decision regarding the risks of the operation and the need to dramatically alter their lifestyles. The indications for banding are the same as the indications for gastric bypass.

- Bariatric operations should not be offered unless a dedicated team is in place for the thorough preoperative evaluation and close long-term follow-up that are required for every patient.

- Banding is considered the safest of all the bariatric operations.

- Twenty percent to 40% of patients getting an adjustable gastric band will need to have a hiatal hernia repair. Small but significant hiatal hernias can be missed on preoperative studies. These are often not diagnosed until the intraoperative test, so the surgeon must be prepared for this inevitable situation.

- Patients should receive prophylaxis against wound infection with an intravenous cephalosporin and against venous thrombosis with sequential compression devices and low-molecular-weight heparin before induction of anesthesia.

♦ Each incision site is preemptively anesthetized with local anesthetic injection.

♦ General anesthesia is required for this operation. An anesthesia team specially trained and equipped for the morbidly obese patient is necessary.

♦ There are currently two devices with approval from the U.S. Food and Drug Administration (FDA) for use in the United States. There are several others being used internationally. The techniques for insertion may differ slightly, but the principles are the same.

♦ Use of the devices requires a formal education and official proctoring process before the bands are made available to the surgeon. This description is not meant to substitute for that qualification process.

STEP 3: OPERATIVE STEPS

1. INCISIONS

♦ Five small incisions are made as diagrammed. Initial entry is made using a 5-mm optically guided bladeless trocar at the left costal margin in the midclavicular line—this will be the main telescope port. The peritoneal cavity is insufflated and the remaining ports are placed under direct internal visualization. The liver retractor is inserted near the xiphoid process. A 5-mm trocar is placed on either side of the midline to be used as the surgeon's working ports. A 15-mm trocar is placed below the left costal margin near the anterior axillary line. The assistant will use this port to expose the esophagogastric area **(Figure 35-1)**.

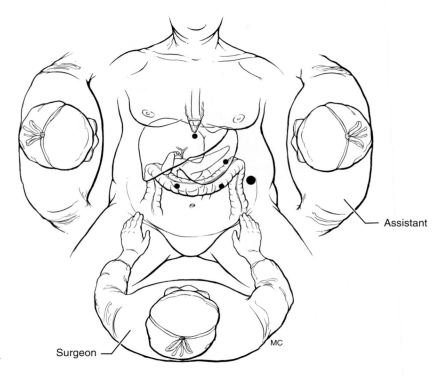

FIGURE 35–1

2. DISSECTION

- The orogastric calibration tube is inserted and watched as it enters the stomach. The balloon is inflated with 15 mL of air or water. The tube is pulled back to identify and test the integrity of the esophagogastric junction. If the balloon slips up into the mediastinum, a hiatal repair should be performed, usually by mobilization of the anterior aspect of the distal esophagus and suturing the anterior aspect of the hiatus. A larger hiatal hernia may require a posterior repair. Once the balloon confirms adequate hiatal repair, it is deflated, and the tube is removed.

- The pars flaccida is the clear membrane covering the caudate lobe and running between the lesser curvature of the stomach and the liver. This membrane is bluntly opened **(Figure 35-2)**.

- The assistant grasps the fat along the lesser curvature and retracts it to the patient's left. This maneuver exposes the right crus of the diaphragm, which should be carefully distinguished from the inferior vena cava. The peritoneum covering the fat just anterior to the lower aspect of the right crus is bluntly opened just enough to allow passage of the 5-mm articulating dissector. The dissector is placed through this opening and should pass without the slightest resistance behind the stomach aiming toward the angle of His **(Figure 35-3)**.

- The band is selected and prepared according to the manufacturer's specifications. The band and tubing are inserted through the 15-mm trocar by grasping the tip of the band buckle and pushing the device through the trocar with the band first. The grasper then releases the band, and the tubing is gently grasped and fed through the trocar, as well. The tip of the tubing is grasped before inserting the tubing all the way through the trocar. The tip of the tube is grasped by the retrogastric grasper or, if using a band passer, fed through the eye at the tip of the instrument **(Figure 35-4)**.

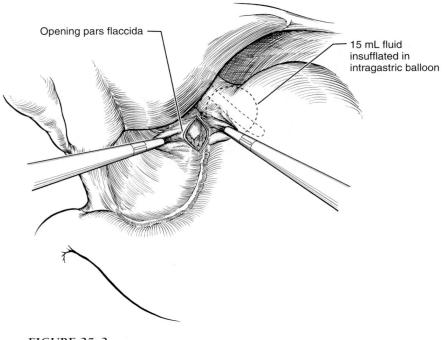

Opening pars flaccida

15 mL fluid insufflated in intragastric balloon

FIGURE 35–2

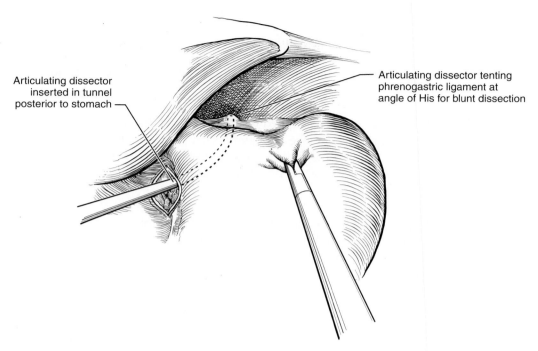

Articulating dissector inserted in tunnel posterior to stomach

Articulating dissector tenting phrenogastric ligament at angle of His for blunt dissection

FIGURE 35–3

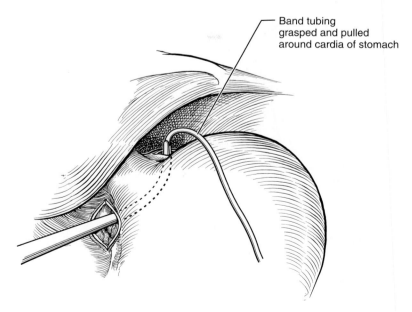

Band tubing grasped and pulled around cardia of stomach

FIGURE 35–4

◆ The retrogastric instrument is withdrawn, pulling the tubing and band into position behind the stomach. There is often significant resistance met as the band passes behind the stomach. The tubing is fed through the band buckle, and the device is closed securely. Each band has an indicator to identify a securely closed band **(Figures 35-5 and 35-6)**.

◆ The fundus of the stomach is then wrapped over the left lateral aspect of the band and secured to the pouch of stomach above the band with a series of interrupted seromuscular 2-0 polyester sutures. Usually three sutures are sufficient. No effort should be made to cover the area around the buckle or the buckle itself **(Figure 35-7)**.

◆ The buckle is lifted to check for underlying tension and then rotated toward the lesser curvature as far as allowable. The tip of the band tubing is grasped and pulled through the 15-mm trocar after the surgeon ensures that the tubing is not knotted. The instruments including the liver retractor are removed, and the pneumoperitoneum is released.

◆ The 15-mm trocar is removed, leaving the band tubing in place. A pocket is created bluntly through the 15-mm port site. The pocket is medial to the incision and at the level of the anterior abdominal fascia. Enough space should be made for the injection port to rest flush against the fascia as far medially as allowable.

◆ Two to four nonabsorbable sutures are placed in the fascia in an orientation consistent with the port being used. The two tails of each suture are clamped together with a hemostat to avoid tangling. The distal few centimeters of the tubing is trimmed and connected to the injection port, which has been prepared according to the manufacturer's specifications. The sutures are threaded through the holes on the injection port and then clamped together again **(Figure 35-8)**.

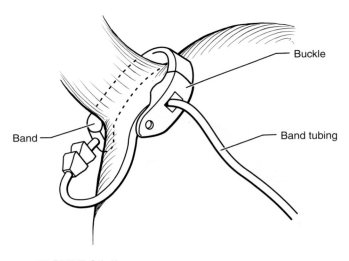

Buckle

Band

Band tubing

FIGURE 35–5

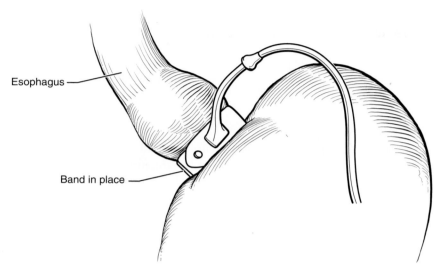

Esophagus

Band in place

FIGURE 35–6

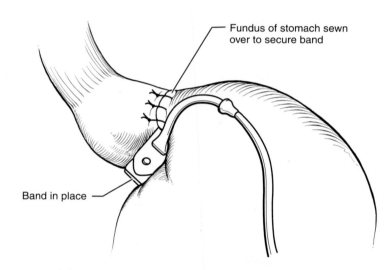

Fundus of stomach sewn over to secure band

Band in place

FIGURE 35–7

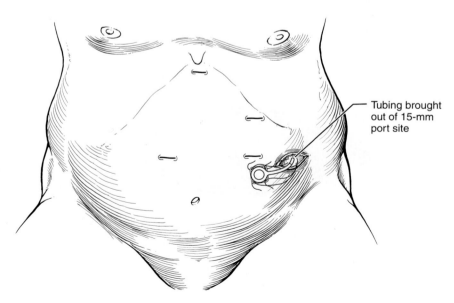

Tubing brought out of 15-mm port site

FIGURE 35–8

- Once all of the sutures are in place, the excess tubing is fed through the fascial opening and into the peritoneal cavity. The port is rested on the fascial surface, and the sutures are tied **(Figure 35-9)**.

3. CLOSURE

- The wounds are inspected for hemostasis. A subcuticular closure with absorbable suture is preferred. The wounds are dressed with tissue adhesives or wound approximation tapes and small bandages.

STEP 4: POSTOPERATIVE CONSIDERATIONS

- A low-potency oral narcotic combination elixir, such as acetaminophen with codeine or hydrocodone/acetaminophen, is usually sufficient for pain management.

- Nausea is a common postoperative complaint that should be effectively managed to avoid retching and possible displacement of the band.

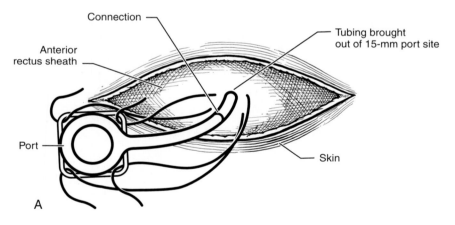

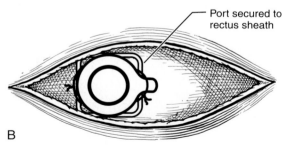

FIGURE 35–9

◆ Patients are offered sugar-free, carbonation-free clear liquids when awake. Advancing the diet to pureed foods is determined by patient progress, but no solid foods are offered for 4 postoperative weeks.

◆ A barium swallow is used to check band position and patency before discharge. It is also helpful to have this early postoperative study for comparison and troubleshooting of problems in the future.

◆ Most patients are observed in the hospital overnight, but outpatient band surgery is becoming more common recently, and is likely to be the most common postoperative management strategy soon.

◆ A dedicated postoperative adjustment and follow-up schedule must be provided to achieve even reasonable results with gastric banding. Weight loss approaches that seen after gastric bypass when patients have access to band adjustments on short notice. The first adjustment is not offered until 6 weeks after the operation.

STEP 5: PEARLS AND PITFALLS

◆ Failure to repair even the smallest hiatal hernia can result in worsening of reflux as the band is inflated, leading to frustrating symptoms and unsatisfactory outcomes.

◆ The position of the bra line and belt line should be kept in mind when selecting the location of the 15-mm trocar to minimize discomfort over the site of the injection port.

◆ The posterior aspect of the distal esophagus and stomach wall are at risk for injury when passing the angled dissector through the retrogastric tunnel. One must be sure no resistance is met when the instrument is inserted and flexed. In addition, there should be no esophageal or gastric tissue when passing the tip of the instrument through the peritoneum at the angle of His. Often the peritoneum overlying the left crus immediately to the left of the angle of His should be bluntly opened before passing the dissector through the pars flaccida window. If this is done, the tip of the dissector will be easily identified.

◆ Once buckled, the band can be quite difficult or impossible to reopen. One should be sure the band is in the appropriate position and will not be too tight before closing it. If the band appears too tight, the underlying fat along the lesser curvature or at the esophagogastric junction may need to be divided with the cautery or ultrasonic shears. Rarely, the band may have to be replaced with a larger size.

◆ Careful needle management and knot tying must be used to avoid sticking any component of the band system. Leaks of the band balloon can be fixed only by replacing the whole system. The needle should remain in view continuously.

CHAPTER 36

MECKEL'S DIVERTICULECTOMY

Dai H. Chung

STEP 1: SURGICAL ANATOMY

- Meckel's diverticulum is an outpouching in the terminal ileum on the antimesenteric border. It exists in approximately 2% of the population but is largely asymptomatic. The frequent presence of ectopic gastric mucosa contributes to its common clinical presentation of brisk gastrointestinal (GI) hemorrhage.

STEP 2: PREOPERATIVE CONSIDERATIONS

- Asymptomatic Meckel's diverticulum is identified during abdominal cavity operation for other unrelated etiology. In general, resection of asymptomatic Meckel's diverticulum should be considered carefully based on the patient's overall condition and initial reasons for laparotomy.

- All symptomatic Meckel's diverticulum should be resected. Massive lower GI tract hemorrhage is its typical presentation, and the diagnosis is determined by scintigraphy with sodium technetium-99m (Tc-99m)-pertechnetate, which localizes ectopic gastric mucosa.

- For Meckel's diverticulitis, its presenting signs and symptoms are generally indistinguishable from acute appendicitis and determined only at operation.

- Preoperative prophylactic antibiotic should be administered intravenously 30 minutes before skin incision.

STEP 3: OPERATIVE STEPS

1. INCISION

- Patient is positioned supine and the right-sided transverse abdominal skin incision is made slightly inferior to the umbilicus (**Figure 36-1**).

◆ For a laparoscopic approach, umbilical trocar incision is made for the laparoscope and two additional small trocar incisions on either side of the abdomen for instrumentation.

◆ Meckel's diverticulum is typically located on the antimesenteric side of the terminal ileum, within 2 to 3 feet from the ileocecal region **(Figure 36-2)**.

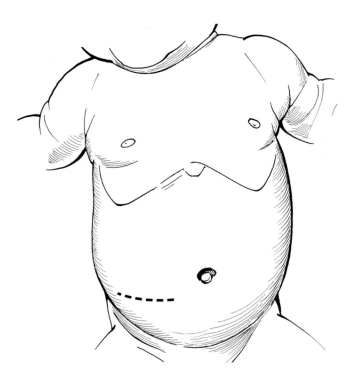

FIGURE 36–1

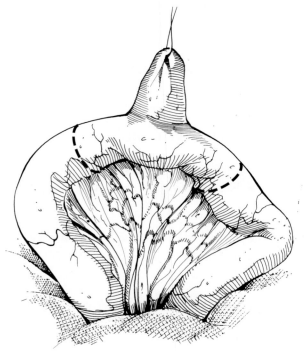

FIGURE 36–2

2. DISSECTION

◆ Segmental resection of ileum incorporating the Meckel's diverticulum is the ideal resection margin, because ectopic mucosa may be present throughout the entire axis of the diverticulum **(Figure 36-3)**. For resection, proximal and distal luminal content flow should be controlled using either gentle placement of bowel clamps or circumferential vessel loops. A stapling device may also be used to perform bowel resection.

◆ Alternatively, wedge resection of the diverticulum is also acceptable, if no abnormal thickening at the base is confirmed. After controlling intraluminal flow, the surgeon resects the diverticulum using a knife or electrocautery **(Figure 36-4)**.

◆ Two-layer anastomosis is preferred using inner running chromic sutures with outer interrupted seromuscular silk stitches **(Figure 36-5)**. For small infants (younger than 6 months), single-layer anastomosis with full-thickness silk sutures is also acceptable. The mesenteric defect should be closed to prevent potential internal hernia.

◆ For a laparoscopic approach, the tip of the Meckel's diverticulum is suspended with a grasper, and an ensdoscopic gastrointestinal anastomosis (GIA) stapler is used to transect at its base. Stapling at 90 degrees to the longitudinal axis of the ileum is ideal to avoid narrowing the lumen **(Figure 36-6)**.

3. CLOSING

◆ Once anastomosis is complete and hemostasis is ensured, abdominal fascia closure is performed in layers using absorbable sutures (3-0 polyglycolic) in a continuous manner.

◆ The skin is reapproximated with a subcuticular stitch of 5-0 absorbable Monocryl suture.

STEP 4: POSTOPERATIVE CARE

◆ Nasogastric tube decompression is seldom necessary.

◆ Patient may be started on an oral clear liquid diet on postoperative day 1 and then gradually advanced to regular diet appropriate for age.

◆ Two doses of postoperative intravenous antibiotics are administered.

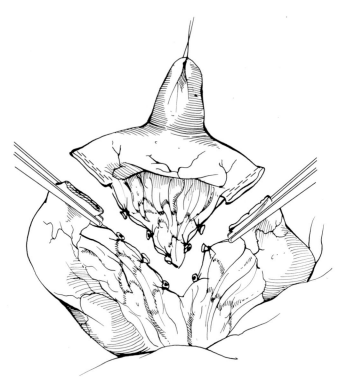

FIGURE 36–3

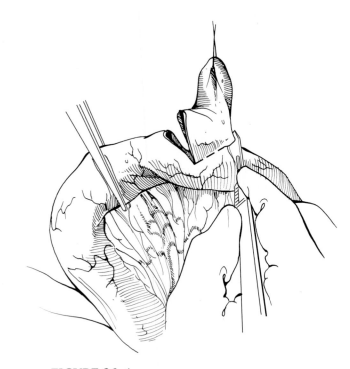

FIGURE 36–4

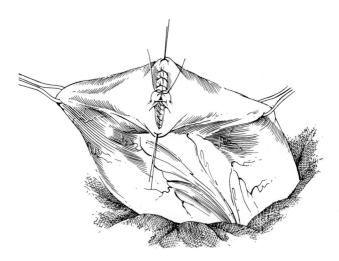

FIGURE 36–5

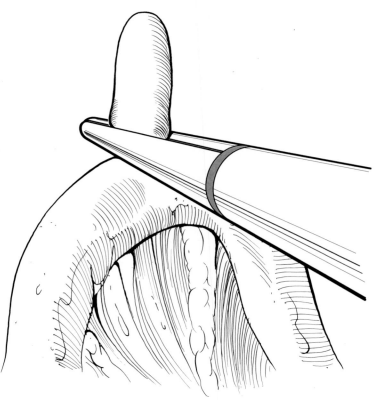

FIGURE 36–6

STEP 5: PEARLS AND PITFALLS

- Adequate resection of Meckel's diverticulum with complete incorporation of any ectopic mucosa is critical to this procedure.

- Laparoscopic approach is gaining popularity; however, it is critical to ensure adequate resection margin at the base.

SELECTED REFERENCES

1. Yahchouchy EK, Marano AF, Etienne JC, Fingerhut AL: Meckel's diverticulum. J Am Coll Surg 2001;192:658-662.
2. Cullen JJ, Kelly KA: Current management of Meckel's diverticulum. Adv Surg 1996;29:207-214.
3. Brown RL, Azizkhan RG: Gastrointestinal bleeding in infants and children: Meckel's diverticulum and intestinal duplication. Semin Pediatr Surg 1999;8:202-209.
4. Rothenberg SS: Laparoscopic segmental intestinal resection. Semin Pediatr Surg 2002;11:211-216.

CHAPTER 37

LAPAROSCOPIC APPENDECTOMY

Arthur P. Sanford

STEP 1: SURGICAL ANATOMY

- ◆ Anatomic relationships of the appendix for laparoscopic appendectomy are identical to those for the open appendectomy.

- ◆ With the limited access and visibility possible through the laparoscope, the serosal landmarks of the colon and appendix become more significant.

STEP 2: PREOPERATIVE CONSIDERATIONS

- ◆ Early diagnosis and expeditious operative intervention for appendicitis prevents the complications of perforation and spillage of purulence.

- ◆ Perform laparoscopic appendectomy after careful consideration with the option of open appendectomy and after assessing the patient, habitus, placement of trocars and scars, and likelihood that you can complete the procedure without needing to convert to an open procedure.

STEP 3: OPERATIVE STEPS

1. INCISION/TROCAR PLACEMENT

- Both the surgeon and assistant/camera operator assume places at the left side of the patient **(Figure 37-1)**.

- Access to the peritoneum begins with a 12-mm umbilical port, placed by either Hasson or Veress technique and insufflated to 15 cm H_2O pressure for placement of the laparoscope.

- Thorough laparoscopic evaluation of the abdomen is undertaken to ensure that it is appropriate to proceed without conversion to an open procedure.

- The patient is placed in enough of the Trendelenburg position to move the intra-abdominal contents out of the lower quadrants of the abdomen.

- Two additional ports are placed under direct visualization from the laparoscope, with a 5-mm port in the left lower quadrant (LLQ) and a 10-mm port in the right upper quadrant (RUQ).

- Transillumination of the abdominal wall prevents injury to the nearby vascular structures.

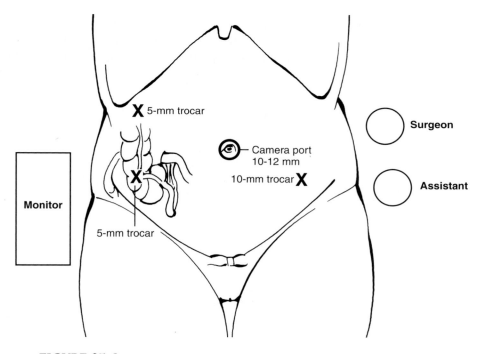

FIGURE 37–1

2. DISSECTION

♦ Use the instruments to expose the cecum and appendix.

♦ It is necessary to dissect the cecum to take down the white line of Toldt and adequately mobilize the base of the appendix and the mesoappendix.

♦ Elevate the cecum and base of the appendix using a laparoscopic Babcock clamp from the RUQ trocar.

♦ Identify the mesoappendix containing the appendiceal artery and pass a curved Maryland dissector through the mesoappendix at the base of the appendix; visualize both sides of the mesoappendix to ensure no other unintended structures are present.

♦ Divide the mesoappendix between the free edge of the mesoappendix and the previously dissected point using an endoscopic stapler, endoscopic clips, or a harmonic scalpel **(Figure 37-2)**.

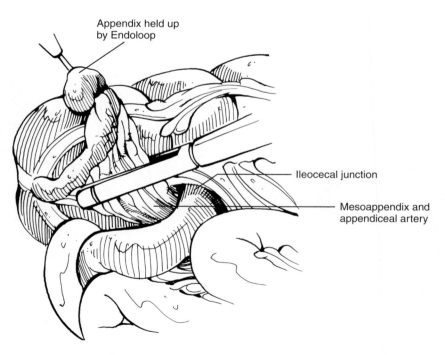

FIGURE 37–2

◆ Ligate the appendical base with either an endoscopic stapler using a tissue load or an Endoloop to prevent spillage of cecal contents (**Figure 37-3**).

◆ Then either place the appendix in an Endobag or retract into the larger RUQ trocar for withdrawal from the abdomen (**Figure 37-4**).

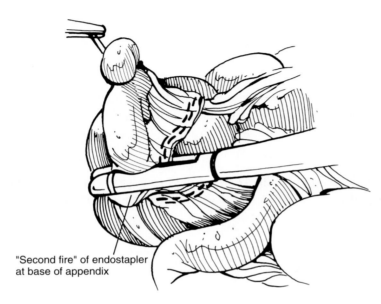

"Second fire" of endostapler
at base of appendix

FIGURE 37–3

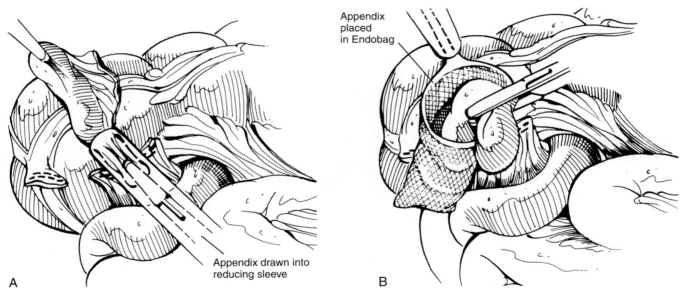

Appendix drawn into
reducing sleeve

Appendix
placed
in Endobag

A

B

FIGURE 37–4

3. CLOSING

◆ Undertake a final inspection for hemostasis before removal of the laparoscope and ports.

◆ Minimize irrigation of the abdomen to a volume that you can completely aspirate to prevent abscess formation.

◆ Remove ports under direct visualization from within the abdomen.

◆ Undertake suture closure for any port greater than 5 mm and the umbilical port.

◆ Apply sterile dressings.

◆ No peritoneal drains are indicated.

STEP 4: POSTOPERATIVE CARE

◆ If placed at operation, nasogastric tube and Foley catheter can be removed immediately postoperatively.

◆ Dietary resumption may begin immediately in the case of acute appendicitis, but if free purulence was found at operation, postoperative ileus mandates awaiting the return of bowel function.

◆ Postoperative antibiotics are not necessary in acute appendicitis but should be continued in the presence of intra-abdominal purulence.

STEP 5: PEARLS AND PITFALLS

◆ Placement of trocars facilitates intra-abdominal manipulation and avoids narrow angles of functional use.

SELECTED REFERENCES

1. Silen W, Cope Z: Cope's Early Diagnosis of the Acute Abdomen, 21st ed. New York, Oxford University Press, 2005, pp 67-83.
2. Lally KP, Cox CS Jr, Andrassy R: The appendix. In Townsend CM, Beauchamp RD, Evers BM, Mattox KL (eds): Sabiston Textbook of Surgery, 17th ed. Philadelphia, Saunders, 2004, pp 1381-1399.

CHAPTER 38

Open Appendectomy

Arthur P. Sanford

STEP 1: SURGICAL ANATOMY

- ◆ The blood supply for the appendix comes from the appendiceal artery, a branch of the ileocolic artery.

- ◆ The location of the appendix in the right lower quadrant (RLQ) is variable, depending on a possible retrocecal position.

- ◆ **Note:** The gravid uterus also displaces the cecum cephalad.

- ◆ To increase exposure of the peritoneal cavity, extend a muscle-splitting incision, lateral to the arcuate line, medially and laterally.

STEP 2: PREOPERATIVE CONSIDERATIONS

- ◆ History, physical examination, laboratory tests, and computed tomography (CT) scan as indicated will identify patients with acute appendicitis for appendectomy.

- ◆ Appropriate preoperative antibiotics should be administered upon confirmation of the diagnosis of appendicitis until operative intervention, with postoperative administration based on operative findings. Coverage should include typical intestinal flora, including gram-negative organisms and anaerobes.

STEP 3: OPERATIVE STEPS

1. INCISION

◆ Identify the midpoint of a line between the umbilicus and right anterior-superior iliac spine. Appropriate skin incision is made at this level **(Figure 38-1)**.

◆ Electrocautery is used to dissect down to the fascia of the external oblique muscle, lateral to the rectus abdominus muscle.

◆ The external oblique fascia is incised along the length of its fibers and spread.

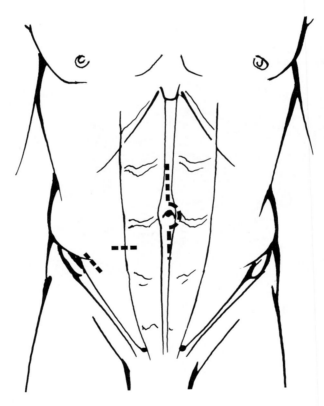

FIGURE 38–1

◆ Blunt dissection can be used to separate the underlying internal oblique and transversus abdominis muscles along the length of their fibers in layers, as well **(Figure 38-2).**

◆ The peritoneum can then be cleaned off and incised.

◆ Peritoneal incision is typically done by elevating the peritoneum between two hemostats and making sure no intra-abdominal contents have been trapped in the operative field.

2. DISSECTION

◆ Once the peritoneum has been entered, the RLQ can be explored to identify the location of the appendix and any associated pathologic findings or abscess.

◆ The small intestine can be retracted medially, allowing identification of the cecum.

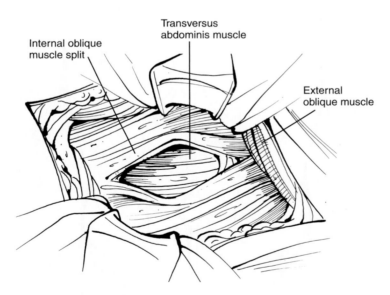

FIGURE 38–2

♦ The taeniae coli converge at the base of the appendix, allowing identification of anatomic landmarks that aid in its removal **(Figure 38-3)**.

♦ Mobilization of the cecum by incision of the lateral, avascular attachments of the right side of the colon may allow better visualization of a retrocecal appendix **(Figure 38-4)**.

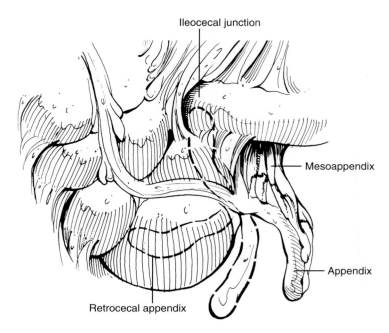

FIGURE 38–3

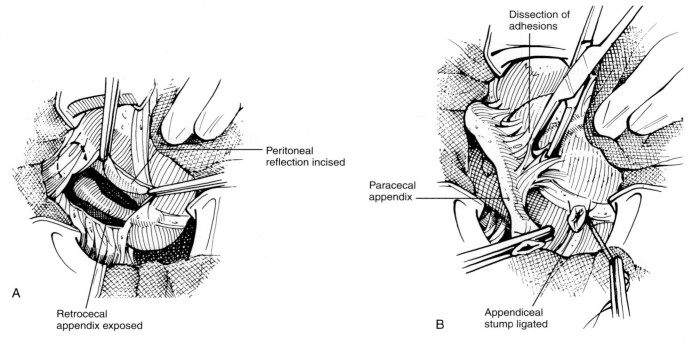

FIGURE 38–4

- The cecum and base of the appendix are brought out of the wound.

- The mesoappendix containing the appendiceal artery is divided and ligated down to the serosa of the appendix where it joins the cecum **(Figure 38-5)**.

- The appendiceal base is crushed at the proposed level of division, and the clamp released and replaced distally. This creates a position to ligate the appendix **(Figure 38-6, A)**.

- The appendiceal stump can be doubly ligated with slowly absorbing suture, or the appendix can be singly ligated with rapidly absorbing suture if it is to be imbricated. The ligature is to obliterate the lumen but not strangulate the short segment of appendix between the ligatures **(Figure 38-6, B)**.

- The mucosa of the appendiceal stump should be obliterated with electrocautery to prevent accumulation of a mucocele.

- Purse-string suture around the appendiceal base or Z stitch can be used to secure the base of the appendix, as well.

3. CLOSING

- Once hemostasis is ensured, the abdomen is closed in layers, starting with the peritoneum (optional); if a muscle-splitting incision has been performed, the internal oblique and transversus abdominis muscles require only loose approximation.

- More attention should be given to closure of the fascia of the external oblique muscle, which will be a strength layer.

- In more corpulent patients, Scarpa's fascia can be loosely approximated.

- If purulent appendicitis was found at exploration, the skin should be left open, or closed in acute appendicitis.

- No intraperitoneal drains are indicated.

- Sterile dressings are applied.

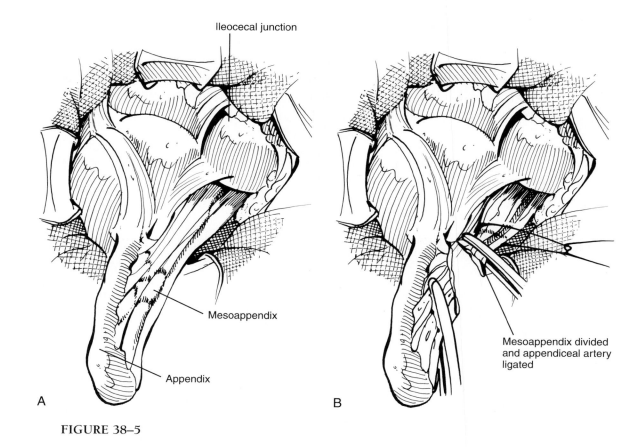

Ileocecal junction

Mesoappendix

Appendix

A

B

Mesoappendix divided
and appendiceal artery
ligated

FIGURE 38–5

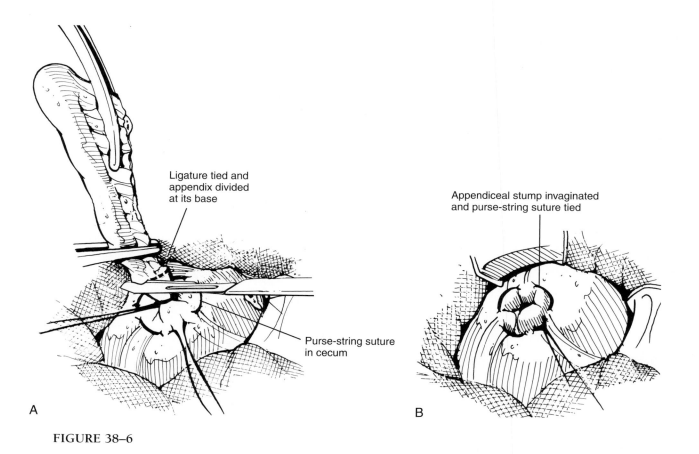

Ligature tied and
appendix divided
at its base

Purse-string suture
in cecum

Appendiceal stump invaginated
and purse-string suture tied

A

B

FIGURE 38–6

STEP 4: POSTOPERATIVE CARE

- ◆ Dietary resumption may begin immediately in the case of acute appendicitis, but if free purulence was found at operation, postoperative ileus mandates awaiting the return of bowel function.

- ◆ Postoperative antibiotics are not necessary in acute appendicitis but should be continued in the presence of intra-abdominal purulence.

STEP 5: PEARLS AND PITFALLS

- ◆ Placement of the skin incision slightly cephalad to the anticipated position of the appendix in its anatomic position will allow easier manipulation of the cecum, once brought out of the RLQ wound.

- ◆ Despite preoperative evaluation, a missed diagnosis (normal appendix at exploration) should include a search for the underlying pathologic condition, including perforated duodenal ulcer, pancreatitis, urinary tract infections or calculi, gynecologic pathologic findings, or Meckel's diverticulum.

SELECTED REFERENCES

1. Silen W, Cope Z: Cope's Early Diagnosis of the Acute Abdomen, 21st ed. New York, Oxford University Press, 2005, pp 67-83.
2. Lally KP, Cox CS Jr, Andrassy R: The appendix. In Townsend CM, Beauchamp RD, Evers BM, Mattox KL (eds): Sabiston Textbook of Surgery, 17th ed. Philadelphia, Saunders, 2004, pp 1381-1399.

CHAPTER 39

INTUSSUSCEPTION

Dai H. Chung

STEP 1: SURGICAL ANATOMY

- Intussusceptions in infants and toddlers occur as a result of invagination of proximal bowel (intussusceptum) into the lumen of the distal bowel (intussuscipiens). It typically involves the ileocolic region of the intestine with variable degree of colonic involvement. The leading point of the intussusception is typically a Peyer's patch in the terminal ileum. Occasionally, Meckel's diverticulum may be the leading point of the intussusception.

STEP 2: PREOPERATIVE CONSIDERATIONS

- Sudden, intermittent, colicky, severe abdominal pain associated with calm, asymptomatic periods in a toddler is characteristic. It is commonly associated with a history of preceding upper respiratory tract infections. A jelly stool is another characteristic of this condition.

- Abdominal radiographs may demonstrate paucity of bowel gas in the right lower quadrant along with soft tissue mass in the upper abdomen representing an intussusceptum.

- When the diagnosis is suspected, hydration status along with presence of acute abdomen (peritonitis, perforation, or obstruction) should be assessed. Ultrasound examination can identify the presence of an intussusception.

- Contrast (or air) enema study can confirm diagnosis and also potentially be therapeutic. Hydrostatic or pneumatic reduction of intussusception is successful in approximately 60% to 95% of cases. A history longer than 24 hours or radiologic evidence of bowel obstruction significantly reduces the likelihood of successful reduction by enema.

- Contrast is instilled through a catheter from a reservoir 100 cm above the patient. Air is delivered at 80 to 150 mm Hg. The criterion for successful reduction is reflux of contrast or air into the terminal ileum.

- After a successful reduction, the child is observed overnight to ensure complete resolution of symptoms and absence of recurrence.

STEP 3: OPERATIVE STEPS

1. INCISION

◆ Operative reduction is necessary for failed enema reduction and/or multiple recurrent intussusceptions.

◆ Preoperative prophylactic intravenous antibiotic should be administered 30 minutes before skin incision.

◆ Patient is positioned supine and the right-sided transverse abdominal skin incision is made slightly inferior to the umbilicus **(Figure 39-1)**. Depending on the degree of intussusception, the incision may be made at the level of or above the umbilicus.

2. DISSECTION

◆ Muscle-splitting technique is used to dissect through external, internal oblique, and transversalis fascia.

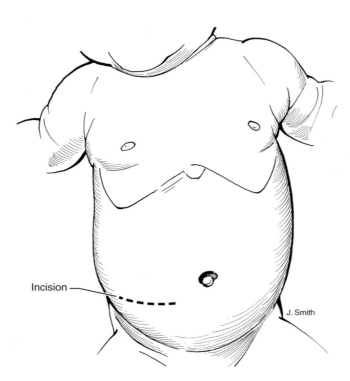

FIGURE 39–1

◆ Bowel loops of intussusception are carefully delivered into the wound and reduction is achieved by gently squeezing the bowel distal to the apex along with gentle pull of proximal bowel to aid with the reduction **(Figure 39-2)**. Traction or strong pulling of intussuscepted bowel should be avoided, because this can easily result in further injury to the bowel.

◆ After reduction, general condition of the intussuscepted terminal ileum should be assessed carefully **(Figure 39-3)**. Occasionally, segmental bowel resection is necessary if reduction cannot be achieved or necrotic bowel is identified after reduction. Commonly, reduced terminal ileum appears dusky and thickened to palpation. Placement of a warm, moist sponge for a few minutes can improve local tissue perfusion, thus, potentially avoiding unnecessary surgical resection.

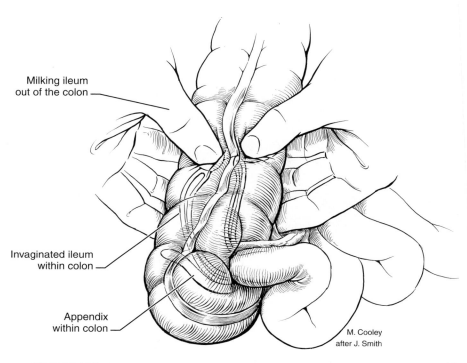

Milking ileum
out of the colon

Invaginated ileum
within colon

Appendix
within colon

M. Cooley
after J. Smith

FIGURE 39–2

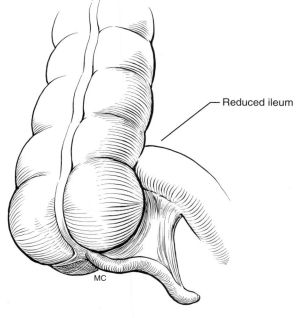

Reduced ileum

MC

FIGURE 39–3

◆ Standard appendectomy should be performed if the adjacent cecal wall is normal **(Figure 39-4)**. In general, inversion appendectomy is not recommended.

3. CLOSING

◆ Once reduction is achieved or resection performed (if required) and hemostasis is ensured, abdominal fascia closure is performed in layers using 3-0 absorbable sutures in continuous manner.

◆ The skin is reapproximated with a subcuticular stitch of 5-0 absorbable suture.

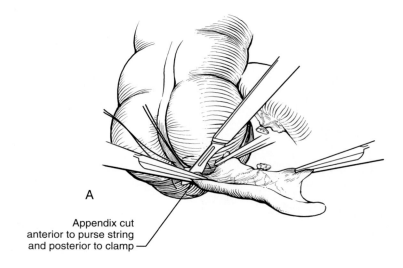

A

Appendix cut
anterior to purse string
and posterior to clamp —

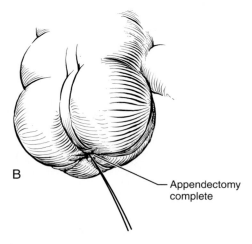

B

— Appendectomy
complete

FIGURE 39–4

STEP 4: POSTOPERATIVE CARE

- ◆ Nasogastric tube decompression is necessary if there were symptoms of bowel obstruction preoperatively.

- ◆ The patient may be started on an oral clear liquid diet with return of bowel function and gradually advanced to regular diet.

- ◆ Two postoperative doses of an intravenous antibiotic are administered.

STEP 5: PEARLS AND PITFALLS

- ◆ Recognition of acute abdomen is critical to prompt surgical management and to avoid unsafe delays and risks to patients with attempts of enema reduction.

- ◆ Intussusception should be reduced by pushing the involved bowel retrogradely, with only gentle pull if necessary.

SELECTED REFERENCES

1. DiFiore JW: Intussusception. Semin Pediatr Surg 1999;8:214-220.
2. Shehata S, El Kholi N, Sultan A, El Sahwi E: Hydrostatic reduction of intussusception: Barium, air or saline. Pediatr Surg Int 2000;16:380-382.

CHAPTER 40

CORRECTION OF MALROTATION WITH MIDGUT VOLVULUS

Carlos A. Angel

STEP 1: SURGICAL ANATOMY

- In patients without malrotation, a broad mesentery and attachments at the cecum and ascending and descending colon prevent volvulation of the small bowel around the superior mesenteric vessels **(Figure 40-1)**. Incomplete rotation of the intestine during fetal development results in lack of these attachments, a very narrow mesentery, and peritoneal bands (Ladd's bands) that place the cecum close to the duodenum. This incomplete rotation may cause obstruction in the second or third portions of the duodenum **(Figure 40-2)**. The absence of peritoneal attachments, in combination with a narrow mesentery and a relatively fixed point to the duodenocecal area, creates the conditions in which the midgut can volvulate (in clockwise fashion) around the superior mesenteric vessels **(Figure 40-3)**. Although most patients present in the neonatal period or in the first year of life with bilious vomiting, this condition may remain asymptomatic until adulthood.

STEP 2: PREOPERATIVE CONSIDERATIONS

- In children younger than 1 year of age, however, bilious vomiting must be considered due to malrotation until proven otherwise. The diagnosis is confirmed by upper gastrointestinal series, barium enema, or sonography. Once this condition is diagnosed, surgical correction should always be treated as an emergency.

- In the presence of midgut volvulus, time is of the essence. Vigorous intravenous resuscitation and broad-spectrum antibiotics are initiated. The stomach is decompressed with an orogastric tube, and a urinary catheter is placed to measure urine output. The operation should not be delayed in an attempt to correct metabolic imbalances, because this is usually futile until the volvulus is managed.

- After thorough gastric suctioning, general endotracheal anesthesia is induced with the patient supine. The abdomen is prepped with povidone-iodine (Betadine) solution.

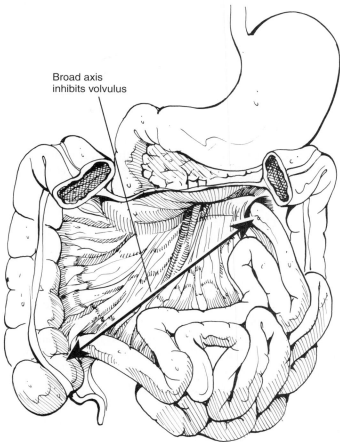

Broad axis
inhibits volvulus

FIGURE 40–1

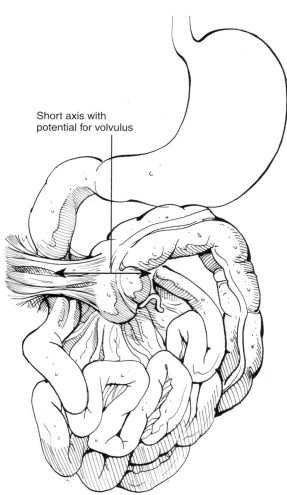

Short axis with
potential for volvulus

FIGURE 40–2

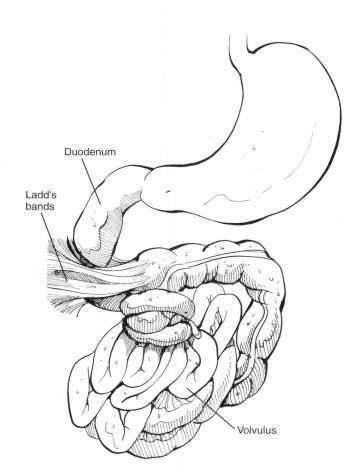

Duodenum

Ladd's
bands

Volvulus

FIGURE 40–3

STEP 3: OPERATIVE STEPS

1. INCISION

♦ A right upper quadrant transverse laparotomy is performed, the muscles are divided in the direction of the incision, and the umbilical vein in the free edge of the falciform ligament is tied with 5-0 silk sutures and divided **(Figure 40-4)**.

2. DISSECTION

♦ The entire bowel is delivered outside the incision to verify the presence or absence of a midgut volvulus (see Figure 40-4). Because, in most cases, the volvulus has twisted clockwise, devolvulation should proceed counterclockwise **(Figure 40-5)**. This maneuver usually produces significant improvement in the appearance of the intestine. Warm compresses can be applied to intestine of questionable viability and left alone for 10 minutes. All intestines that are frankly gangrenous should be removed; intestines of questionable viability should be left behind, and a second-look laparotomy planned in 24 to 36 hours to allow for better demarcation of the segments to be resected. Often during this second-look operation a primary end-to-end anastomosis can be performed. Ladd's bands extend from the cecum and ascending colon, attaching to the anterior surface of the duodenum and across the duodenum to the posterior aspect of the right upper quadrant. These bands are sharply divided **(Figure 40-6)**. To relieve any obstruction, the surgeon must free the duodenum from the Ladd's bands on both its lateral and medial aspects. The duodenum is straightened by division of the ligament of Treitz. Takedown of Ladd's bands results in separation of the duodenum, cecum, and ascending colon and broadening of the mesentery **(Figure 40-7)**. A nasogastric tube is passed to make sure that there is no further obstruction of the duodenal lumen. Because the cecum will ultimately lie in the left upper quadrant, an appendectomy is performed **(Figure 40-8)**. The intestines are retrieved into the abdominal cavity beginning with the duodenum, leaving the duodenum and small bowel on the *right* side and the colon on the *left* side.

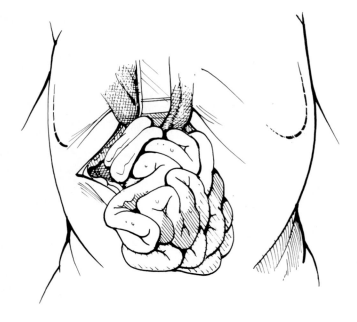

FIGURE 40–4

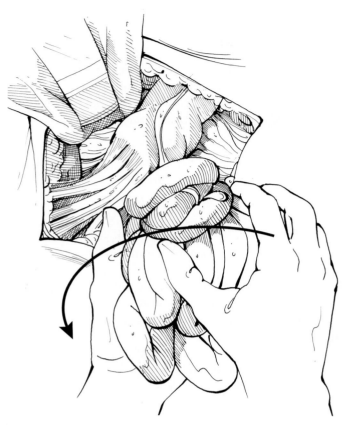

FIGURE 40–5

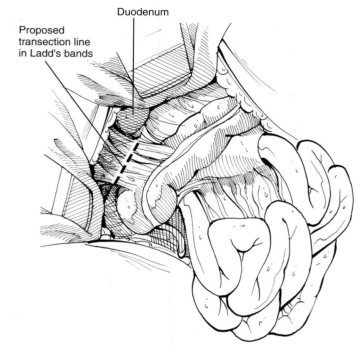

Proposed
transection line
in Ladd's bands

Duodenum

FIGURE 40–6

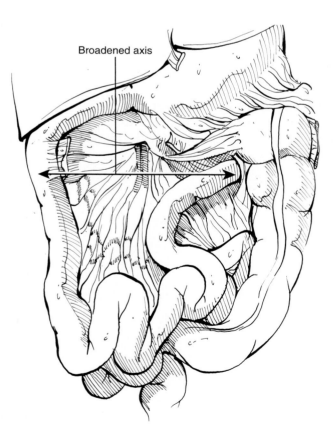

Broadened axis

FIGURE 40–7

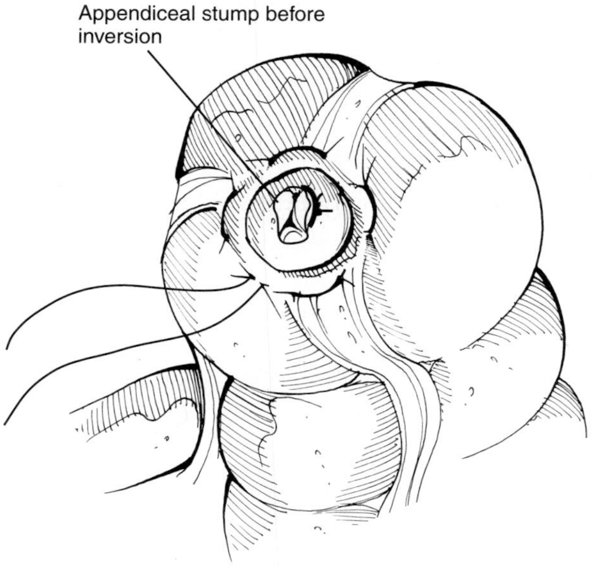

Appendiceal stump before
inversion

FIGURE 40–8

3. CLOSING

◆ The incision is closed in layers with running 5-0 polyglactin sutures on tapered needles. These layers include the peritoneum and posterior rectus fascia, anterior rectus fascia, Scarpa's fascia, and subcutaneous tissue. The skin is infiltrated with 0.25% bupivacaine without epinephrine and closed with a running 6-0 subcuticular absorbable undyed monofilament suture and adhesive strips.

STEP 4: POSTOPERATIVE CARE

◆ Continued monitoring in an intensive care setting and administering intravenous fluids, antibiotics, and analgesics are mandatory during the initial postoperative period. Prolonged ileus or short bowel syndrome may require total parenteral nutrition. The incidence of recurrent volvulus is less than 10%. Ladd's procedure creates enough adhesions, broadens the mesentery, and eliminates the fixed point resulting from bands between the duodenum and cecum so that recurrence of midgut volvulus is unlikely and seldom reported. The risk of small bowel obstruction is not higher than that of any other open abdominal operations. Wound infections or dehiscence are rare in cases in which no intestinal resections are performed. Massive loss of bowel may lead to sepsis, septic shock, and death. In survivors, short bowel syndrome results in dependency on total parenteral nutrition and ultimately in small bowel or multiorgan transplantation.

STEP 5: PEARLS AND PITFALLS

◆ Great attention must be paid at the time of replacing the small bowel in the intestinal cavity. It is very easy to kink or twist the intestinal blood supply, and any signs of venous congestion or intestinal ischemia should prompt the surgeon to immediately exteriorize the bowel, correct any twists or kinks of the mesentery, and resume the process of placing the intestines in order back into the intestinal cavity.

SELECTED REFERENCES

1. Spitz L: Malrotation. In Spitz L, Coran AG (eds): Rob and Smith's Operative Surgery (Pediatric Surgery), 5th ed. London, Chapman & Hall, 1995, pp 341-347.
2. Ashcraft K: Atlas of Pediatric Surgery. Philadelphia, Saunders, 1994, pp 97-101.

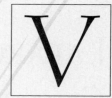

SECTION V

GALLBLADDER

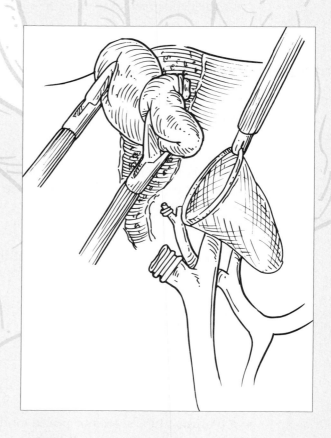

LAPAROSCOPIC AND OPEN CHOLECYSTECTOMY

Taylor S. Riall

STEP 1: SURGICAL ANATOMY

- An understanding of the biliary and hepatic arterial anatomy is critical to performing successful cholecystectomy (laparoscopic or open). The cystic duct joins the common hepatic duct, forming the common bile duct distally. The cystic artery most commonly originates from the right hepatic artery. However, there are many variants in both biliary and hepatic arterial anatomy.

- To avoid common bile duct or hepatic arterial injury during cholecystectomy (laparoscopic or open), it is necessary to identify the cystic duct at its origin from the infundibulum of the gallbladder and to identify the cystic artery as it enters the gallbladder.

STEP 2: PREOPERATIVE CONSIDERATIONS

1. PREPARATION

- The indications for laparoscopic cholecystectomy include symptomatic cholelithiasis, acute cholecystitis, chronic cholecystitis, biliary dyskinesia (low gallbladder ejection fraction), and gallstone pancreatitis.

- Before induction of anesthesia, sequential compression devices should be placed on the lower extremities and patients should be given subcutaneous heparin for venous thromboembolism prophylaxis.

- The patient should be asked to void just before coming to the operating room. If this is not done, a Foley catheter should be placed or a straight catheterization should be performed for bladder decompression.

- A orogastric tube should be placed for decompression of the stomach.

◆ A first-generation cephalosporin should be used for antibiotic prophylaxis, unless the patient is taking therapeutic antibiotics for acute cholecystitis. Clindamycin can be used if the patient has a penicillin allergy.

2. OPERATING ROOM SETUP

◆ The patient is placed supine on the operating room table. Both arms can be out to the side, or the left arm can be tucked.

◆ The surgeon stands on the patient's left side, and the first assistant stands on the patient's right side. If a second assistant is available to hold the camera, he or she stands on the patient's left side below the surgeon.

◆ The video monitors are arranged at the head of the bed on the right and left sides, such that the surgeons and assistants can comfortably view the monitor across from them without having to turn around.

◆ A fluoroscopy table or table with x-ray capability is needed for possible intraoperative cholangiography.

◆ For open cholecystectomy, the patient is supine with both arms extended.

STEP 3: OPERATIVE STEPS

LAPAROSCOPIC CHOLECYSTECTOMY

1. INCISION/PORT PLACEMENT

- The first port is placed in the supraumbilical position. An 11-mm port is used **(Figure 41-1)**.

- Access to the abdominal cavity can be performed using an open (Hasson) or closed (Veress needle) technique.

- For either technique, the supraumbilical area is anesthetized with local anesthetic. A transverse supraumbilical incision is made using a scalpel.

- For the open technique, electrocautery is used to dissect down to the fascia. The fascia is secured with 0 Vicryl sutures, and the peritoneal cavity is opened under direct vision. The trocar is placed directly into the peritoneal cavity and secured with the 0 Vicryl sutures on each side.

- For the closed technique, the Veress needle is inserted blindly into the abdominal cavity after skin incision.

- The surgeons should observe free flow of fluid into the needle to confirm intraperitoneal positioning.

- The initial pressure should be low (<3 mm Hg), confirming intraperitoneal placement. The abdomen is then insufflated to 15 mm Hg.

- The 11-mm trocar can then be placed under direct vision using a zero-degree laparoscope and an optical port.

- After initial port placement, a 30-degree or zero-degree laparoscope can be used. The 30-degree scope can facilitate difficult views but requires a more experienced assistant.

- A 5-mm port is then placed in the right anterior axillary line along the costal margin, between the 12th rib and the iliac crest (see Figure 41-1).

- A second 5-mm port is placed in the midclavicular line. Both of the 5-mm ports should be 2 fingerbreadths below the right costal margin and should be 7 to 10 cm apart (see Figure 41-1).

- The final port is placed in the epigastric region (see Figure 41-1). This port should be placed last and should be positioned after the gallbladder is retracted superiorly **(Figure 41-2)**. This allows the surgeon to place the port in a direct line to the infundibulum. This provides a good line for clip placement and avoids unnecessary torque on the instruments.

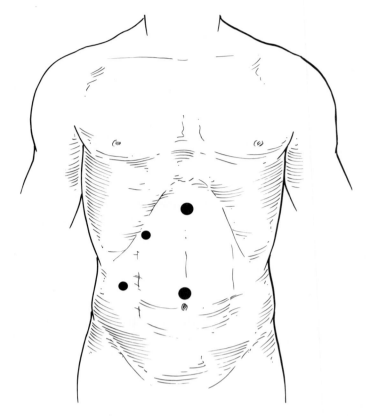

FIGURE 41–1

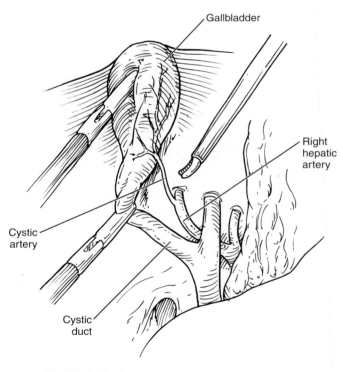

Gallbladder

Right
hepatic
artery

Cystic
artery

Cystic
duct

FIGURE 41–2

2. DISSECTION

- ◆ The patient can be placed in reverse Trendelenburg position to allow the duodenum, stomach, and other intra-abdominal contents to fall away from the dissection field.

- ◆ A 5-mm locking grasper is placed through the most lateral port, and the gallbladder is retracted cephalad, toward the patient's right shoulder (see Figure 41-2).

- ◆ A second grasper is placed through the medial 5-mm port and used to retract the infundibulum of the gallbladder laterally (to the patient's right side) and inferiorly, opening up the triangle of Calot (bounded by the cystic duct, the common hepatic duct, and the liver edge) and better exposing the cystic structures (see Figure 41-2). This can be done by the first assistant or by the operating surgeon.

- ◆ Using a Maryland dissector through the epigastric port, any adhesions between the gallbladder and the omentum, hepatic flexure, stomach, and duodenum are taken down by grasping them close to the gallbladder and peeling them down along the axis of the cystic duct.

- ◆ The dissection of the triangle of Calot is best performed laterally to medially, first exposing the infundibulum–cystic duct junction on the patient's right side, then medially. The cystic duct is circumferentially dissected (see Figure 41-2).

- ◆ The cystic artery, which is usually medial and superior with the infundibulum retracted laterally, is then dissected circumferentially in similar fashion using the Maryland dissector (see Figure 41-2).

- ◆ No structure should be divided until the cystic duct is identified at the cystic duct–infundibulum junction and the cystic artery has been identified and dissected free.

- ◆ At this point, cholangiography can be performed if indicated. **Figure 41-3** demonstrates the placement of a Kumar clamp through the 5-mm port. This clamp is placed entirely across the cystic duct, occluding it and preventing flow of the contrast back into the gallbladder. A cholangiocatheter with a needle tip is then placed through the clamp and into the cystic duct distally. Contrast is injected, and a cholangiogram can be obtained to evaluate the biliary anatomy and rule out any retained stones in the common bile duct.

- ◆ The cystic duct can now be ligated with clips applied with a 10-mm clip applier through the epigastric port. Two clips should be placed distally and one proximally on the duct **(Figure 41-4).**

- ◆ A curved or hook scissors is then used to divide between the most proximal and the two distal clips **(Figure 41-5).**

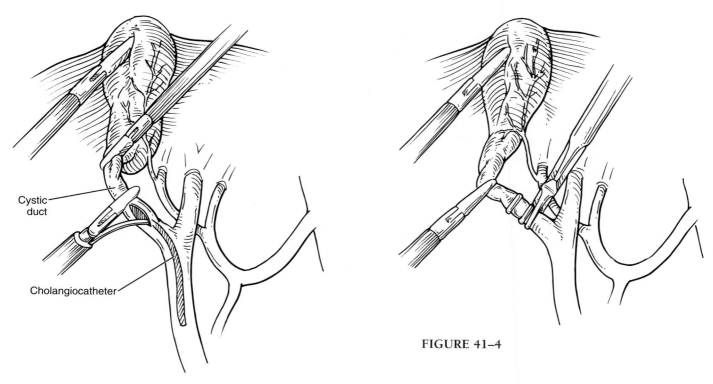

Cystic
duct

Cholangiocatheter

FIGURE 41–3

FIGURE 41–4

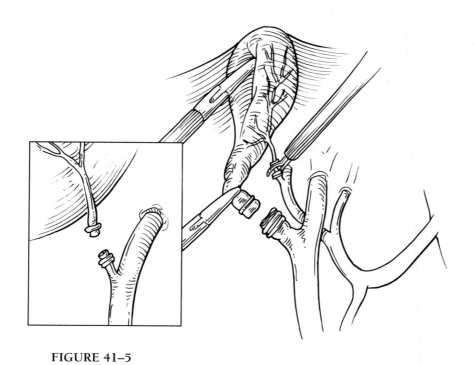

FIGURE 41–5

- The cystic artery is then clipped in similar fashion (see Figure 41-5) and divided with the scissors, leaving two clips on the distal, retained stump.

- The gallbladder is then dissected out of the gallbladder fossa using electrocautery **(Figure 41-6).** The hook cautery is shown here, but the dissection can also be performed with a spatula, the Maryland dissector, or the scissors. This dissection is performed from the infundibulum to the fundus. The graspers in the two 5-mm ports are used to provide traction on the gallbladder, exposing the dissection plane between the gallbladder and the liver.

- Before completely removing the gallbladder from the liver bed, the surgeon can use the gallbladder to retract the liver while inspecting the cystic artery and duct stumps for any signs of bleeding or bile leakage. Any bleeding from the liver bed should also be controlled at this time.

- After removal of the gallbladder, the camera is placed through the epigastric port. A retrieval bag is placed through the umbilical port **(Figure 41-7).** Removal with a retrieval bag is recommended especially if there is spillage of bile or gallstones.

- The gallbladder is placed in the retrieval bag (see Figure 41-7) and removed through the umbilical port. The camera can then be replaced and the camera returned to the umbilical port.

- The patient is returned to a flat, supine position. The field is then irrigated to ensure no bleeding or bile leakage.

3. CLOSING

- The ports are removed under direct vision to make sure there is no bleeding from the port sites.

- The fascia at the two 11-mm ports is usually closed with interrupted 0 Vicryl suture, which can be placed using conventional methods or the laparoscopic suture passer. The fascia at the 5-mm ports does not require closure.

- The skin is then closed with absorbable subcuticular sutures.

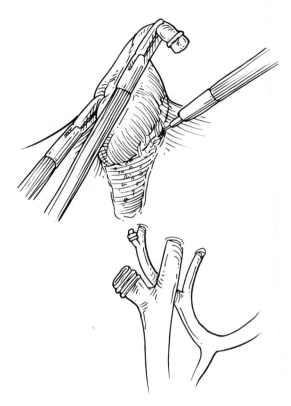

FIGURE 41–6

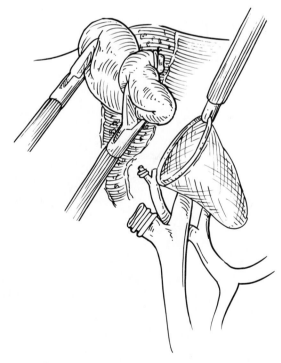

FIGURE 41–7

OPEN CHOLECYSTECTOMY

1. INCISION

♦ The incision for open cholecystectomy is typically made 2 fingerbreadths below the right costal margin, although an upper midline incision can also be used (**Figure 41-8, A**).

♦ Retractors are placed to retract the skin, as well as to retract the liver superiorly (**Figure 41-8, B**).

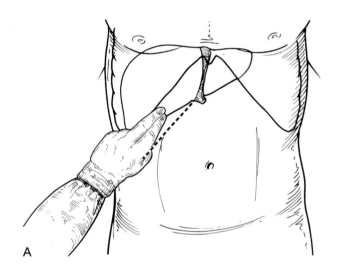

A

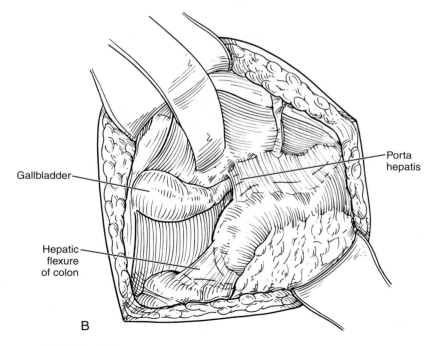

Porta
hepatis

Gallbladder

Hepatic
flexure
of colon

B

FIGURE 41–8

2. DISSECTION

◆ A clamp is placed on the gallbladder fundus and used to retract the gallbladder superiorly **(Figure 41-9)**. A second clamp can be used to retract the infundibulum of the gallbladder laterally (see Figure 41-9), exposing the triangle of Calot.

◆ Ideally, the cystic artery is identified, circumferentially dissected, and ligated (see Figure 41-9) before dissection of the gallbladder out of the gallbladder fossa. As in the laparoscopic case, care should be taken not to injure the right hepatic artery.

◆ The gallbladder is then removed from the gallbladder fossa from the top down using electrocautery **(Figure 41-10)**.

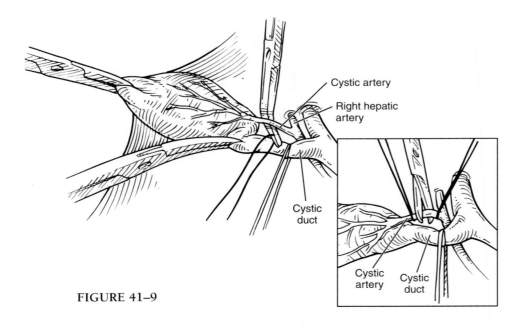

Cystic artery

Right hepatic artery

Cystic duct

Cystic artery   Cystic duct

FIGURE 41–9

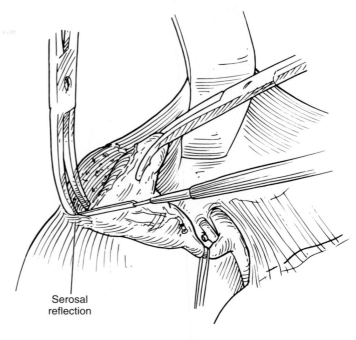

Serosal reflection

FIGURE 41–10

◆ Clamps are placed proximally and distally on the cystic duct. The cystic duct is divided between the clamps (**Figure 41-11, A**), and the gallbladder is removed from the field.

◆ The cystic duct stump is suture ligated using a 3-0 silk suture (**Figures 41-11, B-D**).

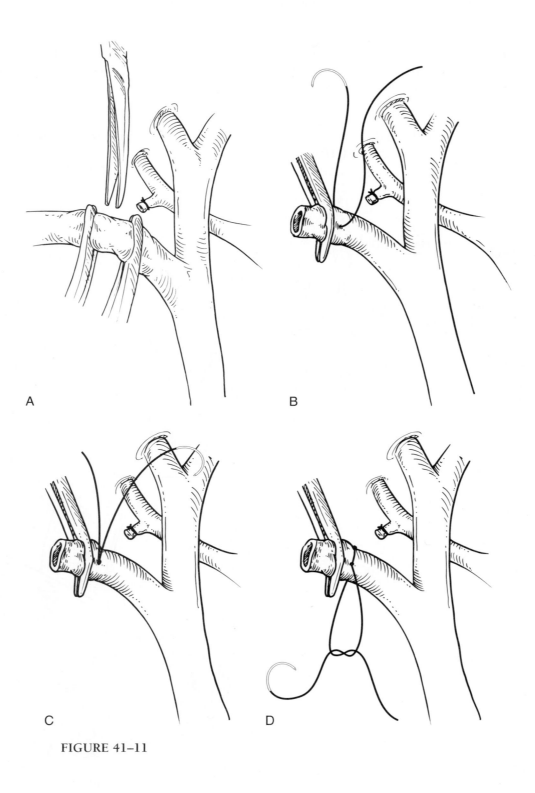

A

B

C

D

FIGURE 41–11

- The cystic duct and cystic artery stumps are examined for any signs of bile leakage or bleeding **(Figure 41-12)**. The abdomen is copiously irrigated with normal saline solution.

3. CLOSING

- The placement of closed suction drains is not always required. They are placed only if bile leakage from the cystic duct stump is expected or observed. If bile leakage is observed, the surgeon must rule out common bile duct injury.

- The fascia is closed in two layers using running or interrupted sutures.

- The skin is then closed with absorbable subcuticular sutures or skin staples.

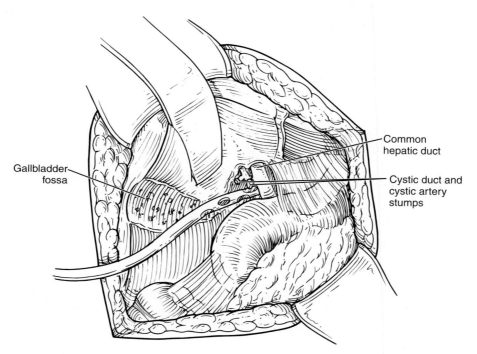

FIGURE 41–12

STEP 4: POSTOPERATIVE CARE (LAPAROSCOPIC AND OPEN CHOLECYSTECTOMY)

- Postoperative complications include hematoma, bleeding, or leakage from the cystic duct stump.

- If a drain is placed operatively, the output should be monitored. If no bilious drainage is observed at 24 to 48 hours, the drain can be removed.

- If bilious drainage is noted, this can initially be managed conservatively with continued observation. Liver function tests should be performed to evaluate for bile duct injury. If drainage persists, endoscopic retrograde cholangiopancreatography (ERCP) is indicated to definitively rule out injury. In addition, a common bile duct stent placed via ERCP will also treat persistent cystic duct leaks in the absence of common bile duct injury.

- Clear liquids can be started immediately postoperatively for both laparoscopic and open cholecystectomy and generally advanced as tolerated. Patients undergoing open procedures may have a longer time to return to regular diet.

- Patients are discharged home the same day after laparoscopic cholecystectomy and 2 to 3 days after open cholecystectomy.

- Longer stay may be necessary in the setting of acute cholecystitis.

- For uncomplicated gallstone disease, antibiotics are not continued postoperatively.

STEP 5: PEARLS AND PITFALLS

- To avoid bile duct injury, it helps to retract the infundibulum of the gallbladder laterally to open up the triangle of Calot and form a 90-degree angle of the cystic duct with the common hepatic duct. Pulling the infundibulum superiorly orients the cystic duct similar to the common bile duct and can lead to injury.

- After dividing the cystic duct and cystic artery, it is useful to begin the dissection of the gallbladder bluntly to make sure there are no ductal structures present.

- A 5-mm port and a 5-mm clip applier can be used at the epigastrium. If this is done, a 5-mm camera will need to be present if a retrieval bag is going to be used to remove the gallbladder, because this comes in only the larger size.

- Cholecystectomy can be performed from the top down in both the laparoscopic and the open settings, although it is more difficult in the laparoscopic setting.

◆ The clips placed on the cystic duct and artery need to completely occlude the lumen. If this is not possible on the cystic duct, an Endoloop can be placed. In this setting, the anatomy should be reviewed to ensure that the cystic duct is ligated and the anatomy has not been incorrectly identified, because the clips are usually large enough to occlude the cystic duct.

◆ Cholangiogram can be performed routinely or selectively, based on the preference of the operating surgeon.

◆ If common bile duct stones are identified, a laparoscopic or open common bile duct exploration can be performed. Alternatively, ERCP can be performed to clear the duct postoperatively.

◆ Multiple previous abdominal surgeries, severe cardiac disease, and severe acute cholecystitis are relative contraindications to laparoscopic cholecystectomy. When a patient has a history of multiple previous abdominal surgeries, an open technique should be used to place the initial umbilical port.

◆ When performing laparoscopic procedures, it is best to convert to an open procedure if (1) there is uncontrolled bleeding; (2) safe laparoscopic access to the abdominal cavity cannot be obtained; (3) the anatomy of the triangle of Calot cannot be clearly delineated; or (4) injury to the common bile duct, small bowel, or any other structure is suspected. This should not be considered a failure.

SELECTED REFERENCES

1. Jones DB, Maithel SK, Schneider BE (eds): Atlas of Minimally Invasive Surgery. Woodbury, Conn, Ciné-Med, 2006, pp 12-39.
2. Cameron JL: Atlas of Surgery, vol 1. Philadelphia, BC Decker, 1990, pp 2-9.
3. Posther KE, Pappas TN: Acute cholecystitis. In Cameron JL (ed): Current Surgical Therapy, 8th ed. Philadelphia, Mosby, 2002, pp 385-391.
4. Hutter MM, Rattner DW: Open cholecystectomy: When is it indicated? In Cameron JL (ed): Current Surgical Therapy, 8th ed. Philadelphia, Mosby, 2002, pp 400-401.

CHAPTER 42

CHOLEDOCHODUODENOSTOMY AND HEPATICOJEJUNOSTOMY

Taylor S. Riall

STEP 1: SURGICAL ANATOMY

- A comprehensive understanding of the biliary, pancreatic, and foregut anatomy is critical before performing any surgical procedure on the biliary tree, pancreatic duct and pancreas, distal stomach, and duodenum.

- **Figure 42-1, A** demonstrates the location of the right subcostal incision 2 fingerbreadths below the right costal margin.

- **Figure 42-1, B** shows the surgical anatomy after placement of retractors on the abdominal wall and liver. In this case the patient had prior cholecystectomy. The common bile duct travels posterior to the first portion of the duodenum and through the head of the pancreas, draining into the ampulla of Vater in the second portion of the duodenum. The hepatic artery lies medial to the common bile duct, and the portal vein is posterior to the common bile duct.

- The diameter of the common bile duct needs to be at least 1.5 to 2.0 cm for a choledochoduodenostomy to be performed successfully. This is usually the case if the procedure is being performed for retained common bile duct stones. Hepaticojejunostomy can be performed in nondilated ductal systems, but it is more difficult.

STEP 2: PREOPERATIVE CONSIDERATIONS

1. PREPARATION

- The indications for side-to-side choledochoduodenostomy include retained common bile duct stones after common bile duct exploration, primary common bile duct stones, and recurrent common bile duct stones. The side-to-side choledochoduodenostomy enables retained or new stones to pass spontaneously. It is especially useful in the setting of distal common bile duct stricture.

◆ The indications for hepaticojejunostomy include benign distal biliary stricture, recurrent cholangitis secondary to a stricture or stone disease, palliation of jaundice in patients with unresectable periampullary cancer, and bile duct injury (usually iatrogenic). With bile duct injuries, the duct is often normal caliber, making the operation more difficult.

◆ The patient is placed supine on the operating room table, with both arms extended.

◆ Subcutaneous heparin is given, and sequential compression devices are used to prevent venous thromboembolism.

◆ A second-generation cephalosporin is used for antibiotic prophylaxis before skin incision and redosed for the first 24 hours.

◆ A Foley catheter is placed to monitor urine output.

◆ A nasogastric (NG) tube is placed to decompress the stomach. This is left in postoperatively.

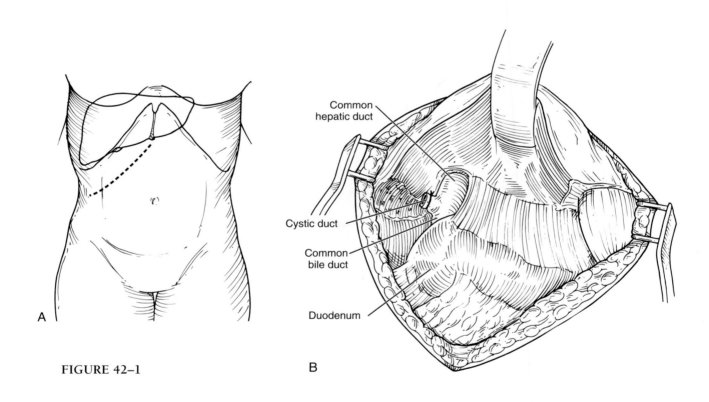

FIGURE 42–1

STEP 3: OPERATIVE STEPS

CHOLEDOCHODUODENOSTOMY

1. INCISION

♦ The operation is performed through a right subcostal incision (see Figure 42-1, A). It can also be done using an upper midline incision.

2. DISSECTION

♦ Patients have often had previous cholecystectomy, and there may be adhesions between the liver and the portal structures. The adhesions are dissected sharply using electrocautery or scissors, or both.

♦ The duodenum and extrahepatic biliary tree are exposed (see Figure 42-1, B).

♦ The duodenum is kocherized out of the retroperitoneum **(Figure 42-2).** This may require mobilization of the hepatic flexure of the colon inferiorly. It is important to completely mobilize the duodenum to perform the choledochoduodenostomy without tension.

♦ The duodenum is sharply dissected off the anterior surface of the distal common bile duct. The common bile duct should be clearly exposed in the anterior and lateral surfaces.

♦ Using a no. 15 blade, an anterior choledochotomy is made in the common bile duct where it courses posterior to the duodenum. The choledochotomy is extended to a length of approximately 2 cm using Potts scissors **(Figure 42-3).** Stones are extracted if present.

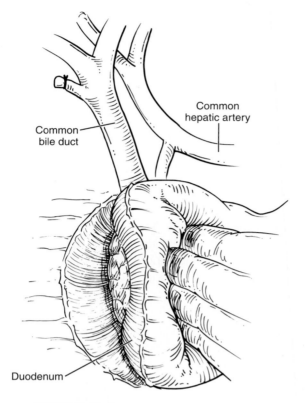

FIGURE 42–2

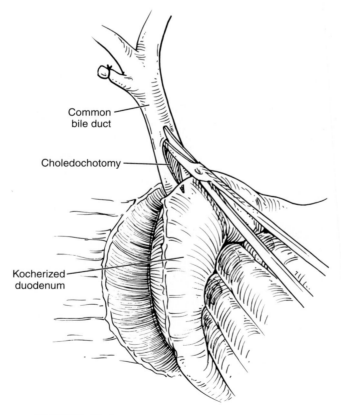

FIGURE 42–3

- A transverse duodenotomy is then performed adjacent to the choledochotomy using electrocautery **(Figure 42-4, A)**.

3. ANASTOMOSIS

- Absorbable 4-0 Vicryl sutures are used to perform a single-layer, side-to-side anastomosis. A stitch is first placed at the inferior apex of the choledochotomy, through the center of the back wall of the duodenotomy with the knots placed on the outside. This apex suture is tied (see Figure 42-4, A).

- Next, lateral stay sutures are placed. They pass from the midpoint of the choledochotomy on each side to the respective end of the duodenotomy. These sutures are not tied and are placed in hemostat clamps **(Figure 42-4, B)**. Holding these stay sutures out laterally nicely aligns the bile duct and duodenum for placement of the remaining sutures.

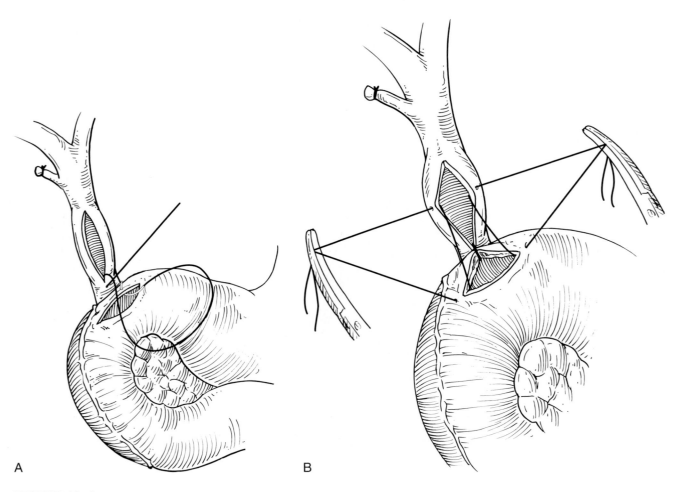

A   B

FIGURE 42–4

◆ The posterior row of sutures is then placed with the knots on the outside **(Figure 42-5).** These can be tied and cut as the surgeon proceeds from the apex stitch to the lateral corner on each side.

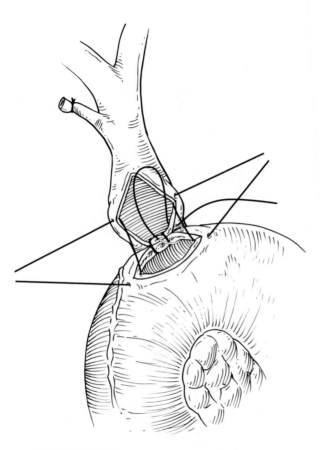

FIGURE 42–5

◆ The anterior row is then completed in similar fashion. An apex stitch is placed from the midpoint of the duodenotomy to the superior apex of the choledochotomy **(Figure 42-6, A)**. The remaining stitches are placed in the anterior bile duct **(Figure 42-6, B)**. To allow for easier suture placement and careful approximation of the bile duct and duodenal mucosa, the anterior sutures are all placed before they are tied down.

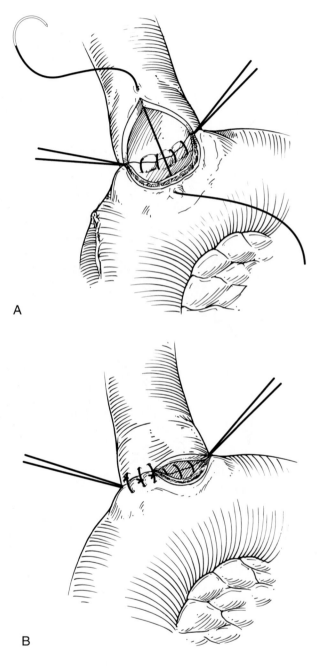

FIGURE 42–6

HEPATICOJEJUNOSTOMY

1. INCISION

- The operation is performed through a right subcostal incision or an upper midline incision **(Figure 42-7).**

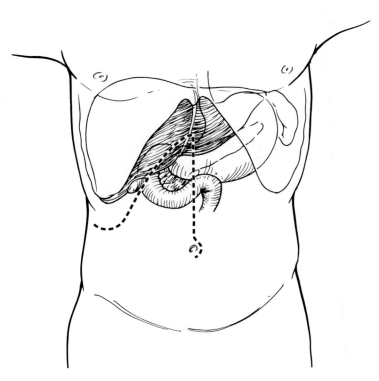

FIGURE 42–7

2. DISSECTION

◆ Patients have often had previous cholecystectomy and there may be adhesions between the omentum and the liver and portal structures. These are dissected sharply using electrocautery or scissors, or both **(Figure 42-8)**.

◆ The common bile duct/common hepatic duct are circumferentially dissected **(Figure 42-9)**. If a biliary stent has been previously placed, it can be palpated in the porta hepatis to help identify the dissection plane. A vessel loop can be placed around the common bile duct, which can facilitate dissection superiorly and inferiorly along the duct. The gallbladder has often already been removed, but if it has not, cholecystectomy should be performed at the same time.

◆ The common hepatic duct is then divided using electrocautery or scissors **(Figure 42-10)**. If a stricture is present, it is critical to divide the bile duct proximal to the stricture.

◆ **Figure 42-11** shows excision of the strictured portion of the extrahepatic biliary tree if present. The insert shows the ligation of the distal common bile duct with running absorbable suture.

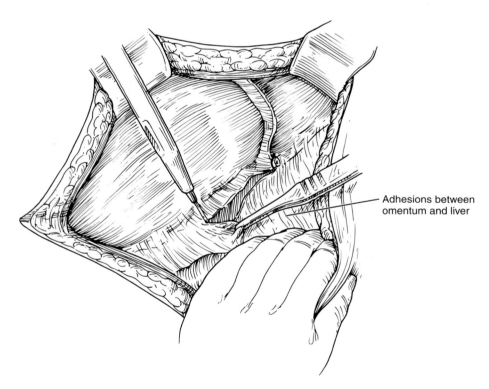

Adhesions between
omentum and liver

FIGURE 42–8

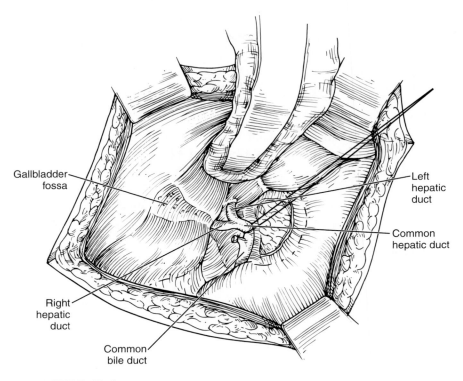

Gallbladder fossa

Left hepatic duct

Common hepatic duct

Right hepatic duct

Common bile duct

FIGURE 42–9

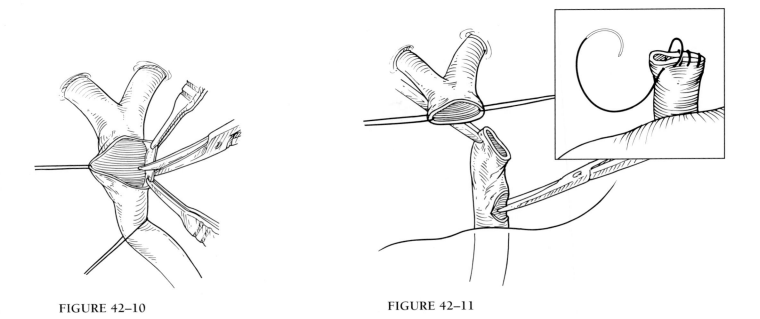

FIGURE 42–10

FIGURE 42–11

◆ After the bile duct has been divided and the distal end oversewn, a Roux-en-Y limb is created. The transverse colon is lifted and the ligament of Treitz is identified. The jejunum is divided distal to the ligament of Treitz at a convenient arcade such that the Roux limb will easily reach the bile duct. An incision is made in the transverse mesocolon above the duodenum and to the right of the middle colic vessels (**Figure 42-12**).

◆ The Roux limb is brought retrocolic through the transverse mesocolon on the right side for the hepaticojejunostomy (**Figures 42-13 and 42-14**).

◆ The staple line of the jejunal limb is oversewn using interrupted 3-0 silk sutures.

3. ANASTOMOSIS

◆ Absorbable 4-0 Vicryl sutures are used to perform a single-layer, end-to-side hepaticojejunostomy.

◆ Before making an enterotomy in the jejunum, the posterior layer of the anastomosis is performed. Two corner sutures are placed first. These sutures go through the jejunum, incorporating the submucosa. They are then placed inside out through the bile duct and secured with hemostats (**Figure 42-15, A**).

◆ The back wall is then placed through the jejunum, incorporating the submucosa, and then through the bile duct with the knots on the inside (**Figure 42-15, B**).

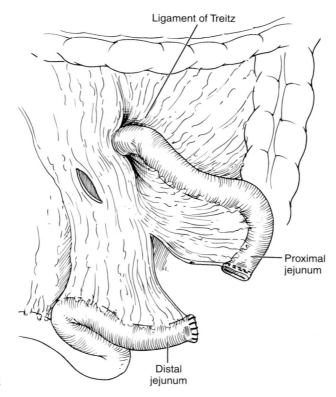

Ligament of Treitz

Proximal jejunum

Distal jejunum

FIGURE 42–12

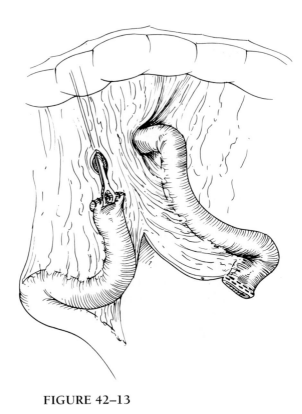

FIGURE 42–13

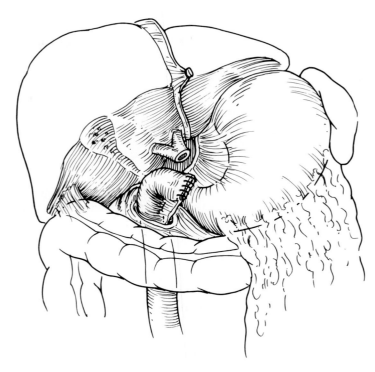

FIGURE 42–14

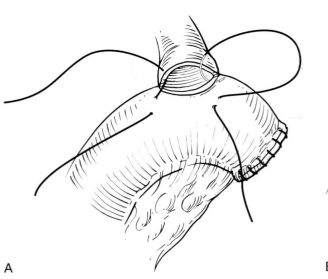

A

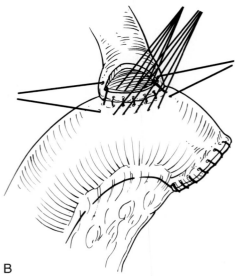

B

FIGURE 42–15

◆ After all the sutures in the posterior row have been placed, the jejunum is telescoped down to the bile duct and all of the sutures are tied, including the corner sutures. The corner sutures are placed back in hemostats and the other sutures are cut.

◆ After tying the posterior row of sutures, the surgeon makes a small enterotomy in the jejunum (**Figure 42-16, A**). If a biliary stent is used, the surgeon places the distal end into the jejunal limb at this point.

◆ The anterior layer of the anastomosis is completed using interrupted 4-0 Vicryl sutures through both the jejunum and the bile duct (**Figure 42-16, B**).

◆ After construction of the hepaticojejunostomy, the surgeon perfoms a standard two-layer end-to-side jejunojejunal anastomosis to restore bowel continuity. The posterior row of interrupted 3-0 silk is shown in **Figure 42-17, A**. The running inner layer of 3-0 Vicryl is shown in **Figure 42-17, B**. This is a running, locking suture in the posterior row and a Connell stitch in the anterior row. **Figure 42-17, C** shows the interrupted layer of 3-0 silk sutures used to complete the anterior row.

◆ **Figure 42-17, D** shows the completed anastomosis. Interrupted 3-0 silk sutures are used to close the mesenteric defect at the jejunojejunal anastomosis (see Figure 42-17, D) and to tack the Roux limb to the transverse mesocolon, where it passes retrocolic to prevent internal herniation.

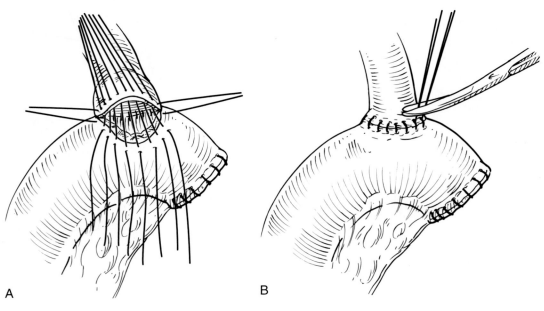

A   B

FIGURE 42–16

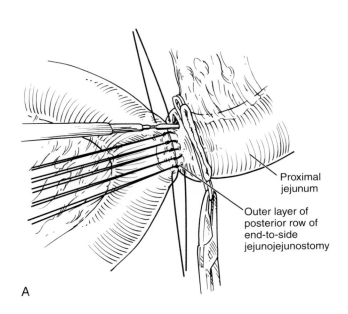

A

Proximal
jejunum

Outer layer of
posterior row of
end-to-side
jejunojejunostomy

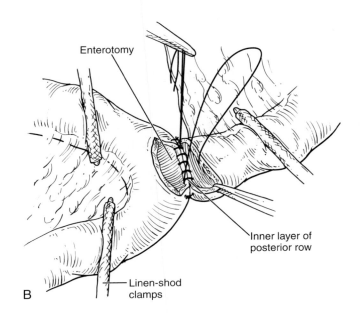

B

Enterotomy

Inner layer of
posterior row

Linen-shod
clamps

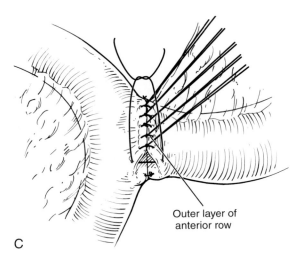

C

Outer layer of
anterior row

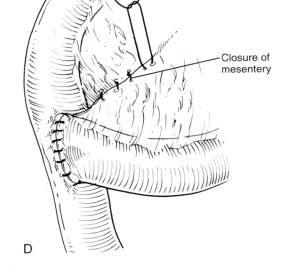

D

Closure of
mesentery

FIGURE 42–17

◆ The completed operation is shown in **Figure 42-18.**

4. CLOSING (CHOLEDOCHODUODENOSTOMY AND HEPATICOJEJUNOSTOMY)

◆ A closed suction drain is used to drain the choledochoduodenostomy or the hepaticojejunostomy in the event of bile leakage.

◆ The fascia is closed in running or interrupted fashion per the preference of the surgeon. Absorbable or permanent sutures can be used.

◆ The skin is closed with skin staples or absorbable subcuticular sutures.

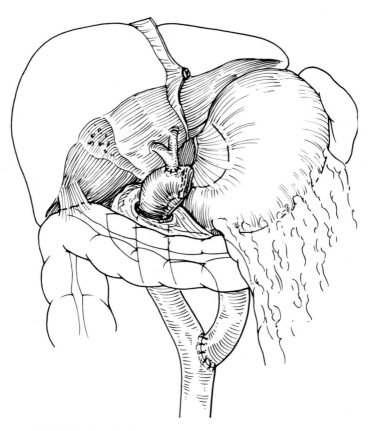

FIGURE 42–18

STEP 4: POSTOPERATIVE CARE (CHOLEDOCHODUODENOSTOMY AND HEPATICOJEJUNOSTOMY)

- Postoperative complications include bile leak, stricture at the hepaticojejunostomy, cholangitis, and hematoma/bleeding.

- If a percutaneous biliary stent was placed before surgery, it should initially be placed to external drainage. Before removal of the drain, the biliary stent should be capped off, internalizing the drainage.

- The output from the operatively placed drain should be monitored. If no bilious drainage is observed after 4 to 5 days (and after internalization of biliary drainage if stent is in place), the drain can be removed.

- If bilious drainage is noted, it can initially be managed conservatively with continued observation. Large leaks may require the placement of a percutaneous biliary drain to divert the bile flow externally while the anastomosis heals, if one was not present preoperatively.

- Biliary stents, if present before surgery or placed after, should be left in place at least 6 weeks before removal.

- An NG tube is kept in place the evening of surgery and removed on postoperative day 1.

- Clear liquids are started in 48 to 72 hours, and the diet is advanced as tolerated.

- The duration of stay is usually 5 to 8 days.

STEP 5: PEARLS AND PITFALLS

- In the past, percutaneous biliary stents were commonly placed before hepaticojejunostomy. Many studies show that infectious complications are increased if a biliary stent is placed preoperatively, presumably caused by bactobilia. However, if cholangitis is present preoperatively, a percutaneous or endoscopic stent is needed to relieve the obstruction and prevent sepsis. Cholangitis is uncommon in malignant obstruction. The data were from patients undergoing pancreaticoduodenectomy and have been extrapolated to hepaticojejunostomy alone.

- Tumors arising at the confluence of the right and left hepatic ducts require resection of the extrahepatic biliary tree, including the confluence, and require bilateral hepaticojejunostomies for reconstruction. In this case, bilateral preoperative stents may make the small anastomoses easier and prevent postoperative stricture formation.

- ◆ Preoperative biliary stents may also be helpful in the event of common bile duct injury to control leakage and make the anastomosis in a normal caliber bile duct easier.

- ◆ In the nondilated bile duct, it is best to perform the enterotomy in the jejunal limb before performing the posterior row of the hepaticojejunostomy to prevent occlusion of the lumen by excess tissue. This is not a problem in dilated bile ducts.

- ◆ With distal common bile duct stricture, malignancy should be considered and ruled out before biliary bypass.

SELECTED REFERENCES

1. Cameron JL: Atlas of Surgery, vol 1. Philadelphia, BC Decker, 1990, pp 28-57.
2. Sohn TA, Yeo CJ, Cameron JL, et al: Do preoperative biliary stents increase postoperative complications? J Gastrointest Surg 2000;4:258-267.
3. Jagannath P, Dhir V, Shrikhande S, et al: Effect of preoperative biliary stenting on immediate outcome after pancreaticoduodenectomy. Br J Surg 2005;92:256-361.
4. Povoski SP, Karpeh MS, Conlon KC, et al: Association of preoperative biliary drainage with postoperative outcome following pancreaticoduodenectomy. Ann Surg 1999;230:131-142.

SPHINCTEROPLASTY

Taylor S. Riall

STEP 1: SURGICAL ANATOMY

◆ A comprehensive understanding of the biliary, pancreatic, and foregut anatomy is critical before performing any surgical procedure on the biliary tree, pancreatic duct, pancreas, distal stomach, or duodenum.

◆ **Figure 43-1** illustrates the normal pancreaticobiliary anatomy. Structures that must be considered during sphincteroplasty include the gallbladder, the common bile duct (CBD), the head of the pancreas, the main and minor pancreatic ducts, the ampulla of Vater (major papilla), the minor papilla, and the duodenum. It is critical to understand the complex relationship of these structures to one another, with the CBD beginning at the confluence of the cystic duct and common hepatic duct. The CBD runs through the head of the pancreas and drains into the duodenum at the ampulla of Vater. In most patients the main pancreatic duct joins the distal CBD before draining into the ampulla of Vater, forming a common channel.

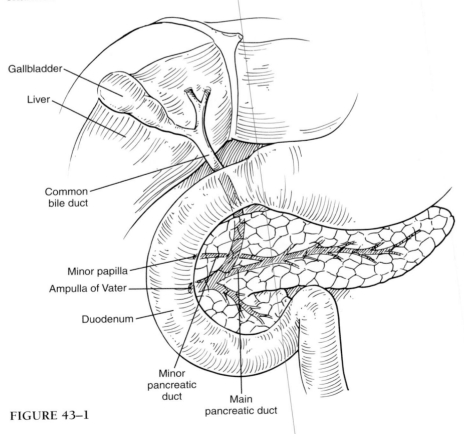

Gallbladder

Liver

Common bile duct

Minor papilla

Ampulla of Vater

Duodenum

Minor pancreatic duct

Main pancreatic duct

FIGURE 43–1

- **Figure 43-2** represents pancreas divisum, the most common congenital anomaly of the pancreatic ductal system. Pancreas divisum occurs in approximately 6% to 7% of healthy patients at autopsy. It occurs in up to 10% to 20% of patients with recurrent acute pancreatitis. Pancreas divisum results from a failure of fusion of the dorsal pancreatic duct and the duct draining the uncinate process and head of pancreas. The result is that the major portion of the drainage of the exocrine pancreas is through the minor papilla, with only the duct to the uncinate process draining to the ampulla of Vater. The role of this anomaly in causing pancreatitis is unclear, but it is thought to be the cause in a small number of patients with recurrent acute pancreatitis, pancreas divisum, and a stenotic minor papilla.

STEP 2: PREOPERATIVE CONSIDERATIONS

- The use of transduodenal sphincteroplasty is controversial in many settings. For many indications it has been replaced by endoscopic sphincterotomy via endoscopic retrograde cholangiopancreatography (ERCP). The decision to perform this operation depends on the surgeon's expertise, the clinical situation, and the expertise of local gastroenterologists.

- Transduodenal sphincteroplasty has been used in a variety of settings. The indications for transduodenal CBD sphincteroplasty include:
  - Calculous disease of the biliary tract not amenable to stone removal via ERCP.
    - Sphincteroplasty should be performed if the surgeon believes there are retained stones after CBD exploration.
    - Sphincterotomy and sphincteroplasty can be used to retrieve stones impacted in the distal CBD that cannot be removed with choledochotomy and CBD exploration.
    - Sphincteroplasty can be used to explore the CBD with a small-caliber duct in which choledochotomy and T-tube placement may be difficult.
  - Treatment of recurrent and acute pancreatitis with ampullary stenosis identified and no other cause of pancreatitis identified; considered a rare indication.
  - The use of sphincteroplasty and pancreatic duct septotomy for postcholecystectomy syndrome remains controversial.
  - CBD sphincteroplasty and pancreatic duct septotomy are often performed with minor papilla sphincteroplasty (see later) to ensure adequate drainage in patients with symptomatic pancreas divisum.

- The indications for minor papilla sphincteroplasty include:
  - Recurrent acute pancreatitis (abdominal pain and hyperamylasemia)
  - Pancreas divisum with no other obvious cause of acute pancreatitis identified

STEP 3: OPERATIVE STEPS

1. INCISION

- The patient is placed supine on the operating table, with both arms extended out to the side.

- A fluoroscopy table or table with radiographic capability is needed for possible intraoperative cholangiography.

- The operation can be performed through a right subcostal or upper midline incision.

- In addition to the abdominal wall being retracted, the liver should be retracted superiorly, exposing the gallbladder, portal structures, and duodenum **(Figure 43-3)**.

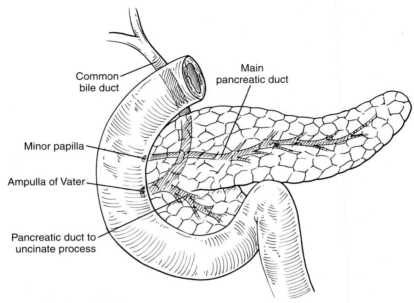

FIGURE 43–2

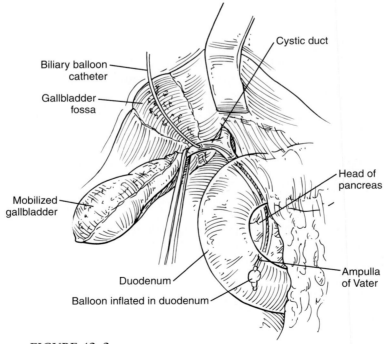

FIGURE 43–3

2. DISSECTION

◆ If the gallbladder is in place, a cholecystectomy is performed by dissecting the gallbladder out of the gallbladder fossa, from the fundus down to the cystic structures (see Figure 43-3). The cystic artery is identified and ligated.

◆ The cystic duct is then opened and a biliary balloon catheter is placed into the CBD from the cystic duct. Cholangiography, if indicated, is easily performed at this point. The catheter should exit into the duodenum at the ampulla of Vater.

◆ At this point the duodenum should be mobilized out of the retroperitoneum using the Kocher maneuver. Then the balloon should be inflated and pulled back flush to the ampulla of Vater and easily palpated (see Figure 43-3).

◆ After palpating the balloon on the biliary catheter, the balloon is advanced into the duodenum. Two 3-0 silk stay sutures are placed to the right and left of where the duodenotomy will be performed. A longitudinal duodenotomy is made at the site of initial palpation right over the ampulla of Vater **(Figure 43-4)**. This can be done with electrocautery.

◆ The surgeon can then place his or her finger in the duodenotomy and palpate the balloon and ampulla of Vater. The duodenotomy is then extended distally for adequate exposure of the ampulla **(Figure 43-5)**.

◆ Absorbable 5-0 sutures are then placed medial and lateral to the exiting biliary catheter at the ampulla of Vater (see Figure 43-5).

◆ Using the biliary catheter for guidance, the surgeon performs a sphincterotomy of the ampulla of Vater using electrocautery (see Figure 43-5). This should be performed slowly, 3 to 4 mm at a time for a total length of 1 to 2 cm. The length of the sphincterotomy will vary depending on the indication.

◆ After the sphincterotomy is performed, the CBD mucosa is approximated to the duodenal mucosa using interrupted 5-0 absorbable sutures. The apex suture is shown in **Figure 43-6**, with several other sutures already in place.

◆ Once the CBD is opened, the pancreatic duct orifice can be identified, and a lacrimal duct probe can be placed into the duct (see Figure 43-6).

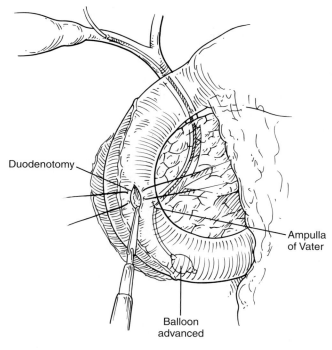

Duodenotomy

Ampulla
of Vater

Balloon
advanced

FIGURE 43–4

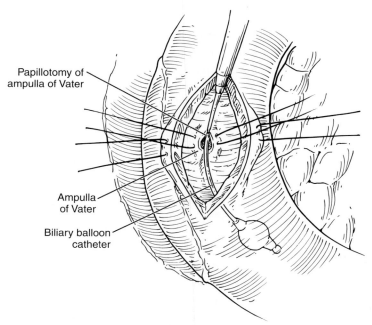

Papillotomy of
ampulla of Vater

Ampulla
of Vater

Biliary balloon
catheter

FIGURE 43–5

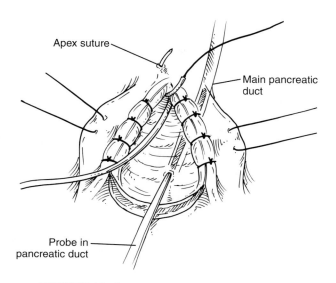

Apex suture

Main pancreatic
duct

Probe in
pancreatic duct

FIGURE 43–6

- To ensure adequate drainage of the pancreatic duct, a pancreatic duct septotomy can be performed over the probe (**Figure 43-7**).

- In the case of pancreas divisum, the duodenotomy may need to be extended proximally on the duodenum to identify the minor papilla. In cases where this is difficult to identify, secretin can be given to stimulate pancreatic secretion and aid in identification.

- The minor papilla is small and can be difficult to cannulate. A small lacrimal duct probe should be used and inserted atraumatically to prevent hematoma at the minor papilla (**Figure 43-8**).

- After cannulation, a papillotomy can be performed over the probe using electrocautery similar to performing the sphincterotomy at the major papilla.

- The pancreatic ductal mucosa is approximated to the duodenal mucosa using 5-0 absorbable suture, similar to the approximation of the CBD to the mucosa after ampulla of Vater sphincteroplasty.

- After the sphincteroplasty is completed, the biliary catheter can be retracted and a cholangiogram performed if necessary.

- The biliary catheter is then removed and the cholecystectomy is completed by ligating the cystic duct distal to the ductotomy made for the biliary balloon catheter, dividing the cystic duct, and removing the gallbladder from the field.

- The duodenotomy is then closed longitudinally in two layers. Care must be taken not to narrow the duodenal lumen. Stay sutures of 3-0 silk are placed at the most proximal and distal points of the duodenotomy. The first layer is performed with absorbable 3-0 suture in Connell fashion (**Figure 43-9**).

- The outer layer is closed in interrupted fashion using 3-0 silk suture (**Figure 43-10**).

- A closed-suction drain is placed to drain the duodenotomy.

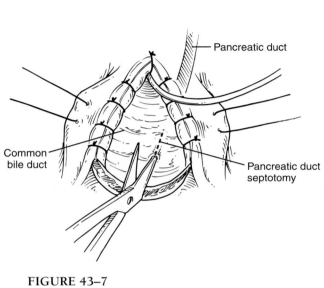

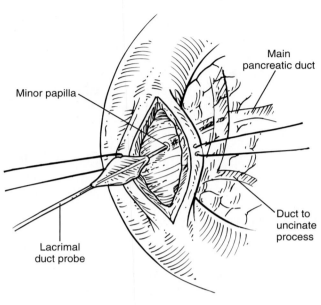

FIGURE 43–7

FIGURE 43–8

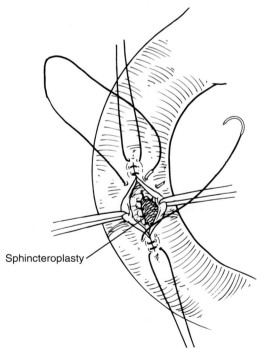

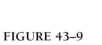

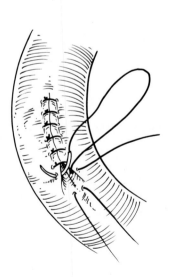

FIGURE 43–9

FIGURE 43–10

3. CLOSING

◆ The closed-suction drain is brought out through the anterior abdominal wall on the right side, with care taken to avoid injury to the epigastric vessels.

◆ After irrigation is completed and hemostasis is ensured, fascial closure is performed per surgeon preference. Running or interrupted and permanent or absorbable sutures may be used per surgeon preference.

◆ The skin is closed with a 4-0 Monocryl subcuticular suture or skin staples.

STEP 4: POSTOPERATIVE CARE

◆ Postoperative complications included hematoma, bleeding, or leakage from the duodenotomy.

◆ The output from the operatively placed drain should be monitored. This fluid may be bilious or amylase-rich if a leak is present at the duodenotomy. If unsure, the drained fluid can be sent for amylase and bilirubin levels, which should be less than three times the current serum levels.

◆ Diet can be quickly advanced to normal by 2 to 4 days postoperative.

◆ The drain should not be removed until the patient is tolerating a regular diet. The regular diet stimulates pancreatic secretion, and duodenal leaks may not be evident until the patient is tolerating a regular diet.

STEP 5: PEARLS AND PITFALLS

◆ It is helpful to place a biliary balloon catheter through the CBD and into the duodenum before making your duodenectomy. This is most easily achieved by inserting the catheter through the cystic duct in a patient who has not had a cholecystectomy, as shown previously.

◆ If the patient has already had a cholecystectomy, the catheter can be placed through a small choledochotomy in the CBD.

◆ If gallstones are obstructing the CBD and the catheter cannot be passed, the incision should be made in the second portion of the duodenum. After the ampulla of Vater is identified, the incision can be elongated.

◆ The ampulla of Vater can be cannulated retrogradely after the ampulla of Vater is identified, because it is easier to perform the sphincterotomy over a probe or catheter.

◆ When attempting to cannulate the minor papilla, take great care not to create a hematoma. If a hematoma forms it may be impossible to cannulate the pancreatic duct at the minor papilla.

SELECTED REFERENCES

1. Mulholland MW, Lillemoe KD, Doherty GM, et al (eds): Greenfield's Surgery: Scientific Principles and Practice, 4th ed. Philadelphia, Lippincott Williams & Wilkins, 2005.
2. Zuidema GD, Yeo CJ, Turcotte J (eds): Shackelford's Surgery of the Alimentary Tract, 5th ed. Philadelphia, Saunders, 2002.
3. Cameron JL (ed): Atlas of Surgery: Gallbladder and Biliary Tract, the Liver, Portasystemic Shunts, the Pancreas, vol 1. Philadelphia, BC Decker, 1990.
4. Cameron JL (ed): Current Surgical Therapy, 8th ed. Philadelphia, Mosby, 2002.

LIVER

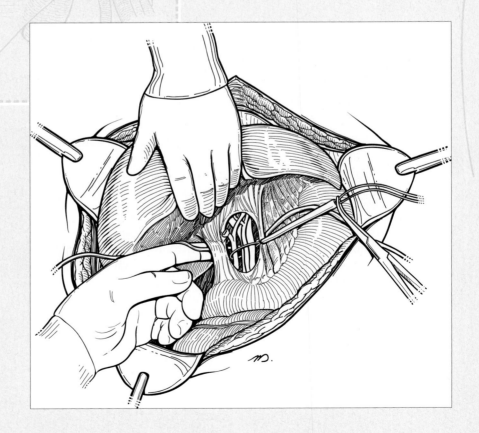

SEGMENTAL HEPATIC RESECTION—LEFT LATERAL SEGMENTECTOMY AND NONANATOMIC RESECTIONS

William H. Nealon

STEP 1: SURGICAL ANATOMY

- The liver is suspended in the right upper quadrant by avascular ligamentous attachments. The falciform ligament is oriented vertically and suspends the liver from the anterior abdominal wall at its inferior limit to the diaphragm just anterior to the vena cava. The left and right triangular ligaments extend in a transverse direction, beginning on the lateral borders of both the left and right liver, coursing along the diaphragm, and terminating at the vena cava where they join the superior extent of the falciform ligament. The triangular ligaments are composed of both anterior and posterior leaflets.

- Based on the intraparenchymal anatomy, the liver is divided into left and right livers, each composed of four segments. The line of demarcation is located several centimeters to the right of the falciform ligament and projects in a line, which transects the gallbladder bed from anterior to posterior (**Figures 44-1 and 44-2**).

- On gross examination, the liver appears to be composed of two discrete lobes. Thus, there is a traditional terminology in which the left and right lobes are defined by the falciform ligament. Resection of one of these is termed a left or right lobectomy. This terminology has largely been replaced by one based on the intraparenchymal vascular and biliary structures (**Figures 44-3 and 44-4**).

- The left liver is served by the left portal vein, left hepatic artery, and left bile duct. It is composed of segments I, II, III, and IV. Segments II and III represent the traditionally termed left lobe. Segment II is located at the surface of the left hemidiaphragm, and segment III occupies the inferior aspect of the left lobe. The boundary between the two extends horizontally approximately midway through the left lobe. Segment I is also called the caudate lobe. It occupies the posterior aspect of the liver in the midline. The segment wraps rather like a collar around the vena cava on its left aspect. This segment is unique for its venous drainage, which is independent of the left or middle hepatic veins and is composed of multiple tiny tributaries between the vena cava and the segment. Segment IV, termed the quadrate lobe, occupies the area between the falciform ligament medially and the gallbladder bed laterally. It is the only segment that has been designated to have two discrete components. IV-A is the anterior half of segment IV, and IV-B is the posterior half. This distinction can be significant in nonanatomic resections (see Figures 44-1 and 44-2).

Hepatic Segments

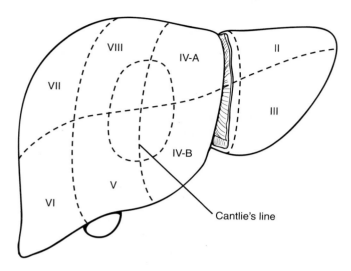

FIGURE 44–1

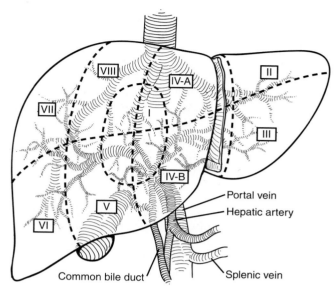

FIGURE 44–2

Left Lobectomy

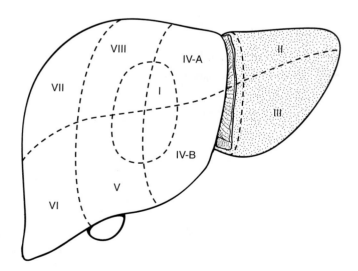

FIGURE 44–3

Left Hepatectomy

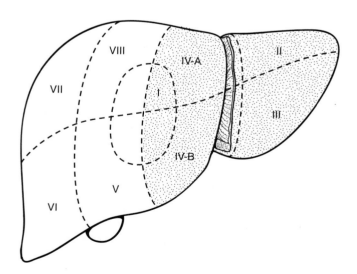

FIGURE 44–4

◆ The right liver is composed of segments V, VI, VII, and VIII. These four are oriented around a horizontal line transecting the right liver at its mid-portion and similarly by a vertical line, which transects the right liver at its mid-portion. Beginning at the inferomedial segment V, the segments follow a clockwise direction, with VI inferolateral, VII superolateral, and VIII superomedial (see Figures 44-1 and 44-2).

◆ Lymphovascular and biliary structures exit the liver through the hepatoduodenal ligament, which courses between the duodenum into the base of segments IV and V—an area that is termed the porta hepatis. The portal triad of microanatomy is matched by the gross anatomic orientation in the hepatoduodenal ligament, composed of hepatic artery, portal vein, and bile duct. Each structure divides into a left and right branch and then arborizes within the liver in a pattern defined by the segments (see Figures 44-1 and 44-2).

◆ Venous drainage of the liver is primarily located at the superior aspect of the liver in the midline in short structures between the vena cava and the liver. The left, middle, and right hepatic veins each enter the vena cava within 2 to 4 cm of one another in a coronal orientation. One or all of these venous elements may be intrahepatic or may have exceedingly short extrahepatic components. This anatomic feature raises considerably the risk of uncontrolled hemorrhage during dissection and resection (see Figure 44-2). In addition to these three venous structures, there are between 2 and 20 tiny tributaries between the posterior surface of the liver and the contiguous vena cava. These must be divided to fully mobilize the right liver.

◆ In discussions of nonanatomic resections, one must recognize that similar principles will be used for essentially all such procedures, and there are a wide variety of examples. In patients with gallbladder cancer, for example, one may choose to perform a complete resection of the gallbladder bed by performing a segment IV, V resection **(Figure 44-5)**, or one may choose to perform an isolated segment IV-B resection **(Figure 44-6)**.

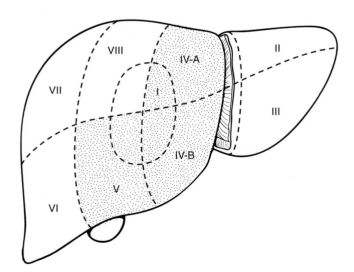

Resection of Segments IV and V

FIGURE 44–5

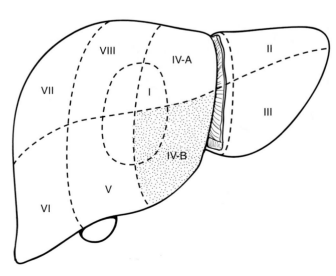

Resection of Segment IV-B

FIGURE 44–6

STEP 2: PREOPERATIVE CONSIDERATIONS

♦ Due to the magnitude of hepatic surgery, one first consideration is the medical status of the patient and likely risk of surgery. Thus one must exclude significant coronary, pulmonary, or renal disease or age and frailty. Of particular concern in relation to hepatic surgery is the underlying hepatic function. Because hepatocellular carcinoma is associated with prior hepatitis and cirrhosis, one must determine first whether cirrhosis exists and second what level of function is apparent. Historically, this was measured by examining synthetic and excretory functions and measures of portal hypertension (serum albumin level, coagulation profile, serum bilirubin level, ascites, and mental status/serum ammonia). More recently, the Model for End-Stage Liver Disease (MELD) score was developed as a means of segregating candidates for liver transplant. This system incorporates prior variables, but has added and places considerable significance to renal function. Particularly when one anticipates a major resection, one must establish that sufficient liver will remain to support life. Unfortunately, this estimate of "hepatic reserve" is even today an inexact science.

♦ Nutritional status, renal function, degree of ascites, and coagulation abnormalities are all factors that may be improved by medical management before surgery. Unfortunately, we have personal experience that such patients may thereby achieve an improved functional grade but appear to carry a risk that exceeds the risk in patients who have had this improved functional status without a need for medical manipulation to achieve it.

♦ In the case of malignancy, one must establish that curative resection is clinically achievable.

STEP 3: OPERATIVE STEPS

1. INCISION

♦ We prefer the inverted L incision. This incision offers the option of extending the horizontal component of the incision either laterally into the right flank or medially across the midline. The vertical component of the incision can be extended toward the xiphoid process. By then placing self-retaining retractors, the exposure of the right upper abdomen is maximized. The incision can be extended if the operative view is inadequate.

2. DISSECTION

♦ First, the concept of nonanatomic resections encompasses wedge resections, which do not require individual segmental dissection. The term also encompasses the many variations on segmental or multisegmental resections.

♦ For wedge resection, most surgeons will use a combination of total inflow occlusion with compression of the hepatoduodenal ligament combined with local compression at the site of resection.

- For segmental resection, although a vast variety of procedures are included in this category, the concept is the same. Vascular control is obtained by dissecting along the hepatoduodenal ligament and accessing and temporarily or permanently occluding the vessels corresponding to that segment or the primary feeding vessel to that segment. To illustrate, we will describe the steps involved in resection of segment VIII **(Figure 44-7)**.

- Inferior to the liver edge, divide the falciform ligament between clamps and tie with heavy silk suture. Cut the sutures at the caudal divided ligament. Place a hemostat on the uncut cephalad end of suture on the divided ligament for use in manipulating the liver during dissection. You will discover the need for a constant balance between retracting the liver cephalad and retracting caudad. Using this tether, you may restore some caudal exposure while the self-retaining retractor suspends the liver toward the diaphragm **(Figure 44-8)**.

- Using electrocautery, the filmy, avascular falciform ligament is incised beginning at its attachment to the anterior abdominal wall and continuing in a cephalad and dorsal direction up to the point of convergence of this ligament with the left and right triangular ligaments. The hepatic veins are visualized at the superior extent of this dissection. Carefully incise the peritoneal surface to clearly define the right and middle hepatic veins. We favor placing a vessel loop around the right and middle hepatic veins at this juncture.

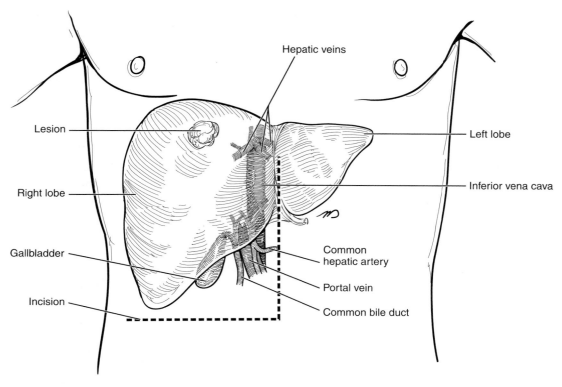

Lesion

Right lobe

Gallbladder

Incision

Hepatic veins

Left lobe

Inferior vena cava

Common hepatic artery

Portal vein

Common bile duct

FIGURE 44–7

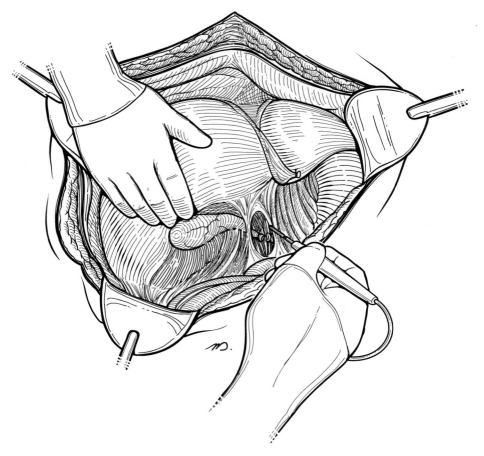

FIGURE 44–8

◆ Divide the anterior and posterior leaflets of the right triangular ligament using electrocautery. It is usually best to first extend the incision of the anterior leaflet from the right lateral margin to the midline. At this point, gentle blunt dissection will separate the diaphragmatic attachments, better revealing the posterior leaflet and facilitating division of this structure. In this fashion, the liver is mobilized to the midline, as well as in a caudal direction **(Figure 44-9)**. With full mobilization, it is possible to bring the liver into the midline, affording a wide access to the entire liver.

◆ Dissect the peritoneum overlying the hepatoduodenal ligament in a transverse direction. After dividing the typically filmy gastrohepatic or lesser omentum medial to the ligament, it is possible to pass your finger or an instrument into the foramen of Winslow and completely encircle the structures contained in the hepatoduodenal ligament. Pass an umbilical tape around the ligament, and using the hooked instrument with a section of rubber tubing create a Rummel loop. This safety measure is performed to permit complete inflow occlusion should this be necessary to control undue hemorrhage if encountered at any time during the procedure. Place a hemostat on the two loose ends of umbilical tape **(Figure 44-10)**.

◆ At approximately the mid-portion of the hepatoduodenal ligament, dissect and isolate the common bile duct laterally and the proper hepatic artery located on the medial edge of the ligament. Place a ¼-inch Penrose drain around the bile duct and a vessel loop around the artery, and use traction on these two structures to reveal the portal vein positioned between and posterior to these two parallel structures. Gently tease the filmy adhesions to isolate all three structures and extend this dissection toward the hilum.

◆ Follow the common bile duct, hepatic artery, and portal vein toward the hilum of the liver, and then isolate and encircle the right branch of each structure. Each of these will follow a course directed toward the gallbladder bed, which rises at approximately a 60-degree angle from the hilum toward the right liver.

◆ Interrupt vascular inflow to the right liver temporarily by placing atraumatic vascular clamps on the right hepatic artery and right portal vein.

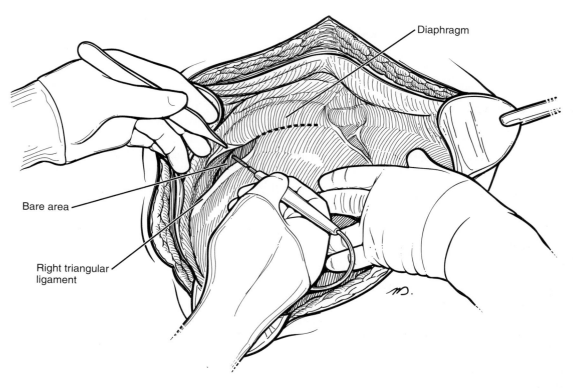

Diaphragm

Bare area

Right triangular
ligament

FIGURE 44–9

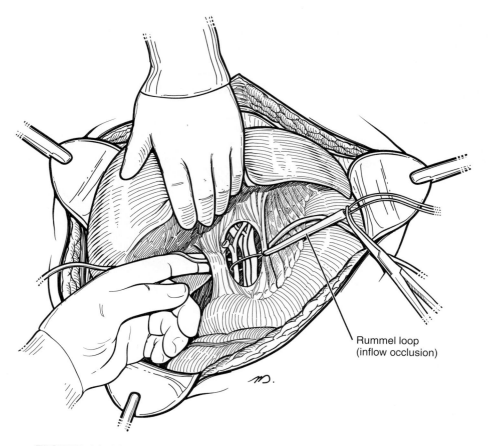

Rummel loop
(inflow occlusion)

FIGURE 44–10

◆ Score the capsule of the liver along the line anatomically consistent with segment VIII. Ultrasound guidance can be very helpful to define anatomy and to target the lesion **(Figure 44-11).**

◆ Perform dissection through the parenchyma of the liver carefully and progressively using the handheld harmonic dissector. The recently available tissue-coagulating instrument, based on radio-frequency energy (Habib device), may be substituted for division of parenchyma but should not be used near major vessels. This instrument is particularly useful in nonanatomic resections because of its effectiveness in controlling hemorrhage during the parenchymal incision (see Figure 44-11).

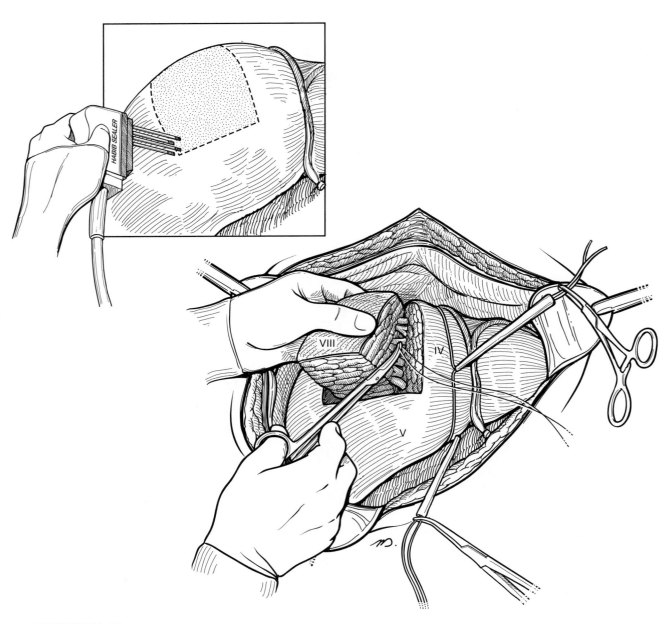

FIGURE 44–11

◆ Using visual inspection, and if necessary ultrasound guidance, identify major intraparenchymal vascular tributaries and branches, and then clamp, divide, and ligate. Biliary radicals, which must be ligated individually, are most difficult to identify at the time of dissection. Failure to ligate these structures results in postoperative bile leaks (see Figure 44-11). The right and middle hepatic veins should be identified and remain undisturbed during the dissection.

◆ Perform ultrasound examination intraoperatively to ensure adequate margin of resection in the case of malignant tumor removal. A 1-cm margin is considered to be adequate, but in major resections, margins are not typically an issue.

◆ Bring out two 10-mm Jackson-Pratt drains through separate stab wounds on the right side of the abdomen and place along the divided edge of the liver (**Figure 44-12**). Some will advocate taking omentum and placing it in the bed of the resected liver to act as a biologic seal for the raw edge of the liver parenchyma.

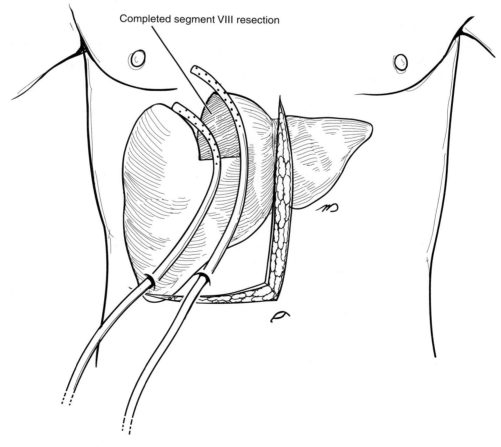

Completed segment VIII resection

FIGURE 44–12

3. CLOSING

◆ Close the abdomen in a standard manner. We favor a horizontal mattress closure (Smead-Jones) with heavy-gauge absorbable suture.

STEP 4: POSTOPERATIVE CARE

◆ In the first 24 hours after surgery, the primary concern is hemorrhage and the related measure of coagulation status. These should be monitored by means of serial measurement of hemoglobin and coagulation factors.

◆ In all major resections, particularly in patients with cirrhosis, one must be vigilant for any signs of hepatic failure. A particularly ominous finding is the progressive rise in bilirubin level with an enzyme pattern that supports neither obstruction nor parenchymal cell death, such as transaminase elevations. The most ominous finding is a plummeting serum glucose level, which reflects the loss of glycogen stores in the liver and by inference the loss of viable liver. Unfortunately, there is little one can do to reverse this pattern of failure. One possible cause is inadequate remaining liver after resection. This can resolve over time as the liver regenerates, which it will do to some degree.

◆ One possibly remediable cause of this progressive demise is thrombus formation in the portal vein. This would seem to be unlikely, because coagulation is typically inadequate in these patients, but we have seen this phenomenon. It is possible that lysis of this clot may restore vital flow.

◆ Sepsis is particularly metabolically taxing to the liver. In the compromised postoperative liver, sepsis can be catastrophic. One should monitor and obtain cultures if necessary to prevent infectious processes from progressing.

◆ Ascites may form, and one must be aware when this phenomenon has occurred and treat as one would normally treat this entity with careful and judicious use of salt-containing intravenous fluids and with diuresis.

◆ Remove drains if no bile is seen in the effluent.

STEP 5: PEARLS AND PITFALLS

- ◆ As with all such major operative procedures, one must exercise extreme care in patient selection.

- ◆ If hemorrhage occurs at any time during the procedure, the liver can be compressed into the spine or into the right flank to gain control, and another capable surgeon can be called for assistance.

- ◆ Before dividing any of the major vascular structures, stop and reconfirm that the proper structure is being divided.

- ◆ If ascites forms and the drains are still in place, excessive electrolyte and fluid loss can occur through actively draining liters of fluid per day. In this setting, the drains (assuming they are not bile tinged) should be removed, and the skin overlying the drain tract should be sutured.

SELECTED REFERENCES

1. Blumgart LH, Belghiti J: Liver resection for benign disease and for liver and biliary tumors. In Blumgart LH (ed): Surgery of the Liver, Biliary Tract and Pancreas, 4th ed. Philadelphia, Saunders, 2007, pp 1341-1388.
2. Liu CL, Fan, ST, Cheung ST, et al: Anterior approach versus conventional approach right hepatic resection for large hepatocellular carcinoma: A prospective randomized controlled study. Ann Surg 2006;244: 194-203.
3. Nanashima A, Sumida Y, Abo T, et al: Anatomic resection of segments 5, 6 and 7 of liver for hepatocellular carcinoma: Prior control of right paramedian Glisson. Hepatogastroenterology 2008;55:1077-1080.
4. Shirabe K, Shimada M, Gio T, et al: Postoperative liver failure after major hepatic resection for hepatocellular carcinoma in the modern era with special reference to remnant liver volume. J Am Coll Surg 1999;188:304-309.

CHAPTER 45

RIGHT HEPATECTOMY

William H. Nealon

STEP 1: SURGICAL ANATOMY

- The liver is suspended in the right upper quadrant by avascular ligamentous attachments. The falciform ligament is oriented vertically and suspends the liver from the anterior abdominal wall at its inferior limit to the diaphragm, just anterior to the vena cava. The left and right triangular ligaments extend in a transverse direction beginning on the lateral borders of both the left and right liver, coursing along the diaphragm, and terminating at the vena cava, where they join the superior extent of the falciform ligament. The triangular ligaments are composed of both anterior and posterior leaflets.

- The liver appears on gross examination to be composed of two discrete lobes. Thus there is a traditional terminology in which the left and right lobes are defined by the falciform ligament. Resection of one of these is termed a left or right lobectomy. This terminology has largely been replaced by one based on the intraparenchymal vascular and biliary structures.

- Based on the intraparenchymal anatomy, the liver is divided into left and right livers, each composed of four segments. The line of demarcation is located several centimeters to the right of the falciform ligament and projects in a line, which transects the gallbladder bed from anterior to posterior **(Figure 45-1)**.

- Using the segmental anatomy, the liver is divided into left liver and right liver. The left liver is served by the left portal vein, left hepatic artery, and left bile duct. It is composed of segments I, II, III, and IV. Segments II and III represent the traditionally termed left lobe. Segment II is attached to the left hemidiaphragm by the left triangular ligament, and segment III occupies the inferior aspect of the left lobe. The boundary between the two extends horizontally, approximately midway through the left lobe. Segment I, also called the caudate lobe, occupies the posterior aspect of the liver in the midline. The segment wraps rather like a collar around the vena cava on its left aspect. This segment is unique for its venous drainage, which is independent of the left or middle hepatic veins and is composed of multiple tiny tributaries between the vena cava and the segment. Segment IV, the quadrate lobe, occupies the area between the falciform ligament medially and the gallbladder bed laterally (see Figure 45-1).

- The right liver is composed of segments V, VI, VII, and VIII. These four are oriented around a horizontal line transecting the right liver at its mid-portion and similarly by a vertical line that transects the right liver at its mid-portion. Beginning at the inferomedial segment V, the segments follow a clockwise direction with VI inferolateral, VII superolateral, and VIII superomedial (see Figure 45-1).

◆ Lymphovascular and biliary structures enter the liver through the hepatoduodenal ligament that courses between the duodenum into the base of segments IV and V, which is termed the porta hepatis. The portal triad of microanatomy is matched by the gross anatomic orientation in the hepatoduodenal ligament, composed of hepatic artery, portal vein, and bile duct. Each structure divides into a left and right branch and then arborizes within the liver in a pattern defined by the segments (see Figure 45-1).

◆ Venous drainage of the liver is primarily located at the superior aspect of the liver in short structures between the vena cava and the liver. The left, middle, and right hepatic veins each enter the vena cava within 2 to 4 cm of one another in a coronal orientation. One or all of these venous elements may be intrahepatic or may have exceedingly short extrahepatic components. This anatomic feature raises considerably the risk of uncontrolled hemorrhage during dissection and resection **(Figure 45-2)**. In addition to these three venous structures, there are between 2 and 20 tiny tributaries between the posterior surface of the liver and the contiguous vena cava. These must be divided to fully mobilize the right liver.

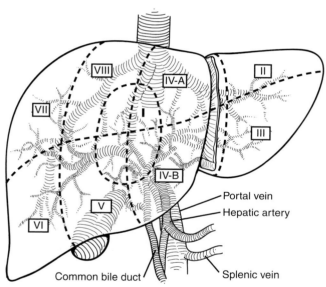

FIGURE 45–1

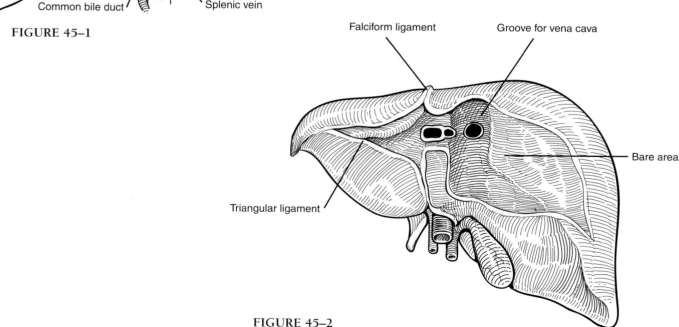

FIGURE 45–2

STEP 2: PREOPERATIVE CONSIDERATIONS

◆ Due to the magnitude of hepatic surgery, one first consideration is the medical status of the patient and likely risk of surgery. Thus one must exclude significant coronary, pulmonary, or renal disease, or age and frailty. Of particular concern in relation to hepatic surgery is the underlying hepatic function. Because hepatocellular carcinoma is associated with prior hepatitis and cirrhosis, one must determine first whether cirrhosis exists and second what level of function is apparent. Historically, this was measured by examining synthetic and excretory functions and measures of portal hypertension (serum albumin level, coagulation profile, serum bilirubin level, ascites, and mental status/serum ammonia). More recently, the Model for End-Stage Liver Disease (MELD) score was developed as a means of segregating candidates for liver transplant. This system incorporates prior variables, but has added and places considerable significance to renal function. Particularly when one anticipates a major resection, one must establish that sufficient liver will remain to support life. Unfortunately, this estimate of "hepatic reserve" is even today an inexact science.

◆ Nutritional status, renal function, degree of ascites, and coagulation abnormalities are all factors that may be improved by medical management before surgery. Unfortunately, we have personal experience that such patients may thereby achieve an improved functional grade but appear to carry a risk that exceeds the risk in patients who have had this improved functional status without a need for medical manipulation to achieve it.

STEP 3: OPERATIVE STEPS

1. INCISION

◆ Several incisions have been proposed. We favor the inverted L incision, with the option to extend the incision vertically in the midline for added exposure, as well as extending farther the horizontal component of the incision either laterally into the right flank or across the midline (**Figure 45-3**).

◆ Placing self-retaining retractors maximizes the exposure of the right upper abdomen. The incision should be extended if the operative view is inadequate.

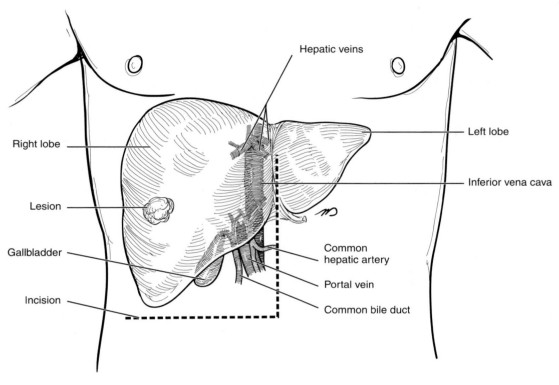

Hepatic veins

Right lobe

Lesion

Gallbladder

Incision

Left lobe

Inferior vena cava

Common
hepatic artery

Portal vein

Common bile duct

FIGURE 45–3

2. DISSECTION

◆ Inferior to the liver edge, divide the falciform ligament between clamps and tie with heavy silk suture. Cut the sutures at the caudal divided ligament. Place a hemostat on the uncut cephalad end of the divided ligament for use in manipulating the liver during dissection. You will discover the need for a constant balance between retracting the liver cephalad and retracting caudad. Using this tether, you may restore some caudal exposure while the self-retaining retractor suspends the liver toward the diaphragm.

◆ Using electrocautery, the filmy, avascular falciform ligament is incised beginning at its attachment to the anterior abdominal wall and continuing in a cephalad and dorsal direction until the point of convergence of this ligament meets the left and right triangular ligaments **(Figure 45-4)**. The hepatic veins are visualized at the superior extent of this dissection. Carefully divide the peritoneal surface to clearly define the right and middle hepatic veins. We favor placing a vessel loop around the right and middle hepatic veins at this juncture **(Figure 45-5)**.

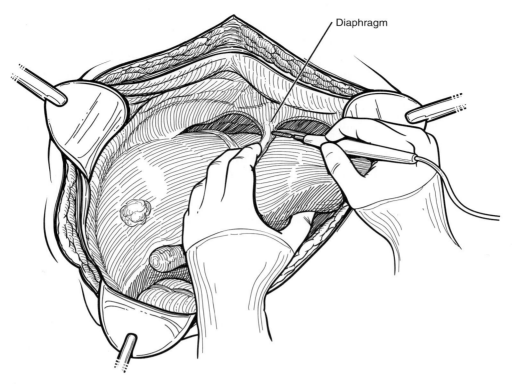

Diaphragm

FIGURE 45–4

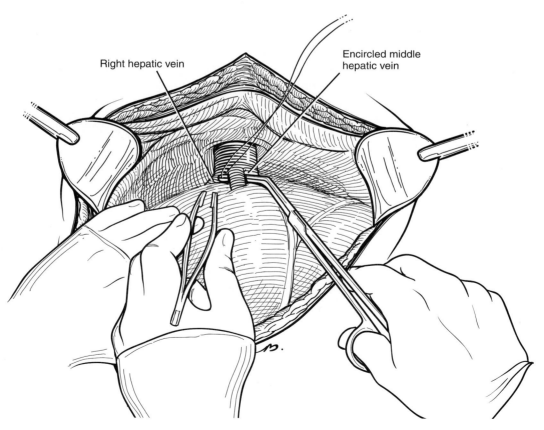

Right hepatic vein

Encircled middle
hepatic vein

FIGURE 45–5

- Divide the anterior and posterior leaflets of the right triangular ligament using electrocautery. It is usually best to first extend the incision of the anterior leaflet from the right lateral margin to the midline. At this point, gentle blunt dissection will separate the diaphragmatic attachments, better revealing the posterior leaflet and facilitating division of this structure. In this fashion, the liver is mobilized to the midline, as well as in a caudal direction **(Figure 45-6)**.

- At the most posterior and medial extent of this dissection, the vena cava is seen, and the small tributaries between the posterior surface of the liver and the vena cava can be visualized. We delay division of these vessels until we have fully dissected the hepatoduodenal ligament. The umbilical tape is used as a tourniquet surrounding the liver parenchyma from the posterior to the anterior surface in the anticipated line of resection. On occasion, this maneuver may be useful to control parenchymal bleeding during division of the right liver (see Figure 45-6).

- The right hepatic and middle hepatic veins will be visible at the superior extent of dissection in the midline. Dissect and place a vessel loop around the right hepatic vein at this time for later division. Because the liver may be displaced either to the left or to the right compared with classic orientation, one must confirm that the vein encircled is in fact the right hepatic vein (see Figure 45-5).

- Dissect the peritoneum overlying the hepatoduodenal ligament in a transverse direction. After dividing the typically filmy gastrohepatic or lesser omentum medial to the ligament, it should be possible to pass your finger or an instrument into the foramen of Winslow and completely encircle the structures contained in the hepatoduodenal ligament **(Figure 45-7)**.

- Pass an umbilical tape around the ligament and, using the hooked instrument with a section of rubber tubing, create a Rummel loop. This safety measure is performed to permit complete inflow occlusion, which may be necessary to control undue hemorrhage if encountered during the procedure. Place a hemostat on the two loose ends of umbilical tape (see Figure 45-7).

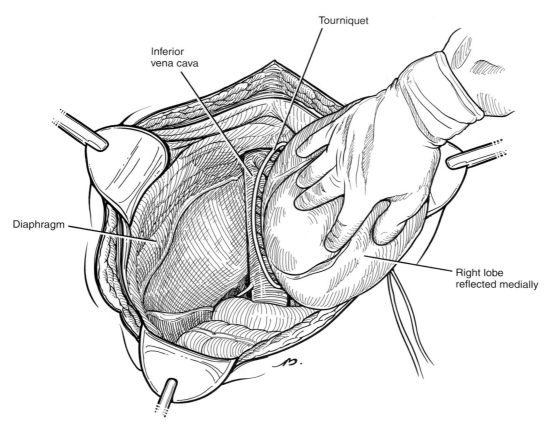

Tourniquet

Inferior
vena cava

Diaphragm

Right lobe
reflected medially

FIGURE 45–6

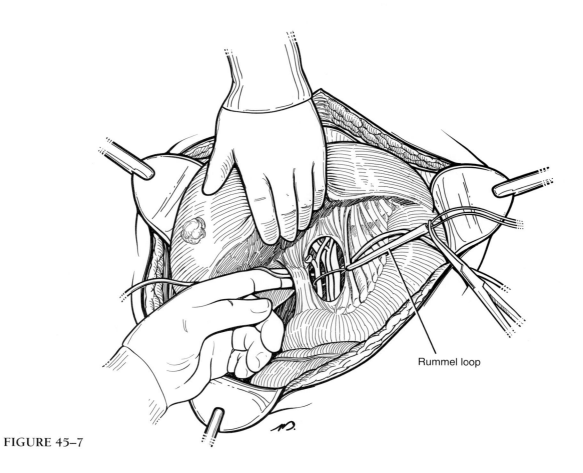

Rummel loop

FIGURE 45–7

- Remove the gallbladder **(Figure 45-8).**

- At approximately the mid-portion of the hepatoduodenal ligament, dissect and isolate the common bile duct laterally; the proper hepatic artery is located on the medial edge of the ligament. Place a ¼-inch Penrose drain around the bile duct and a vessel loop around the artery, and use traction laterally and medially on these two structures to reveal the portal vein, positioned between and posterior to these two parallel structures. Gently tease the filmy adhesions to isolate all three structures toward the hilum **(Figure 45-9).**

- Follow the common bile duct, hepatic artery, and portal vein toward the hilum of the liver, and then isolate and encircle the right branch of each structure. Each of these will follow a course directed toward the cystic plate, deep to the gallbladder bed (see Figure 45-9).

- By retracting the liver to the left, you expose the vena cava. Identify, ligate, and divide multiple small tributaries between the vena cava and the right lobe of the liver, permitting full mobilization of the right liver.

- Interrupt vascular inflow to the right liver by dividing the right hepatic artery between clamps and suture ligating (see Figure 45-9).

- Divide the right branch of the portal vein between clamps. With the clamp in place, a continuous running closure is performed with 5-0 Prolene, beginning at one corner. At the opposite corner, lock the suture. Remove the clamp and place a second layer of continuous suture back to the original corner and tie. Vascular staples may be substituted (see Figure 45-9).

- Divide and suture ligate the right branch of the hepatic duct using absorbable suture (see Figure 45-9).

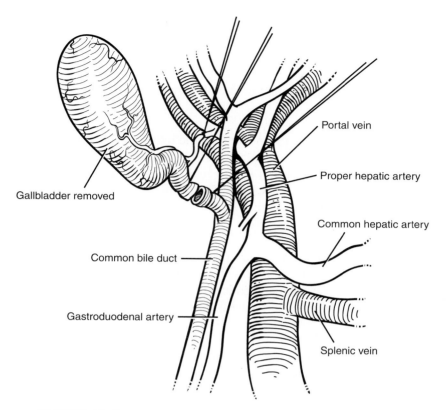

FIGURE 45–8

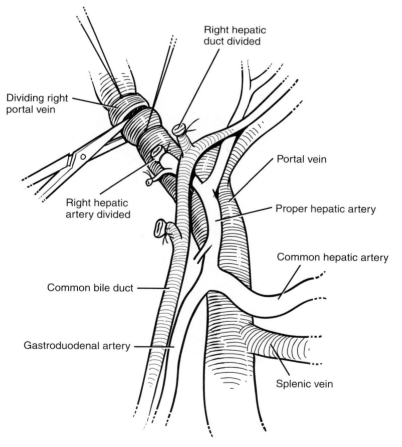

FIGURE 45–9

◆ Once the vascular inflow is interrupted, the anatomic right liver assumes a dark purple hue, giving it a clear demarcation for resection (**Figure 45-10**).

◆ Score the capsule of the liver along the line of demarcation using electrocautery.

◆ Perform dissection through the parenchyma of the liver carefully and progressively using the handheld harmonic dissector (see Figure 45-10). The recently available tissue-coagulating instrument based on radio-frequency energy may be substituted for division of parenchyma but should not be used near major vessels. The normal right lobe may be as deep in its anterior to posterior dimensions as 20 cm. Patience must be exercised (**Figure 45-11**).

◆ Using visual inspection, and if necessary ultrasound guidance, identify major vascular tributaries and branches, and then clamp, divide, and ligate. Biliary radicles, which must be ligated individually, are most difficult to identify at the time of dissection. Failure to ligate these structures results in postoperative bile leaks (**Figure 45-12**).

◆ Perform ultrasound examination intraoperatively to ensure adequate margin of resection in the case of malignant tumor removal. A 1-cm margin is considered adequate, but in major resections margins are not typically an issue.

◆ Extend division of the liver from the anterior to posterior capsule at the level of the vena cava.

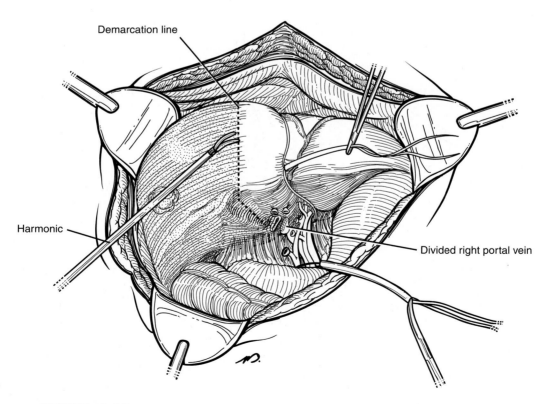

FIGURE 45–10

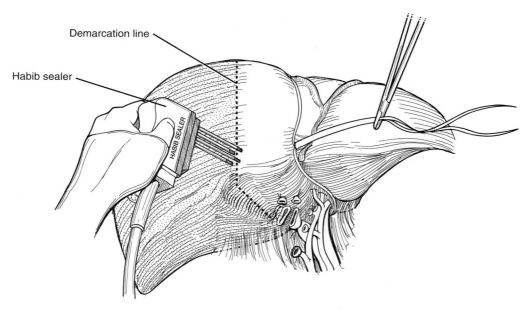

FIGURE 45–11

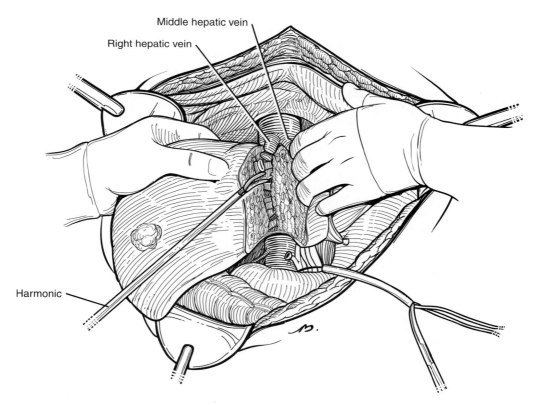

FIGURE 45–12

◆ Carry the dissection from the inferior edge of the liver to the superior edge, terminating at the right hepatic vein. You might encounter tributaries within the parenchyma of the liver before reaching the right hepatic vein. Throughout division of the parenchyma of the liver, repeatedly reorient the specimen to be certain that dissection is not migrating toward the left liver and more importantly toward the major vascular structures necessary for the left liver's viability (**Figure 45-13**, and see Figure 45-12).

◆ Double clamp the right hepatic vein on the vena cava side. Divide the right hepatic vein. Close the stump of the right hepatic vein using running 5-0 Prolene suture in an identical manner to that used on the portal vein (Figure 45-13 and **Figure 45-14**).

◆ Bring out two 10-mm Jackson-Pratt drains through separate stab wounds on the right side of the abdomen and place along the divided edge of the liver. Some will advocate taking omentum and placing it in the right upper quadrant to act as a biologic seal for the raw edge of the liver parenchyma (**Figure 45-15**).

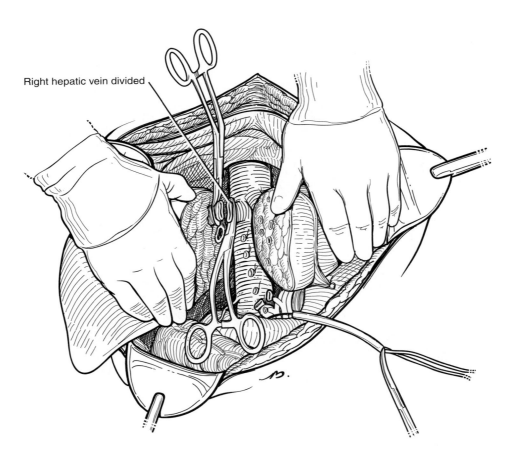

Right hepatic vein divided

FIGURE 45–13

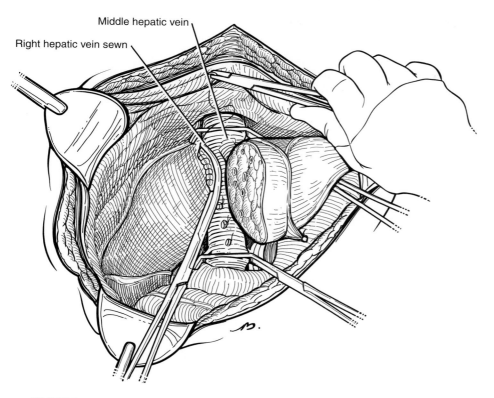

Right hepatic vein sewn

Middle hepatic vein

FIGURE 45–14

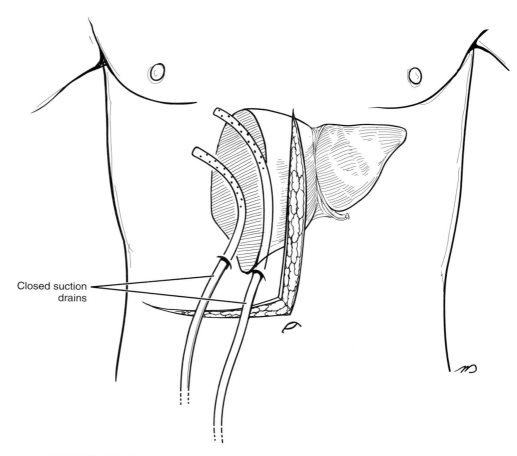

Closed suction drains

FIGURE 45–15

3. CLOSING

- ◆ Close the abdomen in a standard manner. We favor Smead-Jones closure with heavy-gauge absorbable suture.

STEP 4: POSTOPERATIVE CARE

- ◆ In the first 24 hours after surgery, the primary concern is hemorrhage and the related measure of coagulation status. These should be monitored by serial measurement of hemoglobin and coagulation factors.

- ◆ In all major resections, particularly in patients with cirrhosis, one must be vigilant for any signs of hepatic failure. A particularly ominous finding is the progressive rise in bilirubin level with an enzyme pattern that supports neither obstruction nor parenchymal cell death, such as transaminase elevations. The most ominous finding is a plummeting serum glucose level, which reflects the loss of glycogen stores in the liver and by inference the loss of viable liver. Unfortunately, there is little one can do to reverse this pattern of failure. One possible cause is inadequate remaining liver after resection. This can resolve over time as the liver regenerates, which it will do to some degree.

- ◆ One possible remediable cause of this progressive demise is thrombus formation in the portal vein. This would seem to be unlikely, because coagulation is typically inadequate in these patients, but we have seen this phenomenon. It is possible that lysis of this clot may restore vital flow.

- ◆ Sepsis is particularly metabolically taxing to the liver. In the compromised postoperative liver, sepsis can be catastrophic, and one should monitor and obtain cultures if necessary to prevent infectious processes from progressing.

- ◆ Ascites may form, and one must be aware when this phenomenon has occurred and treat as one would normally treat this entity with careful and judicious use of salt-containing intravenous fluids and with diuresis.

- ◆ Remove drains if no bile is seen in the effluent.

- ◆ One preoperative option, which was originally developed for cirrhotic patients with what appeared to be inadequate functional reserve but later applied to all candidates, is embolization of the portal vein. In this manner some degree of the regeneration of lost liver takes place before the stress of surgery is added.

STEP 5: PEARLS AND PITFALLS

- As with all major operative procedures, one must be extremely careful with patient selection.

- If hemorrhage occurs at any time during the procedure, the liver can be compressed into the spine or into the right flank to gain control, and another capable surgeon can be called for assistance.

- Before dividing any of the major vascular structures, stop and reconfirm that the proper structure is being divided.

- If ascites forms and the drains are still in place, excessive electrolyte and fluid loss can occur through actively draining liters of fluid per day. In this setting, the drains (assuming they are not bile tinged) should be removed, and the skin overlying the drain tract should be sutured.

SELECTED REFERENCES

1. Blumgart LH, Belghiti J: Liver resection for benign disease and for liver and biliary tumors. In Blumgart LH (ed): Surgery of the Liver, Biliary Tract and Pancreas, 4th ed. Philadelphia, Saunders Elsevier, 2007, pp 1341-1388.
2. Liu CL, Fan, ST, Cheung ST, et al: Anterior approach versus conventional approach right hepatic resection for large hepatocellular carcinoma: A prospective randomized controlled study. Ann Surg 2006;244: 194-203.

CHAPTER 46

LEFT HEPATIC LOBECTOMY

William H. Nealon

STEP 1: SURGICAL ANATOMY

- The liver is suspended in the right upper quadrant by avascular ligamentous attachments. The falciform ligament is oriented vertically and suspends the liver from the anterior abdominal wall at its inferior limit to the diaphragm just anterior to the vena cava. The left and right triangular ligaments extend in a transverse direction beginning on the lateral borders of both the left and right liver, coursing along the diaphragm, and terminating at the vena cava where they join the superior extent of the falciform ligament. The triangular ligaments are composed of both anterior and posterior leaflets.

- The liver appears on gross examination to be composed of two discrete lobes. Thus there is a traditional terminology in which the left and right lobes are defined by the falciform ligament. Resection of one of these is termed a left or right lobectomy. This terminology has largely been replaced by one based on the intraparenchymal vascular and biliary structures.

- Based on the intraparenchymal anatomy, the liver is divided into left and right livers, each composed of four segments. The line of demarcation is located several centimeters to the right of the falciform ligament and projects in a line that transects the gallbladder bed from anterior to posterior **(Figures 46-1 and 46-2)**.

- Using the segmental anatomy, the liver is divided into left liver and right liver. The left liver is served by the left portal vein, left hepatic artery, and left bile duct. It is composed of segments I, II, III, and IV. Segments II and III represent the traditionally termed left lobe. Segment II is attached to the left diaphragm, and segment III occupies the inferior aspect of the left lobe. The boundary between the two extends horizontally approximately midway through the left lobe. Segment one is also called the caudate lobe. It occupies the posterior aspect of the liver in the midline. The segment wraps rather like a collar around the vena cava on its left aspect. This segment is unique for its venous drainage, which is independent of the left or middle hepatic veins and is composed of multiple tiny tributaries between the vena cava and the segment. Segment IV is also termed the quadrate lobe, and it occupies the area between the falciform ligament medially and the gallbladder bed laterally (see Figure 46-1).

- The right liver is composed of segments V, VI, VII, and VIII. These four are oriented around a horizontal line transecting the right liver at its mid-portion and similarly by a vertical line that transects the right liver at its mid-portion. Beginning at the inferomedial segment V, the segments follow a clockwise direction, with VI inferolateral, VII superolateral, and VIII superomedial (see Figures 46-1 and 46-2).

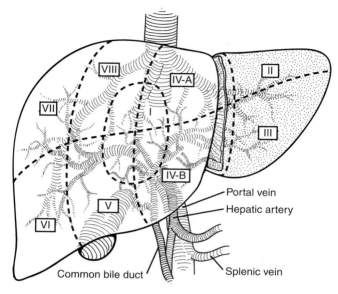

FIGURE 46–1

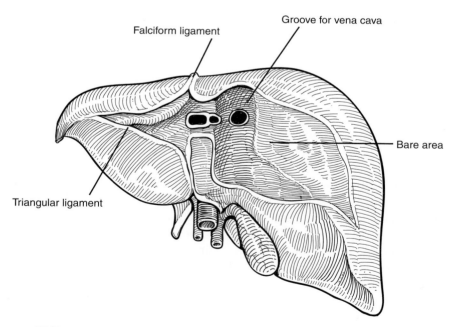

FIGURE 46–2

- Lymphovascular and biliary structures enter the liver through the hepatoduodenal ligament that courses between the duodenum into the base of segments IV and V, which is termed the porta hepatis. The portal triad of microanatomy is matched by the gross anatomic orientation in the hepatoduodenal ligament—composed of hepatic artery, portal vein, and bile duct. Each structure divides into a left and right branch and then arborizes within the liver in a pattern defined by the segments (see Figures 46-1 and 46-2).

- Venous drainage of the liver is primarily located at the superior aspect of the liver in the midline in short structures between the vena cava and the liver. The left, middle, and right hepatic veins each enter the vena cava within 2 to 4 cm of one another in a coronal orientation. One or all of these venous elements may be intrahepatic or may have exceedingly short extrahepatic components. This anatomic feature raises considerably the risk of uncontrolled hemorrhage during dissection and resection (see Figure 46-2). In addition to these three venous structures, there are between 2 and 20 tiny tributaries between the posterior surface of the liver and the contiguous vena cava. These must be divided to fully mobilize the right liver.

INDICATIONS

- Left hepatic lobectomy is performed primarily for the treatment of malignant disease, which includes hepatocellular carcinoma, intrahepatic cholangiocarcinoma, and a variety of metastatic lesions—most commonly of abdominal origin. The best outcomes are achieved in patients with metastatic lesions from carcinoma of the colon and rectum.

- However, the procedure is also performed for benign diseases, such as cystadenoma of the liver, giant hemangioma of the liver, and intrahepatic biliary strictures existing primarily on the left side of the biliary tree, and at times for lesions such as either hepatic adenoma or focal nodular hyperplasia determined to be clinically significant, perhaps because of increasing size.

STEP 2: PREOPERATIVE CONSIDERATIONS

- Due to the magnitude of hepatic surgery, one first consideration is the medical status of the patient and likely risk of surgery. Thus one must exclude significant coronary, pulmonary, or renal disease or age and frailty. Of particular concern in relation to hepatic surgery is the underlying hepatic function. Because hepatocellular carcinoma is associated with prior hepatitis and cirrhosis, one must determine first whether cirrhosis exists and second what level of function is apparent. Historically, this was measured by examining synthetic and excretory functions and measures of portal hypertension (serum albumin level, coagulation profile, serum bilirubin level, ascites, and mental status/serum ammonia). More recently, the Model for End-Stage Liver Disease (MELD) score was developed as a means of segregating candidates for liver transplant. This system incorporates prior variables but has added and places considerable significance to renal function. Particularly when one anticipates a major resection one must establish that sufficient liver will remain to support life. Unfortunately, this estimate of "hepatic reserve" is even today an inexact science.

◆ Nutritional status, renal function, degree of ascites, and coagulation abnormalities are all factors that may be improved by medical management before surgery. Unfortunately, we ha personal experience that such patients may thereby achieve an improved functional de but appear to carry a risk that exceeds the risk in patients who have had this improved functional status without a need for medical manipulation to achieve it.

◆ In the case of malignancy, one must establish that curative resection is clinically achievable.

◆ Routine bowel preparation with both colonic cleansing and antibiotics by the oral route should be performed. Measures should be taken to have blood transfusions available for the operation, and on rare occasions platelets should be available.

STEP 3: OPERATIVE STEPS

1. INCISION

◆ Several incisions can be used with success for the left hepatic resection. We favor the inverted L incision. Added exposure may be achieved in this incision by extending the incision either laterally toward the right flank along the horizontal component of this incision or medially across the midline. In addition, one may improve exposure by extending the vertical component of the incision toward the xiphoid process **(Figure 46-3)**. Some surgeons prefer the bilateral subcostal incision with an option to extend the incision in the midline toward the xiphoid.

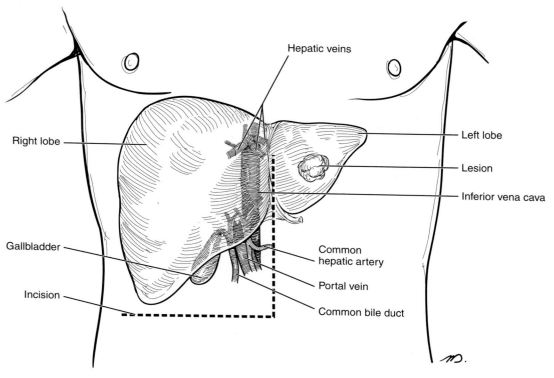

FIGURE 46–3

2. DISSECTION

◆ Divide the falciform ligament and leave a 2-0 silk suture as a stay suture, and place a
hemostat on the silk suture. Carefully incise the avascular plane extending from falciform
ligament back toward the diaphragm using electrocautery after placing the right falciform
beneath the left lobe of the liver **(Figure 46-4)**. In a similar manner under direct vi
incise the left triangular ligament using electrocautery by first cauterizing the anterior
of the left triangular ligament. Second, take the posterior leaflet of the left triangular liga
over toward the vena cava. Anticipate, possibly visualizing, the left hepatic vein as the diss
tion carries close to the vena cava and carefully monitor to prevent any injury to the left
hepatic vein. Carefully divide some of the fiber attachments between the diaphragm and the
superior border of the liver, where the falciform ligament has inserted, and begin to visualize
the vena cava and possibly visualize the middle and left hepatic veins **(Figure 46-5)**.

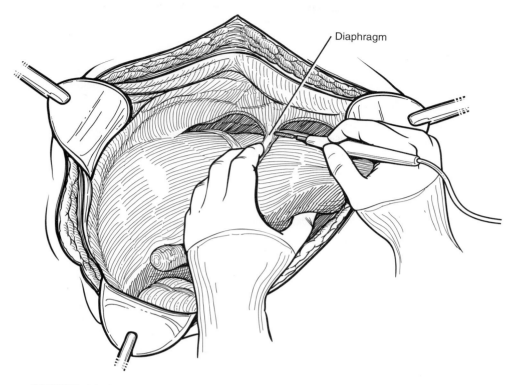

Diaphragm

FIGURE 46–4

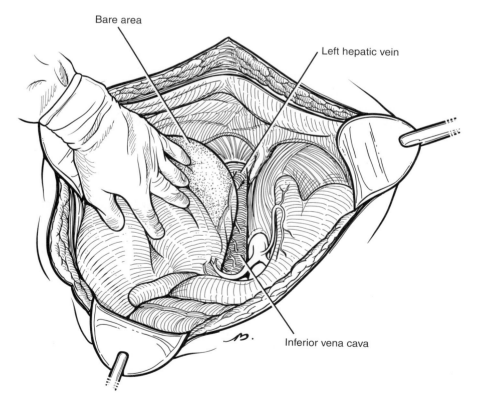

Bare area

Left hepatic vein

Inferior vena cava

FIGURE 46–5

- Place a Rummel loop surrounding the portal triad by incising the peritoneum just medial to the hepatoduodenal ligament. By passing the left hand into the foramen of Winslow, you pass an umbilical tape. This tape is grasped and placed in the hook device, and the umbilical tape is passed through a section of rubber tubing **(Figure 46-6).** Use this step in the event that uncontrolled hemorrhage is encountered during the resection. At this point it is occasionally necessary to use ultrasound for two reasons:
    - To establish that the anticipated line of resection includes the lesion you want to resect
    - To visualize intrahepatic vascular structures, particularly hepatic venous and intrahepatic portions of the portal venous system (see Figure 46-6)

- Next, direct attention to the hepatoduodenal ligament where you must separately identify each of the three major components of the ligament, which include the following:
    - Common bile duct
    - Proper hepatic artery
    - Portal vein

- Encircle the common bile duct with a ¼-inch Penrose drain. Then encircle the proper hepatic artery using vessel loops. By placing lateral traction on the bile duct and medial traction on the artery, you will expose the portal vein, which is situated between these two structures in a slightly deeper plane. By gently teasing the tissues toward the hilum following a horizontal plane along the base of segment IV, you will lower the falciform plate. This provides visualization of the left structures of the portal, arterial, and biliary systems **(Figure 46-7).**

- Establish an acceptable length on each of these structures to ensure careful and safe division.

- Divide the left hilar structures sequentially. Divide the left hepatic duct. You must use nonabsorbable suture, either 3-0 or 4-0 Vicryl or polydioxanone (PDS). Divide the left hepatic artery between clamps and suture ligate using 3-0 silk suture ligature. Divide the portal vein between clamps. Sew the stump of the left portal vein with a continuous running 4-0 Prolene suture (see Figure 46-7).

- After division of all of the left hilar structures, a clear line of demarcation will be seen with purple discoloration of the anatomic left liver. The demarcation crosses the gallbladder bed from anterior to posterior.

- In patients who still have a gallbladder, perform a cholecystectomy in the normal fashion.

- Encircle the left hepatic vein with a vessel loop. It is important to note that at times, with varying sizes of the liver, the left hepatic vein may be situated in a more lateral and inferior location than you might anticipate, and it is vital to establish whether the vein that is first seen in the dissection along the diaphragm is not the middle hepatic vein. It is also vital that you not sacrifice the middle hepatic vein if it is not necessary to do so. Do not divide the hepatic veins until you complete the dissection. However, establish some control of the vein by encircling it.

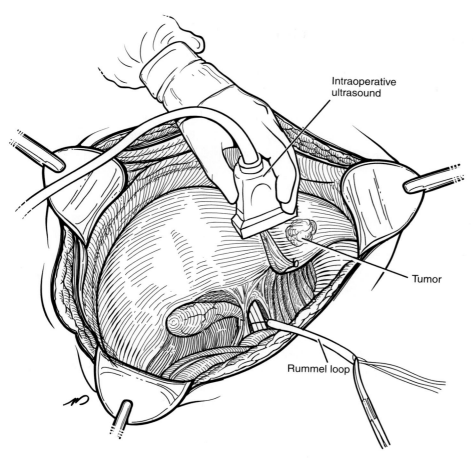

Intraoperative
ultrasound

Tumor

Rummel loop

FIGURE 46–6

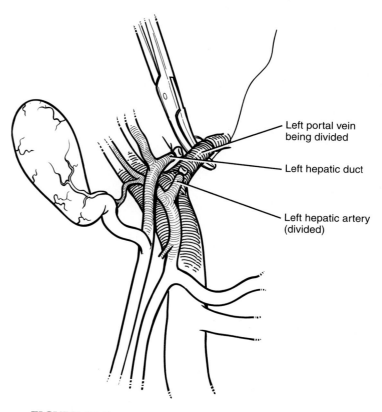

Left portal vein
being divided

Left hepatic duct

Left hepatic artery
(divided)

FIGURE 46–7

◆ Once you establish safety, proceed with the resection. The Habib radio-frequency device may be used for division of parenchyma that is remote from major structures. During division of the parenchyma, you will visualize vascular and biliary structures. When size dictates, these may be divided between clamps and tied **(Figure 46-8)**.

◆ Along the line of demarcation, score the capsule of the liver anteriorly, using electrocautery. Then use a harmonic scalpel to carefully and sequentially divide the liver by layers. Do not permit yourself to establish a deep hole in the liver where control of hemorrhage will be greatly compromised.

◆ During this dissection, divide major portal, arterial, and biliary structures between clamps and suture ligate using 3-0 silk suture ligatures. Slightly blunt clearing of surrounding flaky parenchyma may be achieved using a metal-tipped fine-tip suction apparatus, such as the Frazier tip instrument. As the dissection is carried toward the hilar structures, it is vital to recognize and avoid injury to the right hepatic vessels; failure to do so can result in ischemia of the right liver (see Figure 46-8).

◆ At this point, no more than 0.5 to 2 cm depth of liver remains before you encounter the vena cava. Carry the dissection down to the vena cava, beginning in the inferior border of the liver. The left hepatic vein is typically situated at the diaphragmatic surface of the superior border of the left liver. Once again, note that at times the liver may be rotated, and what appears to be the left hepatic vein may be the middle hepatic vein. Do not divide the vein until all inflow has been reliably interrupted. Typically, the hepatic veins are not divided until the completion of the dissection. Thus stay alert for the identification of the left hepatic vein as the dissection is carried superiorly for the final 0.5 to 2 cm thickness of remaining left liver attached to the right liver **(Figure 46-9)**.

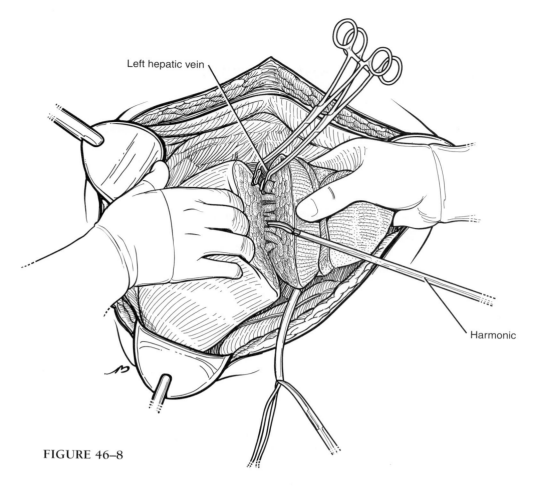

Left hepatic vein

Harmonic

FIGURE 46–8

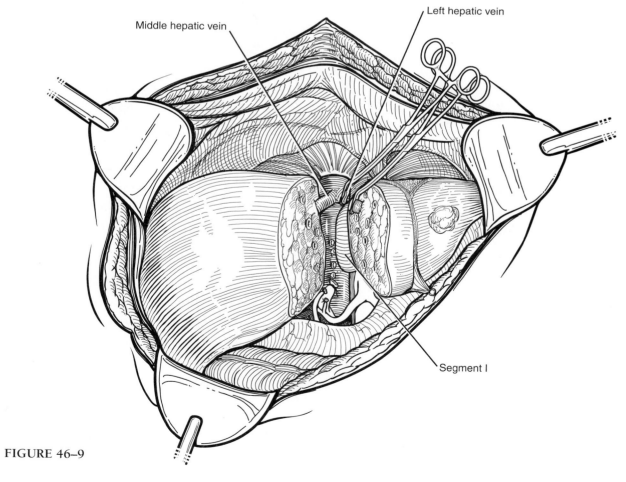

Middle hepatic vein

Left hepatic vein

Segment I

FIGURE 46–9

◆ Division of the left hepatic vein is performed in a manner similar to the division of the left portal vein. Divide it between clamps. Close the open end of the divided vein with the running 4-0 Prolene suture **(Figure 46-10)**.

◆ This step frees the specimen for removal. Perform ultrasound to confirm that resection is adequate and that the anticipated mass has been included in the specimen. The resulting open space is now available for final inspection **(Figure 46-11)**.

◆ Finally, address the large open surface of divided liver. Examine this surface for any large blood vessels that may not have been adequately ligated. In particular, look for biliary structures that must be ligated to prevent postoperative biliary leak. Drain the area with two closed suction drains such as Jackson-Pratt or Blake drains. Place one drain more anteriorly and the other more posteriorly. We prefer to place omentum in the space previously occupied by the left liver **(Figure 46-12)**.

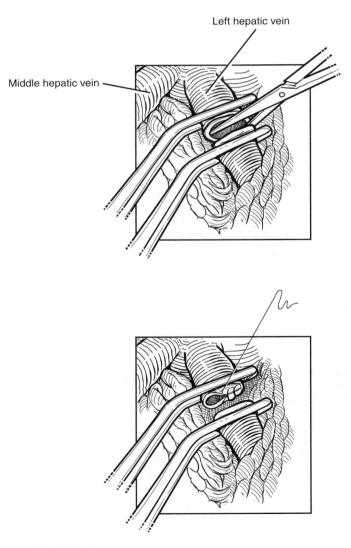

FIGURE 46–10

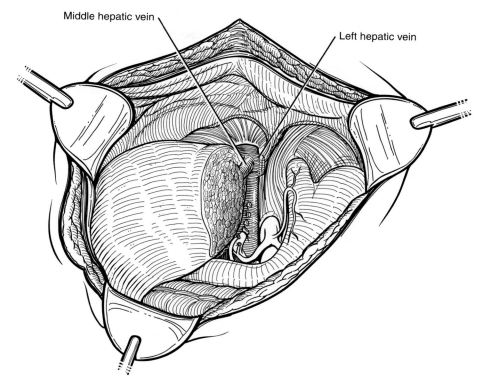

FIGURE 46–11

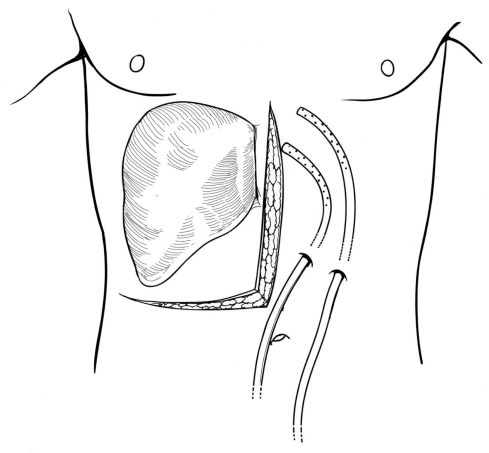

FIGURE 46–12

3. CLOSING

- We close the fascia with an interrupted horizontal mattress suture (Smead-Jones) using heavy-gauge absorbable suture. The skin is reapproximated in the standard fashion.

STEP 4: POSTOPERATIVE CARE

- In the first 24 hours after surgery, the primary concern is hemorrhage and the related measure of coagulation status. These should be monitored by means of serial measurement of hemoglobin and coagulation factors.

- In all major resections, particularly in patients with cirrhosis, one must be vigilant for any signs of hepatic failure. A particularly ominous finding is the progressive rise in bilirubin level with an enzyme pattern that supports neither obstruction (alkaline phosphatase elevation) nor parenchymal cell death (transaminase elevations).

- The most ominous finding is a plummeting serum glucose level, which reflects the loss of glycogen stores in the liver and by inference the loss of viable liver. Unfortunately, there is little one can do to reverse this pattern of failure.

- One possible cause of failure is inadequate liver remaining after resection. This can potentially resolve over time as the liver regenerates, which it will do to some degree. Support of the patient during this marginal period is vital.

- One possible remediable cause of this progressive demise is thrombus formation in the portal vein. This would seem to be unlikely, because coagulation is typically inadequate in these patients, but we have seen this phenomenon. It is possible that lysis of this clot may restore vital flow.

- Sepsis is particularly metabolically taxing to the liver. In the compromised postoperative liver, sepsis can be catastrophic. One should monitor and obtain cultures if necessary to prevent infectious processes from progressing.

- Ascites may form, and one must be aware when this phenomenon has occurred and treat as one would normally treat this entity with careful and judicious use of salt-containing intravenous fluids and with diuresis.

- Remove drains if no bile is seen in the effluent.

STEP 5: PEARLS AND PITFALLS

- As with all such major operative procedures, one must be extremely careful with patient selection.

- If hemorrhage occurs during the procedure, one can compress the liver into the spine or into the right flank to gain control, and always call for assistance from another capable surgeon.

- Before dividing any of the major vascular structures, stop and reconfirm that the proper structure is being divided.

- If ascites forms and the drains are still in place, excessive electrolyte and fluid loss may occur from active draining of liters of fluid per day. In this setting, one must remove the drains (assuming they are not bile tinged) and suture the skin overlying the drain tract.

- In recent years, there has been some enthusiasm for preoperative embolization of the portal vein on the side of the anticipated resection. This may offer some element of ischemia/necrosis of the diseased liver and simultaneous regeneration of the opposite side.

SELECTED REFERENCES

1. Blumgart LH, Belghiti J: Liver resection for benign disease and for liver and biliary tumors. In Blumgart LH (ed): Surgery of the Liver, Biliary Tract and Pancreas, 4th ed. Philadelphia, Saunders, 2007, pp 1341-1388.
2. Sugiyama M, Suzuki Y, Abe N, et al: Modified hanging maneuver with extraparenchymal isolation of the middle hepatic vein in left hepatectomy. J Hepatobiliary Pancreat Surg 2009;16:156-159.
3. Shirabe K, Shimada M, Gion T, et al: Postoperative liver failure after major hepatic resection for hepatocellular carcinoma in the modern era with special reference to remnant liver volume. J Am Coll Surg 1999;188:304-309.

PANCREAS

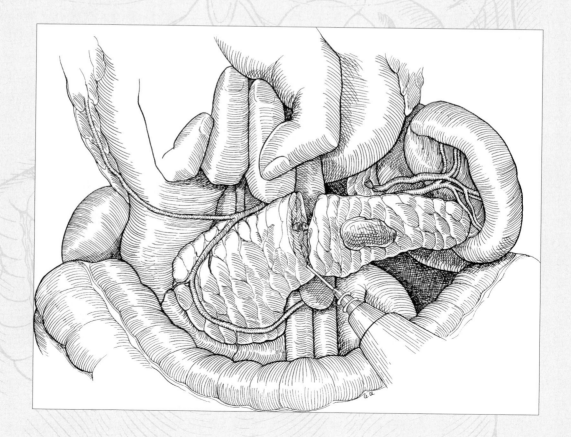

CHAPTER 47

DISTAL PANCREATECTOMY AND SPLENECTOMY

William H. Nealon

STEP 1: SURGICAL ANATOMY

- The term distal pancreatectomy and splenectomy typically refers to any resection beginning at approximately the level of the spine and moving toward the tail of the pancreas and the spleen. The associated anatomy includes the tail of the pancreas. This structure traverses the left lateral boundaries of the retroperitoneum and extends superiorly, finally ending toward the left hemidiaphragm. The tail fits into the concave area formed by the medial aspect of the spleen. The blood supply to the tail of the pancreas is provided by the splenic artery and vein.

- The splenic artery **(Figure 47-1)** traverses the superior border of the body and tail of the pancreas. There are many small branches between the artery and the body and tail of the pancreas, which must be addressed should one choose to preserve the spleen after distal pancreatectomy.

- The splenic vein is located on the posterior surface of the pancreas, and as it runs medially, it joins the superior mesenteric vein to form the portal vein. From the body of the pancreas out toward the tail, the splenic vein can be anticipated to maintain its position behind the body of the pancreas until it reaches the hilum of the spleen. Once again, very small tributaries will likely be encountered between the body and tail of the pancreas and splenic vein—these must be addressed should one choose to preserve the spleen during a distal pancreatectomy.

- The spleen is attached on its lateral and superior borders to the retroperitoneum, connecting the peritoneal serosa to the visceral serosa. Posterior to the spleen and the tail of the pancreas is the left kidney and the left adrenal gland. These may be encountered during dissection. The stomach is situated anterior to the body and tail of the pancreas, and there are vascular branches between the fundus of the stomach and the spleen. These vessels are termed "short gastric vessels." The transverse colon and, in particular, the transverse mesocolon may be apposed to these tissues, and the dissections of these structures away from the spleen and the body and tail of the pancreas are necessary to complete the resection. The splenic flexure of the colon typically will be mobilized during this dissection (see Figure 47-1).

INDICATIONS

◆ Distal pancreatectomy with or without splenectomy may be used for treatment of benign and malignant lesions. Benign lesions may include an inflammatory mass or infected pseudocyst. Distal pancreatectomy may be required for individuals who have sustained what has been termed "disconnected duct syndrome," with a complete separation of the ductal system in the tail of the pancreas from the head and body of the pancreas. This may be found after episodes of necrotizing pancreatitis, as well as after trauma in which typically the injury to the pancreatic duct is where the body of the pancreas traverses the spine. Distal pancreatectomy may be used for premalignant lesions, such as intraductal papillary mucinous neoplasms (IPMN). Similarly, mucinous cystic neoplasms are typically located in the tail of the pancreas and are also considered to be premalignant lesions. These are also candidates for resection. Patients may have neuroendocrine tumors, which are not clearly malignant. These may include insulinoma or vasoactive intestinal peptide (VIP)oma, and at times resection of the tail of the pancreas is performed to remove these. Malignant lesions, such as primary carcinoma of the pancreas and metastatic tumors to the pancreas, most notably renal cell carcinoma, may require distal pancreatectomy. Among lesions in this category are primary adenocarcinoma of the pancreas, malignant mucinous cysts, malignant neuroendocrine tumors, and metastic lesions in the tail of the pancreas.

◆ The question of preserving the spleen is always mentioned when discussing distal pancreatectomy, although often the decision for including a splenectomy is made at the time of the operation, depending on the anatomy encountered and the amount of distortion of planes created by the underlying disease. There is general agreement that malignancies be uniformly accompanied by splenectomy to ensure adequate margins. For benign disease, particularly for lesions such as IPMN, in which the pancreas is essentially normal, it should be possible to safely resect the tail of the pancreas without including the spleen.

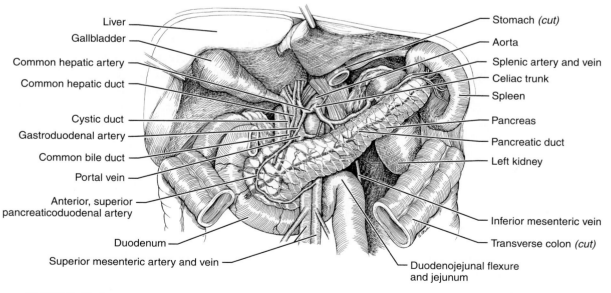

FIGURE 47–1

STEP 2: PREOPERATIVE CONSIDERATIONS

◆ As with all major abdominal surgery, one needs to consider the patient's American Society of Anesthesiologists (ASA) status and relative risk of operation. Specific to this operation are a number of features. First, because the density of beta cells may be far greater in the tail of the pancreas than in the body and the head, there is a heightened risk of insulin dependence after distal pancreatectomy. Surprising to some, the risk of insulin dependency is greater after distal pancreatectomy than it is after a resection of the head of the pancreas. It is important to advise the patient of this risk preoperatively. If the patient has an associated diagnosis of chronic pancreatitis or borderline diabetes, certainly the risk of developing insulin dependence is higher.

◆ The second issue is the possibility of a splenectomy and the need to address the issue of postsplenectomy sepsis. This entity is now relatively easily managed by obtaining vaccines for the encapsulated organisms that are responsible for postsplenectomy sepsis. These are pneumococcus, meningococcus, and *Haemophilus influenzae*. There are two choices for administering these vaccines. The first is to administer them a minimum of 2 weeks before the operative procedure. The strategy is that the immune status will be sufficient to mount an antibody response to the antigens before surgery. If the decision to administer vaccines is delayed until it is clear that the patient has had a splenectomy, then the vaccines may need to be administered postoperatively. Because of the proven changes in immune capabilities early after major surgery, the recommendation is to wait a minimum of 4 weeks after surgery to administer the vaccines. These vaccines should be administered at 5-year intervals for life, and the patient should be advised of this issue before surgery. It is well known that a patient with a splenectomy may also develop thrombocytosis after surgery, and this should be monitored carefully.

◆ Finally, particularly in patients with a normal pancreas, there is a chance that postoperative pancreatitis may develop, and enzymes should be followed for evidence of acute inflammation in the early postoperative period. It is possible to assume some of these changes are simply related to the stress of operation. One must exercise a high level of suspicion in this regard.

◆ Perhaps the most nettlesome postoperative issue in these patients is the frequency of pancreatic fistula after resection of the tail of the pancreas. There are those who have suggested routinely using preoperatively placed pancreatic ductal stents to prevent this. This is certainly not practiced widely. In any event, it is important to advise patients that this eventuality is seen in as many as 25% of patients who have undergone resection of the tail of the pancreas. This compares poorly with the 15% risk of pancreatic fistula after pancreaticoduodenectomy.

STEP 3: OPERATIVE STEPS

◆ Preoperative bowel prep and intravenous antibiotics at the time of the incision are both recommended. The characteristic bowel preparation is bowel cleansing combined with oral neomycin and erythromycin for three doses before the surgery. Intravenous antibiotics are generally second-generation cephalosporins or something similar.

1. INCISION

◆ We use the left subcostal incision with a horizontal shaping of the subcostal incision at the midline to facilitate extending to the right subcostal if necessary. We similarly create a horizontal direction to the incision as we pass beneath the costal margin laterally, again to facilitate extending an incision if necessary. In general, with the exception of markedly obese patients, one can perform this operation safely with the relatively minimal incision in the left subcostal region **(Figure 47-2)**.

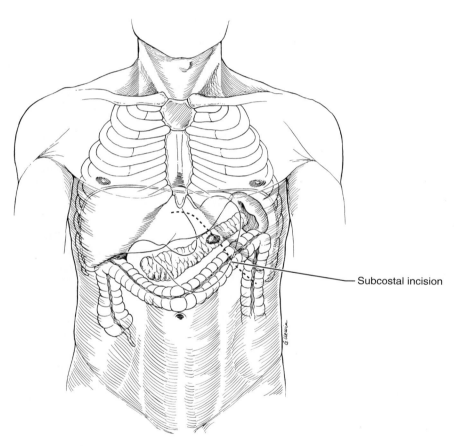

Subcostal incision

FIGURE 47–2

2. DISSECTION

◆ Upon entering the abdomen, the general evaluation of the abdomen may be necessary, particularly if malignancy is being treated. Specifically, one should look for evidence of peritoneal seeding or any evidence of hepatic metastasis. It is also usually possible to palpate the lesion whether benign or malignant through the omentum in the left upper quadrant.

◆ The lesser sac is entered by grasping the gastrocolic omentum and reflecting superiorly and anteriorly. This reveals the posterior surface of the omentum as it attaches to the transverse mesocolon. Using electrocautery and beginning well to the left of the spine, it is possible to dissect the attachments between the omentum and the transverse colon. There is characteristically some amount of adhesion between the appendices epiploicae and the transverse mesocolon, and these must be carefully separated until the lesser sect can be entered **(Figure 47-3)**. At times in patients who have had previous significant pancreatitis, this plane may be impossible to traverse. As the omentum is mobilized along the transverse colon, the necessary window into the lesser sac will depend on the size of the patient and the size of the lesion. It is certainly possible to extend the dissection well over to the right of the midline if necessary to establish a wider entry into the lesser sac. Upon entering the lesser sac in this fashion, it is possible to reflect the stomach superiorly and anteriorly, revealing the anterior surface of the body of the pancreas. The omentum dissection can be carried to the left, mobilizing the splenic flexure of the colon in this fashion. It may be helpful to reflect the splenic flexure of the colon inferiorly to delineate the inferior border of the spleen and the inferior border of the tail of the pancreas. After this amount of dissection, it is hoped that one should have fully visualized the lesion and determined exactly what amount of body of the pancreas may need to be removed for adequate excision. If it is not possible to fully identify the lesion at this point, it may be necessary to use an ultrasound probe to facilitate identification. This is commonly needed when exploring for benign neuroendocrine tumors, such as insulinoma or gastrinoma (see Figure 47-3).

◆ At this point, an option is available for defining and dissecting the splenic artery on the superior border of the pancreas. This maneuver may facilitate control of hemorrhage if one anticipates encountering significant hemorrhage during the dissection of the spleen and the tail of the pancreas. This can simply be done with an atraumatic vascular clamp if one is not certain that the spleen will need to be removed and serves as a control for hemorrhage (see Figure 47-3).

◆ Next, attention is directed to the left hemidiaphragm in the left upper quadrant of the abdomen. The peritoneal attachments, lateral to the spleen, are incised using electrocautery, and this permits beginning of the mobilization of the spleen and the tail of the pancreas toward the midline. One may continue medially along the superior border of the spleen. As one turns the dissection in an inferior direction on the medial (hilar) aspect of the spleen, one encounters the short gastric vessels **(Figure 47-4)**.

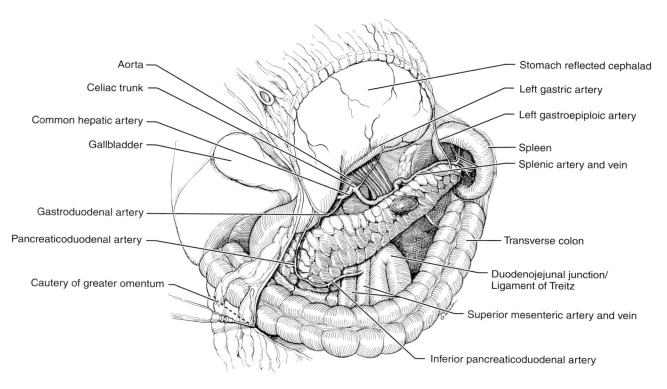

Aorta

Celiac trunk

Common hepatic artery

Gallbladder

Gastroduodenal artery

Pancreaticoduodenal artery

Cautery of greater omentum

Stomach reflected cephalad

Left gastric artery

Left gastroepiploic artery

Spleen

Splenic artery and vein

Transverse colon

Duodenojejunal junction/
Ligament of Treitz

Superior mesenteric artery and vein

Inferior pancreaticoduodenal artery

FIGURE 47–3

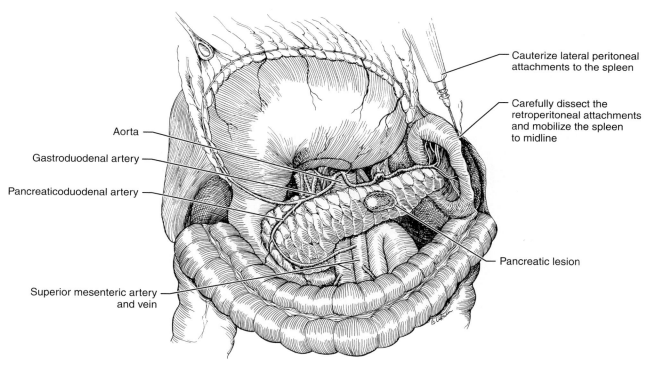

Aorta

Gastroduodenal artery

Pancreaticoduodenal artery

Superior mesenteric artery
and vein

Cauterize lateral peritoneal
attachments to the spleen

Carefully dissect the
retroperitoneal attachments
and mobilize the spleen
to midline

Pancreatic lesion

FIGURE 47–4

◆ Careful dissection of the retroperitoneum will permit mobilization between the kidney and the adrenal glands posteriorly and the spleen and the tail of the pancreas anteriorly. After this has been done, there is typically a vascular attachment at the inferior border of the pancreas between the spleen and the splenic flexure of the colon. This should be divided between clamps and tied using 3-0 or 2-0 silk ties. At the same time, the vascular attachments between the greater curvature of the stomach at the fundus and the spleen, the short gastric vessels, are divided between clamps and tied using 2-0 and 3-0 silk ties. Caution should be taken not to place a tie on the wall of the stomach, because this may result in a necrosis of the greater curvature. After this amount of mobilization, it should be possible to separate completely the spleen and the tail of the pancreas from its retroperitoneal attachments further toward the midline. Typically this dissection is carried until one has reached a minimum of 3 cm medial to the mass that is anticipated for resection **(Figure 47-5)**.

◆ At this point, the decision needs to be made regarding preservation of the spleen. If no plans are made to preserve the spleen, it should be possible to separate and ligate the splenic artery and the splenic vein. One must always divide the artery before dividing the vein to prevent any engorgement and bleeding of the spleen that would result from dividing the vein first **(Figure 47-6)**.

◆ If one is planning on preserving the spleen, then the small vascular attachments between the splenic artery and the tail of the pancreas and body of the pancreas and between the splenic vein and the body and tail of the pancreas must be carefully divided and tied using 3-0 silk ties. It is during this dissection that one may conclude that a splenectomy is safer than the hemorrhage that could at times result from this dissection in a patient who has had a significant history of pancreatitis **(Figure 47-7)**.

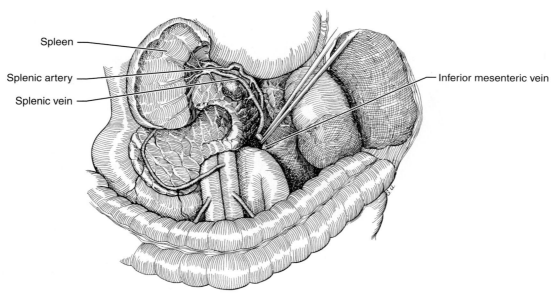

Spleen

Splenic artery

Splenic vein

Inferior mesenteric vein

FIGURE 47–5

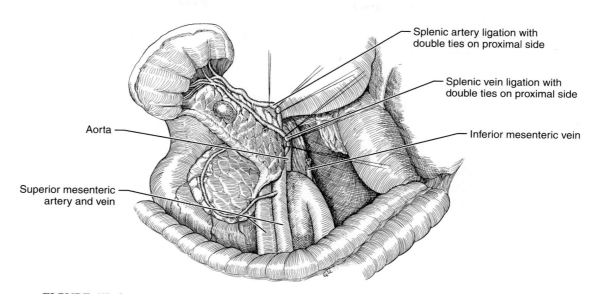

Splenic artery ligation with double ties on proximal side

Splenic vein ligation with double ties on proximal side

Aorta

Inferior mesenteric vein

Superior mesenteric artery and vein

FIGURE 47–6

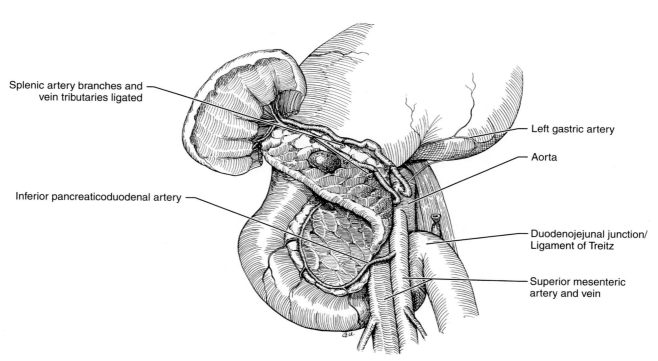

Splenic artery branches and vein tributaries ligated

Left gastric artery

Aorta

Inferior pancreaticoduodenal artery

Duodenojejunal junction/ Ligament of Treitz

Superior mesenteric artery and vein

FIGURE 47–7

◆ At this point, one should have separated the tail of the pancreas from the splenic artery and vein or should have divided the splenic artery and vein, and the only remaining attachments should be the parenchyma of the pancreas. We prefer a fish mouth opening to the body of the pancreas. This involves angling at approximately 45 degrees toward the head of the pancreas, along the anterior border of the body of the pancreas to approximately half the depth of the body of the pancreas. We then go to 90 degrees in the opposite direction, again with a 45-degree angulation, and incise toward the tail of the pancreas. This permits apposing the ends of the divided pancreas in the hopes of preventing a pancreatic fistula **(Figure 47-8)**.

◆ At this point, one must carefully identify the pancreatic duct. This may be accomplished by gently massaging the body of the pancreas and expressing pancreatic juice through the pancreatic duct. In certain patients, particularly patients with a normal pancreas, the pancreatic duct can be quite miniscule. The duct is ligated with a 4-0 Prolene stitch **(Figure 47-9)**.

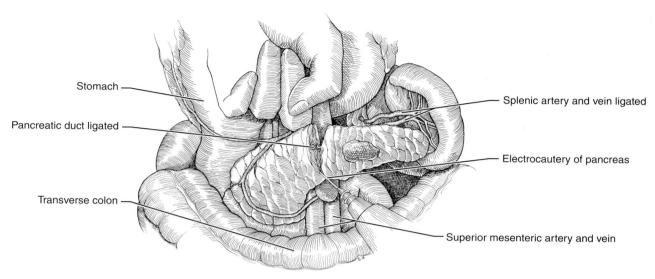

Stomach

Pancreatic duct ligated

Transverse colon

Splenic artery and vein ligated

Electrocautery of pancreas

Superior mesenteric artery and vein

FIGURE 47–8

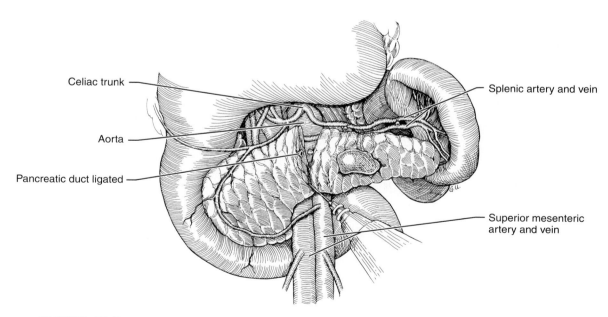

Celiac trunk

Aorta

Pancreatic duct ligated

Splenic artery and vein

Superior mesenteric artery and vein

FIGURE 47–9

◆ After the pancreatic duct is ligated, the anterior and posterior portions of the fish mouth created by dividing the body of the pancreas are reapproximated using interrupted 2-0 Prolene
sutures. After this is completed, the area is irrigated and two drains are placed in the retroperitoneum, just lateral of the divided body of the pancreas. This closure is identical for
patients who have had splenectomy or splenic preservation (**Figures 47-10 through 47-13**).

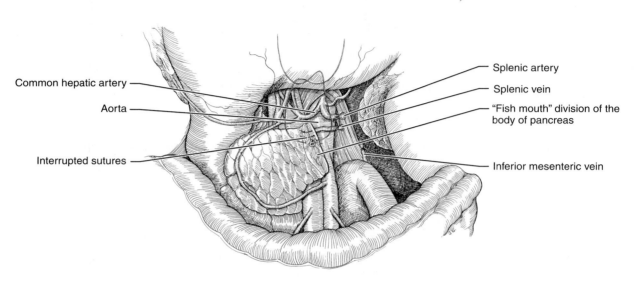

FIGURE 47–10

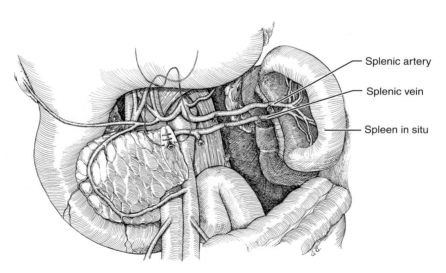

FIGURE 47–11

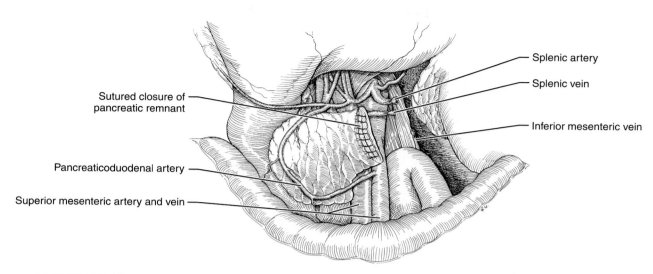

Splenic artery

Splenic vein

Sutured closure of
pancreatic remnant

Inferior mesenteric vein

Pancreaticoduodenal artery

Superior mesenteric artery and vein

FIGURE 47–12

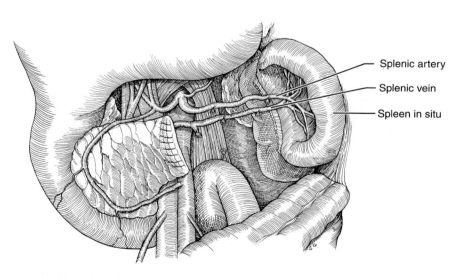

Splenic artery

Splenic vein

Spleen in situ

FIGURE 47–13

3. CLOSING

◆ The abdomen and skin are closed in the usual fashion. The drains are placed to closed bulb suction.

STEP 4: POSTOPERATIVE CARE

◆ Monitor blood glucose and urine glucose.

◆ Monitor amylase and lipase levels to detect postoperative pancreatitis.

◆ Monitor platelet count to detect postoperative thrombocytosis.

◆ One may consider keeping a nasogastric tube in place after this procedure. There has traditionally been a concern that a dilated stomach may undermine the sutures along the short gastric vessels. More recent practice has endorsed very brief use of such tubes.

◆ Monitor the drain outputs, and particularly examine them for amylase levels beginning on day 4 or after a regular diet has been resumed to detect pancreatic fistula.

STEP 5: PEARLS AND PITFALLS

◆ It is important to recognize that all significant vascular inflow to the spleen comes along the splenic artery. For that reason, early isolation of the splenic artery may well maintain control in the event that significant hemorrhage occurs during the attempted resection. Particularly with postinflammatory changes, the dissection along the spleen and the tail of the pancreas may be fraught with potential hemorrhage, and much of this can be prevented by taking early control of the splenic artery.

◆ Although we do not currently recommend additional measures preoperatively, one should be prepared for the possibility of pancreatic fistula, and we therefore take very seriously the ligation of the divided main pancreatic duct in the pancreatic remnant. We particularly make an effort to have good tissue apposition by the closure of our body of the pancreas. It is also quite important to remove the drains after this operation only when one is certain that they have been functioning and that they no longer have any significant output. It is unfortunately well known that one may remove a drain because he or she believes the drain outputs have ceased when they have simply stopped because of drain failure. In this event, one may require interventional radiology to help with proper drainage.

SELECTED REFERENCES

1. Blumgart LH, Belghiti J: Liver resection for benign disease and for liver and biliary tumors. In Blumgart LH (ed): Surgery of the Liver, Biliary Tract and Pancreas, 4th ed. Philadelphia: Saunders, 2007, pp 1341-1388.
2. Sugiyama M, Suzuki Y, Abe N, et al. Modified liver hanging maneuver with extraparenchymal isolation of the middle hepatic vein in left hepatectomy. J Hepatobiliary Pancreat Surg 2009;16:156-159.
3. Shirabe K, Shimada M, Gion T, et al. Postoperative liver failure after major hepatic resection for hepatocellular carcinoma in the modern era with special reference to remnant liver volume. J Am Coll Surg 1999;188:304-309.

CHAPTER 48

BEGER AND FREY PROCEDURES

William H. Nealon

STEP 1: SURGICAL ANATOMY

- All pancreatic surgery requires an understanding of the anatomic relationships in the lesser sac. After either an upper midline or a bilateral subcostal (chevron) incision, one enters the lesser sac by dissecting along the avascular plane at the points of attachment of the gastrocolic omentum to the transverse colon. The proper plane is between the anterior and posterior leaflets. This is my favored point of entry. The alternative entry is by dividing and ligating, in a transverse direction, the vascular structures embedded in the omentum while preserving the gastroepiploic vessels located along the greater curvature of the stomach.

- Upon entering the lesser sac, one will encounter varying amounts of inflammatory adhesions between the posterior wall of the stomach and the anterior surface of the pancreas. Considerable dense adhesions may be encountered in the background of chronic pancreatitis.

- The pancreas is essentially encased in a sandwich of major blood vessels. The vena cava and aorta occupy the posterior surface in the midline. The splenic artery courses along the superior surface from the aorta toward the tail. The splenic vein occupies the posterior superior surface of the body and tail of the pancreas. It meets the superior mesenteric vein, which is oriented vertically in the groove created by the uncinate process in the posterior aspect of the head of the pancreas and the right lateral and anterior components of the head. The confluence of these two veins constitutes the portal vein, which traverses the uncinate groove encased by the head of the pancreas and emerges to join the bile duct and the hepatic artery in the hepatoduodenal ligament.

- The superior mesenteric artery is located in a plane posterior and slightly medial to the superior mesenteric vein. The common hepatic artery, a branch of the celiac trunk (along with the splenic artery and left gastric artery), courses along the superior border of the head of the pancreas to join the hepatoduodenal ligament. Its first branch is the typically miniscule right gastric artery. Just distal is the more substantial gastroduodenal artery, which emerges at a right angle to the hepatic artery from its inferior surface and courses beneath the pylorus, and after sending the right gastroepiploic artery in the plane between the inferior aspect of the pylorus and the superior surface of the head of the pancreas, the gastroduodenal artery pierces the head of the pancreas.

- The anterior superior and the posterior superior pancreaticoduodenal arteries also arise from branches of the gastroduodenal artery. These arteries form an arch medial to the C-loop of the duodenum, and they collateralize with branches of the anterior and posterior inferior pancreaticoduodenal arteries, which are branches of the superior mesenteric artery. Small branches from these arteries provide blood supply to the duodenum. Both the Beger and Frey procedures include division of these anterior vessels. Preservation of the posterior arcade ensures viability of the duodenum.

◆ Key anatomic features in pancreatic head resections and in the Beger and Frey procedures are the network of tributaries projecting between the superior mesenteric vein/portal vein confluence and the uncinate process. These tributaries are located at the right lateral aspect of the veins. These tiny veins exit the pancreas at the mid-portion of the groove in which the major veins reside.

◆ The pancreas is entirely retroperitoneal, and therefore operative procedures will require mobilization of the pancreas from its retroperitoneal position. The plane lateral to the C-loop of the duodenum is incised in nearly all procedures; this plane is avascular, and its mobilization is termed the Kocher maneuver. This exposes the vena cava and aorta, and it permits "bimanual palpation" of the head of the pancreas. The dissection may be easily extended to the fourth portion of the duodenum and the ligament of Treitz (see Figure 48-3).

◆ The inferior border of the body of the pancreas is also avascular, although the inferior mesenteric vein may be encountered to the right of the spine.

◆ Peritoneum overlies the hepatoduodenal ligament. Dissection reveals the triad in gross anatomic terms, which corresponds to the microscopic portal triad—with portal venous, hepatic arterial, and biliary structures. The common bile duct is located in an anterior lateral position, and the hepatic artery is anterior medial. The portal vein is positioned in the posterior groove created by the apposition of these anterior structures (see Figure 48-5).

◆ On the inferior border of the pancreatic head, just where the duodenum dives beneath the superior mesenteric vein and artery, one may dissect the peritoneum and visualize the superior mesenteric vein as it passes superiorly beneath the head of the pancreas.

◆ The main pancreatic duct originates in the tail of the pancreas and traverses the length of the pancreas to exit in the duodenum through both main ampulla (Vater) and the accessory ampulla, which is located more proximally in the duodenum. The main pancreatic duct (Wirsung) and the minor or accessory duct (Santorini) fuse during fetal development at what is termed the genu or "knee" of the duct.

INDICATIONS

◆ The indication for surgery in all patients with chronic pancreatitis is essentially the same. The most common indication for surgery is chronic unremitting abdominal pain.

◆ A second indication for surgery in chronic pancreatitis is episodes of recurrent, acute exacerbations, either alone or combined with constant pain.

- Some element of biliary stricture results either in jaundice, which is rare, or in some element of bile duct dilation. This can be confirmed by extremely high circulating levels of alkaline phosphatase in the blood.

- Poor nutrition and inability to adequately process nutrients because of exocrine or endocrine insufficiency, as well as the pain associated with eating, is an additional indication for surgery.

STEP 2: PREOPERATIVE CONSIDERATIONS

- It is vital to establish the significance of the pain associated with chronic pancreatitis to be certain that this person's pain is of sufficient magnitude to warrant major operation.

- The patient must be carefully scrutinized for current nutritional status, as well as the proper medical management of either exocrine or endocrine dysfunction, which is often associated with this disease. Surgery should be delayed until nutritional status has been stabilized.

- Some amount of counseling regarding narcotic dependence should be initiated preoperatively in these patients.

- Specific discussion should be made regarding the goals of resuming normal activities, stopping ethanol abuse, and resuming employment. It is incumbent upon the pancreatic surgeon to participate in this form of rehabilitation of these patients to ensure satisfactory outcomes for the goals of this operation.

- If a patient has finally reached very high narcotic requirements to manage his or her pain preoperatively, the management of the postoperative pain in these patients can be a daunting task. We have found significant improvements when we perform this procedure with an epidural catheter in place. We have found that even high doses of intravenous narcotics failed to properly manage the pain in these patients in the postoperative period.

- We have experience with improving narcotic effectiveness by placing patients on epidural access some days ahead of surgery and using a pure bupivacaine analgesic. If this can be achieved, the patient may have some freedom of his or her endorphin receptors by the time surgery is undertaken.

- We perform bowel preparation and colonic cleansing in all patients preoperatively.

- A single dose of preoperative intravenous antibiotic prophylaxis is administered using a second-generation cephalosporin.

STEP 3: OPERATIVE STEPS

1. INCISION

◆ We prefer a midline incision for this procedure. The incision is taken from the xiphoid process to just above the umbilicus. Self-retaining retractors are used to establish exposure **(Figure 48-1).**

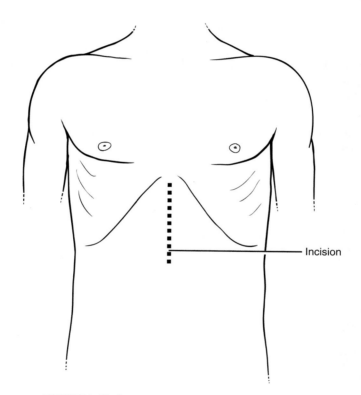

Incision

FIGURE 48–1

2. DISSECTION

◆ The gastrocolic omentum is separated from its attachments along the transverse mesocolon in the avascular plane by using electrocautery. We find it easiest to enter this plane beginning well to the left of the spine. After entering the lesser sac, the omentum is dissected free of its attachments to the hepatic flexure of the colon and toward the cecum if necessary. This permits access to the lesser sac, and any adhesions between the posterior wall of the stomach and the anterior surface of the body and head of the pancreas are carefully dissected **(Figure 48-2)**.

◆ Any of the fatty tissues or adhesions overlying the body and head of the pancreas are carefully cleared to visualize the anterior surface of the pancreas. You will see a bundle of fatty tissue inferior to the pylorus. The right gastroepiploic vessels are within this bundle. These should not be divided at this time. Often a branch can be seen traversing between this bundle and vessels on the inferior border of the pancreas. These can be divided safely between clamps.

◆ At this point, the duodenum and the head of the pancreas are mobilized from their posterior attachments in the retroperitoneum by dividing the peritoneum lateral to the C-loop of the duodenum. This dissection is then carried out toward the left beneath the head of the pancreas. The superior vena cava and the aorta can be identified posteriorly during the dissection. After adequate dissection, you may bimanually palpate the head of the pancreas **(Figure 48-3)**.

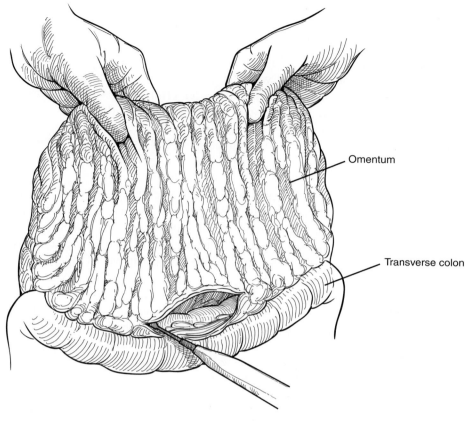

Omentum

Transverse colon

FIGURE 48–2

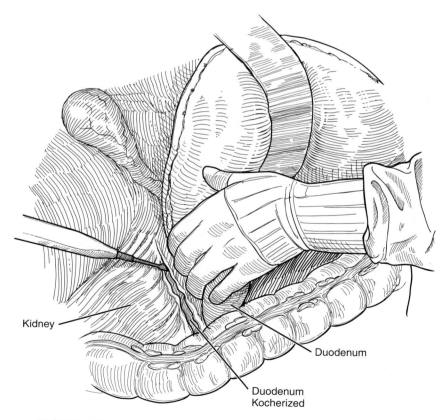

Kidney

Duodenum

Duodenum
Kocherized

FIGURE 48–3

BEGER PROCEDURE

◆ Both the Beger and Frey procedures will use all of the previous steps. The steps unique to each one will now be reviewed, with the Beger procedure first. In many ways the Beger procedure can be viewed as a modification of a resection (pancreaticoduodenectomy)—in other words, a lesser resection. The Frey procedure can be looked upon as a modification of a drainage procedure (Puestow)—in other words, an extended drainage. By virtue of this fact, the two procedure are surprisingly similar.

◆ The inferior border of the pancreas is mobilized beginning to the left of the spine and working toward the head of the pancreas. This is categorized as a vascular plane; however, as the dissection carries toward the insertion of the superior mesentery vein, one must exercise considerable caution because of the variable number of venous tributaries to the mesenteric vein or even piercing beneath the pancreas to the splenic vein (**Figure 48-4**).

◆ The third and fourth portions of the duodenum are carefully dissected, and as one approaches the terminal portions of the C-loop of the duodenum as it courses beneath the mesenteric vessels, the superior mesenteric vein can be easily identified as it courses along the root of the mesentery. A plane can now be established posterior to the head of the pancreas and anterior to the superior mesenteric vein directed toward the hepatoduodenal ligament.

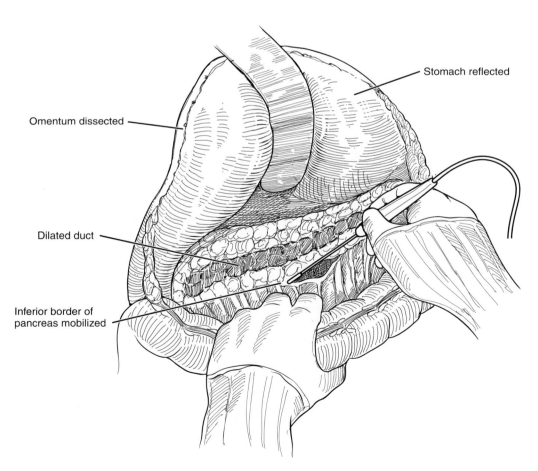

Omentum dissected

Stomach reflected

Dilated duct

Inferior border of
pancreas mobilized

FIGURE 48–4

◆ The peritoneum overlying the hepatoduodenal ligament is next dissected and the common bile duct is encircled with a ¼-inch Penrose drain. Similarly, the proper hepatic artery is encircled by a vessel loop. Place traction laterally on the bile duct and medially on the hepatic artery. In this fashion, you will visualize the portal vein between these two structures, but in a deeper plane. It is now possible to establish a plane between the previously dissected superior mesenteric vein on the inferior border of the pancreas and the portal vein in the hepatoduodenal ligament (**Figure 48-5**).

◆ Carefully divide the vascular attachments along the superior border of the pancreas to the left of the portal vein. Follow the hepatic artery to the point that it diverts in a right angle. At just this point, you will identify the gastroduodenal artery. Divide between clamps, tie, and suture ligate (**Figure 48-6**).

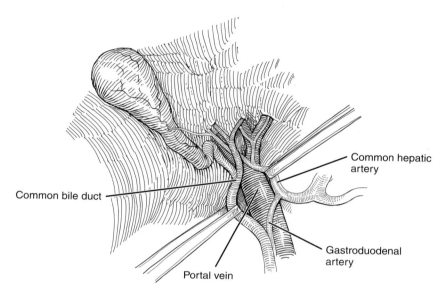

Common hepatic artery

Common bile duct

Gastroduodenal artery

Portal vein

FIGURE 48–5

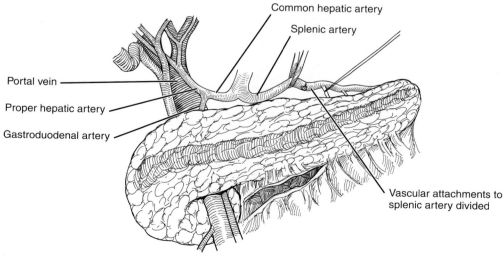

Common hepatic artery

Splenic artery

Portal vein

Proper hepatic artery

Gastroduodenal artery

Vascular attachments to splenic artery divided

FIGURE 48–6

- Division of the gastroduodenal artery permits skeletonization of a perhaps 2-to 3-cm area along the superior border of the head of the pancreas. A line drawn between this plane and the area of dissection along the superior mesenteric vein constitutes the planned line of division of the neck of the pancreas **(Figure 48-7)**.

- Place 2-0 Prolene sutures on the superior and inferior border of the body of the pancreas, both to the left and the right of the anticipated incision site. This is useful both for manipulation of the head of the pancreas during the remaining dissection and to control some of the intraparenchymal vessels. Divide the pancreas using a scalpel and obtain a margin of tissue for biopsy, because chronic pancreatitis may harbor an associated carcinoma **(Figure 48-8)**.

- Then place 2-0 Prolene sutures in a circular fashion on the inner border of the C-loop of the duodenum between the duodenum and the head of the pancreas. These are placed essentially in a continuous fashion, although they are interrupted. These continue from the pylorus on the superior aspect around to the region of the superior mesenteric vein. Both the anterior superior and the anterior inferior vessels are ligated **(Figure 48-9)**. After gaining significant control of hemorrhage with these 2-0 Prolene sutures, one can now begin to excavate the head of the pancreas.

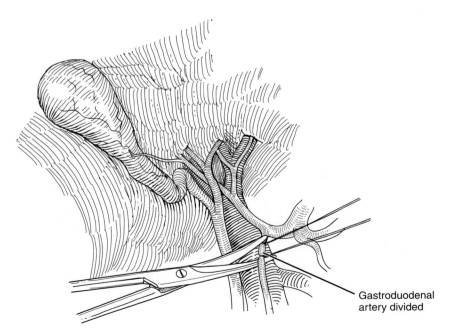

Gastroduodenal
artery divided

FIGURE 48–7

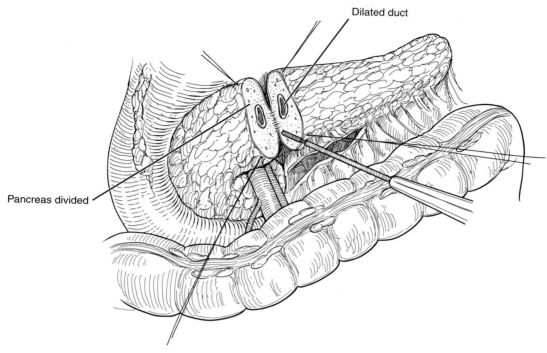

FIGURE 48–8

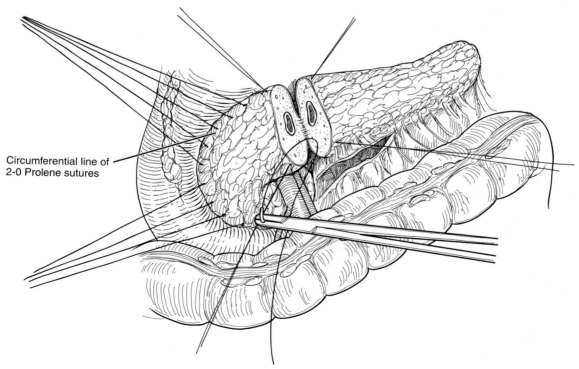

FIGURE 48–9

- Electrocautery or cold knife is used to carefully divide the mass in the head of the pancreas, all the while using bimanual palpation to ensure a thickness in the posterior plane of 5 to 10 mm (**Figures 48-10 and 48-11**).

- Carefully examine the area at the second portion of the duodenum during the excavation to identify the intrapancreatic portions of the bile duct. Optimally, any encasement of the bile duct by the inflammatory mass can be released. This may be sufficient to resolve a bile duct stricture and thereby negate the need for a separate bilioenteric anastomosis (see Figure 48-10).

- At times, there may be entry into the bile duct during this dissection, and in this case, either perform a hepaticojejunostomy or simply include the bile duct within the anastomosis to the jejunum in the excavated head of the pancreas.

- Care should be taken when encountering hemorrhage, which can be quite brisk during this dissection. Apply 3-0 silk suture ligature at all times to control this hemorrhage. Postoperative bleeding is a known complication of this procedure. Once the mass is excised, palpate once again to confirm the thickness of the posterior shell. Complete the placement of the 2-0 Prolene sutures along the border of the uncinate process beneath the superior mesenteric vein/portal vein complex (see Figure 48-11).

- In the case of patients with a dilated main pancreatic duct, one may then perform a longitudinal incision along the main pancreatic duct, as is often done in a Puestow type of procedure. It should be noted that the original description of the Beger procedure did not include this longitudinal pancreaticojejunostomy, but it is now commonplace to combine this portion of the procedure. This addition further exemplifies the similarities between the Beger and the Frey procedures.

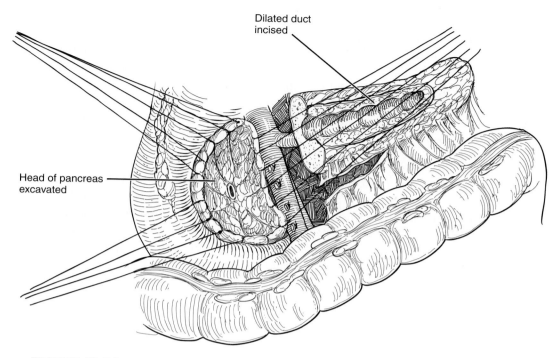

Dilated duct
incised

Head of pancreas
excavated

FIGURE 48–10

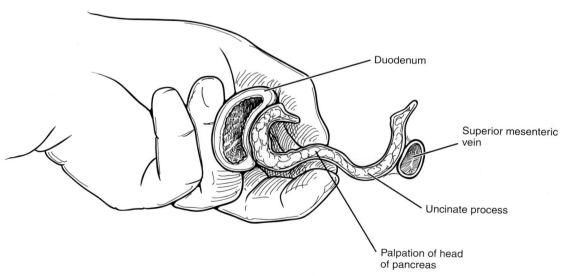

Duodenum

Superior mesenteric
vein

Uncinate process

Palpation of head
of pancreas

FIGURE 48–11

◆ After fully excavating the head of the pancreas, establishing hemostasis, and making a longitudinal incision where appropriate in the main pancreatic duct, a limb of jejunum is chosen approximately 15 cm distal to the ligament of Treitz. The mesentery is divided between clamps, and the jejunum is divided using a gastrointestinal anastomosis (GIA) stapling device **(Figure 48-12)**. A rent is made in the transverse mesocolon to the left of the middle colic vessels. The limb of jejunum is brought up into the lesser sack and placed in a side-to-side fashion with the divided jejunum aligned toward the head of the pancreas **(Figure 48-13)**.

◆ A side-to-side pancreaticojejunostomy is performed using the previously placed 2-0 Prolene sutures, which encircle the excavated head and whose needles were left in place after being tied. Place a posterior suture line first. Open the jejunum and complete the anterior suture line again using the 2-0 Prolene sutures. A separate pancreaticojejunostomy is performed between the divided tail of the pancreas and the same limb of jejunum. This anastomosis is performed using 3-0 silk interrupted sutures **(Figure 48-14)**.

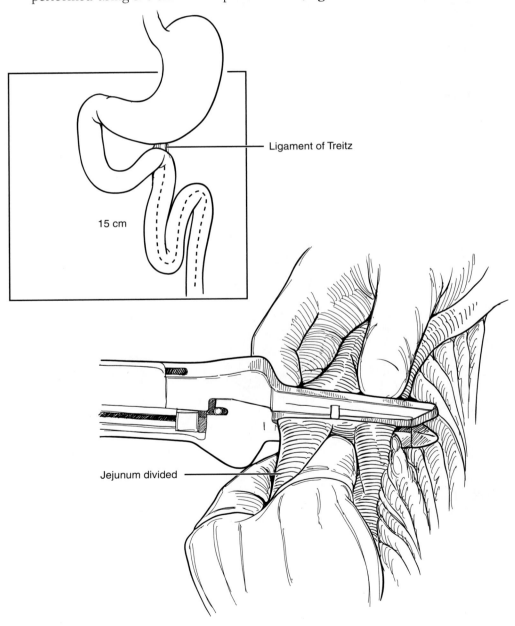

Ligament of Treitz

15 cm

Jejunum divided

FIGURE 48–12

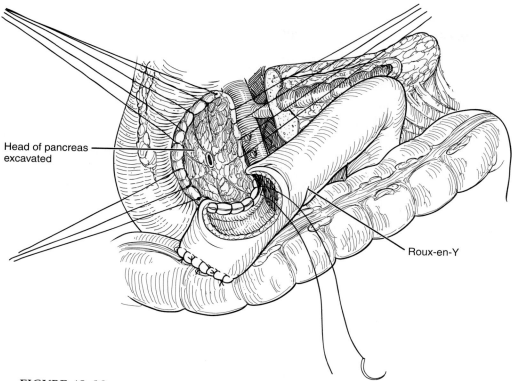

Head of pancreas
excavated

Roux-en-Y

FIGURE 48–13

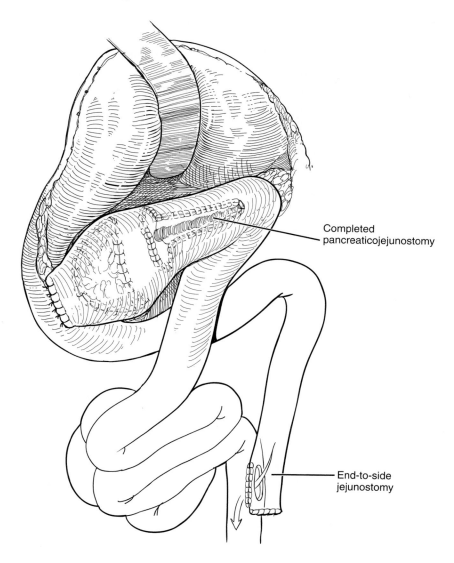

Completed
pancreaticojejunostomy

End-to-side
jejunostomy

FIGURE 48–14

- If the bile duct has been opened, a separate anastomosis with this jejunal limb to the opened bile duct can be performed using interrupted 4-0 Vicryl sutures. We prefer a separate hepaticojejunostomy over an attempt at this type of closure within the head of the pancreas.

- The rent in the transverse mesocolon where the limb of jejunum traverses is fixed in place using interrupted 3-0 silk stitch. Next, approximately 40 cm distal to the pancreaticojejunostomy, a side-to-side jejunojejunostomy is performed in two layers, using an outer layer of interrupted 3-0 silk stitch and an inner layer of running locking 3-0 Vicryl stitch posteriorly, which converts to a Connell type of stitch anteriorly. If the bile duct has been entered or sewn, a closed suction drain is placed in the foramen of Winslow and brought out in a separate stab wound on the right side of the abdomen. We do not place a drain across the pancreaticojejunostomy (see Figure 48-14).

FREY PROCEDURE

- Once again, the procedure description begins after mobilization of the head of the pancreas and bimanual palpation. Once again, the lesser sac is entered and the Kocher maneuver performed **(Figures 48-15 and 48-16).**

- Palpate the anterior surface of the body of the pancreas, searching for the dilated main pancreatic duct. This is typically easily done by palpating along the very hard texture of the pancreas usually seen in chronic pancreatitis and searching for an area of softer tissue with a feel not unlike that of a palpable vein under the skin. Often the duct seems to be oriented more toward the superior aspect of the body. This is an acquired skill, and even an experienced pancreatic surgeon will at times be challenged to find the duct (see Figure 48-15). After adequately determining the presence of the main pancreatic duct, a 20-gauge angiocatheter is passed into the duct where crystal clear fluid should be encountered.

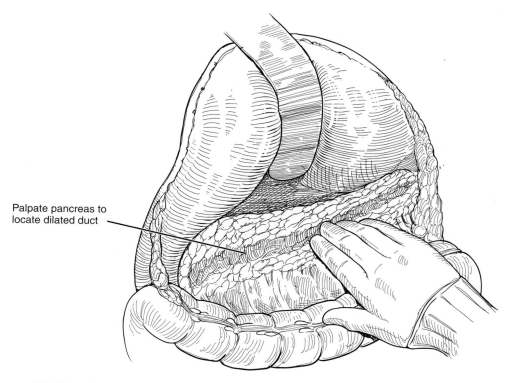

Palpate pancreas to
locate dilated duct

FIGURE 48–15

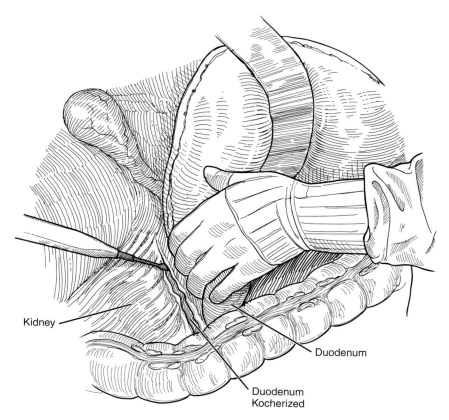

Kidney

Duodenum

Duodenum
Kocherized

FIGURE 48–16

♦ At this point, we often place a catheter using water manometry; we measure the pressure within the main pancreatic duct. Electrocautery is then used to follow the tract of the angiocatheter down into the main pancreatic duct where a larger amount of clear fluid should be encountered. A long narrow hemostat such as a tonsil clamp is used to probe the duct to demonstrate the proper direction to continue the longitudinal incision. Extend the incision toward the tail of the pancreas. It is not necessary to extend through the entire tail, but one should ascertain that no high-grade strictures remain. Similarly, extend the incision toward the head of the pancreas. In contrast to the classic Puestow procedure, one need not extend fully into the duct as it dives deeper into the parenchyma of the head, because this will be excavated later **(Figure 48-17)**.

♦ Place a circumferential line of 2-0 Prolene sutures along the border between the medial aspects of the C-loop of the duodenum and the head of the pancreas. Tie each suture as you proceed, and leave the needles on the sutures. Be careful to avoid needlesticks. The line of sutures begins at the level of the neck of the pancreas on the superior border, typically close to the pylorus. The line of sutures terminates at the neck of the pancreas in the inferior border. This suture line will finally join the suture line in the longitudinal pancreaticojejunostomy **(Figure 48-18)**. Identify the anterior superior and the anterior inferior pancreaticoduodenal arteries, divide, and ligate.

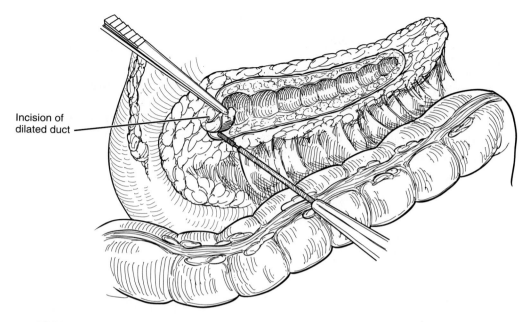

FIGURE 48–17

Incision of
dilated duct

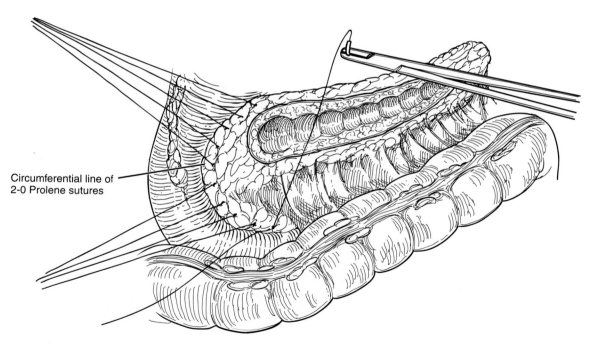

FIGURE 48–18

Circumferential line of
2-0 Prolene sutures

◆ Electrocautery is used to excavate the head of the pancreas through the majority of the inflammatory mass that has developed as the result of chronic pancreatitis. The amount of tissue will vary widely **(Figure 48-19)**. Perform bimanual palpation of the head of the pancreas frequently during the excavation to ensure a minimum thickness of 5 mm in the posterior rim of the excavated pancreatic head **(Figure 48-20)**. Care must be taken to suture ligate any bleeding intraparenchymal vessels. Further care should be taken at the level of the second portion of the duodenum to avoid injury to the intrapancreatic portion of the bile duct. The options regarding the bile duct during this procedure are identical to the precepts exercised during the Beger procedure.

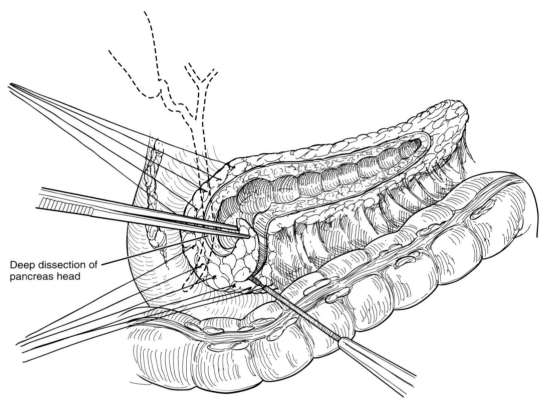

Deep dissection of
pancreas head

FIGURE 48–19

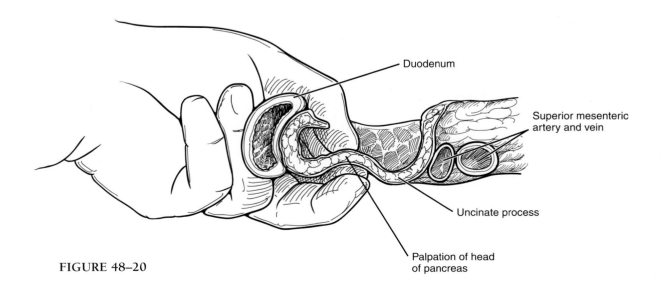

Duodenum

Superior mesenteric
artery and vein

Uncinate process

Palpation of head
of pancreas

FIGURE 48–20

◆ A limb of jejunum is now chosen approximately 15 cm distal to the ligament of Treitz. The limb is divided using a GIA stapling device, and the mesentery is divided between clamps in a vertical fashion toward the root of the mesentery to provide adequate length while preserving viability. A rent is made in the transverse mesocolon, and the distal end of the divided jejunum is brought through the rent and placed in the lesser sac where a side-to-side pancreaticojejunostomy is performed in one layer using interrupted 3-0 silk stitch. The divided end of the jejunum is placed toward the left of the patient, and the posterior row of silk sutures is placed before the jejunum is opened **(Figure 48-21).** The suture line extends from the open duct along the body and tail of the pancreas over toward the excavated head where the rim along the medial border of the C-loop of the duodenum is sewn to the jejunum, using the previously placed Prolene sutures.

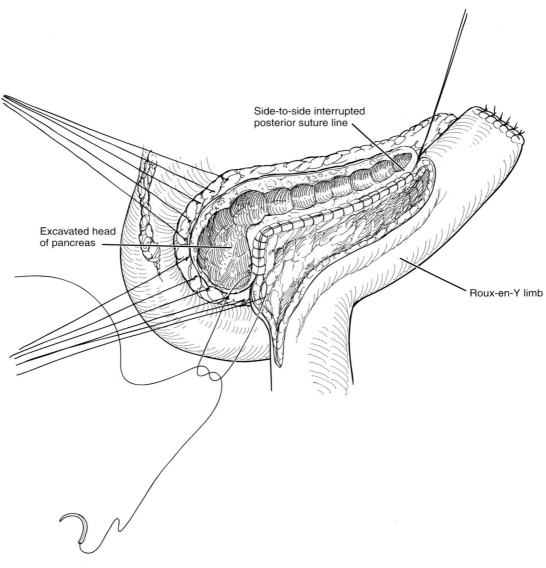

Side-to-side interrupted posterior suture line

Excavated head of pancreas

Roux-en-Y limb

FIGURE 48–21

◆ After placing the posterior row of sutures and tying, open the jejunum. Ensure proper alignment because an excessively large jejunotomy will result in a distorted anastomosis. To this end, we also place a first suture on the anterior row directly in the middle of the incision in the pancreas and directly in the middle of the open jejunotomy. We similarly split the closure at the halfway point between the left and right corners of the incisions and this mid-portion suture. Tie as you go. In this manner, the closure will be symmetrical. Finally, further interrupted silk sutures are placed to fill the gaps that remain in the anterior suture line **(Figure 48-22).**

◆ After completion of this anastomosis, the rent and transverse mesocolon are fixed to the limb of jejunum using 3-0 silk stitch; and finally, 40 cm distal to the pancreaticojejunostomy, a jejunojejunostomy is performed in a side-to-side fashion in two layers with an outer layer of interrupted 3-0 silk stitch and inner layer of running locking 3-0 Vicryl stitch posteriorly, which converts to a Connell type of stitch anteriorly. The mesentery defect between these two limbs is reapproximated using 3-0 silk stitch (see Figure 48-22).

◆ We do not use drains. The fascia is closed in the usual fashion. The skin is closed using subcuticular stitch.

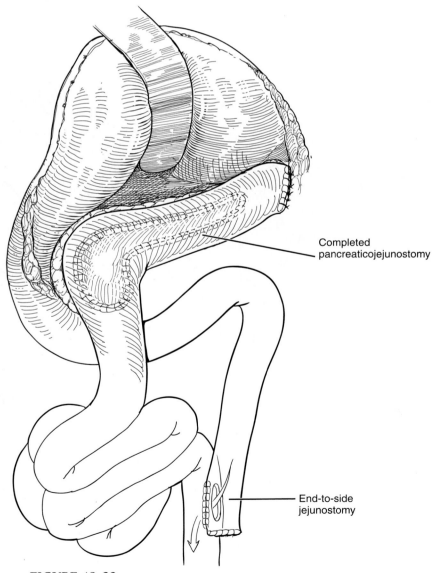

Completed pancreaticojejunostomy

End-to-side jejunostomy

FIGURE 48–22

STEP 4: POSTOPERATIVE CARE

- The patient will be monitored for adequate analgesia. This can be quite challenging in patients who have had large doses of narcotics preoperatively. Assuming we have used intraoperative epidural anesthesia, this problem is less significant because analgesia is better achieved with this modality.

- In the first 24 hours, we monitor for hemorrhage and hyperglycemia. Glycosuria may be mistaken for euvolemia.

- A nasogastric tube is used, and this is removed on the first postoperative day and a liquid diet is begun. If tolerated, this is advanced to a regular diet.

- During the first 3 to 5 days postoperatively, we monitor for evidence of endocrine or exocrine insufficiency and treat these as necessary with either enzyme supplementation or insulin. It should be noted that the actual degree of functional derangement will not be fully appreciated until the patient has resumed a full diet and is tolerating food well.

- The process of reducing and finally eliminating narcotic use will require weeks or months of effort after discharge.

STEP 5: PEARLS AND PITFALLS

- We have added the use of the interrupted 2-0 Prolene around the circumference of the head of the pancreas in the Frey procedure. We use a large needle and make an effort to place sutures deeply to achieve adequate hemostasis. Ischemia to the duodenum is extremely unlikely.

- The actual amount of tissue removed during the excavation will differ based on the size of the inflammatory mass preoperatively.

- Note that the significant difference between the two procedures is that the body of the pancreas is not divided in the Frey procedure as it is in a Beger procedure. Avoiding this step will make less likely any significant encounter with the superior mesenteric vein/portal vein complex. In the inflammatory changes, which are seen in chronic pancreatitis, the plane between the pancreas and these delicate structures is treacherous and therefore best avoided. Comparisons of outcome in these procedures have been identical in large series.

- Because an amount of pancreatic parenchyma has been removed, one can anticipate a percentage of patients who will sustain functional derangements as a result of this procedure.

SELECTED REFERENCES

1. Di Sebastiano P, Di Mola F, Friess H: Management of chronic pancreatitis: Conservative, endoscopic and surgical. In Blumgart LH (ed): Surgery of the Liver, Biliary Tract and Pancreas, 4th ed. Philadelphia, Saunders, 2007, pp 728-740.
2. Buchler M, Friess H, Bittner R, et al: Duodenum preserving pancreatic head resection: Long term results. J Gastrointest Surg 1997;1:13-19.
3. Frey CF, Amikura K: Local resection of the head of the pancreas combined with longitudinal pancreatico-jejunostomy in the management of patients with chronic pancreatitis. Ann Surg 1994;220:492-507.

CHAPTER 49

PYLORUS-SAVING PANCREATICODUODENECTOMY

William H. Nealon

STEP 1: SURGICAL ANATOMY

- ◆ All pancreatic surgery requires an understanding of the anatomic relationships in the lesser sac. After either an upper midline or a bilateral subcostal (chevron) incision, one enters the lesser sac by dissecting along the avascular plane at the points of attachment of the gastrocolic omentum to the transverse colon **(Figure 49-1)**. The proper plane is between the anterior and posterior leaflets. This is my favored point of entry. The alternative entry is by transversely dividing and ligating the vascular structures embedded in the omentum while preserving the gastroepiploic vessels located along the greater curvature of the stomach.

- ◆ Upon entering the lesser sac, one will encounter varying amounts of adhesions between the posterior wall of the stomach and the anterior surface of the pancreas. These fetal adhesions do not imply prior inflammatory events. Considerable dense adhesions may be encountered in pathologic states.

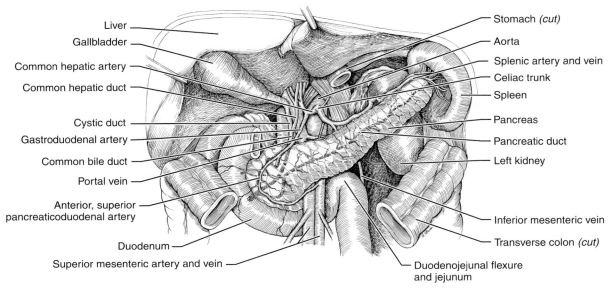

FIGURE 49–1

- The pancreas is essentially encased in a sandwich of major blood vessels. The vena cava and aorta occupy the posterior surface in the midline. The splenic artery courses along the superior surface from the aorta toward the tail. The splenic vein occupies the posterior superior surface of the body and tail of the pancreas. It meets the superior mesenteric vein, which is oriented vertically in the groove created by the uncinate process in the posterior aspect of the head of the pancreas and the right lateral and anterior components of the head. The confluence of these two veins constitutes the portal vein, which traverses this uncinate groove and emerges to join the bile duct and the hepatic artery in the hepatoduodenal ligament (see Figures 49-1, 49-3, and 49-4).

- The superior mesenteric artery is located in a plane posterior and slightly medial to the superior mesenteric artery. The common hepatic artery, another branch of the celiac trunk (along with the splenic artery and left gastric artery), courses along the superior border of the head of the pancreas to join the hepatoduodenal ligament. Its first branch is the typically miniscule right gastric artery. Just distal is the more substantial gastroduodenal artery, which emerges at a right angle to the hepatic artery from its inferior surface and courses beneath the pylorus. After sending the right gastroepiploic artery in the plane between the inferior aspect of the pylorus and the superior surface of the head of the pancreas, the gastroduodenal artery pierces the head of the pancreas (see Figures 49-4 and 49-5).

- The anterior superior and the posterior superior pancreaticoduodenal arteries also arise from branches of the gastroduodenal artery. These arteries form an arch medial to the C-loop of the duodenum, and they collateralize with branches of the anterior and posterior inferior pancreaticoduodenal arteries, which are branches of the superior mesenteric artery. Small branches from these arteries provide blood supply to the duodenum (see Figures 49-3 through 49-6).

- Key anatomic features in pancreatic head resections are the network of tributaries projecting between the superior mesenteric vein/portal vein confluence and the uncinate process. These tributaries are located at the right lateral aspect of the veins. These tiny veins exit the pancreas at the mid-portion of the groove in which the major veins reside (see Figure 49-12).

- Viewed in cross-sectional imaging, the uncinate process forms a C-shaped structure. The terminal posterior extent of the uncinate process projects in a medial direction as a ligamentous structure and contains a variable number of arterial branches from the superior mesenteric artery, which project at right angles to the major artery and provide blood supply to the uncinate process. Division of the tiny venous tributaries and the arterial branches are key steps in respective procedures. This uncinate margin is the most problematic in managing malignant tumors in the head of the pancreas (see Figure 49-13).

- The pancreas is entirely retroperitoneal, and therefore operative procedures will require mobilization of the pancreas from its retroperitoneal position. The plane lateral to the C-loop of the duodenum is incised in nearly all procedures; this plane is avascular, and its mobilization is termed the Kocher maneuver. This exposes the vena cava and aorta, and it permits "bimanual palpation" of the head of the pancreas. The dissection may be easily extended to the fourth portion of the duodenum and the ligament of Treitz (see Figure 49-3).

- The inferior border of the body of the pancreas is also avascular, although the inferior mesenteric vein may be encountered to the right of the spine (see Figure 49-4).

- Peritoneum overlies the hepatoduodenal ligament. Dissection reveals the triad in gross ana-tomic terms, which corresponds to the microscopic portal triad—with portal, hepatic arte-rial, and biliary structures. The common bile duct is located in an anterior lateral position, and the hepatic artery is anterior medial. The portal vein is positioned in the posterior groove created by the apposition of these anterior structures (see Figure 49-5).

- Although lymph nodes may be seen at a wide array of locations, there is a constant lymph node in the groove created by the lateral border of the second portion of the duodenum and the hepatoduodenal ligament. Dissection of this lymph node is necessary to fully visu-alize the proximal hepatic artery. Other common sites of lymph nodes are on the lateral aspect of the mid-portion of the hepatoduodenal ligament, in the fibrovascular bundle sur-rounding the right gastroepiploic complex, and on the superior border of the confluence of the head and body of the pancreas. Beneath this lymph node one finds the origins of the common hepatic artery and the splenic artery.

- On the inferior border of the pancreatic head, just where the duodenum dives beneath the superior mesenteric vein and artery, one may dissect the peritoneum and visualize the supe-rior mesenteric vein as it passes in a superior direction beneath the head of the pancreas.

- The ligament of Treitz is a significant anatomic structure, and it can be accessed by lifting the transverse colon and omentum in an anterior direction. The ligament can be seen to the left of the spine.

- The main pancreatic duct originates in the tail of the pancreas and traverses the length of the pancreas to exit in the duodenum through both main ampulla (Vater) and the accessory ampulla, which is located more proximally in the duodenum. The main pancreatic duct (Wirsung) and the minor or accessory duct (Santorini) fuse during fetal development at what is termed the genu or "knee" of the duct.

STEP 2: PREOPERATIVE CONSIDERATIONS

- Establishment of the indications for pancreatic resection depends on imaging; pathologic confirmation; establishment that curative intent can be applied; and assessment of the medical status of the patient, including nutritional state.

- In the case of cancer, it is not unusual to proceed to resection without pathologic confirma-tion. In this case, a very experienced pancreatic surgeon must make that determination based on strong evidence by imaging that malignant disease exists.

- Resectability of pancreatic cancer in the head must be founded on the presence of meta-static disease (typically in the liver, but potentially many remote sites, as well) and the pres-ence of what has been termed "locally advanced" disease. In the case of adenocarcinoma of the head of the pancreas, local invasion and/or encasement of the superior mesenteric artery or vein are the primary elements that establish this clinical stage. In several large series, local extension is responsible for establishment of unresectability in half of those deemed not to be operative candidates.

- Both chronic pancreatitis and cystic neoplasms such as intraductal papillary mucinous neoplasm (IPMN) are nonmalignant diagnoses that are treated appropriately with radical resection. Because pancreatic cancer may masquerade as chronic pancreatitis or coexist with it, a confirmation of that distinction is not possible. Suspicions to favor chronic pancreatitis are the presence of glandular calcification, the presence of a pancreatic mass in the absence of clinical jaundice, and the chronicity of symptoms. We favor making a strong effort to confirm the diagnosis of IPMN before proceeding to resection.

- Because of the magnitude of the operative procedure, care must be taken to exclude significant cardiac, pulmonary, and renal disease and to determine the presence of diabetes mellitus. Nutritional needs must also be addressed before surgery.

STEP 3: OPERATIVE STEPS

1. INCISION

- Midline/xiphoid to some distance below the umbilicus **(Figure 49-2)**

- Self-retaining retractor such as Thompson retractors

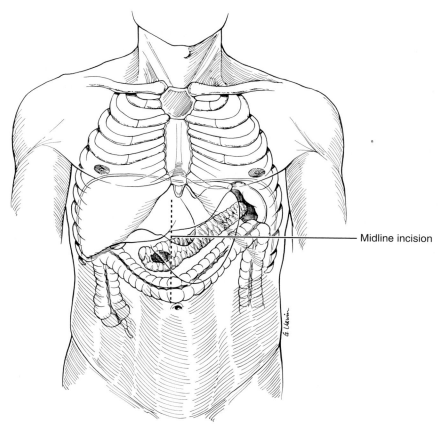

Midline incision

FIGURE 49–2

2. DISSECTION

◆ Perform an extended Kocher maneuver, combining mobilization of the duodenum through to the fourth portion (ligament of Treitz) with mobilization of the hepatic flexure, which is reflected inferiorly **(Figure 49-3)**.

◆ Separate the gastrocolic omentum from its avascular attachment to the transverse colon. Begin the dissection to the left of the spine, and extend the dissection to the cecum. Care must be taken to avoid simply creating a window through both leaflets of the omentum. Identification of the posterior wall of the stomach confirms access to the lesser sac.

◆ Mobilize the inferior border of pancreas beginning at the midline and progressing to the right **(Figure 49-4)**.

◆ The superior mesenteric vein will become apparent to the right of the spine passing over the third portion of the duodenum on the inferior aspect of the dissection. On the superior edge of the divided retroperitoneal plane, the superior mesenteric vein courses beneath the pancreas. Establish this plane posterior to the head of the pancreas and anterior to the superior mesenteric vein/portal vein confluence (see Figure 49-4).

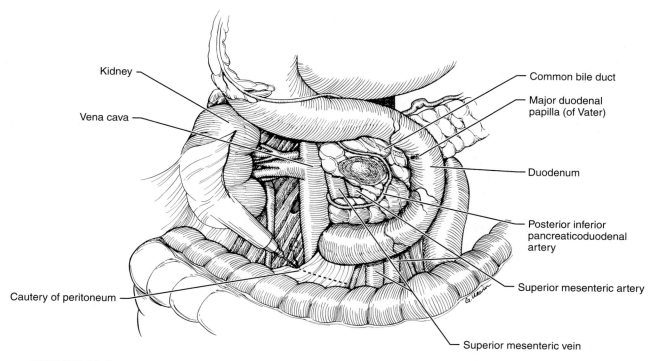

Kidney

Vena cava

Cautery of peritoneum

Common bile duct

Major duodenal papilla (of Vater)

Duodenum

Posterior inferior pancreaticoduodenal artery

Superior mesenteric artery

Superior mesenteric vein

FIGURE 49–3

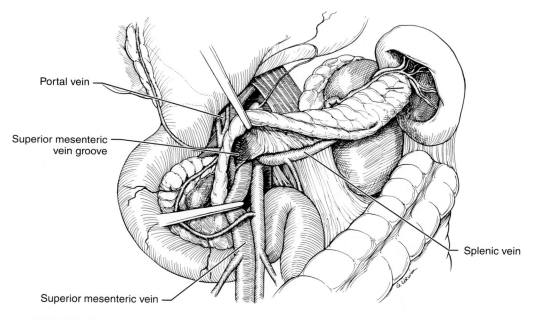

Portal vein

Superior mesenteric vein groove

Splenic vein

Superior mesenteric vein

FIGURE 49–4

◆ Incise the peritoneum, which envelops the hepatoduodenal ligament in a transverse direction, beginning in the distal third of this structure. Isolate and encircle, with vessel loops, the common bile duct and the proper hepatic artery and distract these vessels medially and laterally to reveal the portal vein (**Figure 49-5**).

◆ Establish a plane, if possible, extending from the previously dissected inferior plane of dissection where the superior mesenteric vein courses beneath the head of the pancreas and current plane in the hepatoduodenal ligament where the portal vein has been identified. There is a dense layer of connective tissue overlying the portal vein, and this must be carefully incised to reach the proper plane. Carefully dissecting this plane from the superior aspect permits "meeting in the middle" with the inferior dissection. Pass a ½-inch Penrose drain along this newly established plane and place clamps separately on each end of the drain (**Figure 49-6**).

◆ Follow the proper hepatic artery toward the celiac trunk. The proper hepatic artery travels in a generally transverse direction and takes a right-angle turn directed cephalad. At this right angle, the gastroduodenal artery continues along the same direction as the proper hepatic artery. Thus one must identify the common hepatic artery to avoid misidentifying the proper hepatic artery for the gastroduodenal artery. Dissect the gastroduodenal artery free and double loop it with a silk suture, but do not tie (**Figure 49-7**).

◆ At this point, resectability is established and, if determined, then resection is undertaken. In spite of the fact that 1 or 2 hours of dissection may already have been completed, nothing has been done to this point in the operation that requires reconstruction.

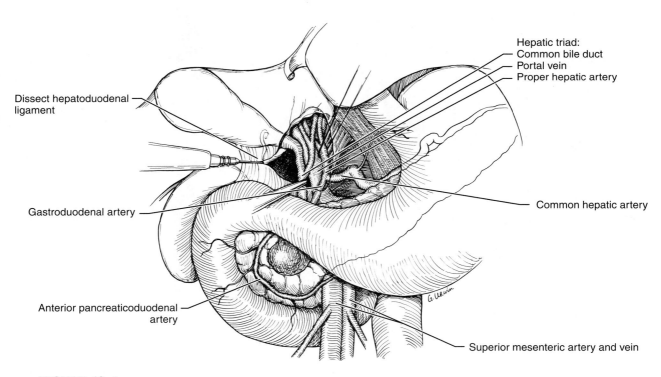

FIGURE 49–5

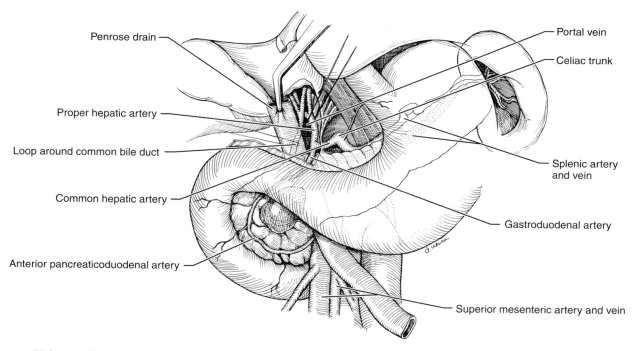

Penrose drain

Proper hepatic artery

Loop around common bile duct

Common hepatic artery

Anterior pancreaticoduodenal artery

Portal vein

Celiac trunk

Splenic artery and vein

Gastroduodenal artery

Superior mesenteric artery and vein

FIGURE 49–6

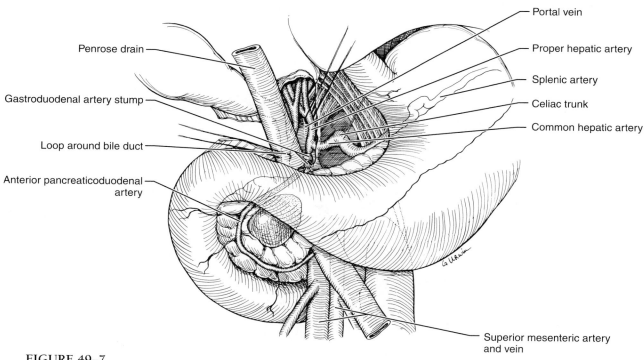

Penrose drain

Gastroduodenal artery stump

Loop around bile duct

Anterior pancreaticoduodenal artery

Portal vein

Proper hepatic artery

Splenic artery

Celiac trunk

Common hepatic artery

Superior mesenteric artery and vein

FIGURE 49–7

- Dissect the gallbladder free of the gallbladder bed, and dissect the cystic duct/common duct confluence. The gallbladder will be included in the en bloc specimen. If it is tense with bile it may be decompressed to maximize visualization.

- Divide the common hepatic duct just proximal to the insertion of the cystic duct. In an operation for malignancy, send a margin of bile duct for frozen section examination. Place a medium clip on the actual (proximal) margin **(Figure 49-8)**.

- Divide and suture ligate the gastroduodenal artery. Soft tissue attachments between the superior aspect of the head of the pancreas and the retroperitoneal structures are quite dense. Several broad, flat lymph nodes overlie the arterial structures (the celiac trunk, common hepatic artery, and splenic artery root). Include the lymph nodes with the specimen (see Figure 49-8). The head of the pancreas will finally be freely mobile for a transverse distance of 3 to 5 cm. The medial aspect of the portal vein is visualized. The anticipated dividing line for most resections approximates the line nearly vertical along the medial border of the superior mesenteric vein/portal vein confluence **(Figure 49-9)**.

- Dissect and divide/ligate the right gastroepiploic arteriovenous bundle approximately 3 cm proximal to the pylorus along the greater curvature. This will include an important lymph node region. Dissect the lymphovascular bundle distally until it separates from the pylorus and remains a part of the specimen (see Figure 49-9).

- Ligate and divide the right gastric artery.

- After skeletonizing the proximal duodenum, divide the duodenum using the gastrointestinal anastomosis (GIA) stapler and reflect the stomach superiorly. This permits a broad, unobstructed view of the entire operative field including the entire pancreas **(Figure 49-10)**.

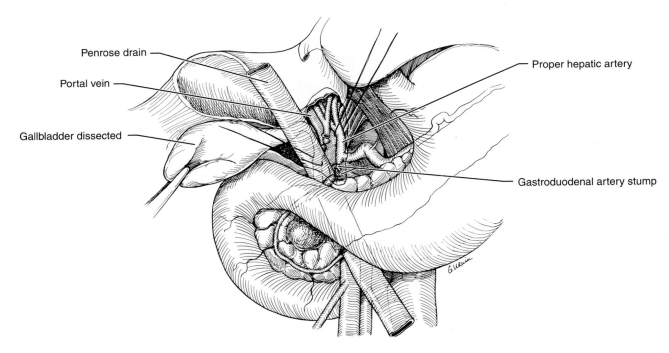

FIGURE 49–8

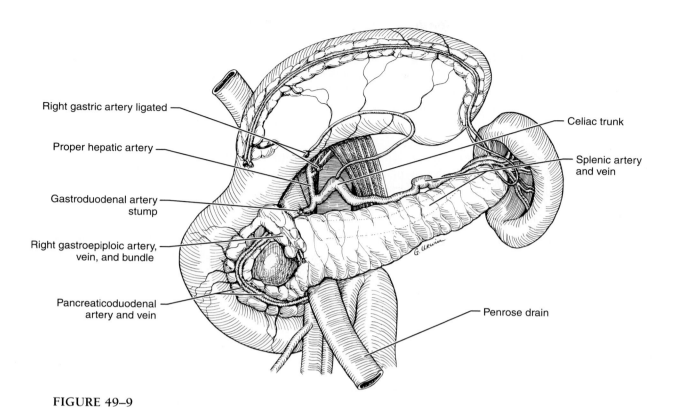

Right gastric artery ligated

Proper hepatic artery

Gastroduodenal artery stump

Right gastroepiploic artery, vein, and bundle

Pancreaticoduodenal artery and vein

Celiac trunk

Splenic artery and vein

Penrose drain

FIGURE 49–9

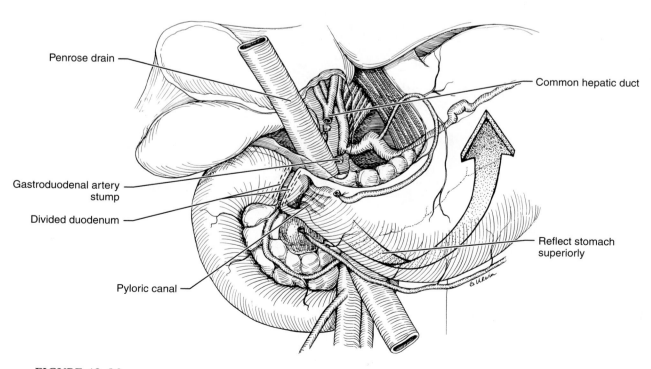

Penrose drain

Gastroduodenal artery stump

Divided duodenum

Pyloric canal

Common hepatic duct

Reflect stomach superiorly

FIGURE 49–10

◆ Having established a horizontal plane along the superior and the inferior border of the pancreas, now place 2-0 Prolene sutures on the inferior and superior border of the body of pancreas to the left and right of the anticipated line of resection of the body of the pancreas. Use a large needle such as CT-1. These sutures are intended to occlude the intraparenchymal arteries, which course longitudinally along the superior and inferior borders of the pancreas. Hemorrhage during the division of the pancreas may thereby be prevented **(Figure 49-11)**.

◆ Divide the pancreas with a scalpel and send a 2-mm margin for frozen section analysis. Mark the "actual" margin by placing a medium clip on the pancreatic duct on the side of the divided pancreas oriented toward the tail of the pancreas.

◆ Reflect the divided body and head of the pancreas toward the right, revealing the superior mesenteric vein/portal vein confluence. Divide the short tributaries between the uncinate process and the superior mesenteric vein and portal vein in continuity using 3-0 silk suture **(Figure 49-12)**.

◆ Divide the final attachment between the uncinate process and the superior mesenteric artery between clamps and ligate after visualizing the course of the superior mesenteric artery. From superior to inferior, the superior mesenteric artery courses downward and toward the right. Thus, if one carries the dissection in a strictly vertical direction, there is a risk that the superior mesenteric artery may be inadvertently divided **(Figure 49-13)**.

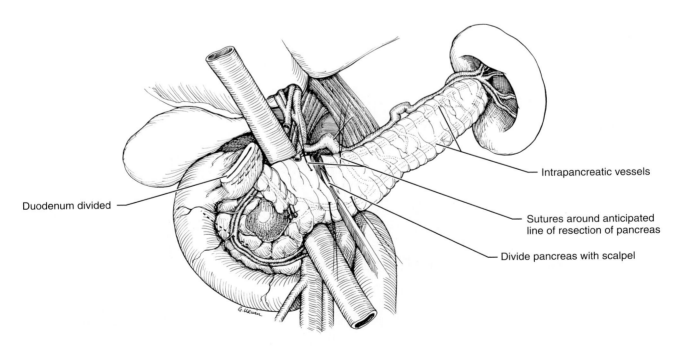

Duodenum divided

Intrapancreatic vessels

Sutures around anticipated line of resection of pancreas

Divide pancreas with scalpel

FIGURE 49–11

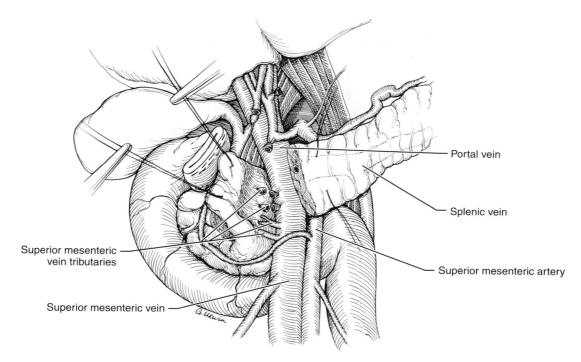

Portal vein

Splenic vein

Superior mesenteric
vein tributaries

Superior mesenteric artery

Superior mesenteric vein

FIGURE 49–12

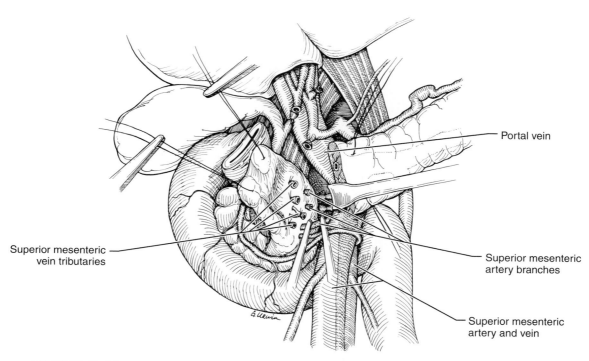

Portal vein

Superior mesenteric
vein tributaries

Superior mesenteric
artery branches

Superior mesenteric
artery and vein

FIGURE 49–13

◆ Redirect attention to below the transverse mesocolon. Divide the mesentery of the jejunum between clamps beginning approximately 15 cm distal to the ligament of Treitz and extending the ligation proximally. Divide the jejunum using the GIA stapling device **(Figure 49-14)**. Divide the avascular elements of the ligament using electrocautery. When the vascular attachments between the duodenojejunal junction and the superior mesenteric artery and vein have been divided, pass the limb of jejunum beneath the artery and vein through the prior site of the ligament of Treitz. This places the jejunum in the same plane in which all prior dissection has taken place (see Figure 49-14, *inset*).

◆ Divide the final vascular attachments between the duodenojejunal junction and the superior mesenteric artery between clamps and ligate. Remove the specimen **(Figure 49-15)**.

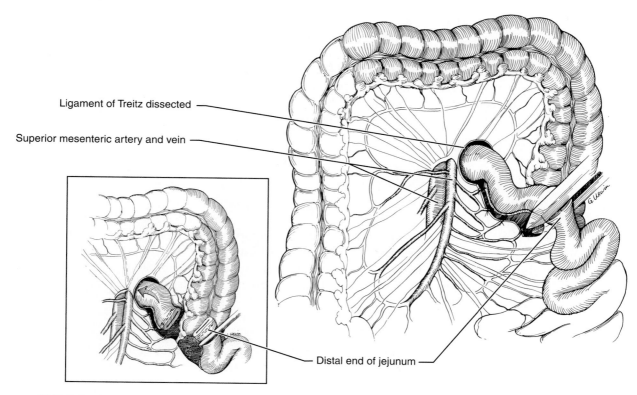

Ligament of Treitz dissected

Superior mesenteric artery and vein

Distal end of jejunum

FIGURE 49–14

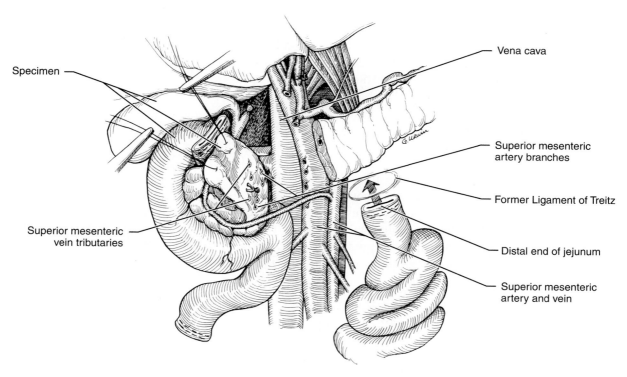

Specimen

Superior mesenteric
vein tributaries

Vena cava

Superior mesenteric
artery branches

Former Ligament of Treitz

Distal end of jejunum

Superior mesenteric
artery and vein

FIGURE 49–15

3. RECONSTRUCTION

◆ Pass the distal divided limb of jejunum beneath the prior site of the ligament of Treitz, and position it directly opposite the pancreatic remnant oriented from the divided end of the pancreas to the side of the jejunal limb. The limb will fall into the right upper quadrant in the area where the hepaticojejunostomy will be performed **(Figure 49-16)**.

◆ Identify the pancreatic duct. Make an incision from the anterior surface of the pancreas down to the duct (1.5 cm in length).

◆ Perform an end-to-side pancreaticojejunostomy in a single layer using interrupted 3-0 silk suture. The anterior surface of the jejunum will drape over the 1.5-cm incision in the duct. Place the sutures in the pancreatic parenchyma using a broad passage of the needle to ensure adequate "purchase" and to avoid tearing parenchyma while tying the sutures (see Figure 49-16).

◆ Perform an end-to-side hepaticojejunostomy using a single layer of interrupted 4-0 polydioxanone (PDS) suture on an RB-1 needle. Use absorbable suture (see Figure 49-16).

◆ Fix the limb of jejunum in place as it passes beneath the prior site of the ligament of Treitz using an interrupted 3-0 silk stitch.

◆ Perform a duodenojejunostomy in an antecolic fashion 40 cm distal to the hepaticojejunostomy. The anastomosis is performed in two layers with an outer layer of interrupted 3-0 silk suture and an inner layer of running locking 3-0 Vicryl suture posteriorly, which is converted to a Connell type of stitch anteriorly **(Figure 49-17)**.

◆ Irrigate the peritoneal cavity with warm, sterile saline.

◆ Place two 10-mm Jackson-Pratt drains:
  ◆ Place one through a stab wound on the left side of the abdomen, and position it posterior to the pancreaticojejunostomy and posterior to the hepaticojejunostomy.
  ◆ Place the other through a stab wound on the right side of the abdomen, and position it anterior to the hepaticojejunostomy and anterior to the pancreaticojejunostomy.
  ◆ The drains are fixed in place using drain fixation sutures of 2-0 silk stitch.

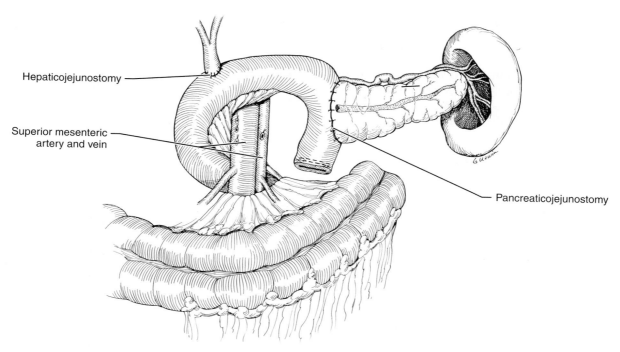

Hepaticojejunostomy

Superior mesenteric artery and vein

Pancreaticojejunostomy

FIGURE 49–16

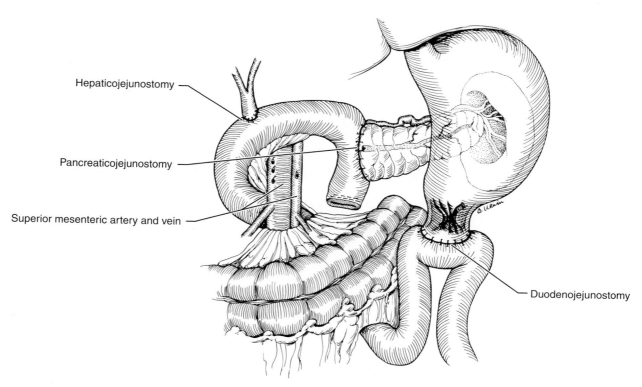

Hepaticojejunostomy

Pancreaticojejunostomy

Superior mesenteric artery and vein

Duodenojejunostomy

FIGURE 49–17

4. CLOSING

◆ Reapproximate the fascia using heavy-gauge Vicryl suture. We favor the Smead-Jones technique. Reapproximate the skin and apply dressings. Place drains to close and bulb suction.

STEP 4: POSTOPERATIVE CARE

◆ In the first 24 hours, the primary concerns are hemorrhage (including monitoring coagulation status) and hyperglycemia. Unexpected glucose intolerance after resection and after the stress of surgery may manifest only as brisk urine output and be interpreted as a sign of euvolemia. Hemoglobin stability must be documented before close, and interval evaluations may be stopped.

◆ Delayed gastric emptying is common, and one must establish low nasogastric tube output before removal (<150 mL per 8 hours). Most can be removed on postoperative day 1.

◆ Drains must be monitored for volume and character. On postoperative day 3, these should be tested for amylase and bilirubin content. Evidence of biliary or pancreatic fistula is managed by continued drainage.

◆ Intravenous antibiotics are stopped after 24 hours.

◆ Diet is resumed as tolerated. If diet is tolerated and drain output is low and devoid of enzymes or bile, the drains may be removed.

◆ Pain control progresses from epidural to patient-controlled analgesia versus oral narcotics.

◆ Once the patient is tolerating diet, is ambulating, and has pain controlled by oral agents, he or she is discharged home.

◆ We rarely require more than 1 day in a critical care setting.

STEP 5: PEARLS AND PITFALLS

- It is best to understand the potential for challenging anatomy. These circumstances include patients with prior pancreatic surgery, patients with chronic inflammation (chronic pancreatitis), patients with prior acute pancreatitis (seen in 37% of patients with IPMN), and patients with tumor close to or invading the superior mesenteric vein and artery.

- If severe hemorrhage is encountered beneath the head of the pancreas in the superior mesenteric vein/portal vein or if it is encountered after division of the pancreas, several measures should be considered:
  - Call for experienced help.
  - Isolate and control the portal vein, superior mesenteric vein, and splenic vein, and place either vessel loops or vascular clamps.
  - Compression should always offer time to establish control and obtain help.
  - Mobilize the pancreas to achieve the best exposure available.
  - One potentially useful maneuver is to pass Fogarty catheters into the lumen of each vein.
  - If some length of vein is lost, it is possible to mobilize the vein to permit as much as a 3-cm defect to be repaired primarily.

SELECTED REFERENCES

1. Katz MH, Wang H, Fleming J, et al: Long-term survival after multidisciplinary management of resected pancreatic adenocarcinoma. Ann Surg Oncol 2009;16:836-847.
2. Kow AW, Chan SP, Earnest A, et al: Striving for a better operative outcome: 101 pancreaticoduodenectomies. HPB (Oxford) 2008;10:464-471.
3. Katz MH, Fleming JP, Pisters PW, et al: Anatomy of the superior mesenteric vein with special reference to the surgical management of first order branch involvement at pancreaticoduodenectomy. Ann Surg 2008;248:1094-1102.

CHAPTER 50

PANCREATICOJEJUNOSTOMY (PUESTOW)

William H. Nealon

STEP 1: SURGICAL ANATOMY

- The head of the pancreas is surrounded by the C-loop of the duodenum laterally. It is fully evaluated after mobilizing the duodenum and head of the pancreas from its retroperitoneal location.

- The right gastroepiploic artery and vein are located in the space between the pylorus of the stomach and the head of the pancreas.

- The anterior superior and the anterior inferior pancreaticoduodenal artery and vein parallel the course of the C-loop of the duodenum, and they are located 1 to 2 mm onto the lateral aspect of the head of the pancreas.

- The body and tail of the pancreas are located posterior to the stomach and can be accessed by dividing the gastrocolic omentum.

- In chronic pancreatitis the transverse mesocolon may be adherent to the anterior and inferior border of the pancreas.

- The dilated pancreatic duct may be palpated in the mid-portion of the body and head of the pancreas running longitudinally **(Figure 50-1)**.

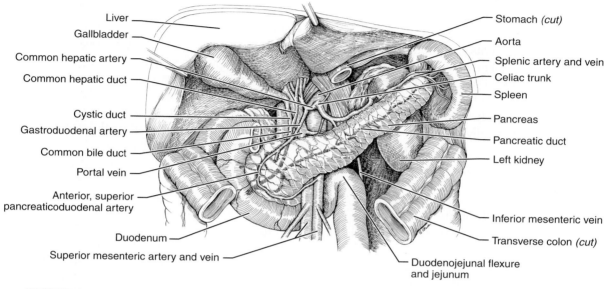

Liver

Gallbladder

Common hepatic artery

Common hepatic duct

Cystic duct

Gastroduodenal artery

Common bile duct

Portal vein

Anterior, superior
pancreaticoduodenal artery

Duodenum

Superior mesenteric artery and vein

Stomach *(cut)*

Aorta

Splenic artery and vein

Celiac trunk

Spleen

Pancreas

Pancreatic duct

Left kidney

Inferior mesenteric vein

Transverse colon *(cut)*

Duodenojejunal flexure
and jejunum

FIGURE 50–1

STEP 2: PREOPERATIVE CONSIDERATIONS

- Indications: This procedure is indicated only in patients with chronic pancreatitis.
  - The primary indication for operation in chronic pancreatitis is chronic unremitting abdominal pain. This operation is restricted to patients who have evidence of pancreatic ductal dilation, and most agree that the dilation should be 7 mm or greater in diameter. The secondary but well-recognized indication is recurring acute exacerbations of chronic pancreatitis. We have identified three categories of patients: patients who have chronic unremitting abdominal pain only; patients with recurring acute exacerbations only; and patients with both manifestations of chronic pancreatitis. Typically some element of dependence on narcotic analgesics to manage the pain is anticipated.
  - Important considerations in preoperative planning for a Puestow procedure include establishing the nutrition status of the patient. Typically patients with this diagnosis present with functional derangements including endocrine and exocrine dysfunction. They also typically have pain worsened by meals, and for that reason nutritional deficits are common. It is therefore vital to determine the nutritional status of patients.
  - Pertinent to functional derangements, it is important to maximize the replacement therapy for patients with functional derangements. This includes insulin therapy for patients who have glucose intolerance and enzyme replacement for patients who have pancreatic malabsorption.
  - The most common cause of splenic vein thrombosis is chronic pancreatitis. It is important to determine those patients who have either splenic vein thrombosis or portal vein thrombosis as a complication of their chronic pancreatitis. These may result in left-sided portal hypertension or in cavernous transformation in the area of the head of the pancreas. These findings can greatly worsen the outcomes in operations for this disease because of the potential of significant hemorrhage during operation.
  - One must also consider the two associated complications of chronic pancreatitis in addition to pancreatic ductal dilation, which may be seen. First, common bile duct dilation occurs because of the narrowing of the distal bile duct created by the fibrotic mass in the head of the pancreas. This can be seen in 30% to 50% of patients with chronic pancreatitis.
  - Finally, one must be cognizant of the possibility of duodenal narrowing caused by chronic pancreatitis. This complication is seen in less than 5% of patients, but it must be recognized as a possible complication. Each of these may require a simultaneous operative intervention during the primary operation for the drainage of the pancreatic duct.
  - All patients undergo bowel preparation with a cathartic combined with oral antibiotic doses of neomycin and erythromycin. Finally, a dose of intravenous antibiotics is administered within 1 hour of the skin incision.

STEP 3: OPERATIVE STEPS

1. INCISION

◆ We favor a midline incision for this procedure. Historically, many have advocated bilateral subcostal incision, but we have recently modified this approach for many pancreatic operative procedures and we favor a midline incision (**Figure 50-2**).

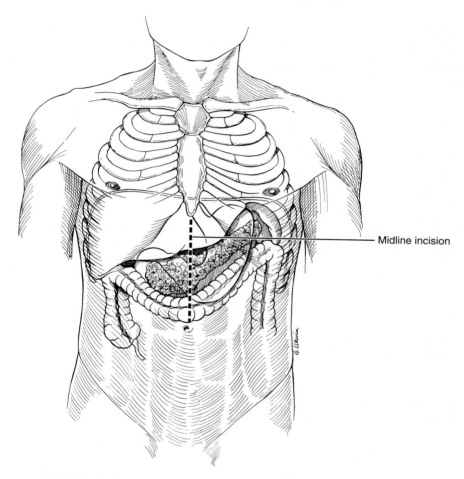

Midline incision

FIGURE 50–2

2. DISSECTION

◆ After entering the abdomen, the surgeon performs a general evaluation of the peritoneal cavity as a routine.

◆ A Kocher maneuver is performed by incising the peritoneum lateral to the C-loop of the duodenum. After mobilizing the duodenum and head of the pancreas medially one can readily palpate the head and neck of the pancreas **(Figure 50-3)**.

◆ The lesser sac is entered by dividing the attachments in the avascular plane between the gastro-colic omentum and the transverse colon. This is accomplished by grasping the omentum and reflecting it anteriorly and superiorly, exposing the posterior aspect of the attachment between the omentum and the transverse colon. Electrocautery is used to divide the peritoneal attachments beginning approximately 5 cm to the left of the spine and continuing the dissection toward the right. In this area, it is possible to establish the plane that leads to the lesser sac. The transverse mesocolon will be displaced inferiorly, and the posterior wall of the stomach will be displaced superiorly. There may be attachments to the appendices epiploicae of the transverse colon, which need to be carefully separated **(Figure 50-4)**.

◆ After establishing entry into the lesser sac, the opening may be extended to the right well beyond the midline to facilitate a wide view of the lesser sac. There are typically a number of adhesions between the posterior wall of the stomach and the anterior surface of the body of the pancreas, and these can be lysed safely **(Figure 50-5)**.

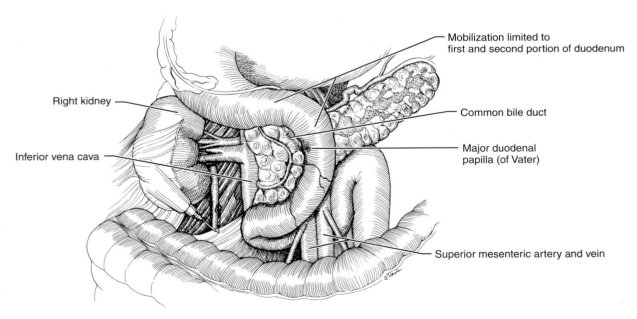

Right kidney

Inferior vena cava

Mobilization limited to first and second portion of duodenum

Common bile duct

Major duodenal papilla (of Vater)

Superior mesenteric artery and vein

FIGURE 50–3

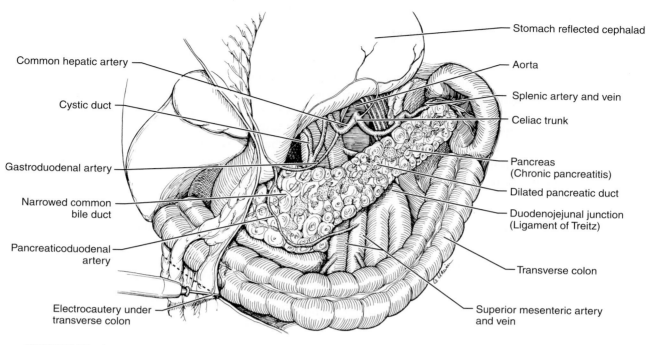

Stomach reflected cephalad

Common hepatic artery

Cystic duct

Gastroduodenal artery

Narrowed common bile duct

Pancreaticoduodenal artery

Electrocautery under transverse colon

Aorta

Splenic artery and vein

Celiac trunk

Pancreas (Chronic pancreatitis)

Dilated pancreatic duct

Duodenojejunal junction (Ligament of Treitz)

Transverse colon

Superior mesenteric artery and vein

FIGURE 50–4

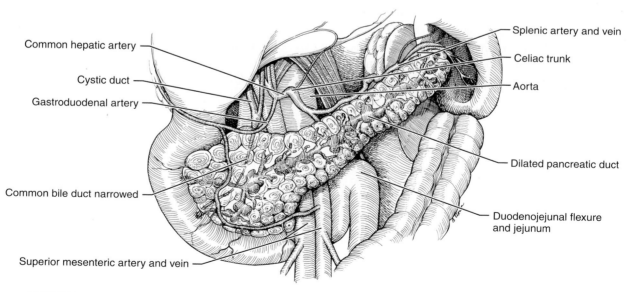

Common hepatic artery

Cystic duct

Gastroduodenal artery

Common bile duct narrowed

Superior mesenteric artery and vein

Splenic artery and vein

Celiac trunk

Aorta

Dilated pancreatic duct

Duodenojejunal flexure and jejunum

FIGURE 50–5

- After a wider entry into the lesser sac is established, the tissues overlying the body and head of the pancreas are carefully dissected free.

- The somewhat thickened fatty structure just inferior to the pylorus is the location of the right gastroepiploic artery and vein. It is at times necessary to divide these structures in performing the pancreaticojejunostomy. Very often there is an anterior branch between the right gastroepiploic artery and superior mesenteric vein or the superior mesenteric artery, which courses along the anterior surface of the body/head of the pancreas. It is advised and safe to divide this arterial connection between clamps as one clears the head of the pancreas (see Figure 50-5).

- In most cases, it is possible to palpate the dilated main pancreatic duct. This should be done with the fingertips and at times by using bimanual palpation by passing the left hand beneath the head of the pancreas. Typically the firm texture of a chronic pancreatitis pancreas is easily distinguished from what feels like a canyon through the course of the main pancreatic duct. Typically in chronic pancreatitis, the duct is displaced more anteriorly and therefore is easier to palpate **(Figure 50-6)**.

- After the location of the pancreatic duct is satisfactorily established, a 20-gauge angiocatheter is passed into the duct, and the clear pancreatic juice is identified (see Figure 50-6).

- We will often perform manometry simply to take note of the presence of high pressures in the main pancreatic duct, which at times have served some predictive value in the success of relieving pain in this operation.

- After the location of the duct with the catheter is established, electrocautery is used to open down along the angiocatheter tract into the pancreatic duct. Typically, the pancreatic duct has a reddish smooth surface, which distinguishes it from false passages within the parenchyma of the pancreas. Care should be taken not to enter through the lobulated texture of the pancreas into a false passage. After the duct is established, a tonsil clamp can be used to probe both toward the tail and toward the head of the pancreas, and the electrocautery follows the hemostat's opened blades **(Figure 50-7)**.

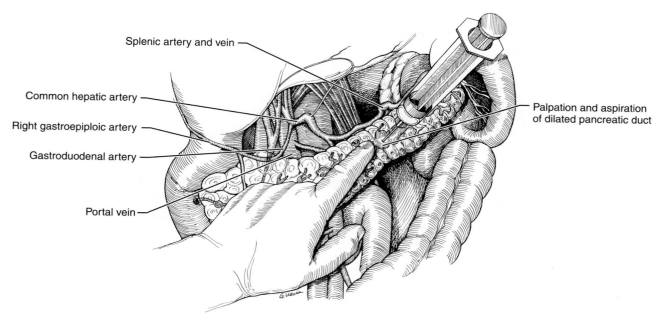

Splenic artery and vein

Common hepatic artery

Right gastroepiploic artery

Gastroduodenal artery

Portal vein

Palpation and aspiration of dilated pancreatic duct

FIGURE 50–6

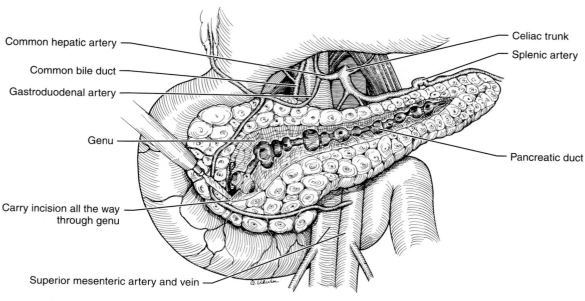

Common hepatic artery

Common bile duct

Gastroduodenal artery

Genu

Carry incision all the way through genu

Superior mesenteric artery and vein

Celiac trunk

Splenic artery

Pancreatic duct

FIGURE 50–7

- It is vital to continue the incision in the main pancreatic duct past the genu of the duct. This portion of the main pancreatic duct courses both inferiorly and posteriorly. Thus the depth of incision into pancreatic parenchyma is considerably greater in this portion of the dissection, and the risk of hemorrhage during this dissection is higher. One should be prepared to perform a suture ligature should one encounter any major bleeding during this dissection. Data confirm that an adequate incision in the main pancreatic duct must include a deep incision into the uncinate process in the head of the pancreas. Suture ligation of these parenchymal arteries is mandatory to prevent postoperative hemorrhage.

- After this incision is completed, identify an area of proximal jejunum approximately 15 cm past the ligament of Treitz. The mesentery is divided between clamps in a vertical fashion down toward the spine. After acceptable mobility of the limb of jejunum, a GIA stapling device is placed across the jejunum, and the jejunum is divided **(Figure 50-8)**.

- The distal segment of the divided jejunum is passed through a rent in the transverse mesocolon and placed side-to-side against the body of the pancreas, with the divided end of jejunum directed toward the left **(Figure 50-9)**.

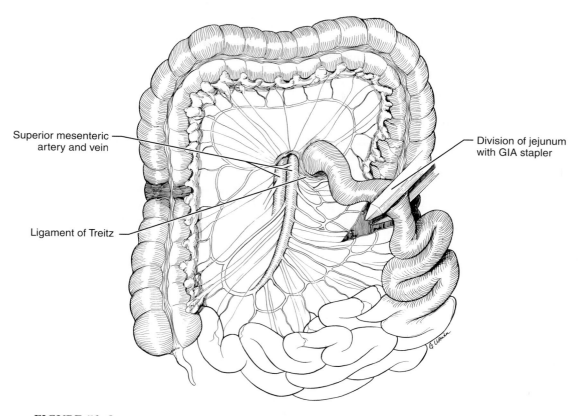

Superior mesenteric
artery and vein

Division of jejunum
with GIA stapler

Ligament of Treitz

FIGURE 50–8

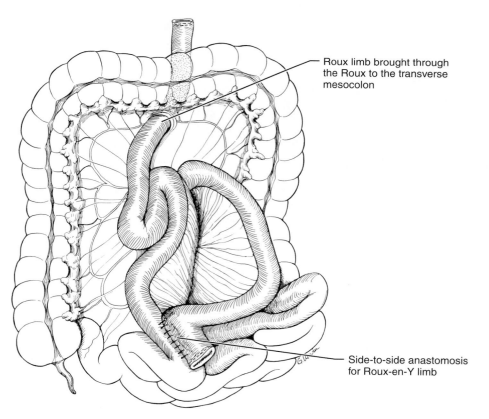

Roux limb brought through
the Roux to the transverse
mesocolon

Side-to-side anastomosis
for Roux-en-Y limb

FIGURE 50–9

◆ A side-to-side pancreaticojejunostomy is performed in one layer using interrupted 3-0 silk stitch. The inferior suture line is placed before the jejunum is opened, and these sutures are tied. After the jejunum is opened, the superior row of sutures in the pancreaticojejunostomy is completed by placing a corner stitch to the left and right boundaries and by placing a stitch midway through the longitudinal incision in the body of the pancreas and midway through the incision in the jejunum **(Figure 50-10).** Immediately tying the sutures on the superior suture line prevents any mismatch in size between the jejunal incision and the pancreatic duct incision. It should be noted that typically the jejunum tends to open much larger than one can anticipate, so care should be taken to place the inferior sutures in the jejunum somewhat closer than they are placed in the inferior aspect of the incision in the wall of the pancreas. After the middle suture on the superior suture line is placed, sutures are placed that bisect the area to the left and right. Finally, individual sutures are placed as appropriate to complete the anastomosis **(Figures 50-11 and 50-12).**

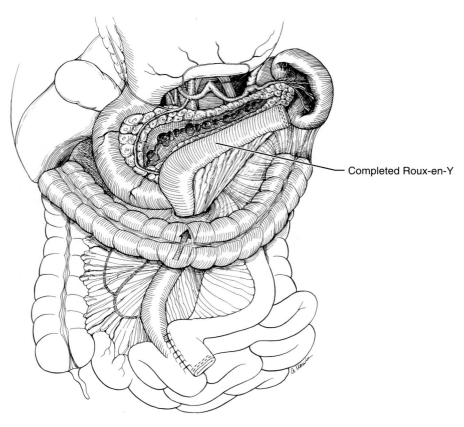

Completed Roux-en-Y

FIGURE 50–10

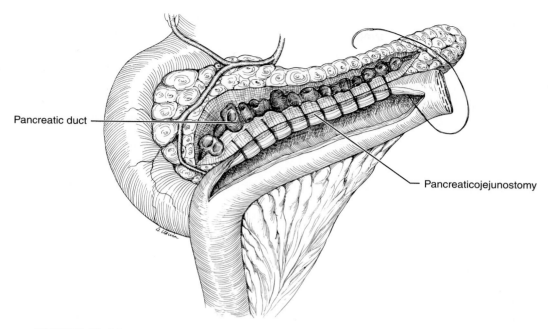

Pancreatic duct

Pancreaticojejunostomy

FIGURE 50–11

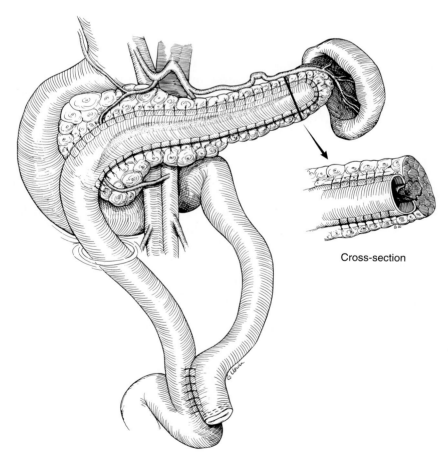

Cross-section

FIGURE 50–12

3. CLOSING

◆ At completion of the pancreaticojejunostomy, the limb of jejunum is fixed in place as it traverses the transverse mesocolon with an interrupted 3-0 silk stitch. Finally, 40 cm distal to the pancreaticojejunostomy, a side-to-side jejunojejunostomy is performed in two layers, with an outer layer of interrupted 3-0 silk stitch and an inner layer of running locking 3-0 Vicryl stitch posteriorly, which converts to a Connell type of stitch anteriorly (see Figure 50-12).

◆ We do not use drains. The fascia is reapproximated in the normal fashion, and the skin is closed using subcuticular suture.

STEP 4: POSTOPERATIVE CARE

◆ Patients will have had a nasogastric tube placed. This is removed on the first postoperative day. The patient starts with a clear liquid diet, and if tolerated, this is advanced to a regular diet.

◆ Care should be taken in the immediate postoperative period to monitor blood glucose, because these patients often have borderline insufficiency or frank diabetes, and for that reason the stress of surgery may result in significant hyperglycemia.

◆ The only significant postoperative complication that can be anticipated in the first 24 to 48 hours is hemorrhage. For that reason, one should carefully monitor hemoglobin levels. Once these have proved to be stable, it is not necessary to continue to monitor these.

STEP 5: PEARLS AND PITFALLS

◆ It can be challenging to find the pancreatic duct in some patients. Although the duct is easily palpable in most, it is not in some. On rare occasions, it may be necessary to perform a vertical incision in the mid-portion of the anterior surface of the body of the pancreas as a means of searching for the actual pancreatic duct. Care should be taken not to extend this incision to either the superior or the inferior border of the pancreas. It is also often possible to express some of the pancreatic juice by massaging either the anterior surface of the tail of the pancreas or the anterior surface of the head of the pancreas. The pancreatic juice is crystal clear and should be easily recognized during this palpation.

◆ As mentioned during the operative procedure, the mismatch between the opening in the jejunum and the opening in the pancreatic duct can be problematic. Care should be taken to limit the size of the opening in the jejunum until one can be certain that it is does not greatly exceed the length of the opening in the main pancreatic duct.

◆ It is not uncommon to have associated bile duct stricture in patients undergoing Puestow procedure, and consideration should be given to the possible need for a hepaticojejunostomy at the same time as the pancreaticojejunostomy.

◆ One may typically encounter stones either within the main pancreatic duct or easily palpable in some of the dilated side branches. We advocate removing these stones when possible. Instruments such as Fogarty catheters and some instruments typically used for biliary lithiasis may be helpful in this event.

SELECTED REFERENCES

1. Katz MH, Wang H, Fleming JB, et al. Long-term survival after multidisciplinary management of resected pancreatic adenocarcinoma. Ann Surg Oncol 2009;16:836-847.
2. Kow AW, Chan SP, Earnest A, et al. Striving for a better operative outcome: 101 Pancreaticoduodenectomies. HPB (Oxford) 2008;10:464-471.
3. Katz MH, Fleming JB, Pisters PW, et al. Anatomy of the superior mesenteric vein with special reference to the surgical management of first-order branch involvement at pancreaticoduodenectomy. Ann Surg 2008;248:1098-1102.

CHAPTER 51

Pseudocysts—Cystogastrostomy, Cystoduodenostomy, and Cystojejunostomy

William H. Nealon

STEP 1: SURGICAL ANATOMY

- All pancreatic surgery requires an understanding of the anatomic relationships in the lesser sac (see Figure 47-1). After either an upper midline or a bilateral subcostal (chevron) incision, one enters the lesser sac by dissecting along the avascular plane at the points of attachment of the gastrocolic omentum to the transverse colon. The proper plane is between the anterior and posterior leaflets. This is my favored point of entry. The alternative entry is by transversely dividing and ligating the vascular structures embedded in the omentum while preserving the gastroepiploic vessels located along the greater curvature of the stomach.

- Upon entering the lesser sac, one will encounter varying amounts of adhesions between the posterior wall of the stomach and the anterior surface of the pancreas. These fetal adhesions do not imply prior inflammatory events. Considerable dense adhesions may be encountered in pathologic states.

- The pancreas is essentially encased in a sandwich of major blood vessels. The vena cava and aorta occupy the posterior surface in the midline. The splenic artery courses along the superior surface from the aorta toward the tail. The splenic vein occupies the posterior superior surface of the body and tail of the pancreas. It meets the superior mesenteric vein, which is oriented vertically in the groove created by the uncinate process in the posterior aspect of the head of the pancreas and the right lateral and anterior components of the head. The confluence of these two veins constitutes the portal vein, which traverses this uncinate groove and emerges to join the bile duct and the hepatic artery in the hepatoduodenal ligament.

- The superior mesenteric artery is located in a plane posterior and slightly medial to the superior mesenteric vein. The common hepatic artery, another branch of the celiac trunk (along with the splenic artery and left gastric artery), courses along the superior border of the head of the pancreas to join the hepatoduodenal ligament. Its first branch is the typically miniscule right gastric artery. Just distal is the more substantial gastroduodenal artery, which emerges at a right angle to the hepatic artery from its inferior surface and courses beneath the pylorus, and after sending the right gastroepiploic artery in the plane between the inferior aspect of the pylorus and the superior surface of the head of the pancreas, the gastroduodenal artery pierces the head of the pancreas.

◆ The anterior superior and the posterior superior pancreaticoduodenal arteries also arise from branches of the gastroduodenal artery. These arteries form an arch medial to the C-loop of the duodenum, and they collateralize with branches of the anterior and posterior inferior pancreaticoduodenal arteries, which are branches of the superior mesenteric artery. Small branches from these arteries provide blood supply to the duodenum.

◆ Key anatomic features in pancreatic head resections are the network of tributaries projecting between the superior mesenteric vein/portal vein confluence and the uncinate process. These tributaries are located at the right lateral aspect of the veins. These tiny veins exit the pancreas at the mid-portion of the groove in which the major veins reside.

◆ Viewed in cross-sectional imaging, the uncinate process forms a C-shaped structure. The terminal posterior extent of the uncinate process projects in a medial direction as a ligamentous structure and contains a variable number of arterial branches from the superior mesenteric artery that project at right angles to the major artery and provide blood supply to the uncinate process. Division of the tiny venous tributaries and the arterial branches are key steps in respective procedures. This uncinate margin is the most problematic in managing malignant tumors in the head of the pancreas.

◆ The pancreas is entirely retroperitoneal, and therefore operative procedures will require mobilization of the pancreas from its retroperitoneal position. The plane lateral to the C-loop of the duodenum is incised in nearly all procedures, and this plane is avascular and its mobilization is termed the Kocher maneuver. This exposes the vena cava and aorta and it permits "bimanual palpation" of the head of the pancreas. The dissection may be easily extended to the fourth portion of the duodenum and the ligament of Treitz .

◆ The inferior border of the body of the pancreas is also avascular, although the inferior mesenteric vein may be encountered to the right of the spine.

◆ Peritoneum overlies the hepatoduodenal ligament. Dissection reveals the triad in gross anatomic terms, which corresponds to the microscopic portal triad—with portal, hepatic arterial, and biliary structures. The common bile duct is located in an anterior lateral position, and the hepatic artery is anterior medial. The portal vein is positioned in the posterior groove created by the apposition of these anterior structures.

◆ Although lymph nodes may be seen at a wide array of locations, there is a constant lymph node in the groove created by the lateral border of the second portion of the duodenum and the hepatoduodenal ligament. Dissection of this lymph node is necessary to fully visualize the proximal hepatic artery. Other common sites of lymph nodes are on the lateral aspect of the mid-portion of the hepatoduodenal ligament, in the fibrovascular bundle surrounding the right gastroepiploic complex, and on the superior border of the confluence of the head and body of the pancreas. Beneath this lymph node one finds the origins of the common hepatic artery and the splenic artery.

◆ On the inferior border of the pancreatic head, just where the duodenum dives beneath the superior mesenteric vein and artery, one may dissect the peritoneum and visualize the superior mesenteric vein as it passes in a superior direction beneath the head of the pancreas.

◆ The ligament of Treitz is a significant anatomic structure, and it can be accessed by lifting the transverse colon and omentum in an anterior direction. The ligament can be seen to the left of the spine.

◆ The main pancreatic duct originates in the tail of the pancreas and traverses the length of the pancreas to exit in the duodenum through both main ampulla (Vater) and the accessory ampulla, which is located more proximally in the duodenum. The main pancreatic duct (Wirsung) and the minor or accessory duct (Santorini) fuse during fetal development at what is termed the genu or "knee" of the duct.

◆ It should be understood that pseudocysts can form at any location including sites quite remote from the pancreas itself. Thus certain pseudocysts may involve anatomy not included in this review.

INDICATIONS

◆ The indication for operation in pseudocysts is somewhat complex.

◆ First, one must confirm that the pseudocyst has persisted long enough to be certain that the cyst will not simply spontaneously resolve.

◆ Although not uniformly accepted, there is literature suggesting that only symptomatic pseudocysts should be treated. Thus one indication for surgery is symptoms (daily pain or difficulty eating, or recurrent attacks of acute pain).

◆ The generally stated indication for surgery or some form of intervention is the development of the complications of pseudocysts (obstruction of intestine or bile duct, hemorrhage into the pseudocysts, infection in the pseudocysts, and rupture of the pseudocysts). Rupture of a pseudocyst will present as ascites, an entity termed pancreatic ascites. A ruptured pseudocyst should be suspected when this entity is identified.

◆ An additional indication may be rapid expansion in a pseudocyst.

◆ An important distinction that should be made in the preoperative evaluation is the possibility that a cyst actually represents a neoplastic cyst. In this case, suspicions may be raised by the fact that a cyst has septations; a cyst has what appears to be wall thickening within the cyst; and the patient may have an elevation in the tumor marker, which is known as CA 19-9. Particularly in the setting of acute pancreatitis, one cannot automatically exclude a cystic neoplasm, because 37% of patients with a diagnosis of intraductal papillary mucinous neoplasm (IPMN) present with pancreatitis. In the event that a neoplastic cyst is suspected, then preoperative aspiration, typically by means of endoscopic ultrasound, is useful. This cyst fluid should be examined for the presence of mucin confirmed by mucicarmine staining, measured for carcinoembryonic antigen (CEA) level, and sent for cytopathologic evaluation.

STEP 2: PREOPERATIVE CONSIDERATIONS

◆ We strongly advocate identification of the pancreatic ductal anatomy before intervention for pseudocyst, and we have published several papers delineating the reasons. One particularly significant reason to evaluate the ductal anatomy is to help direct the choice of modality to treat the pseudocyst. At this time, there is literature supporting three separate modalities to treat pseudocysts (surgery, endoscopy, and interventional radiology). Our data suggest that certain ductal injuries will make the likely success of these nonoperative modalities unacceptably low. We also advocate defining ductal anatomy to recognize the possible coexistence of a diagnosis of chronic pancreatitis, which should be addressed with operative procedures intended to treat that diagnosis rather than simply treating the cyst.

◆ We generally advocate a cystojejunostomy over the use of cystogastrostomy. There are strong data to suggest that a very large cyst has a high likelihood of sepsis after cystogastrostomy, and there are softer data suggesting that cystogastrostomy has a higher risk of postoperative hemorrhage compared with cystojejunostomy.
  ◆ If one is considering a cystogastrostomy, cross-sectional imaging is vital to confirm a fusion of the plane between the pseudocyst and the posterior wall of the stomach. Cross-sectional imaging will also confirm a close adherence between the pseudocyst and duodenum if a cystoduodenostomy is considered. Finally, cross-sectional imaging may help in directing dissection for entering a cyst for cystojejunostomy. For example, the presence of a cyst posteriorly toward the tail of the pancreas may be best addressed by traversing the transverse mesocolon in order to access the cyst. If the cyst is posterior to most of the parenchyma of the pancreas, it may be necessary to dissect beneath the pancreas rather than to incise through normal pancreatic parenchyma to access the cyst.
  ◆ Be sure that your imaging is recent. In the event that a month or more has elapsed since the last imaging, there is a possibility that the cyst has changed or disappeared entirely.

◆ We perform a bowel preparation and a colonic cleansing in all patients.

◆ Within 1 hour of surgery, a single intravenous dose of a second-generation cephalosporin is given.

STEP 3: OPERATIVE STEPS

1. INCISION AND EXPOSURE

◆ We use an upper abdominal midline incision, although subcostal or transverse incisions may be preferable depending on the location of the cyst and the anticipated mode of bypass. We use self-retaining retractors to afford visualization.

2. DISSECTION

Cystogastrostomy

◆ When the decision is made to proceed with cystogastrostomy, the operative procedure is fairly simple **(Figure 51-1)**. Two stay sutures of 3-0 silk stitch are placed in the anterior wall of the stomach after palpating the cyst to confirm the incision will be placed exactly over the primary palpable body of the pseudocyst. After these two sutures are placed on the superior and inferior margin of the anticipated gastrotomy, electrocautery is used to perform an anterior gastrotomy for a length of approximately 8 cm. After this is done, one can easily palpate the connection between the pseudocyst and the posterior wall of the stomach **(Figure 51-2)**.

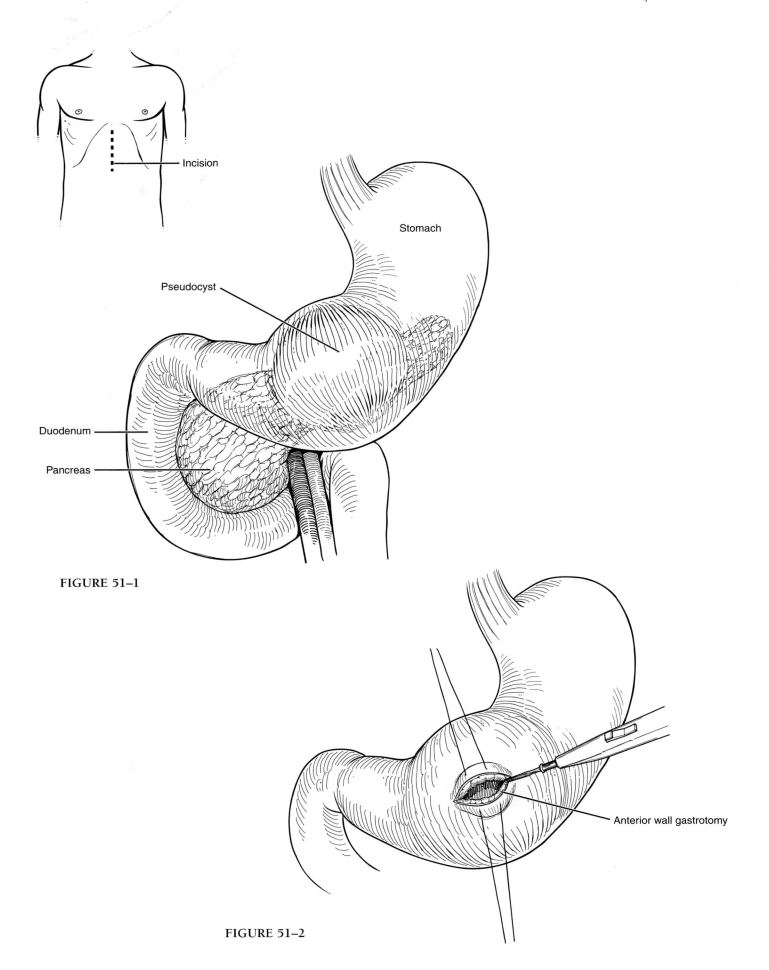

Incision

Stomach

Pseudocyst

Duodenum

Pancreas

FIGURE 51–1

Anterior wall gastrotomy

FIGURE 51–2

◆ At this point, a 20-gauge angiocatheter is placed into the cyst to confirm that cyst fluid will be encountered **(Figure 51-3)**. Finally, electrocautery is used to begin an entryway through the posterior wall of the stomach into the cyst. We then take a long, delicate hemostat such as the Seurat clamp and gently place it through the posterior wall of the stomach and through the anterior wall of the cyst. Typically a large amount of fluid will be evacuated. In most cases, this will result in fairly significant collapse of the pseudocyst. At this point of entry, a larger orifice can be made, and at the same time a biopsy of the wall of the cyst can be obtained **(Figure 51-4)**. This should be sent for frozen section analysis to confirm that it is not a neoplastic cyst. We finally work with approximately 3-cm-diameter entry into the cyst. Next, 2-0 Prolene sutures are used in a running fashion to complete the connection between the cyst and posterior wall of the stomach **(Figure 51-5)**. After this is complete, one evacuates any solid material within the cyst and irrigates the cyst. For all cysts, we believe it is vital to evacuate as much of this debris as possible. Any hemorrhage encountered in the wall of the cyst or in the gastric wall should be suture ligated to prevent postoperative hemorrhage.

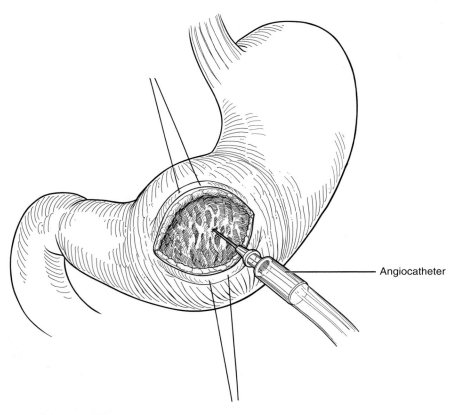

Angiocatheter

FIGURE 51–3

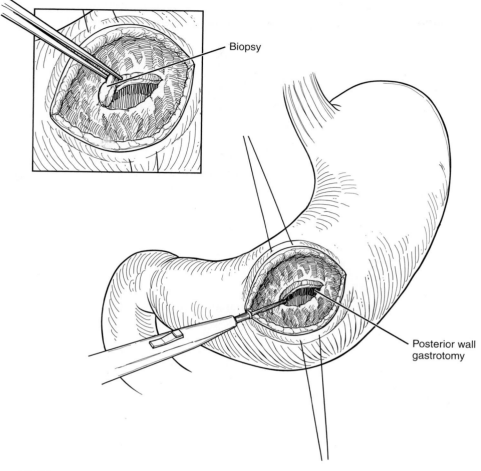

FIGURE 51–4

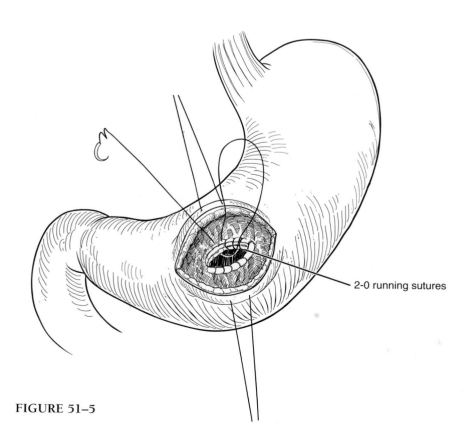

FIGURE 51–5

◆ We often will take a culture of the fluid in the cyst on the chance that the cyst fluid has been colonized (which is common) and the patient develops signs of sepsis in the postoperative period.

◆ The anterior gastrotomy is then closed in two layers with an outer layer of interrupted 3-0 silk stitch and an inner layer of a Connell type of absorbable suture, such as polydioxanone (PDS) or Vicryl. Lembert sutures of 3-0 silk are placed at the two corners of the gastrotomy, tied, and left long on a hemostat for traction. Two 3-0 Vicryl sutures are placed and tied at each corner with the knot on the inside. A Connell type of running inverted stitch is used, starting at each corner and meeting in the middle of the gastrotomy and tied **(Figure 51-6)**. Finally, an interrupted 3-0 silk stitch is used in an interrupted fashion to complete the anterior layer of the gastrotomy closure **(Figure 51-7)**.

◆ We do not use drains. The peritoneal cavity is irrigated.

◆ Fascia is reapproximated in the normal fashion, and subcuticular sutures are placed in the skin.

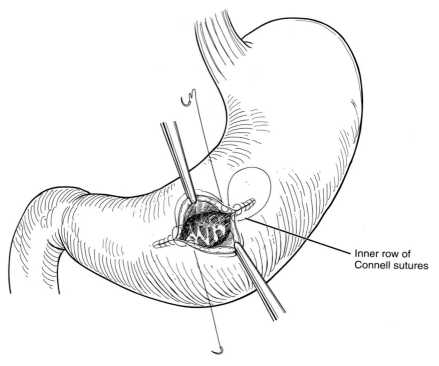

Inner row of
Connell sutures

FIGURE 51–6

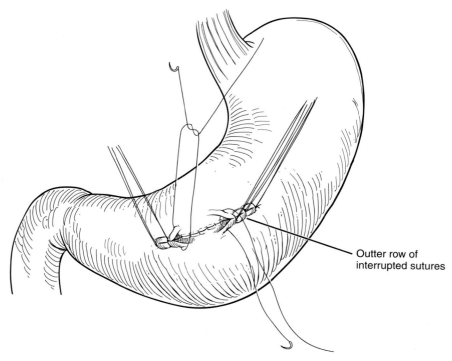

Outter row of
interrupted sutures

FIGURE 51–7

Cystoduodenostomy

◆ If preoperative evaluation convinces the surgeon that a cystoduodenostomy is best, we again use a midline incision **(Figure 51-8)**. The dissection is carried out by entering the lesser sac. This can typically be done by separating the gastrocolic omentum from its attachments along the transverse colon. Obviously, this technique is restricted to patients with pseudocysts located in the head of the pancreas, abutting the medial wall of the duodenum **(Figure 51-9)**.

◆ In the event the adhesions resulting from the acute pancreatitis and the pseudocyst have made entry into the lesser sac unfeasible, one may simply divide the omental attachments overlying the head of the pancreas between clamps. Care should be taken to avoid injury to the right gastroepiploic arteries and to the vessels of the transverse mesocolon, should this access point be chosen. At this point, one should be able to palpate the pseudocyst **(Figure 51-10)**. Throughout this discussion it should be made clear that the extent of adhesions will dictate much of this dissection. If inflammatory adhesions are excessive, then alternative approaches must be sought. I would also caution that simply finding the pseudocyst may be challenging, and intraoperative ultrasound may be useful.

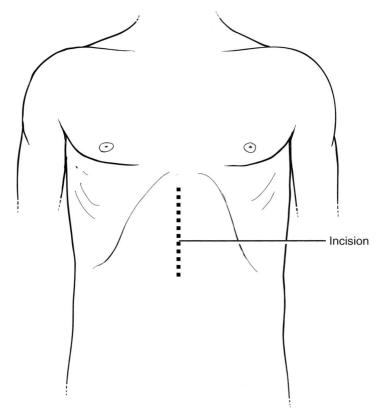

Incision

FIGURE 51–8

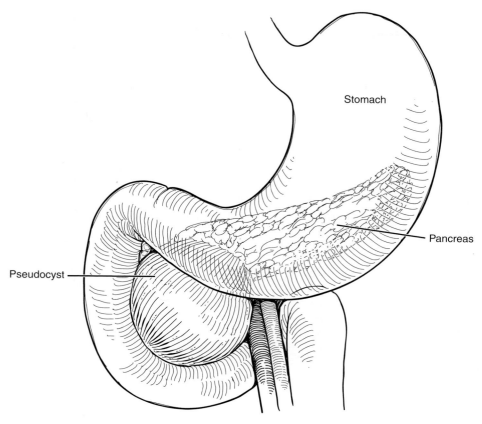

FIGURE 51–9

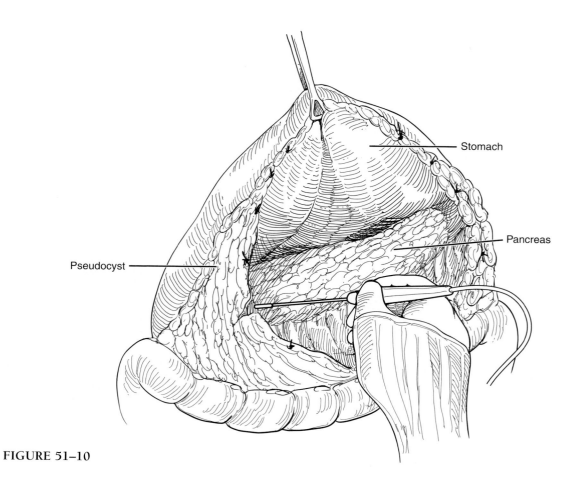

FIGURE 51–10

◆ We then perform a Kocher maneuver by incising the peritoneum along the line outlining the lateral border of the C-loop of the duodenum and mobilizing the duodenum and the head of the pancreas toward the left, teasing the loose the areolar tissue in the retroperitoneum. This permits bimanual palpation of the head of the pancreas and permits the surgeon to ascertain the exact location of the cyst **(Figure 51-11)**. Having ascertained the area of the duodenum most closely approximating the location of the cyst, the surgeon performs a duodenotomy. Stay sutures of 3-0 silk stitch are placed well away from the margin of the duodenum to the head of the pancreas, and after these have been placed, a longitudinal incision is made in the duodenum for the length of approximately 4 cm **(Figure 51-12)**. With proper palpation, one can confirm the area of the posterior wall of the duodenum as it abuts the cyst. At this point, we place an angiocatheter into the cyst and confirm that cyst fluid aspirates **(Figure 51-13)**. We then use electrocautery to carefully dissect through the posterior wall of the duodenum into the cyst. We excise a small portion of the wall of the cyst and send for frozen section analysis to exclude a neoplasm **(Figure 51-14)**.

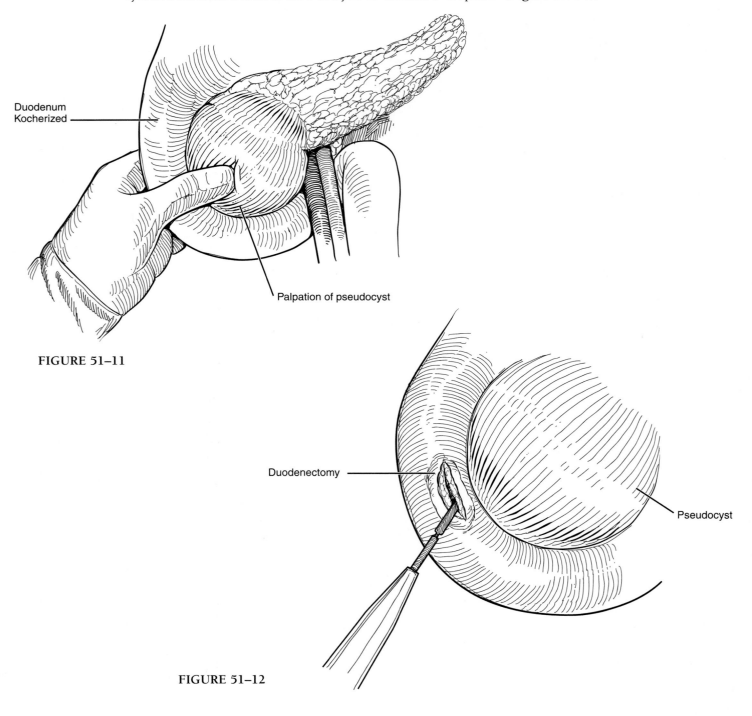

Duodenum Kocherized

Palpation of pseudocyst

FIGURE 51–11

Duodenectomy

Pseudocyst

FIGURE 51–12

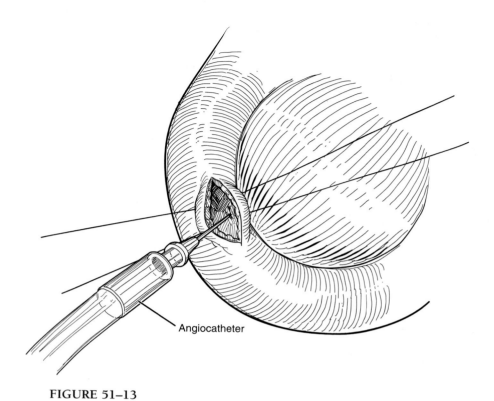

Angiocatheter

FIGURE 51–13

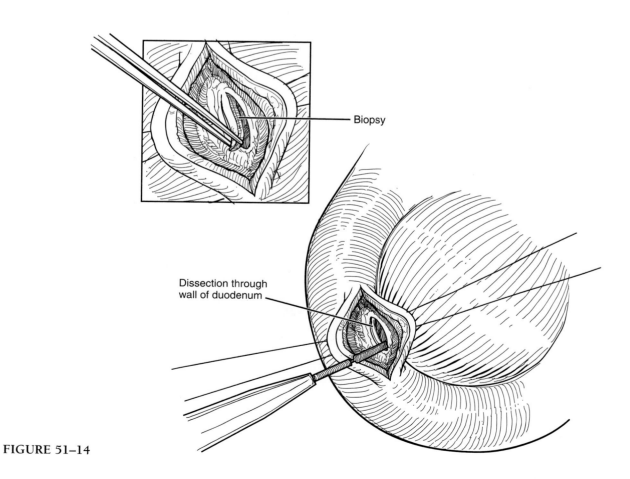

Biopsy

Dissection through
wall of duodenum

FIGURE 51–14

◆ We then open the cyst for a diameter of approximately 2 cm and place 3-0 Prolene sutures in a running fashion circumferentially around the duodenotomy into the cyst **(Figure 51-15)**. In a cross-sectional view, one can see the orientation of the cystoduodenostomy to the pancreas and duodenum **(Figure 51-16)**. Any solid material in the cyst is removed. We again obtain culture of the cyst fluid.

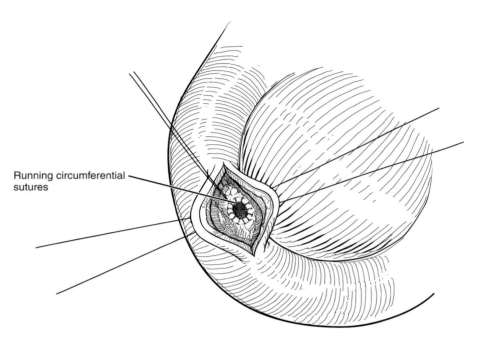

Running circumferential
sutures

FIGURE 51–15

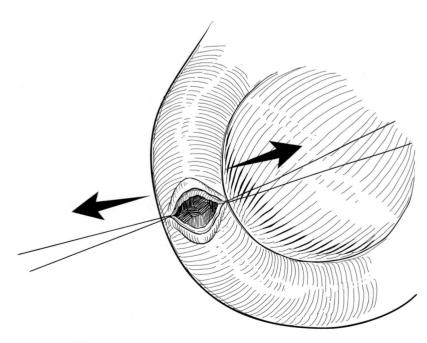

FIGURE 51–16

◆ After this has been done, the longitudinal incision in the duodenum is closed in a transverse fashion similar to a technique of closure first described by Heineke and Mikulicz in their description of a pyloroplasty. This closure is performed in two layers with an outer layer of interrupted 3-0 silk stitch and an inner layer of a Connell type of stitch. Just as in the closure of the gastrotomy, the running absorbable suture line is again taken from each corner and tied in the middle. In this anastomosis, however, the superior and the inferior extent of the duodenotomy are sutured together at the midpoint of the transverse closure. To start, place a Lembert-type stitch with 3-0 silk at exactly the midpoint of the duodenotomy on both the lateral and the medial edges. These will be the new corners. Complete the Connell sutures and then place interrupted silk sutures to complete the closure **(Figures 51-17 and 51-18)**. At completion, the closure should look to be at right angles to the course of the duodenum. This is performed to prevent any significant narrowing of the duodenum after the duodenotomy.

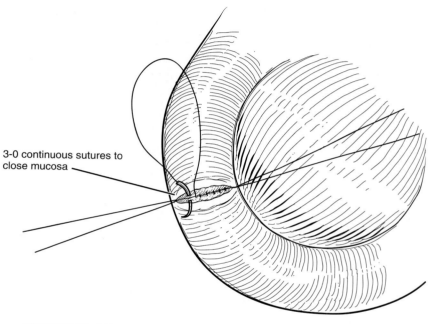

3-0 continuous sutures to close mucosa

FIGURE 51–17

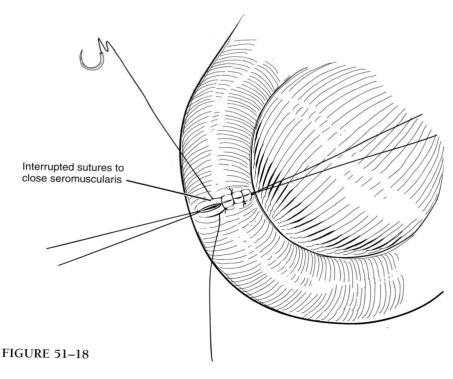

Interrupted sutures to close seromuscularis

FIGURE 51–18

Cystojejunostomy

- When the decision is made to proceed to a cystojejunostomy (our procedure of choice), a Roux-en-Y reconstruction is required. Although this reconstruction can be used for pseudocysts and any number of locations it really is the only option for pseudocyst in the mid-pancreas without any clear shared plane with the posterior wall of the stomach **(Figure 51-19)**.

- Once again, we typically perform this procedure by entering the lesser sac. This is achieved by dividing the attachments between the gastrocolic omentum and the transverse colon. We begin this dissection to the left of the spine and extend it over to the hepatic flexure **(Figure 51-20)**. If this access point is achievable, one may expose the anterior surface of the pancreas, and in most cases, the pseudocyst will be identified and palpable in this area. Care should be taken if extensive adhesions are encountered between the posterior wall of the stomach and the pseudocyst. However, it is not necessary to completely skeletonize the cyst **(Figure 51-21)**. Once an acceptable exposure of the cyst has been performed in the lesser sac, one may then place an angiocatheter into the cyst to confirm the presence of cyst fluid. Finally, an incision for a length of approximately 3 cm is performed transversely, and a large amount of fluid typically is removed.

- Any solid material in the cyst is removed and cultures are routinely obtained.

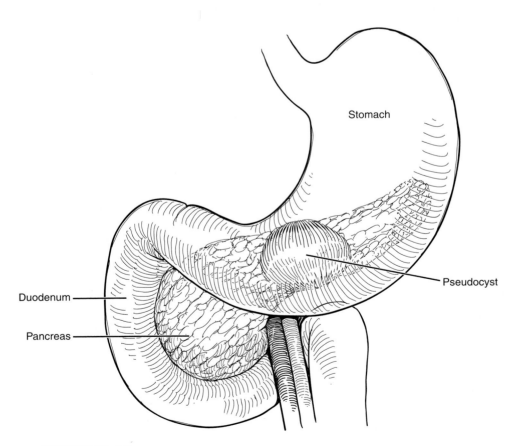

FIGURE 51–19

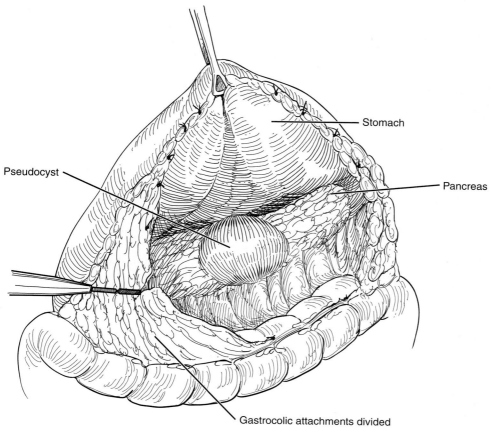

Pseudocyst

Stomach

Pancreas

Gastrocolic attachments divided

FIGURE 51–20

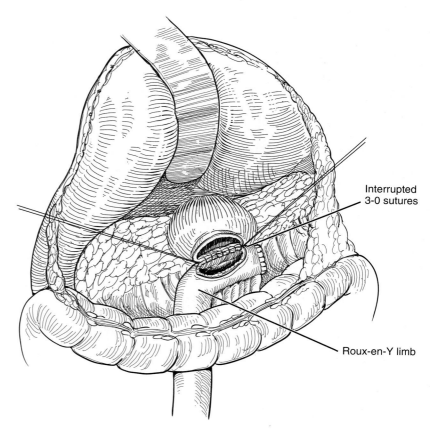

Interrupted
3-0 sutures

Roux-en-Y limb

FIGURE 51–21

◆ An area is chosen in the proximal jejunum approximately 15 cm distal to the ligament of Treitz. This is divided using a gastrointestinal anastomosis (GIA) stapling device, and mesentery is divided vertically toward the base of the mesentery to provide adequate length of jejunum to reach the pseudocyst. The distal end of the divided jejunum is brought up to the opening in the pseudocyst (see Figure 51-21). A single layer of 3-0 silk interrupted suture is used to first attach the jejunum to the inferior border of the open cyst before incising the jejunum (see Figure 51-21), and subsequently the anterior edge is similarly closed **(Figure 51-22).**

◆ After this has been completed, a jejunojejunostomy is performed approximately 40 cm distal to the cystojejunostomy in a side-to-side fashion in two layers, with an outer layer of interrupted 3-0 silk stitch and an inner layer of running locking 3-0 Vicryl stitch on the posterior wall. This is converted to a Connell type of stitch anteriorly. The rent in the mesentery, if one was used, is then reapproximated using 3-0 silk stitch, and any mesentery defect created by the jejunojejunostomy limb is reapproximated using 3-0 silk stitch (see Figure 51-22).

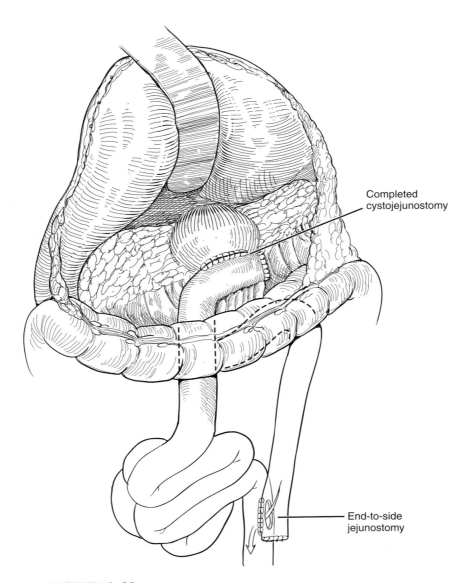

Completed cystojejunostomy

End-to-side jejunostomy

FIGURE 51–22

♦ In the event that one cannot easily access the lesser sac, we will occasionally resort to an incision through the transverse mesocolon into the cyst. We will at times use intraoperative ultrasound to facilitate this access point (**Figure 51-23**).

♦ After adequately palpating through the transverse mesocolon, one will use an angiocatheter to confirm the access to the cyst and, by palpation, will determine that there are no significant mesenteric vessels in the line of dissection. In this case, some of the fat of the mesentery may be carefully divided, and after palpating the wall of the cyst, one may make an incision into the cyst following the path of the angiocatheter. A length of approximately 3 cm is achieved.

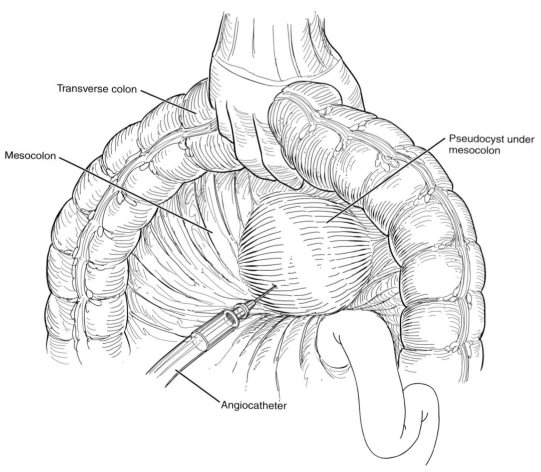

FIGURE 51–23

◆ Once again a limb of jejunum is chosen approximately 15 cm distal to the ligament of Treitz. The limb of jejunum is brought to the incision in the cyst, and a side-to-side anastomosis is begun to approximate the jejunum to the cyst **(Figure 51-24)**. Again, a cystojejunostomy is performed in one layer using interrupted 3-0 silk stitch. If not yet performed, a biopsy is taken of the wall of the cyst and sent for frozen section evaluation (see Figure 51-24).

◆ Although we do not advocate a two-layer anastomosis to the pseudocyst, this variation has been described. In this case, both layers will be nonabsorbable suture. The inner layer is placed, and then a second layer of interrupted 3-0 silk is placed. Finally, the entire two-layer anastomosis is completed **(Figure 51-25)**.

◆ No drains are applied. The fascia is closed in the normal fashion. The skin is closed using subcuticular stitches.

STEP 4: POSTOPERATIVE CARE

◆ Pain management may be a significant issue in some patients, and this at times will require epidural analgesia.

◆ Patients should be monitored for hemorrhage or for glucose intolerance in the first 24 hours.

◆ A nasogastric tube will typically be used but will be removed on the first day. Liquid diet will be advanced to regular diet.

◆ We do not advocate continued antibiotics, although it should be understood that many reports on the surgical management of pseudocysts quote rather high rates of complications, many infectious. So certainly a level of surveillance for signs of infection should be used.

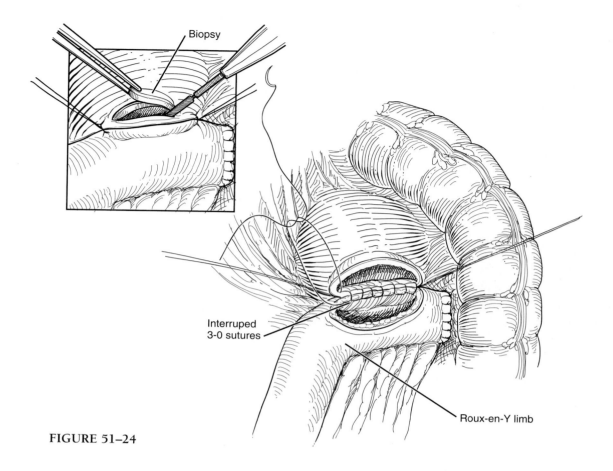

Biopsy

Interruped
3-0 sutures

Roux-en-Y limb

FIGURE 51–24

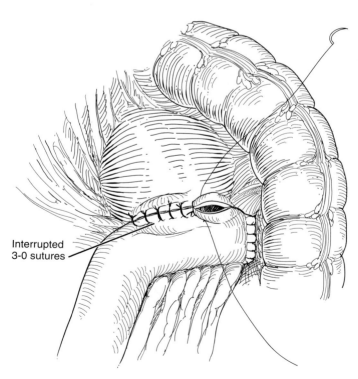

Interrupted
3-0 sutures

FIGURE 51–25

STEP 5: PEARLS AND PITFALLS

◆ As stated before, we advocate several precepts in arriving at the decision to proceed to intervention.

◆ We particularly point out the significance of time since development of the pseudocyst. The literature on nonoperative modalities often describes interventions earlier than 4 weeks after the initial event. The reason to avoid such a decision early is that the texture of the pseudocyst will be unsuitable for holding a suture. We further believe that a percentage of these patients will have complete resolution of the pseudocyst if given enough time to do so.

◆ Once the decision is made to proceed to intervention, we advocate obtaining pancreatic ductal anatomy defined by either endoscopic retrograde cholangiopancreatography (ERCP) or magnetic resonance cholangiopancreatography (MRCP). We have developed a system to categorize the ductal changes seen in patients with pseudocyst; and type II (stricture), type III (complete obstruction), and type IV (chronic pancreatitis) are likely best managed by surgery, whereas type I (normal duct) is ideally suited to nonoperative interventions.

◆ We advocate cystojejunostomy and infrequently use cystoduodenostomy.

◆ Be prepared that some pseudocysts will be difficult to locate during operation. Intraoperative ultrasound can be very helpful in this situation. If in doubt, always aspirate with a fine needle before attempting to incise the wall of the presumed pseudocyst.

◆ We have published the observation that persistent fluid collections after acute necrotizing pancreatitis are often rigid-walled and irregular in contour. These have been called "organized pancreatic necrosis," although the terminology is still evolving. Because of the rigid wall, these fluid collections will not collapse when drained. In our experience, this has resulted in a higher frequency of postoperative infection and in a prolonged period before all symptoms resolve. If you are managing such patients, the radiographs will always be read as pseudocyst, and the surgeon must be prepared to make that distinction based on the history of each individual patient.

SELECTED REFERENCES

1. Nealon WH, Walser E: Main pancreatic ductal anatomy can direct choice of modality for treating pancreatic pseudocysts (surgery vs. percutaneous drainage). Ann Surg 2002;235:751-758.
2. Nealon WH, Walser E: Duct drainage alone is sufficient in the operative management of pancreatic pseudocysts in patients with chronic pancreatitis. Ann Surg 2003;237:614-622.
3. Nealon WH, Bhutani M, Riall TS, et al: A unifying concept: Pancreatic ductal anatomy both predicts and determines the major complications resulting from pancreatitis. J Am Coll Surg 2009;208:790-799.

SPLEEN

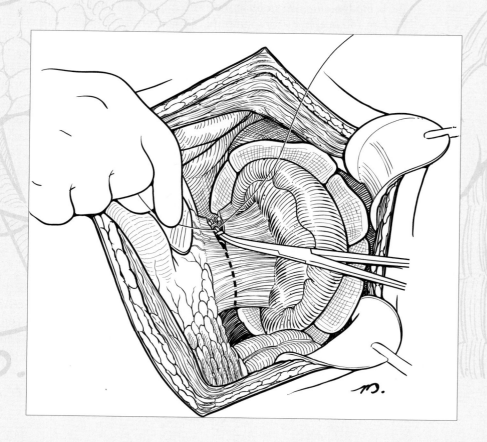

CHAPTER 52

SPLENECTOMY/SPLENIC REPAIR

William J. Mileski

STEP 1: SURGICAL ANATOMY

◆ The vascular supply of the spleen is composed primarily of the splenic artery and vein and the short gastric vessels. Primary anatomic consideration in treating spleen injuries is related to mobilization of the retroperitoneal attachments of the spleen, the splenocolic, splenorenal, and splenophrenic ligaments (**Figures 52-1 and 52-2**).

STEP 2: PREOPERATIVE CONSIDERATIONS

◆ Nonoperative management of spleen injuries is applicable to most patients who present in *hemodynamically stable* condition, and the diagnosis of injury is most often made as a result of computed tomographic (CT) scanning. Under these conditions the success rates for nonoperative therapy is very high, more than 80% in most modern series. Bed rest in the intensive care unit (ICU) should be prescribed, serial complete blood counts obtained, and serial abdominal examinations performed in an ICU for 24 to 48 hours. Hemodynamic deterioration or the development of peritonitis is typically considered indications to alter to an operative treatment mode. Some centers have reported success in controlling hemorrhage from both liver and spleen injuries with angioembolization, but this requires prompt availability of the interventional radiologists, which may not be applicable in many situations. There is no clear definition of what transfusion requirement merits abandonment of nonoperative treatment or how far to allow the hemoglobin to fall in these cases before transfusion and/or operative intervention. In most instances, however, persistent hemorrhage is manifest in the first 24 hours, with progressive reduction in hemoglobin levels at 6, 12, and 18 hours after injury or episodes of hypotension. The development of peritonitis is another clear indication for operative intervention.

◆ Because most patients with spleen injuries who undergo surgery are those who present hemodynamically unstable with severe hemorrhage or have failed attempts at nonoperative management, the approach to surgery is generally of an emergent nature and requires direct and rapid control of hemorrhage. The torso should be widely prepped and draped, and a generous midline incision carried from the xiphisternum to just above the pubis. The use of fixed self-retaining retractors (e.g., Upper Hand, Omni-Tract, Thompson, or Buchwalter) can aid in retraction of the costal margin and exposure.

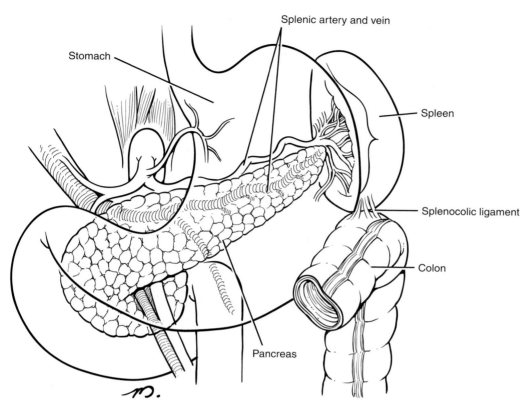

FIGURE 52–1

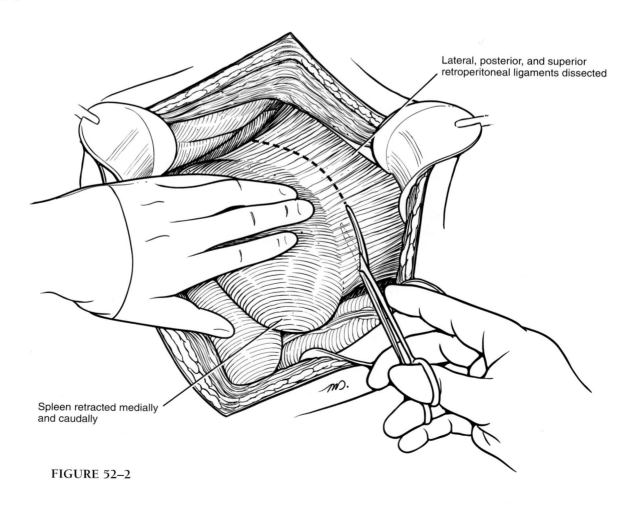

FIGURE 52–2

◆ In some patients, opening of the peritoneum may result in decompression of a degree of tamponade and result in severe hypotension; temporary compression of the aorta at the diaphragmatic hiatus, either manually with an aortic compression device or with the end of a small Richardson retractor, can provide temporization while the anesthesiologists restore intravascular volume. Upon evacuation of the hemoperitoneum, the right upper and left upper quadrants of the abdomen can be initially packed with laparotomy pads and the source of hemorrhage determined.

STEP 3: OPERATIVE STEPS

1. INCISION AND MOBILIZATION OF THE SPLEEN

◆ Through a midline incision the spleen is retracted caudally and medially by the surgeon's left hand, and the assistant retracts the abdominal wall laterally (see Figure 52-2).

2. DISSECTION

◆ The lateral, posterior, and superior retroperitoneal attachments are rapidly released by sharp dissection with a long Metzenbaum scissor (see Figure 52-2).

◆ A retropancreatic/prenephric plane can then be manually dissected, allowing the spleen to be retracted anteriorly and medially into the midline incision **(Figure 52-3)**.

◆ Active bleeding can be easily controlled with manual compression of the splenic hilum or application of vascular clamps to the hilum. If clamps are used, it is important to exercise care to avoid injury to the tail of the pancreas, which may be close by.

◆ Several laparotomy pads should be packed behind the spleen to tamponade bleeding and support the spleen while the lesser sac is opened on the proximal aspect of the greater curve of the stomach, and the short gastric vessels are ligated. While ligating the short gastric vessels, care should be taken to avoid incorporating the gastric wall in the ligatures, which can later lead to necrosis and a gastric fistula. At this point the spleen can be freely mobilized along with the tail of the pancreas to the midline **(Figure 52-4)**.

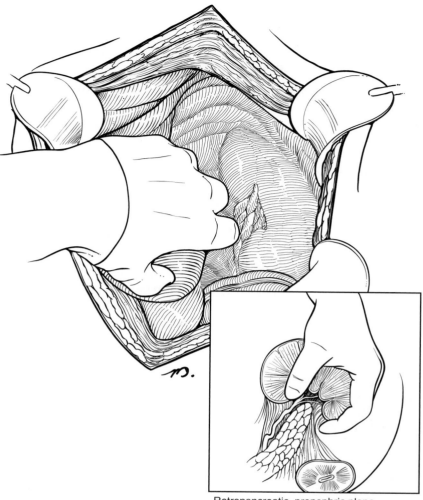

Retropancreatic, prenephric plane
of dissection manually dissected

FIGURE 52-3

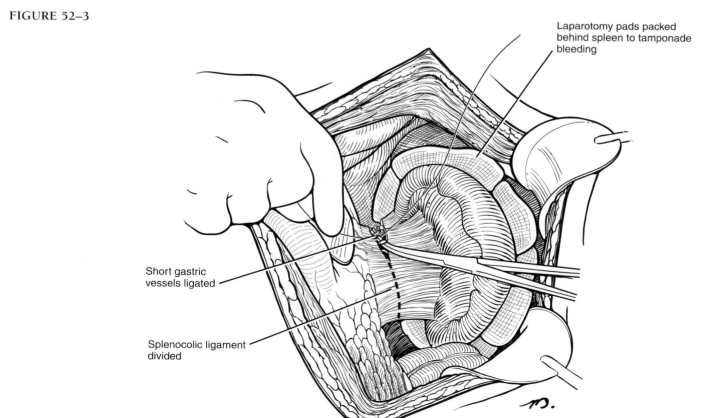

Laparotomy pads packed
behind spleen to tamponade
bleeding

Short gastric
vessels ligated

Splenocolic ligament
divided

FIGURE 52-4

◆ After the spleen is mobilized to the midline, it can be rapidly determined whether the injury has active hemorrhage that will require splenectomy or is a more modest injury amenable to splenorrhaphy or mesh wrapping. If the patient is hypotensive, coagulopathic, acidotic, or hypothermic or has multiple other injuries that contribute to or are worsened by ongoing hemorrhage (closed head injury), the decision to control hemorrhage by splenectomy is straightforward and should be made rapidly **(Figure 52-5)**.

◆ In patients who respond to control of the bleeding and resuscitation, splenorrhaphy remains an option. This can be accomplished with topical hemostatic agents, suture ligature with or without pledgets, and in some cases, wrapping of the spleen in absorbable mesh **(Figure 52-6)**.

◆ The splenic fossa should be carefully examined for hemorrhage and possible injury to the pancreas before closing. If there is evidence of or reasonable concern for possible injury to the pancreas, a closed suction drain should be left in the splenic bed **(Figure 52-7)**.

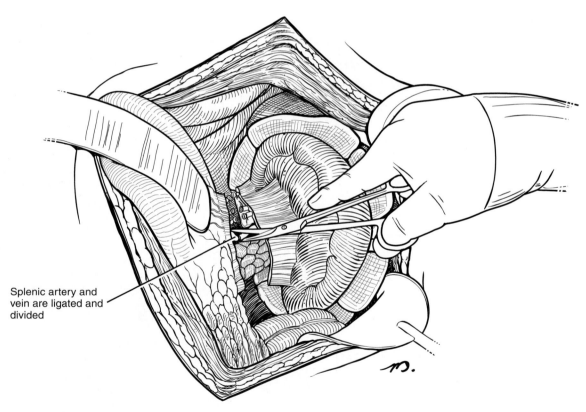

Splenic artery and
vein are ligated and
divided

FIGURE 52–5

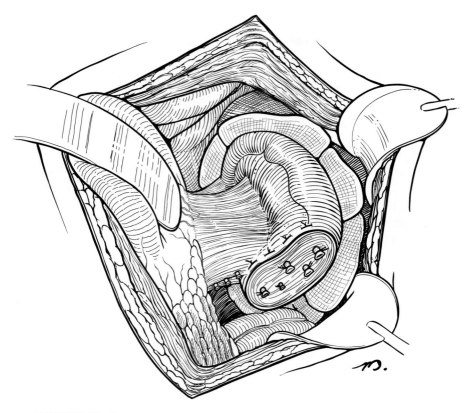

FIGURE 52–6

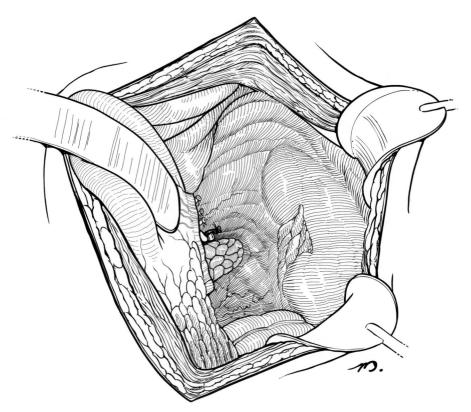

FIGURE 52–7

3. CLOSING

♦ Although nonoperative management is successful in more than 80% of patients with spleen injuries, rapid emergent operative treatment may be required.

♦ It cannot be overemphasized that nonoperative treatment is applicable only when the patient is hemodynamically stable. Patients who have evidence of significant hemoperitoneum, including significant free fluid surrounding loops of small intestine; those with contrast blush on the CT scan; those taking anticoagulants (warfarin [Coumadin], clopidogrel [Plavix]); those with portal hypertension; those with multiple injuries that may increase the risk from hemorrhage or intracranial injury; and the elderly are at increased risk of ongoing hemorrhage and failure of nonoperative treatment.

♦ When operative intervention is indicated, exposure and full mobilization of the spleen are essential to either splenorrhaphy or splenectomy.

STEP 4: POSTOPERATIVE CARE

♦ A nasogastric tube is continued in place until evidence of effective gastric emptying is clearly present. Incentive spirometry and pulmonary toilet are important to limit postoperative atelectasis and pneumonia. Prophylaxis for deep venous thrombosis (DVT) with fractionated heparin may begin on postoperative day 1. In the patients who undergo splenectomy, immunization against pneumococcus, meningococcus, and *Haemophilus influenzae* should be administered before discharge from the hospital.

STEP 5: PEARLS AND PITFALLS

♦ Pancreatic fistula may occur following splenectomy as a result of pancreatic trauma or iatrogenic injury. Careful inspection of the tail of the pancreas and taking care to avoid pancreatic injury while ligating the vasculature of the spleen are the best preventative measures. If there is concern that the tail of the pancreas might be damaged at the time of surgery, a closed suction drain should be left and effluent assayed for amylase and lipase levels before the drain is removed.

♦ Gastric fistula following splenectomy is a recognized complication that can be avoided by careful ligation of the short gastric vessels without including any of the gastric serosa, or if necessary imbricating the short gastric ligatures.

♦ Overwhelming postsplenectomy sepsis may occur.

◆ The spleen contributes to immune competence in a variety of ways, including opsonization and phagocytosis. Asplenic patients are at increased risk of overwhelming postsplenectomy infection from encapsulated bacteria, such as *Streptococcus pneumoniae, Neisseria meningitidis,* and *H. influenzae.* Following splenectomy patients should be counseled regarding the increased susceptibility to infections and vaccinated against these potential infections with Prevnar, Menactra, and ActHIB before discharge from the hospital.

SELECTED REFERENCES

1. Starnes S, Klein P, Magagna L, Pomerantz R: Computed tomographic grading is useful in the selection of patients for nonoperative management of blunt injury to the spleen. Am Surg 1998;64:743-648;748-749 [discussion].
2. Cocanour CS, Moore FA, Ware DN, et al: Delayed complications of nonoperative management of blunt adult splenic trauma. Arch Surg 1998;133:619-624;624-625 [discussion].
3. Ochsner MG: Factors of failure for nonoperative management of blunt liver and splenic injuries. World J Surg 2001;25:1393-1396.

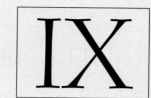

COLON

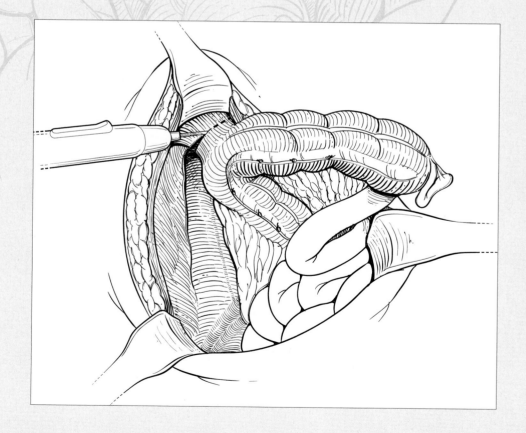

CHAPTER 53

PORT PLACEMENT FOR COLON OPERATIONS

Michael D. Trahan

STEP 1: SURGICAL ANATOMY

- ◆ It is useful to review the anatomy of the abdominal musculature when planning a laparoscopic operation.

STEP 2: PREOPERATIVE CONSIDERATIONS

- ◆ Laparoscopic colonic surgery is usually performed with the patient in the modified lithotomy position. The lower extremities should not be flexed so much as to interfere with movement of the long laparoscopic instruments **(Figure 53-1)**. When tucking the upper extremities, protect the hand from entrapment in the movement of the bed surfaces.

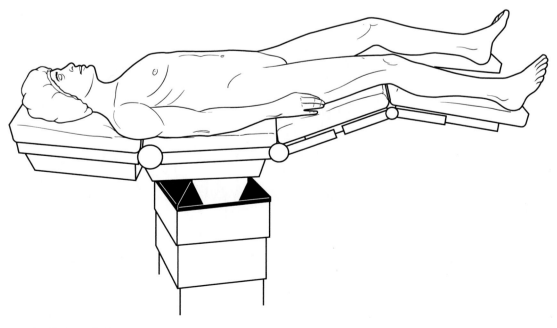

FIGURE 53–1

◆ The principle of triangulation of the operative target should be kept in mind as the plan for port placement is developed. In general, the surgeon should position the operative target between himself or herself and the monitor screen. For a sigmoid colectomy, the surgeon stands at the patient's right and the monitor is at the foot **(Figure 53-2)**. The surgeon should move from the patient's right to the left or between the legs as needed to comfortably reach the target.

◆ An optically guided bladeless trocar is the best selection for the initial port to be inserted. The optical guidance is provided by an end-viewing laparoscope. This port is usually placed at or near the umbilicus but may be placed elsewhere in patients who are expected to have midline adhesions.

◆ The size, selection, and number of the remaining ports are subject to much variability depending on the planned procedure, size and type of anticipated instruments, patient's body habitus, and surgeon's preference.

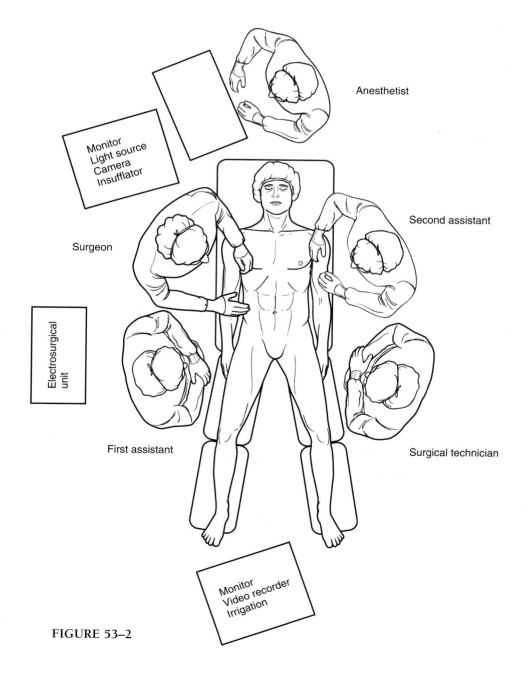

FIGURE 53–2

STEP 3: OPERATIVE STEPS

1. INCISION

- The site of each incision should be preemptively anesthetized with a local anesthetic injection to include the skin and peritoneum.

- The incisions should be just large enough to accommodate the trocar without tension on the skin as the trocar is inserted.

2. DISSECTION

- Five 10- to 12-mm ports are used. One port is near the umbilicus. One port is in each of the abdominal quadrants lateral to the rectus muscles **(Figure 53-3)**.

- A 10- to 12-mm port is near the umbilicus. A 5- or 10-mm port is in the left lower quadrant. A 10- to 12-mm port is in right lower quadrant. A 5- or 10-mm port is in the left upper quadrant **(Figure 53-4)**.

- A 10- to 12-mm port is near the umbilicus. A 10- to 12-mm port is in the right lower quadrant. A 5- or 10-mm port is in the right upper quadrant. A 5- or 10-mm port is in the left lower quadrant **(Figure 53-5)**.

- Four 10- to 12-mm ports are used. One port is near the umbilicus. One port is in each of the mid-clavicular lines at the level of the umbilicus. One port is in the right mid-clavicular line, 10 to 15 cm inferior to the other **(Figure 53-6)**.

3. CLOSING

- Bladeless trocar port sites up to and including 12 mm do not typically need to be closed at the fascial level.

- Transabdominal laparoscopic suture passers provide a quick and relatively simple way to close small abdominal fascial incisions, especially through a deep abdominal pannus.

- If no suture passer is available, larger port site fascial defects should be closed with transabdominal suture externally after appropriate retraction of the skin and subcutaneous tissue.

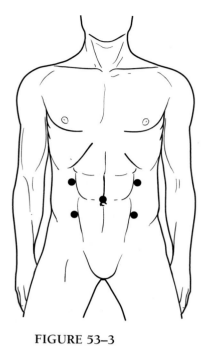

FIGURE 53–3

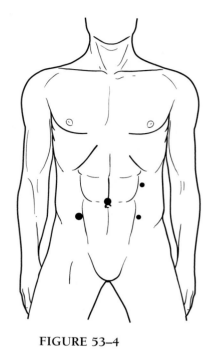

FIGURE 53–4

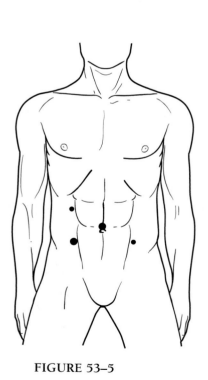

FIGURE 53–5

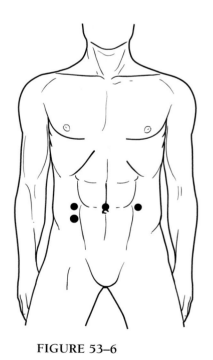

FIGURE 53–6

STEP 4: POSTOPERATIVE CONSIDERATIONS

- Postoperative care is provided consistent with the primary disease process and extent of the operation.

STEP 5: PEARLS AND PITFALLS

- The initial optical entry should be made away from sites expected to have adhesions. In a patient with extensive prior surgical history, the open insertion technique may be preferred.

- Each subsequent trocar entry should be made with direct internal visualization, avoiding the epigastric vessels and the large subcutaneous vessels identified by transillumination.

- One should not hesitate to use additional trocars if needed to improve exposure and the safety of the operation.

- Hand-assisted laparoscopic surgery (HALS) is the approach favored by many. The hand port should be located at the proposed site of specimen extraction.

SELECTED REFERENCES

1. Ludwig KA, Lee WY: Laparoscopic partial colectomy. In Soper NJ, Swanstrom LL, Eubanks WS (eds): Mastery of Endoscopic and Laparoscopic Surgery, 2nd ed. Philadelphia, Lippincott Williams & Wilkins, 2005, pp 436-448.
2. Baig MK, Wexner SD: Laparoscopic-assisted abdominoperineal resection. In Soper NJ, Swanstrom LL, Eubanks WS (eds): Mastery of Endoscopic and Laparoscopic Surgery, 2nd ed. Philadelphia, Lippincott Williams & Wilkins, 2005, pp 449-458.
3. Fowler DL, Sonoda TS, McGinty J: Laparoscopic subtotal and total colectomy. In Soper NJ, Swanstrom LL and Eubanks WS (eds): Mastery of Endoscopic and Laparoscopic Surgery, 2nd ed. Philadelphia, Lippincott Williams & Wilkins, 2005, pp 459-469.

CHAPTER 54

DIVERTING END COLOSTOMY WITH MUCOUS FISTULA OR HARTMANN'S POUCH

Dennis C. Gore

STEP 1: SURGICAL ANATOMY

- ◆ Normal-appearing colon (usually sigmoid/descending colon) proximal to diseased bowel

STEP 2: PREOPERATIVE CONSIDERATIONS

- ◆ Indications:
  - ◆ Relief of colonic obstruction
  - ◆ Complete diversion of fecal stream

- ◆ Anesthesia: general

- ◆ Position: supine

STEP 3: OPERATIVE STEPS

1. INCISION

◆ Midline laparotomy **(Figure 54-1)**

2. DISSECTION

◆ Mobilize the segment of colon chosen for colostomy, usually just proximal to the obstruction or other diseased lesion. For the transverse colon, this entails incising the attachments to the omentum with either electrocautery or scissors.

◆ For sigmoid, descending, or ascending colon, incise the avascular lateral ligaments to the peritoneum.

◆ With blunt forceps dissection, create an opening through the mesentery. Place a gastrointestinal anastomosis (GIA) stapler through this aperture and engage the stapler **(Figure 54-2).**

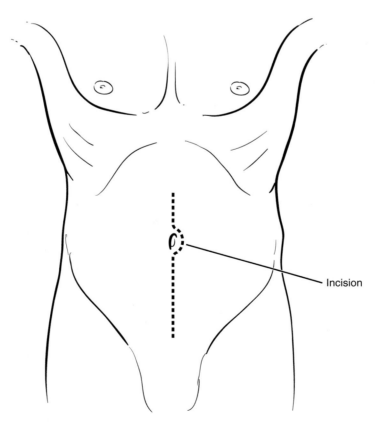

Incision

FIGURE 54–1

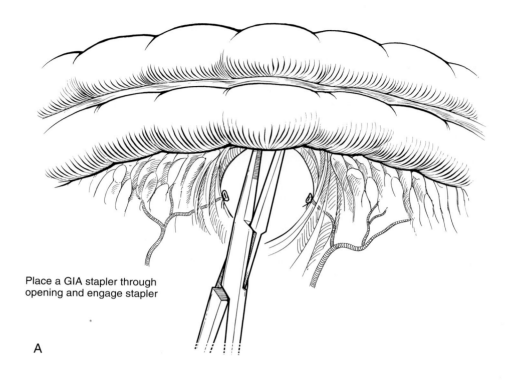

Place a GIA stapler through
opening and engage stapler

A

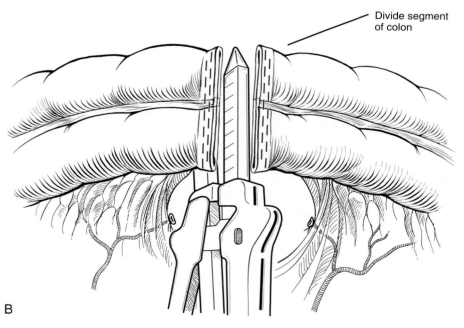

Divide segment
of colon

B

FIGURE 54–2

◆ Using forceps clamps and 3-0 silk ligatures, incise the colonic mesentery from the colostomy site at a sufficient distance so that the two ends of the severed colon can be retracted through the abdominal wall.

◆ Grasp the skin at the site chosen for colostomy, usually just lateral to the rectus abdominis muscle in the right or left lower quadrants, retract the skin, and incise with scalpel or electrocautery, creating a circular opening **(Figure 54-3)**.

◆ Use electrocautery to make a cruciate incision through the abdominal wall and peritoneum **(Figure 54-4)**.

◆ Manually insert at least two fingers through the colostomy site.

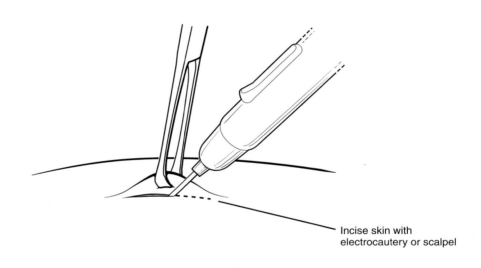

Incise skin with
electrocautery or scalpel

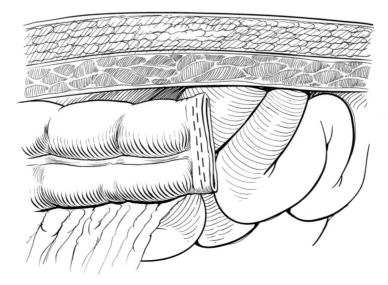

FIGURE 54–3

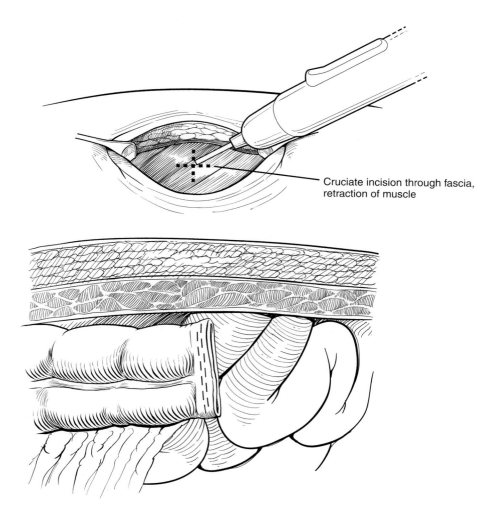

Cruciate incision through fascia, retraction of muscle

FIGURE 54–4

◆ Place two Babcock clamps through the colostomy site, grasp the end of the proximal colon, and retract the colon end through the abdominal wall with at least 4 cm of colon exteriorized (**Figure 54-5**).

◆ Place several 3-0 Vicryl sutures in simple, interrupted fashion to secure the colon to the anterior abdominal fascia.

◆ Use multiple 3-0 silk sutures in a Lembert fashion to buttress the staple line of the distal colon end, thereby creating Hartmann's pouch (**Figure 54-6**).

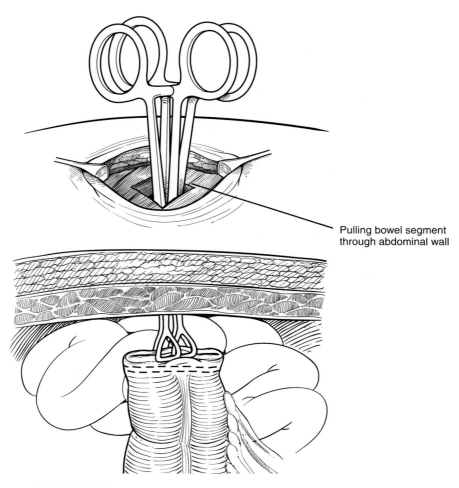

Pulling bowel segment through abdominal wall

FIGURE 54–5

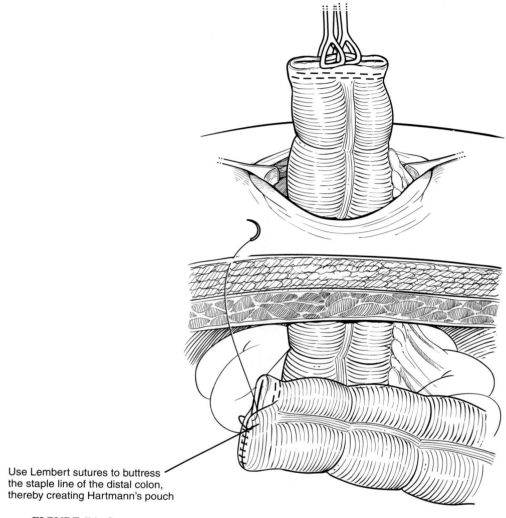

Use Lembert sutures to buttress the staple line of the distal colon, thereby creating Hartmann's pouch

FIGURE 54–6

◆ Complete any further procedures within the abdomen, irrigate copiously, and then close the midline abdominal incision.

◆ Cover the midline wound with antiseptic-impregnated gauze.

◆ Use electrocautery to excise the stapled end of the colon, leaving 2 cm exteriorized from the abdominal wall. Use 4-0 Vicryl sutures or judicious electrocautery to secure hemostasis along the bowel end **(Figure 54-7)**.

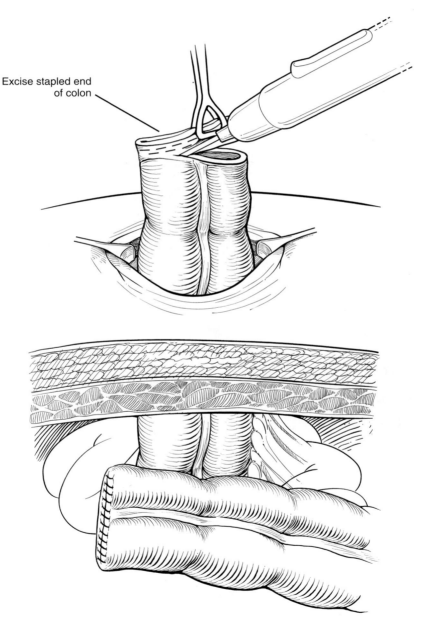

Excise stapled end of colon

FIGURE 54–7

◆ Use several 3-0 Vicryl sutures in simple, interrupted fashion to circumferentially secure edges of the colostomy to skin **(Figures 54-8 and 54-9)**.

◆ If you have a concern that the distal colonic segment is obstructed, creating a closed-loop obstruction, exteriorize the distal colonic segment in the same manner as the end colostomy, which creates a mucous fistula.

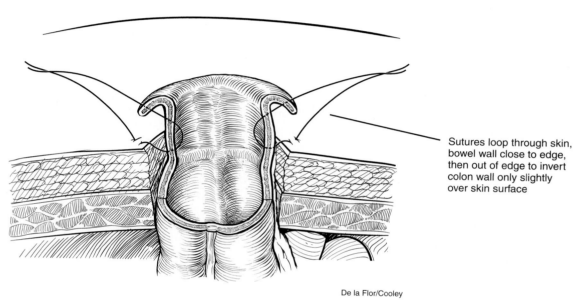

Sutures loop through skin, bowel wall close to edge, then out of edge to invert colon wall only slightly over skin surface

De la Flor/Cooley

FIGURE 54–8

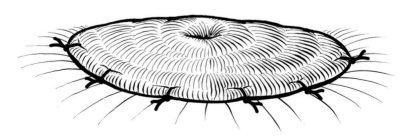

FIGURE 54–9

3. CLOSING

- Routine

STEP 4: POSTOPERATIVE CARE

- Routine ostomy care

STEP 5: PEARLS AND PITFALLS

- It is essential that the colon is straight and free of tension without any restriction on the mesentery to ensure adequate blood supply to the very end of the colostomy.

- Before closure of the abdomen, use suture to close any rents in the mesentery that may be a nidus for future internal herniation. Take care not to occlude the colonic blood supply.

BROOKE ILEOSTOMY

Dennis C. Gore

STEP 1: SURGICAL ANATOMY

♦ Normal-appearing small bowel just proximal to diseased

STEP 2: PREOPERATIVE CONSIDERATIONS

♦ Indications: complete diversion of enteric sulcus

♦ Anesthesia: general

♦ Position: supine

STEP 3: OPERATIVE STEPS

1. INCISION

♦ Midline laparotomy **(Figure 55-1)**

2. DISSECTION

♦ Mobilize free the segment of small intestine chosen, usually as distally as feasible.

♦ With blunt forcep dissection, create an opening through the mesentery, place a gastrointestinal anastomosis (GIA) stapler through this aperture, and engage the stapler **(Figure 55- 2)**.

♦ Using forceps clamps and 3-0 silk ligatures, incise the small bowel mesentery from the enterotomy site for a sufficient distance so that the enterotomy can be retracted through the abdominal wall.

627

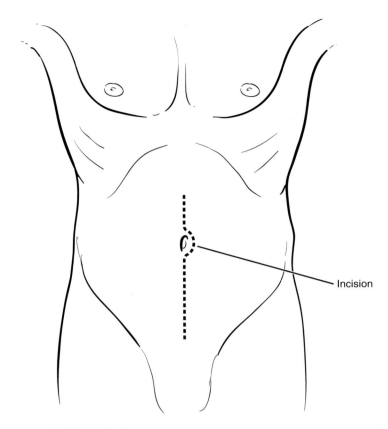

Incision

FIGURE 55–1

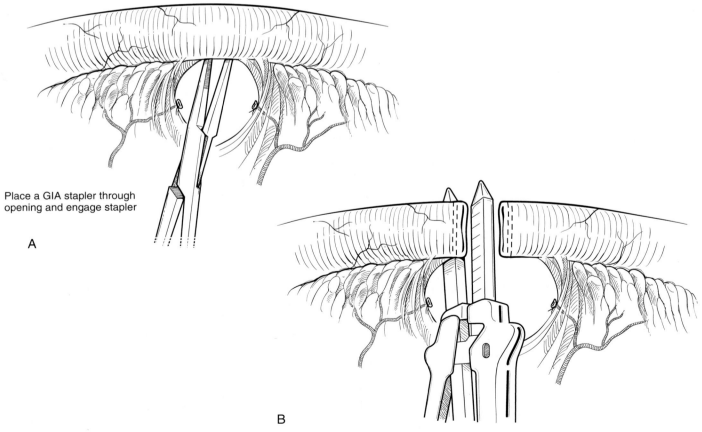

Place a GIA stapler through
opening and engage stapler

A

B

FIGURE 55–2

◆ Grasp the skin at the site chosen for the enterostomy (usually just lateral to the rectus abdominis muscle in the right or left lower quadrant), retract the skin, and incise with scalpel or electrocautery, thus creating a circular opening **(Figure 55-3).**

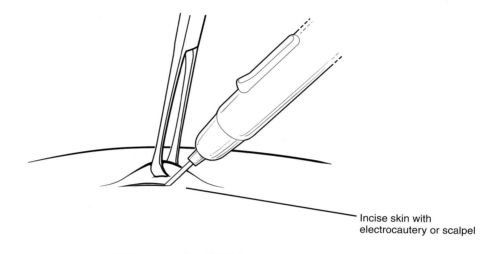

Incise skin with
electrocautery or scalpel

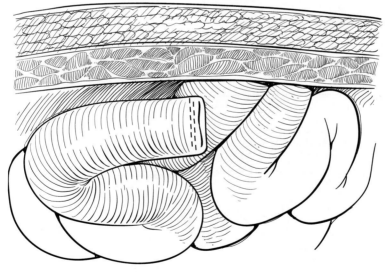

FIGURE 55–3

◆ Use electrocautery to make a cruciate incision through the abdominal wall and peritoneum **(Figure 55-4)**.

◆ Manually insert at least two fingers through the enterostomy site.

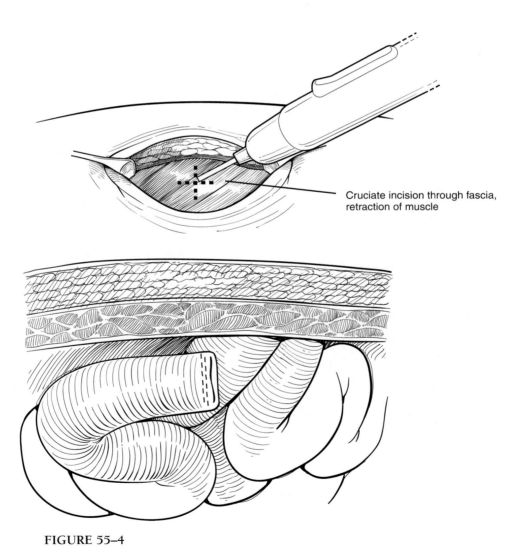

Cruciate incision through fascia, retraction of muscle

FIGURE 55–4

◆ Place two Babcock clamps through the enterostomy site, grasp the end of the proximal bowel, and retract the bowel segment through the abdominal wall with at least 6 cm of bowel exteriorized (**Figure 55-5**).

◆ Place several 3-0 Vicryl sutures in a simple, interrupted fashion to secure the bowel to the anterior abdominal fascia.

◆ Complete any further procedures within abdomen, irrigate copiously, and close the midline abdominal wound.

◆ Cover the midline wound with antiseptic-impregnated gauze.

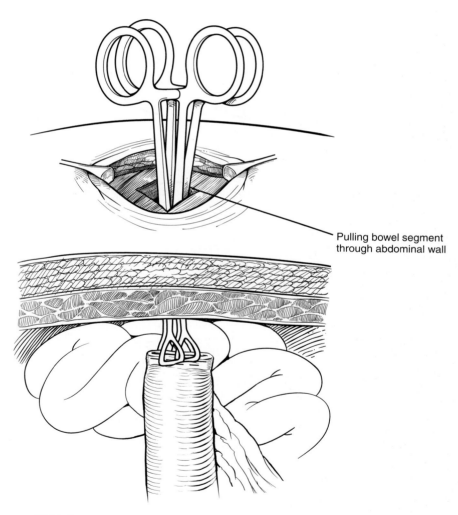

Pulling bowel segment through abdominal wall

FIGURE 55–5

- Use electrocautery to excise the stapled end of bowel, leaving approximately 4 cm exteriorized (**Figure 55-6**).

- Use 4-0 Vicryl sutures or judicious electrocautery to secure hemostasis along bowel end.

- Place several 3-0 Vicryl sutures through first the skin edge, then through the bowel wall just exterior to the abdominal opening, and then through the edge of the enterotomy. Use multiple sutures circumferentially around the enterostomy. As these sutures are closed and tied, the end of the bowel should invert (**Figures 55-7 and 55-8**).

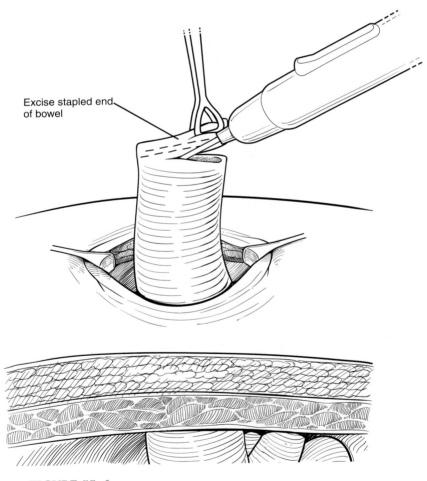

Excise stapled end of bowel

FIGURE 55–6

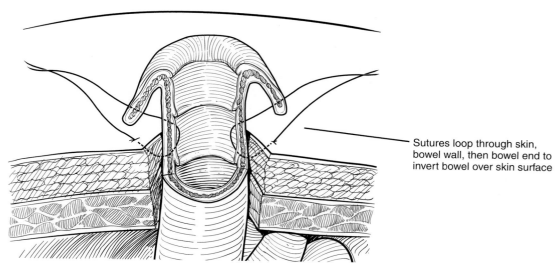

Sutures loop through skin, bowel wall, then bowel end to invert bowel over skin surface

FIGURE 55–7

Brooke ileostomy

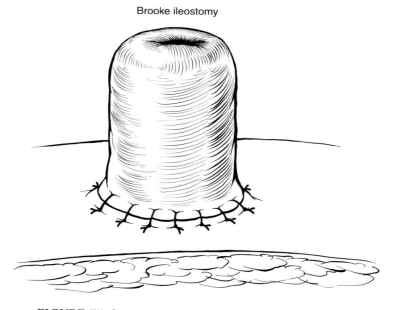

FIGURE 55–8

3. CLOSING

◆ Routine

STEP 4: POSTOPERATIVE CARE

◆ Provide routine ostomy care.

◆ Replace fluids lost from ileostomy intravenously with lactated Ringer solution or other crystalloid solution until the patient's oral intake is sufficient. An antimotility agent is sometimes required to reduce ileostomy output.

STEP 5: PEARLS AND PITFALLS

◆ Adequate blood supply to the enterostomy is essential; supply is aided by maintaining a tension-free placement and ensuring that the mesentery is free of restriction.

◆ The Brooke ileostomy should be of sufficient length from the abdominal wall so that enteric sulcus will fall easily into the ostomy bag with minimal skin contact.

CHAPTER 56

LOOP COLOSTOMY

Dennis C. Gore

STEP 1: SURGICAL ANATOMY

- Normal-appearing colon (usually transverse colon) proximal to diseased bowel

STEP 2: PREOPERATIVE CONSIDERATIONS

- Indications:
  - Relief of colonic obstruction
  - Partial diversion of fecal stream

- Anesthesia: general

- Position: supine

STEP 3: OPERATIVE STEPS

1. INCISION

- The most common colonic segments for placement of loop colostomy are the transverse colon or sigmoid colon. For transverse colostomy, the incision is placed just lateral to the rectus abdominis muscle, most often on the right upper abdomen. For a sigmoid colostomy, the incision is placed in the left lower quadrant, just lateral to the rectus abdominis muscle.

2. DISSECTION

◆ Retract the loop of colon through the incision **(Figure 56-1)**.

◆ Use forceps to bluntly dissect the opening through the mesentery at the loop apex (see Figure 56-1).

◆ Place a plastic or glass rod through the aperture in the mesentery, position the rod transverse to the incision, and thereby prevent retraction of the colon loop back into the abdomen **(Figures 56-2 and 56-3)**.

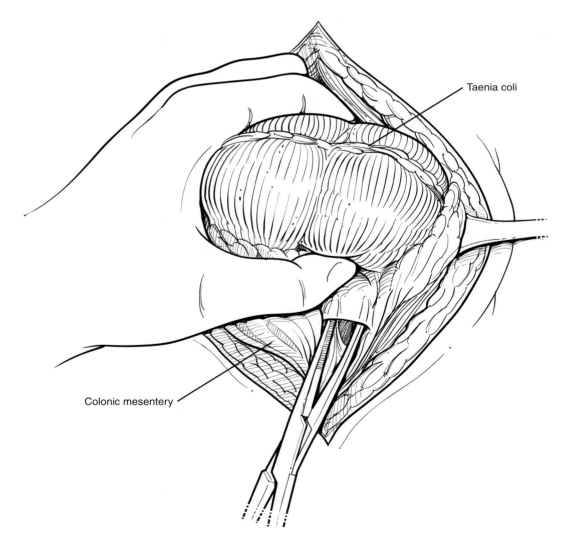

Taenia coli

Colonic mesentery

FIGURE 56–1

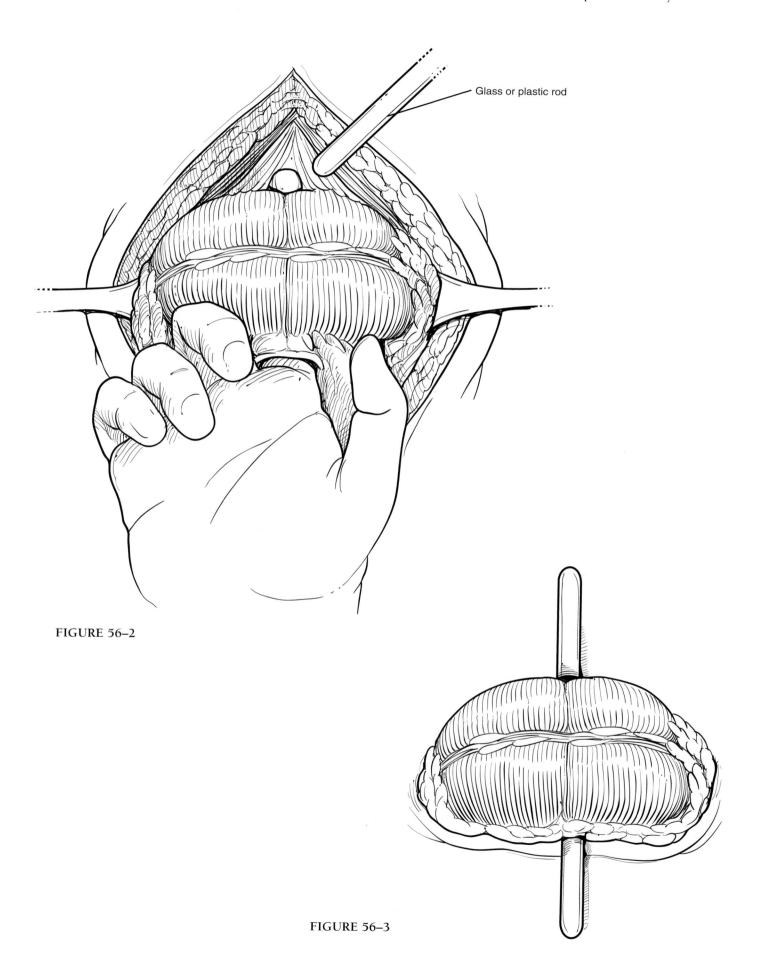

Glass or plastic rod

FIGURE 56–2

FIGURE 56–3

◆ Secure the rod in place by attaching tube catheter to each end of the rod circling over the colon **(Figure 59-4)**.

◆ The colotomy is performed with electrocautery along the taenia coli **(Figure 56-5)**.

◆ Edges of the colotomy are secured to the edges of the incision with multiple 3-0 Vicryl sutures **(Figure 56-6)**.

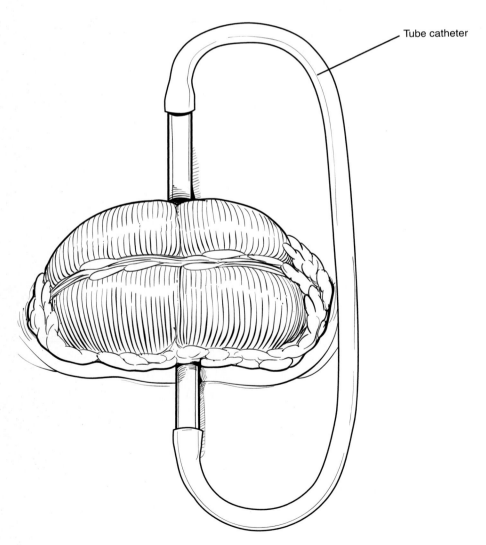

Tube catheter

FIGURE 56–4

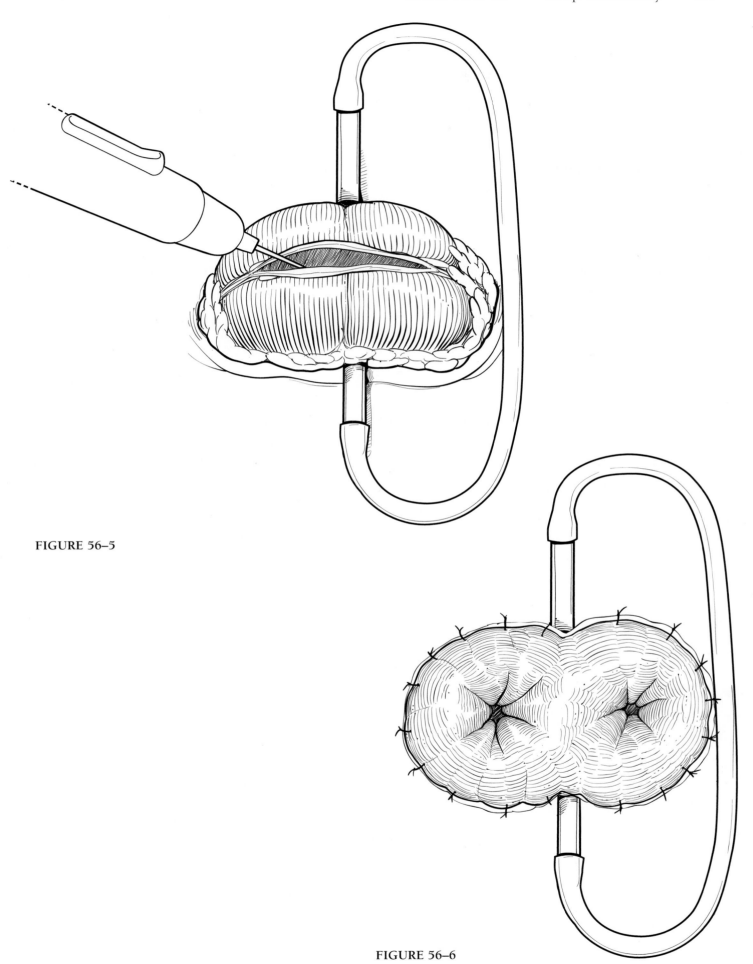

FIGURE 56–5

FIGURE 56–6

3. CLOSING

◆ Routine

STEP 4: POSTOPERATIVE CARE

◆ Provide routine ostomy care.

◆ The plastic rod can be removed once the surgical site has healed, which is usually approximately 2 weeks.

STEP 5: PEARLS AND PITFALLS

◆ Omentum and pericolic fat precludes solid healing of the colostomy to the incision. It is best to trim fat. However, use caution and vigilance in ensuring hemostasis on retracted omentum and mesenteric fat.

CHAPTER 57

STOMA TAKEDOWN: TAKEDOWN OF LOOP COLOSTOMY OR ILEOSTOMY

Valerie P. Bauer

STEP 1: SURGICAL ANATOMY

- The surgeon should be familiar with the anatomy of the double-barrel or looped stoma.

- Fascial closure of the abdominal wall after stoma takedown requires knowledge of the anatomy of the fascial relationship to the rectus abdominis muscle. Below the arcuate line, the posterior wall of the rectus sheath is absent, and the rectus muscle lies on thin transversalis fascia. Thus recognition and closure of the anterior rectus fascia is significantly important in preventing postoperative incisional hernia in patients with stomas below the umbilicus.

STEP 2: PREOPERATIVE CONSIDERATIONS

- Reestablishment of intestinal continuity should take into consideration the original condition for which the diversion was created. Appropriate preoperative imaging and diagnostic studies should be obtained to establish the safety of reversal.

- Wrapping the stoma with Seprafilm, a sodium hyaluronate–based bioresorbable membrane that prevents adhesions during the initial surgery, allows for easier takedown later, and a midline incision should be avoided.

- Informed consent should include potential complications, such as anastomotic stricture or leak, bowel obstruction, wound infection at the former stoma site, intra-abdominal wound infection, hematoma, injury to adjacent bowel or mesentery, incisional hernia, and the need for re-creation of the ostomy.

- The type of bowel preparation is determined by the location of the stoma and the surgeon's preference.
  - Loop ileostomy requires clear liquid the day before and a bottle of magnesium citrate the night before surgery.
  - Loop colostomy requires clear liquid the day before and Fleet enema before surgery. Mechanical bowel preparation is no longer favored for this procedure.

- Appropriate preoperative parenteral antibiotics are administered within 1 hour before cut time, according to the Physician Quality Reporting Initiative (PQRI) measures defined for elective colorectal operations. We use ertapenem (Invanz) 1 g intravenously (IV) without re-dosing, because it has 24-hour duration of action.

- Patients who have been taking steroids preoperatively should receive a stress dose of hydro-cortisone 100 mg IV before the operation. This should be continued postoperatively and tapered accordingly.

STEP 3: OPERATIVE STEPS

- The patient is placed supine on the operating table with arms outstretched on armboards.

- After general endotracheal anesthesia is administered, a Foley catheter is placed along with sequential compression devices on the lower extremities.

- The ostomy appliance is removed and the abdomen is shaved as needed with clippers.

- The abdomen is prepped and draped, and a 2-0 Vicryl suture is used to close the proximal loop of the stoma **(Figure 57-1)**.

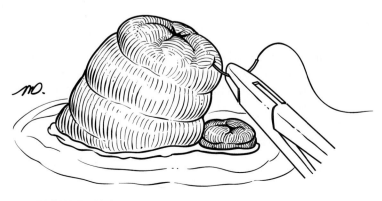

FIGURE 57–1

◆ A no. 15 blade knife is used to make an elliptical incision parallel to the skin lines but staying close to the edge of the ostomy. The incision is carried vertically down to the anterior abdominal fascia **(Figure 57-2)**. Figure 57-2 shows an elliptical incision through the skin.

◆ Once the white line of fascia is identified, it is retracted away from the plane of dissection. The knife is drawn gently toward the bowel circumferentially and the peritoneum is cut **(Figure 57-3)**. Figure 57-3 shows a circumferential dissection around the stoma.

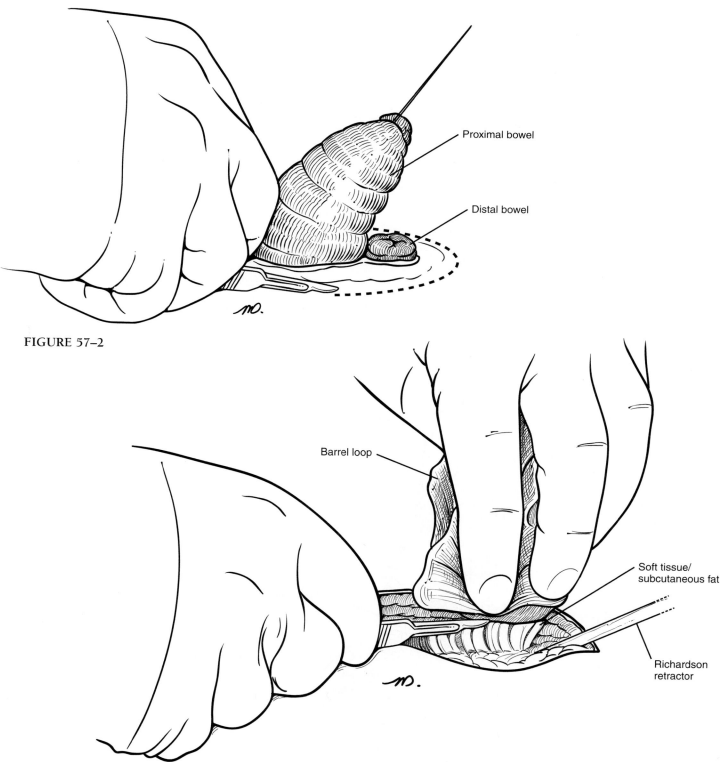

FIGURE 57–2

FIGURE 57–3

◆ As the stoma is lifted up, care is taken to ensure that the mesentery is not cut or ripped. Excess traction can cause tears leading to unrecognized intra-abdominal bleeding **(Figure 57-4)**. A Richardson retractor is used for circumferential exposure to free the stoma.

◆ A finger is placed beneath the incision and passed against the abdominal wall. Small adhesions are freed **(Figure 57-5)**.

◆ The mesentery is fanned out, scored, and divided using hemostats clamps and 2-0 Vicryl suture **(Figure 57-6)**.

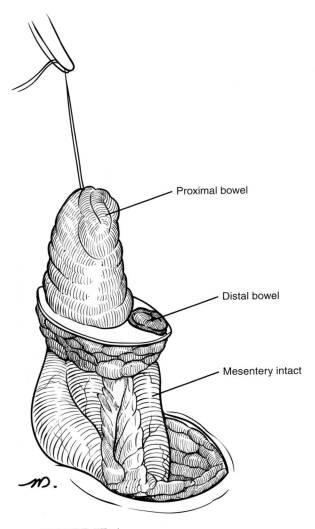

Proximal bowel

Distal bowel

Mesentery intact

FIGURE 57–4

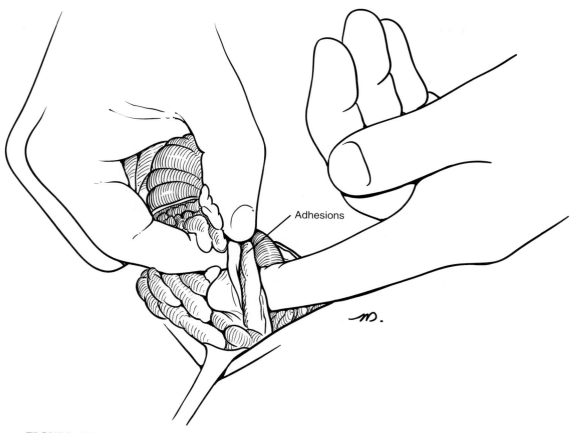

FIGURE 57–5

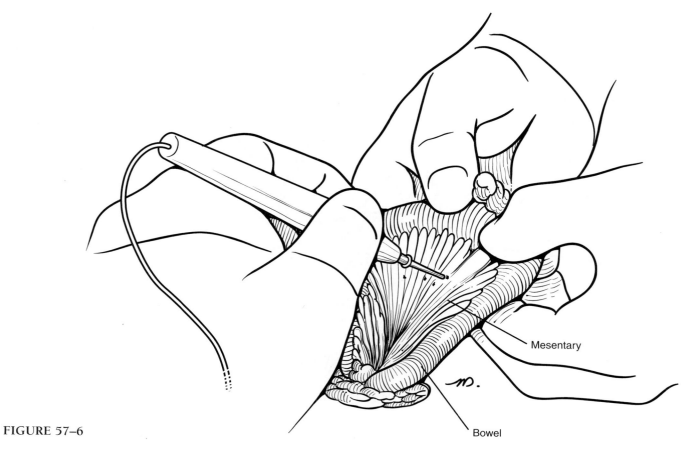

FIGURE 57–6

- The serosal edge of the bowel is cleaned and Ochsner clamps are placed from the antimesentric border to the mesentery in oblique fashion **(Figure 57-7).**

- The field is prepared for opening the bowel. Every measure should be taken to prevent fecal or enteral spillage into the abdominal cavity. A blue towel is folded and placed on the field, which will contain contaminated instruments: a metal pool sucker, Allys bowel clamps, and sponge stick. Moist laparotomy pads are packed around the stoma.

- A no. 10 blade knife is used to divide the bowel **(Figure 57-8).** Allys clamps are placed on the antimesenteric and mesenteric side of each lumen **(Figure 57-9).** The proximal limb is held open with the Allys clamps and the pool sucker is placed into the lumen triangulating the bowel. A bulb syringe with saline is used to irrigate the lumen, taking care not to touch open colon with the tip of the syringe or spill saline over the edge of the lumen.

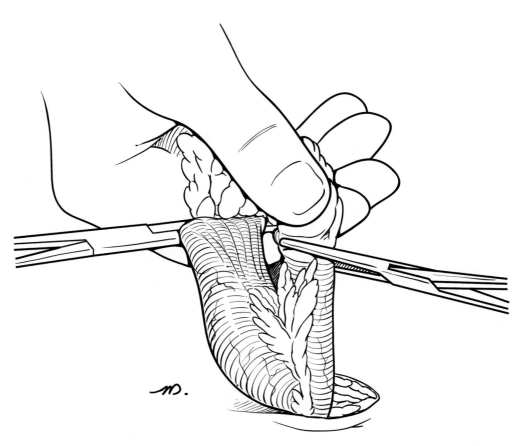

FIGURE 57–7

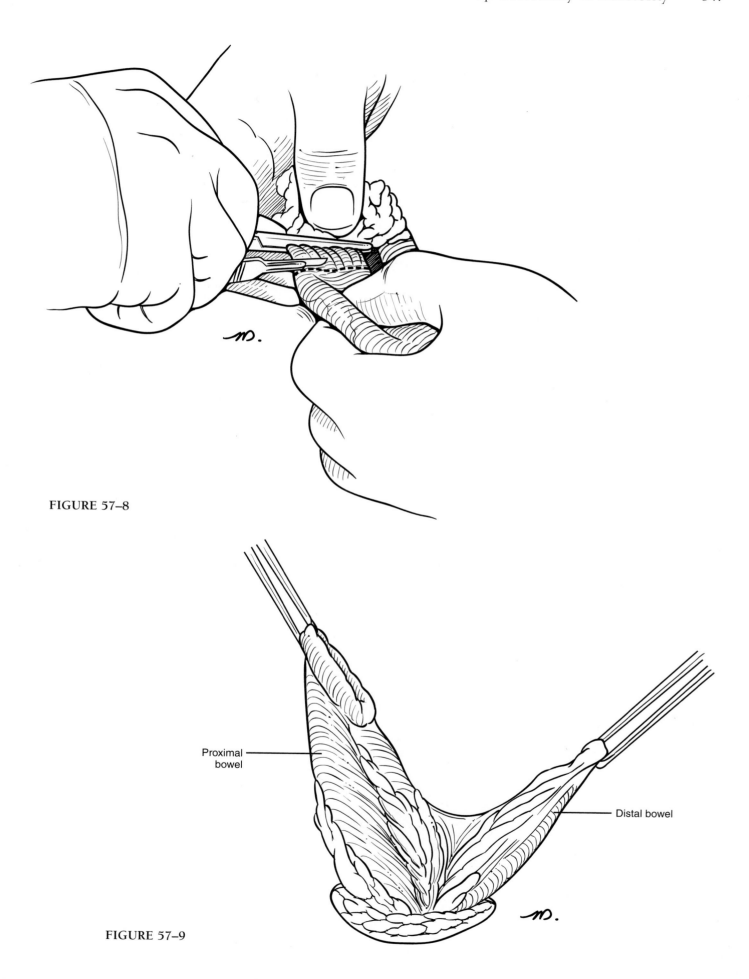

FIGURE 57–8

Proximal bowel

Distal bowel

FIGURE 57–9

◆ The antimesenteric and mesenteric borders of each lumen are lined up.

◆ A double-armed 4-0 Maxon monofilament suture is used to create a single-layered running anastomosis **(Figure 57-10)**. The serosal edge is grasped and the mucosa and submucosal edges are reapproximated. This is done by placing the knot on the outer portion of the bowel at the antimesenteric border. One arm of suture is passed under the knot and used to complete half of the anastomosis, as is the other arm on the other side. The suture line is inspected for integrity.

◆ The completed anastomosis is dropped back into the abdominal cavity **(Figure 57-11)**.

◆ Surgical gloves are changed and the anterior rectus fascia is reapproximated using 0 polydioxanone (PDS) in figure-of-eight interrupted sutures.

◆ The subcutaneous skin is irrigated with bacitracin antibiotic.

◆ A nylon vertical mattress suture is used to loosely close the skin, followed by placement of Telfa wicks between each suture **(Figure 57-12)**. A dry dressing is placed over the wicks and changed as needed. The wicks, however, are not removed until the patient leaves the hospital.

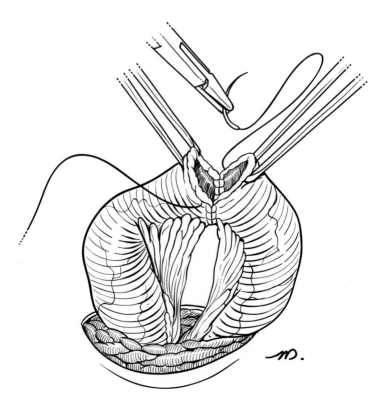

FIGURE 57–10

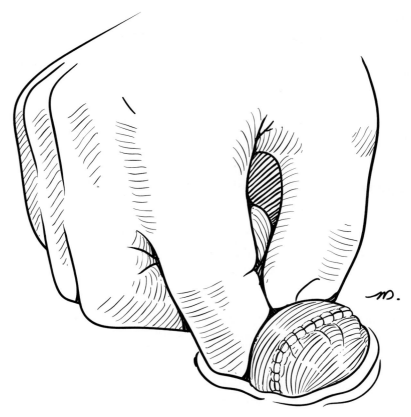

FIGURE 57–11

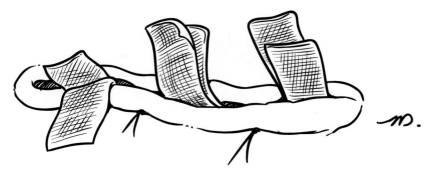

FIGURE 57–12

STEP 4: POSTOPERATIVE CARE

- Adherence to a postoperative colorectal clinical pathway ensures standardization of care.

- Nasogastric decompression is not necessary unless vomiting and postoperative ileus or obstruction occurs.

- Adequate pain control is achieved using patient-controlled algesia.

- Stress ulcer prophylaxis, such as famotidine (Pepcid) 20 mg IV every 12 hours, should be used in patients with prior peptic ulcer disease (PUD), gastroesophageal reflux disease (GERD), or symptoms to suggest disease.

- All patients should receive prophylaxis for deep venous thrombosis (DVT), using sequential compression devices while in bed and heparin 5000 U subcutaneously every 8 hours or enoxaparin 40 mg subcutaneously every morning. Dosing schedules according to PQRI quality measures may begin preoperatively, or, as we practice, within 24 hours from the operation after morning laboratory test results are back, to ensure there is no significant drop in hemoglobin level to suggest postoperative bleeding.

- Adequate intravenous fluid should be administered with monitoring of urine output via urimeter on the Foley bag. The Foley catheter may be removed on postoperative day 1.

- The diet may be limited to ice chips and sips of water in the postanesthesia care unit and on postoperative day 1. Return of bowel function is measured by the frequency and pitch of bowel sounds, lack of abdominal distention, and the patient's subjective will to eat. A clear liquid diet may be offered as sips of clear liquids without carbonation and without a straw to minimize buildup of air in the intestine. This may be advanced ad lib as bowel function returns.

- Early ambulation is crucial for aid in return of bowel function. Patients should be instructed to walk multiple times a day beginning on postoperative day 1.

- The incision site should be checked on postoperative day 1 and daily thereafter to ensure absence of infection. Wicks should be removed before the patient leaves the hospital.

STEP 5: PEARLS AND PITFALLS

- ◆ Soft tissue infection can occur to varying degrees, with necrotizing fasciitis as the worst case scenario. The ostomy site should be loosely closed and meticulous attention paid to the appearance of the wound postoperatively. In addition, anastomotic leak may present in part as a soft tissue infection.

- ◆ Wrapping a temporary ileostomy or colostomy with Seprafilm allows for easier takedown later. This consideration should be made during the initial surgery.

SELECTED REFERENCES

1. Zeng Q, Yu Z, You J, Zhang Q: Efficacy and safety of Seprafilm for preventing postoperative abdominal adhesion: Systematic review and meta-analysis. World J Surg 2007;31:2125-2131;2132 [discussion].
2. QualityNet: Site index. Available at www.qualitynet.org.
3. Itani KM, Wilson SE, Awad SS, et al: Ertapenem versus cefotetan prophylaxis in elective colorectal surgery. N Engl J Med 2006;355:2640-2651.
4. Beck DE, Opelka FG: Perioperative steroid use in colorectal patients: Results of a survey. Dis Colon Rectum 1996;39:995-999.
5. Law WL, Bailey HR, Max E, et al: Single-layer continuous colon and rectal anastomosis using monofilament absorbable suture (Maxon): Study of 500 cases. Dis Colon Rectum 1999;42:736-740.

CHAPTER 58

Right Hemicolectomy

Celia Chao

STEP 1: SURGICAL ANATOMY

- The right colon begins at the ileocecal valve, includes the right (ascending colon) hepatic flexure, and ends at the mid-transverse colon; the appendix is present at the inferior aspect of the cecum. The blood supply to this area comes from the superior mesenteric artery through its ileocolic, right colic, and right branches of the middle colic arteries. The lymphatics to the right colon follow its arterial blood supply. A minimum of 12 lymph nodes within the mesentery is considered an adequate resection when performing a right hemicolectomy for cancer.

STEP 2: PREOPERATIVE CONSIDERATIONS

- Indications: Colon resection is performed for benign diseases, such as diverticulitis, ischemic colitis, volvulus, polyposis, bleeding from arteriovenous malformation, trauma, inflammatory bowel disease, and curative treatment or palliation of malignant tumors of the colon and rectum. The extent of resection is based on the vascular supply of the specific location of the tumor. Tumors at the hepatic flexure or on the proximal transverse colon can be resected with an extended right hemicolectomy, which involves additionally taking the blood supply and transverse colon to the left of the middle colic artery.

- Preoperative planning: In clinical practice throughout North America, an adequate mechanical bowel preparation is generally considered desirable the day before surgical resection. Preoperatively, intravenous antibiotics must be administered before the skin incision. A preoperative dose of subcutaneous heparin (5000 U) or a low-molecular-weight heparin is recommended to prevent deep venous thrombosis. Before induction of general anesthesia, pneumatic compression boots are placed on both lower extremities and continued postoperatively until the patient ambulates on the first postoperative day.

- Anesthesia: General anesthesia is used.

STEP 3: OPERATIVE STEPS

1. INCISION

◆ A midline incision (**Figure 58-1**) is made, and a Thompson retractor is placed to retract the anterior abdominal wall and increase exposure in the region of the right colon.

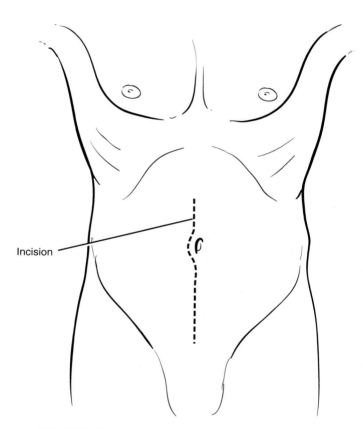

Incision

FIGURE 58–1

2. DISSECTION

◆ A standard exploration of the intra-abdominal cavity is performed to determine the extent of disease and resectability. The peritoneal surface, liver, porta hepatis, mesenteric nodes, and ovaries are examined. The right colon is mobilized from its retroperitoneal attachments by incising the white line of Toldt (**Figure 58-2**).

◆ The cecum and ascending colon are retracted medially, exposing the right ureter and gonadal vessels. Continuing superiorly along this retroperitoneal plane, the hepatocolic ligament is divided to release the hepatic flexure (**Figure 58-3**).

◆ Posteriorly, the duodenum is identified and separated from the colon. The omentum is mobilized off the transverse colon by dissecting along an avascular plane (**Figure 58-4**).

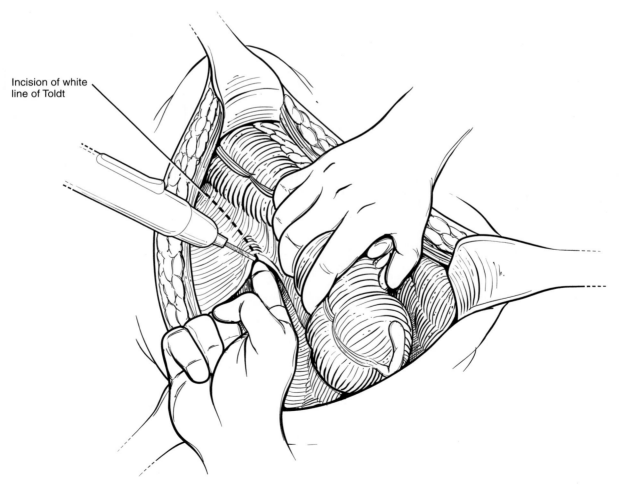

Incision of white
line of Toldt

FIGURE 58–2

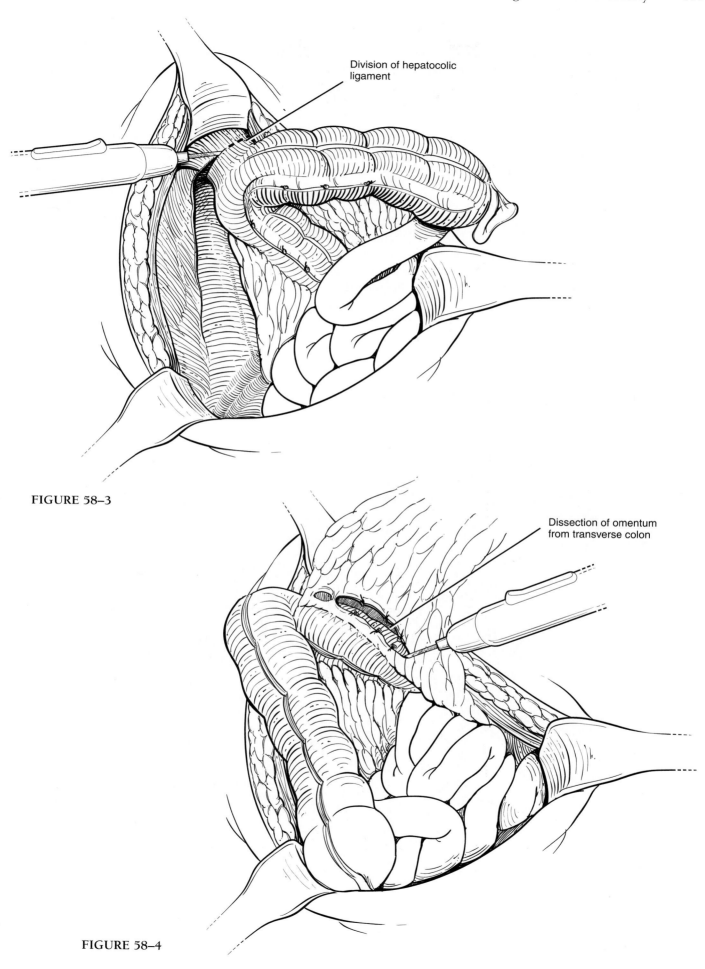

Division of hepatocolic
ligament

FIGURE 58–3

Dissection of omentum
from transverse colon

FIGURE 58–4

◆ If the omentum is adherent or close to the tumor, that portion of the omentum can be removed en bloc with the resected colon. The points of transection of the terminal ileum and transverse colon are decided based on the mesenteric blood supply **(Figure 58-5).**

◆ Using a gastrointestinal anastomosis (GIA) stapler, transect the terminal ileum 10 to 15 cm from the ileocecal valve for lesions involving the cecum and approximately 5 cm for lesions distal to the cecum **(Figure 58-6).**

◆ The transverse colon is divided in similar fashion with the GIA stapler just to the right of the middle colic artery. The peritoneum to the mesentery is scored with electrocautery; the vessels, and not the surrounding fatty tissue, can be more easily clamped and tied. The mesentery corresponding to the points of resection are divided to the origins of the ileocolic and right colic arteries to ensure adequate removal of the node-bearing tissue in the mesentery.

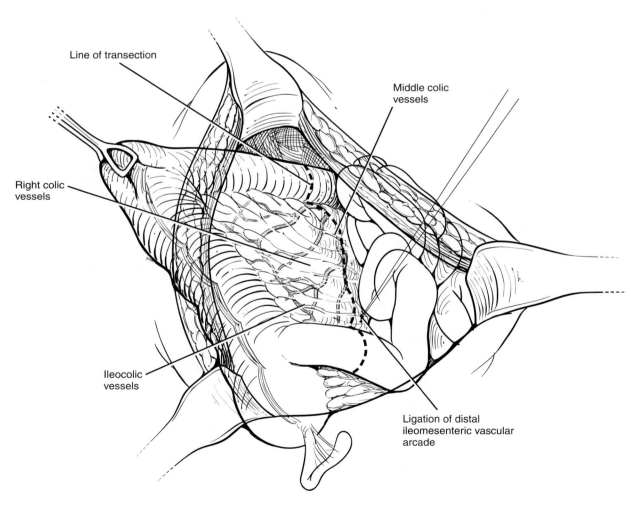

Line of transection

Middle colic
vessels

Right colic
vessels

Ileocolic
vessels

Ligation of distal
ileomesenteric vascular
arcade

FIGURE 58–5

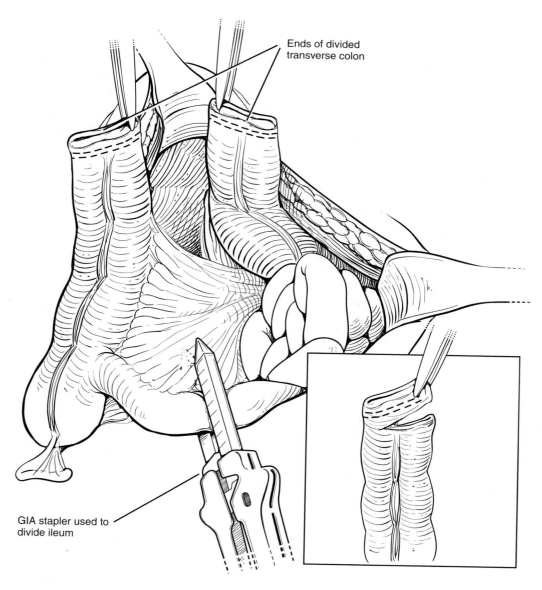

Ends of divided
transverse colon

GIA stapler used to
divide ileum

FIGURE 58–6

◆ Creation of continuity between the terminal ileum and transverse colon can be performed using either a hand-sewn or a stapled technique. A standard end-to-end (**Figures 58-7 through 58-10**) or side-to-side anastomosis (**Figures 58-11 and 58-12**) are then performed.

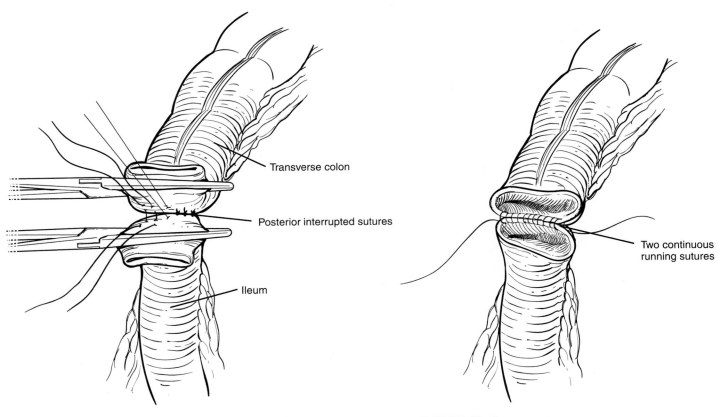

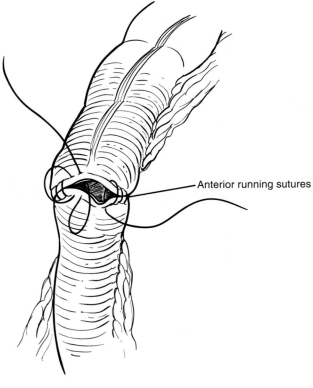

Transverse colon

Posterior interrupted sutures

Ileum

FIGURE 58–7

Two continuous running sutures

FIGURE 58–8

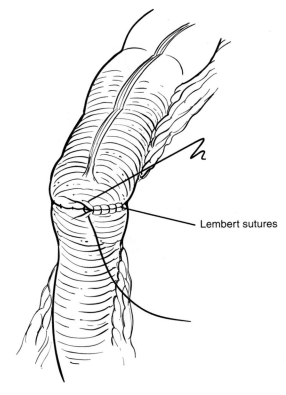

Anterior running sutures

FIGURE 58–9

Lembert sutures

FIGURE 58–10

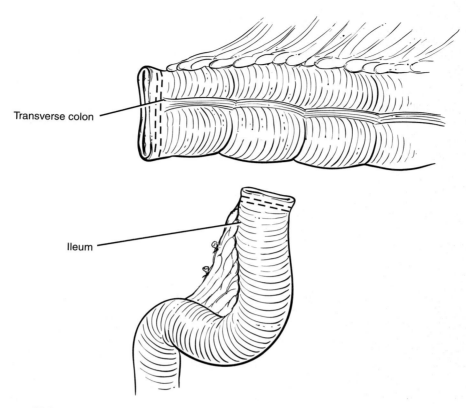

Transverse colon

Ileum

FIGURE 58–11

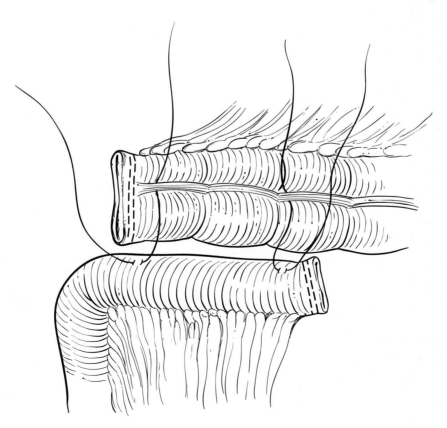

FIGURE 58–12

◆ The two ends of bowel are aligned for the anastomosis so that their respective mesenteries are not twisted. Both the hand-sewn and stapled techniques are acceptable and have been shown to have equivalent functional results. A hand-sewn anastomosis is standardly performed in two layers: a posterior Lembert layer (see Figure 58-7); an inner full-thickness (a good seromuscular bite with a small ridge of mucosa) running continuous layer using absorbable sutures beginning posteriorly and continuing anteriorly as a Connell inverting suture (see Figures 58-8 and 58-9); and finally, an outer row of interrupted Lembert seromuscular stitches, using nonabsorbable sutures (see Figure 58-10).

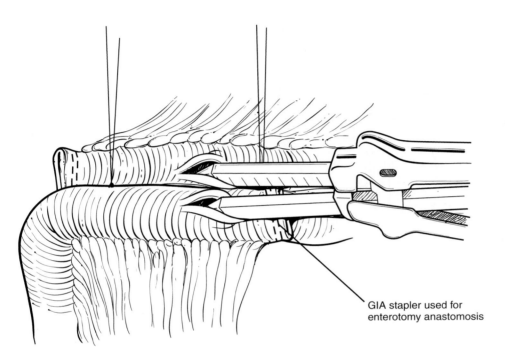

GIA stapler used for enterotomy anastomosis

FIGURE 58–13

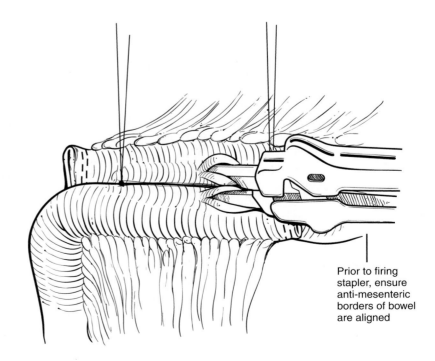

Prior to firing stapler, ensure anti-mesenteric borders of bowel are aligned

FIGURE 58–14

◆ The arms of the GIA stapler are then inserted into each bowel lumen (the ileum and transverse colon), and the antimesenteric borders of the bowel are aligned. Two silk stay sutures are useful to assist with the alignment—one proximal, near the cut edge of bowel, and the other distal, beyond the length of the staple line. The stapled anastomosis is performed by first creating colotomies near the stapled ends of the bowel **(Figures 58-13 and 58-14)**. After firing the GIA stapler, check the mucosa of the bowel along the staple line for bleeding. The resultant ileocolostomy is closed with a TA-55 stapler or by using a single layer of absorbable suture incorporating full thickness of bowel wall in a running continuous fashion **(Figures 58-15 and 58-16)**.

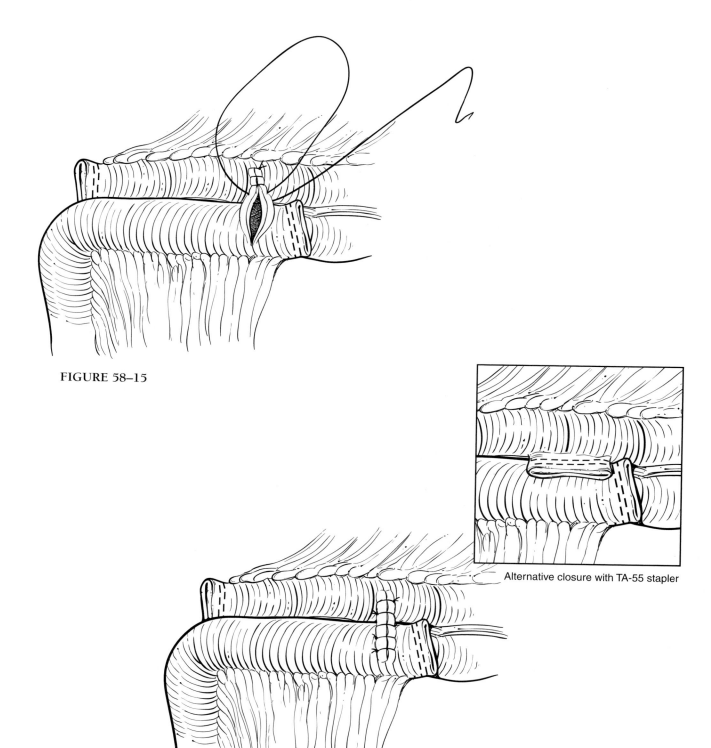

FIGURE 58–15

Alternative closure with TA-55 stapler

FIGURE 58–16

◆ Reapproximating the mesenteric defect must be performed with care to ensure that the underlying vessels supplying the bowel are not compromised. This can be sutured using a continuous absorbable stitch **(Figure 58-17)**.

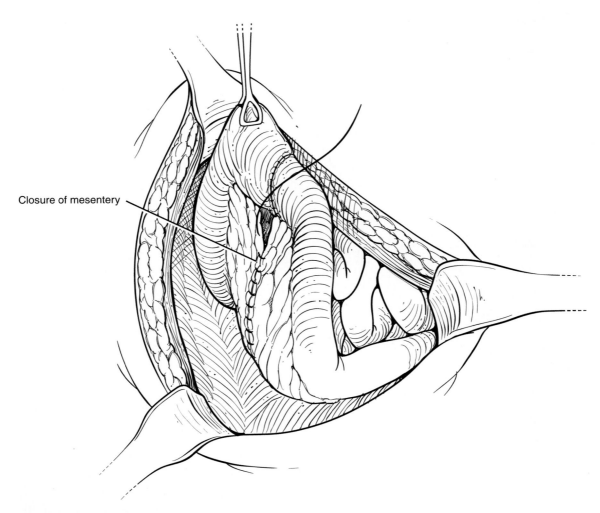

Closure of mesentery

FIGURE 58–17

3. CLOSING

◆ The abdominal cavity is irrigated with copious warm saline. The omentum can be overlaid on top of the newly formed anastomosis. After ensuring hemostasis, sponge counts, and instrument counts, close the abdomen using a no. 1 polydioxanone (PDS) suture. The subcutaneous tissue is irrigated again and the skin is closed with skin clips (see Figure 58-17).

STEP 4: POSTOPERATIVE CARE

◆ A nasogastric tube is generally not required for a routine right hemicolectomy. Patients can generally tolerate sips of clear liquids and progress to a regular diet over the next few postoperative days.

STEP 5: PEARLS AND PITFALLS

◆ Be careful of injury to retroperitoneal structures such as the duodenum and right ureter.

◆ When performing the operation for cancer, it is important to ensure that the pathologists process and look at an adequate number of lymph nodes. This will ensure more accurate nodal staging, which is essential for the decision to treat with adjuvant chemotherapy.

SELECTED REFERENCES

1. Wille-Jørgensen P, Rasmussen MS, Andersen BR, Borly L: Heparins and mechanical methods for thromboprophylaxis in colorectal surgery. Cochrane Database Syst Rev 2004(4):CD001217.
2. Stahl TJ, Gregorcyk SG, Hyman NH, et al: Practice parameters for the prevention of venous thrombosis. Dis Colon Rectum 2006;49:1477-1483.
3. Docherty JG, McGregor JR, Akyol AM, et al: Comparison of manually constructed and stapled anastomoses in colorectal surgery. Ann Surg 1995;221:176-184.
4. LeVoyer TE, Sigurdson ER, Hanlon AL, et al: Colon cancer is associated with increasing number of lymph nodes analyzed: A secondary survey of intergroup trial INT-0089. J Clin Oncol 2003;21:2912-2919.

CHAPTER 59

RIGHT COLECTOMY (LAPAROSCOPIC-ASSISTED)

Valerie P. Bauer

STEP 1: SURGICAL ANATOMY

- The surgeon must be familiar with the fascial attachments of the ascending colon, which can be used for countertraction during laparoscopic resection. The white line of Toldt is the lateral peritoneal attachment of the ascending colon to the abdominal wall and serves as a guide during surgical mobilization.

- The ascending colon is covered by peritoneum on the anterior and lateral sides. The retrocecal and inferior cecal recesses mark the attachment of the cecum to the retroperitoneum. Division of the peritoneum here allows entry behind the cecum and dissection of the fine areolar tissue called the fascia of Toldt. Beneath this plane lie Gerota's fascia and the right kidney. Care should be taken to avoid lifting this structure along with the colon, especially when the areolar plane is fibrotic or densely adhesive (as seen in desmoplastic reactions). In addition, the right ureter lies beneath this plane and parallel to the gonadal vessels and thus should be avoided.

- The second portion of the duodenum is exposed during the retroperitoneal dissection and should be swept downward, away from the posterior wall of the colon.

- The inferior vena cava lies medially in the retroperitoneal plane and should be avoided during the retroperitoneal dissection.

- The main blood supply to the ascending colon is the ileocolic and right colic arteries.

STEP 2: PREOPERATIVE CONSIDERATIONS

- Indications for laparoscopic right colectomy are the same as for conventional operations. The decision to chose this operative approach depends on the skill and experience of the surgeon. Laparoscopic surgery traditionally has been used to treat conditions on an elective basis but has expanded to include selective emergent situations, such as those seen in penetrating abdominal trauma and repair of endoscopically created perforations. Other indications include:

- ◆ Benign polyps or lesions not amenable to endoscopic resection
- ◆ Malignant lesions located in the appendix, cecum, ascending colon, and hepatic flexure
- ◆ Crohn's disease of the terminal ileum and ascending colon
- ◆ Cecal volvulus

- ◆ The hand-assisted technique allows for use of one hand in the abdomen while maintaining pneumoperitoneum. Advantages include preservation of tactile sensation and ease of dissection and should be considered for potentially difficult cases such as those having anticipated adhesions or inflammatory conditions as in cancer and inflammatory bowel disease (IBD). Operative times are shorter and the benefits of the laparoscopic approach are preserved.

- ◆ Informed consent should address such complications as anastomotic stricture or leak, bowel obstruction, wound infection at the port sites, intra-abdominal infection, hematoma, injury to adjacent bowel or mesentery, injury to adjacent structures such as the ureter and great vessels, port site hernias, and the need for creation of an ostomy.

- ◆ Preoperative evaluation of the patient's comorbidities should be obtained, including determination of nutritional status, evidence of anemia, and cardiac risk factors. Appropriate laboratory and cardiac evaluations should be obtained.

- ◆ Patients undergoing resection for malignant or potentially malignant pathologic conditions should have preoperative staging computed tomography (CT) scan of the chest, abdomen, and pelvis, with oral and intravenous (IV) contrast, and a baseline carcinoembryonic antigen (CEA) level drawn. In addition, a complete colonoscopy should be performed to confirm location of the lesion and to rule out synchronous lesions.

- ◆ Aspirin, other blood thinners, and vitamin E should be stopped for 10 days before the procedure.

- ◆ A mechanical bowel preparation may be given based on the surgeon's preference.

- ◆ An accepted parenteral antibiotic is given within 1 hour of the incision to prevent surgical site infection on colorectal cases in accordance with the Surgical Care Improvement Project (SCIP) guidelines. Ertapenem is given once a day and covers the 24-hour postoperative period.

- ◆ Prophylaxis for thrombophlebitis is administered either preoperatively or within 24 hours from surgery in accordance with the SCIP guidelines.

- ◆ Patients on steroids preoperatively should get a stress dose of IV hydrocortisone 100 mg before the operation. This should be continued postoperatively and tapered accordingly.

- Implementing a postoperative colorectal pathway facilitates timely recovery and decreased length of hospital stay. The pathway is reviewed with the patient to outline expectations for ambulation and pain control after surgery. It is imperative that patients understand the importance of ambulation on postoperative return of bowel function.

STEP 3: OPERATIVE STEPS

1. POSITIONING

- The patient is placed supine on the operating table on a deflated bean bag covered with two hospital sheets.

- After general endotracheal anesthesia is administered, a Foley catheter is placed along with sequential compression devices on the lower extremities.

- Depending on the surgeon's preference, the patient may remain supine or be placed in low lithotomy using Allen stirrups. Lithotomy allows for additional mobility for the assistant or the surgeon, should an alternative position be needed.

- The arms are padded and tucked so that the top sheet comes over and underneath the bottom sheet. Care is taken to ensure that all IV lines are padded away from the skin to prevent pressure necrosis. The hands are placed in slightly flexed position with circular roll to prevent intraoperative movement.

- Abdominal and pubic hair is clipped off as needed.

- A warmer is placed appropriately to ensure normothermia during the surgery.

- An orogastric tube is placed by the anesthesia team for the duration of the procedure, to be removed upon completion of the procedure.

- The surgeon will stand on the patient's left, with the assistant between the legs or next to the surgeon on the left.

- Monitors are placed on the upper and lower right side of the patient.

2. INCISION

- The abdomen is prepped and draped in standard fashion according to the surgeon's preference.

- Using a marking pen, mark the midline from pubic symphysis to xiphoid process to aid midline entry if rapid conversion to an open procedure is needed.

- The laparoscopic instruments are positioned accordingly on the operative field to include a 30-degree laparoscope, two insufflation tubing devices attached to CO_2 tanks, electrocautery, suction, and consideration for harmonic scalpel or LigaSure device.

- Port placement
  - Hand-assisted laparoscopic technique
    - A vertical midline incision is made 1 cm less than the width of the hand. I prefer to carry the incision through the center of the umbilicus, which will make up for the difference in length.
    - The abdomen is entered sharply. The midline fascia is divided beyond the limit of the skin incision both proximally and distally. Visible adhesions are taken down in standard fashion.
    - The GelPort (Applied Medical) is used by placing the Alexis retractor into the wound and rotating the outer ring inward, thus tightening the fit. A 5-mm blunt-tipped port is placed through the GelPort, which is attached to the outer ring. Insufflation is initiated on high flow to 15 mm Hg.
    - The left hand is introduced through the GelPort and the laparoscope through the 5-mm port.
    - A 12-mm port is placed in the upper midline.
    - The patient is placed in steep Trendelenburg position and airplaned to the right.
  - Conventional technique
    - The Veress needle or Hassan technique may be used to access the abdomen below the umbilicus. A 12-mm port is placed in the left upper quadrant and a 5-mm port is placed at the upper midline. A second 5-mm port may be placed in the right lower quadrant for traction.

- The liver is visualized and inspected along with the peritoneal cavity for evidence of metastatic disease. Laparoscopic intraoperative ultrasound may be performed at this time.

3. DISSECTION

◆ The small bowel is retracted to the left upper abdominal cavity. The cecum is pushed upward to expose the inferior and retrocecal recesses where the cecum attaches to the retroperitoneum **(Figure 59-1).** A subtle fine white line may be visible, marking the location where electrocautery incision is made. This is extended proximally and medially toward the root of the ascending colon mesentery, just to the right of the superior mesenteric artery.

◆ The ileocolic artery is isolated and divided. A high ligation is performed at its origin of the superior mesenteric artery for oncologic resection **(Figure 59-2).** Before ligation, the vessels are lifted off the retroperitoneal plane and the pedicle skeletonized. The right ureter should be visualized before ligation of the pedicle. The pedicle is taken using an endoscopie gastrointestinal anastomosis (GIA) vascular load stapling device.

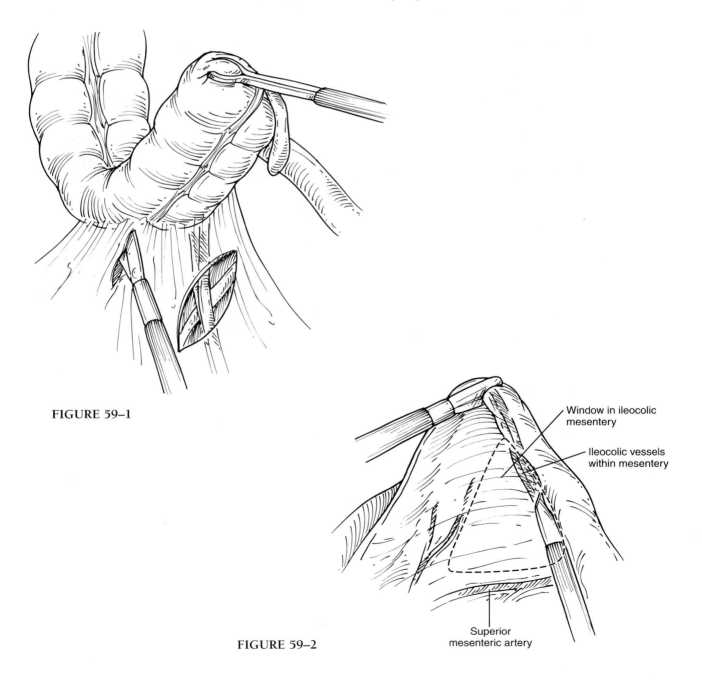

FIGURE 59–1

Window in ileocolic mesentery

Ileocolic vessels within mesentery

Superior mesenteric artery

FIGURE 59–2

◆ The ascending colon and mesentery are further dissected off the retroperitoneum **(Figure 59-3)**.
  ◆ In the hand-assisted technique, this is done by "walking" the left index and second finger up the posterior surface toward the liver. The lateral peritoneal attachment is maintained for countertraction.
  ◆ In the conventional technique, the trochar is used to bluntly create this pocket while the colon is held up in countertraction with atraumatic graspers.

◆ The duodenum is identified and swept downward **(Figure 59-4)**. Similarly, the right kidney is maintained posterior to the plane of dissection.

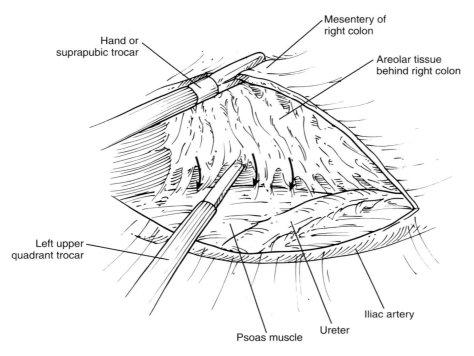

FIGURE 59–3

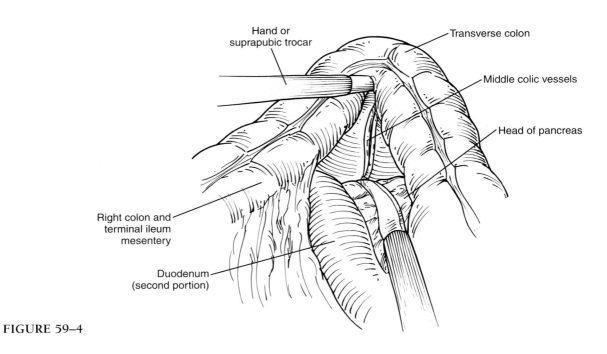

FIGURE 59–4

◆ The right colic artery, if present, is isolated and divided, as is the hepatic branch of the middle colic artery.

◆ The lateral attachment is divided and dissection is carried around the hepatic flexure, taking the hepatocolic ligaments down **(Figure 59-5, A)**. The gastrocolic ligament is detached from the transverse colon just distal to the point where the colon will be divided **(Figure 59-5, B)**. For an oncologic resection, the omentum should be resected with the specimen, taking care to preserve the gastroepiploic artery.

◆ The mesentery is divided to the point of vascular demarcation of the transverse colon.

◆ Pneumoperitoneum is reversed and the mobilized segment is exteriorized.

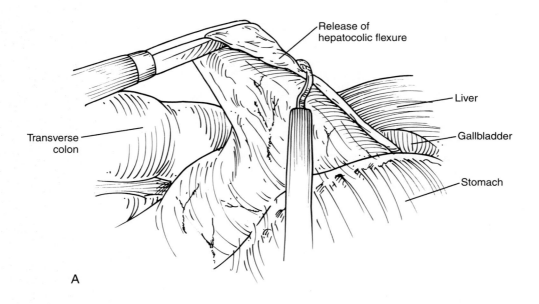

A

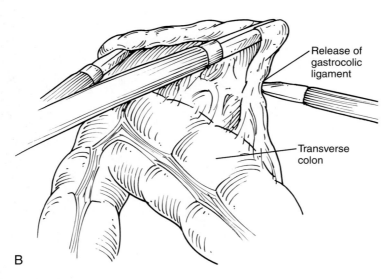

B

FIGURE 59–5

- The mesentery to the terminal ileum is clamped, divided, and ligated to a point 5 to 15 cm away from the ileocecal valve. The mesentery is similarly cleared from the transverse colon.
  - Hand-sewn end-to-end anastomosis:
    - An Ochsner bowel clamp is placed obliquely on the small bowel to make up for the size difference between the small bowel and colon lumen.
    - An Ochsner bowel clamp is placed perpendicularly on the transverse colon.
    - The specimen is transected and removed from the table (**Figure 59-6**).
    - The two ends of bowel are positioned so that the antimesenteric and mesenteric ends are aligned.
    - Both lumens are inspected and irrigated, taking care to maintain sterile technique and minimize fecal spillage.
    - A double-armed 4-0 Maxon monofilament suture is used to create a single-layered running anastomosis. The serosal edge is grasped and the mucosa and submucosal edges are reapproximated. This is done by placing the knot on the outer portion of the bowel at the antimesenteric border. One arm of suture is passed under the knot and used to complete half of the anastomosis, as is the other arm on the other side. The suture line is inspected for integrity.
  - Stapled side-to-side anastomosis:
    - The exteriorized segment is laid out so that the antimesenteric limb of the small bowel is aligned with the antimesenteric limb of the transverse colon. A stay stitch using 2-0 Vicryl suture may be used to maintain alignment.
    - A colotomy and enterotomy are made on the antimesenteric side over the proximal and distal resection lines using Bovie electrocautery.

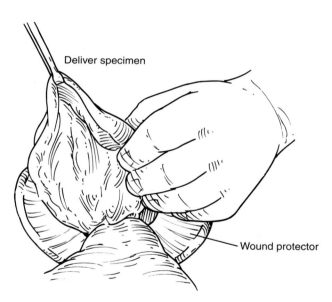

Deliver specimen

Wound protector

FIGURE 59–6

- A 75-mm blue load linear GIA stapling device is introduced through each opening, and a common wall is created between the two, taking care to ensure that the mesentery is away from the staple line.
- The linear stapler is reloaded and fired perpendicularly to the staple line, closing the colostomy and releasing the specimen from the field **(Figure 59-7).**
- The staple line is inspected for integrity. It is our preference to place a 2-0 Vicryl stitch between the colon and ileum to take tension off the staple line. The intersection of the staple line may also be reinforced with a figure-of-eight stitch, because this is a natural weak point.

- The mesenteric defect may be closed according to the surgeon's preference.

- The completed anastomosis is dropped back into the abdominal cavity.

- Surgical gloves are changed, and the Alexis wound retractor is removed. It is our preference to place Seprafilm over the midline incision to minimize postoperative adhesions. The abdomen is reapproximated using 0 polydioxanone (PDS) in figure-of-eight interrupted sutures.

- The subcutaneous skin is irrigated with bacitracin antibiotic (50,000 U in 1 L saline).

- Staples are used to close skin. A small umbilical bolster is created by placing a bacitracin-soaked cotton ball wrapped in Adaptic into the umbilical depression. This is left in place during the hospital stay and removed before discharge home.

- The orogastric tube is removed before extubation, provided there is no extensive lysis of adhesions or indication for maintenance of a nasogastric tube postoperatively.

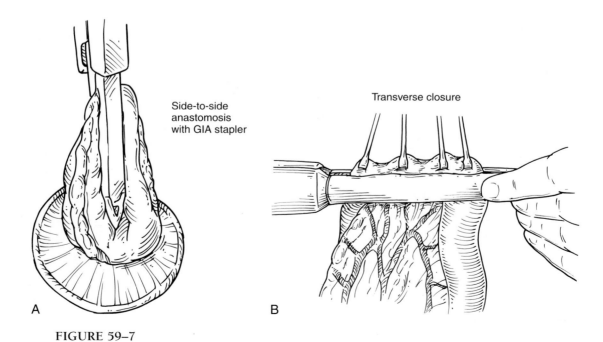

Side-to-side
anastomosis
with GIA stapler

Transverse closure

A   B

FIGURE 59–7

STEP 4: POSTOPERATIVE CARE

◆ Adherence to a postoperative colorectal clinical pathway ensures standardization of care and facilitates timely discharge from the hospital.

◆ Adequate pain control is achieved using patient-controlled analgesia. Use of a nonopioid analgesic such as ketorolac (Toradol) should be considered. In our protocol, this is administered on postoperative day 1, provided there are no contraindications such as renal insufficiency, and given on a scheduled basis of 15 mg intravenously every 8 hours for 9 doses. Patients are transitioned to an oral analgesic on postoperative day 2.

◆ Consideration for stress ulcer prophylaxis should be made for patients with symptoms or history of gastroesophageal reflux disease (GERD) or peptic ulcer disease (PUD).

◆ All patients should receive prophylaxis for deep venous thrombosis, consisting of sequential compression devices while in bed, and heparin 5000 U subcutaneously every 8 hours or enoxaparin 40 mg subcutaneously every morning, starting within 24 hours after surgery.

◆ Adequate IV fluid should be administered with monitoring of urine output. The Foley catheter may be removed on postoperative day 1.

◆ The diet may be limited to ice chips and sips of water in the postanesthesia care unit. A clear liquid diet is started on postoperative day 1. Return of bowel function is measured by the frequency and pitch of bowel sounds, lack of abdominal distention, amount of belching, presence of nausea and vomiting, and the patient's subjective will to eat. Diet may be advanced ad lib as bowel function returns.

◆ Early ambulation is crucial for aid in return of bowel function. Patients should be instructed to walk multiple times a day beginning on postoperative day 1.

◆ The dressing over the incision site is removed on postoperative day 2, and the incision is checked daily thereafter to ensure absence of infection. The umbilical bolster remains in place until the patient is discharged from the hospital.

STEP 5: PEARLS AND PITFALLS

◆ The use of SCIP approved prophylactic antibiotic for colorectal surgery, ertapenem (Invanz) 1 g intravenously, before surgery, requires only a single dose for 24-hour coverage. Furthermore, it lasts for the duration of the procedure and does not require additional dosing.

◆ The hepatic flexure suspensory ligaments should be divided with caution, because there are often large veins here. Careful dissection and the use of energy ligatures should strongly be considered to avoid uncontrollable bleeding and subsequent conversion to open laparotomy.

- Smaller lesions in the colon should be marked with tattoo ink for confirmation of location, which will assist in removal of the primary lesion with adequate 5-cm margin and areas of lymphatic drainage.

- Placement of Seprafilm under the midline incision minimizes adhesions on reentry for subsequent operations. This should be considered, especially for indications such as Crohn's disease and colon cancer.

SELECTED REFERENCES

1. Tinley HS, Constantinides VA, Heriot AG, et al: Comparison of laparoscopic and open ileocecal resection for Crohn's disease: A meta-analysis. Surg Endosc 2007;20:1036-1044.
2. Kaban GK, Novitsky YW, Perugini RA, et al: Use of laparoscopy in evaluation and treatment of penetrating and blunt abdominal injuries. Surg Innov 2008;15:26-31.
3. Kang JC, Chung MH, Yeh CC, et al: Hand assisted laparoscopic colectomy versus open colectomy: A prospective randomized study. Surg Endosc 2004;18:577-581.
4. Itani KMF, Wilson SE, Awad SS, et al: Ertapenem versus cefotetan prophylaxis in elective colorectal surgery. N Engl J Med 2006;355:2640-2651.
5. Guidelines from the Joint Commission on Surgical Care Improvement Project Core Measurement Set. Available on Internet: www.jointcommission.org/PerformanceMeasurement.
6. Law WL, Bailey HR, Max E, et al: Single-layer continuous colon and rectal anastomosis using monofilament absorbable suture (Maxon): Study of 500 cases. Dis Colon Rectum 1999;42:736-740.
7. Max E, Sweeney WB, Bailey HR, et al: Results of 1,000 single-layer continuous polypropylene intestinal anastomoses. Am J Surg 1991;162:461-467.
8. Zeng Q, Yu Z, You J, Zhang Q: Efficacy and safety of Seprafilm for preventing postoperative abdominal adhesion: Systematic review and meta-analysis. World J Surg 2007; 31:2125-2131;2132 [discussion].

CHAPTER 60

LEFT AND SIGMOID COLECTOMY

Celia Chao

STEP 1: SURGICAL ANATOMY

- The left colon begins at the mid-transverse colon and includes the splenic flexure, left (descending) colon, and sigmoid colon. The marginal artery of Drummond provides a vascular anastomosis between the superior and inferior mesenteric arteries. The blood supply to the left colon is derived from the inferior mesenteric artery. The first branch, the left colic artery, supplies the splenic flexure and descending colon. The sigmoid arteries and the superior rectal artery are the most distal branches of the inferior mesenteric artery and supply the sigmoid colon. The lymphatics follow its arterial blood supply. A minimum of 12 lymph nodes within the mesentery is considered an adequate resection when performing a left hemicolectomy or sigmoidectomy for cancer.

STEP 2: PREOPERATIVE CONSIDERATIONS

- Indications: Tumors of the left colon can be resected with a left hemicolectomy, which involves sacrificing the inferior mesenteric blood supply, along with its branches (left colic artery and sigmoid arteries), which supply the splenic flexure to the proximal sigmoid colon. Tumors of the sigmoid colon can be removed with a sigmoid resection, encompassing the distal descending colon and the sigmoid colon, sacrificing the sigmoid and superior rectal arteries **(Figure 60-1)**.

- Preoperative planning: Evaluation of the entire colorectal lumen is necessary to rule out synchronous lesions before surgical intervention. This can be accomplished with either colonoscopy or barium enema, assuming that the patient does not have an obstructing or near-obstructing lesion. An adequate mechanical bowel preparation is generally performed the day before surgical resection, but is not considered necessary. Preoperatively, intravenous antibiotics must be administered before the skin incision. A preoperative dose of subcutaneous heparin (5000 U) or a low-molecular-weight heparin is recommended to prevent deep venous thrombosis. Before induction of general anesthesia, pneumatic compression boots are placed on both lower extremities and continued postoperatively until the patient ambulates on the first postoperative day. A Foley catheter is placed after induction of general anesthesia. Stress ulcer prophylaxis may be given until the patient tolerates oral intake.

- Anesthesia: General anesthesia is used.

STEP 3: OPERATIVE STEPS

1. INCISION

♦ A midline incision is made. A Thompson retractor is used to retract the abdominal wall, particularly the left costal margin, which is necessary to facilitate adequate exposure of the splenic flexure.

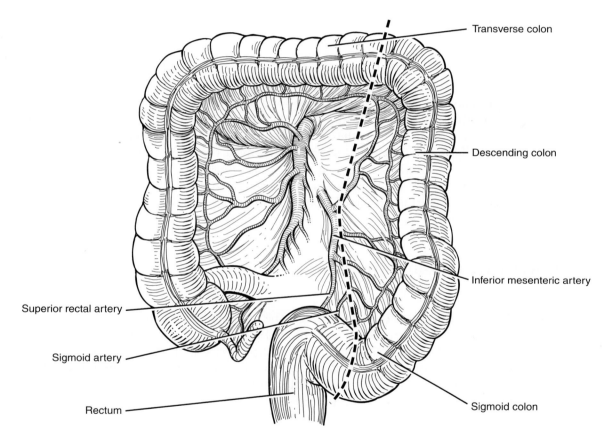

Transverse colon

Descending colon

Inferior mesenteric artery

Superior rectal artery

Sigmoid artery

Sigmoid colon

Rectum

FIGURE 60–1

2. DISSECTION

◆ An intra-abdominal exploration is performed to determine the extent of disease and resect-ability. The small bowel is packed and tucked away to the right upper quadrant of the ab-dominal cavity. The left colon is mobilized from its retroperitoneal attachments by incising the white line of Toldt **(Figure 60-2)**.

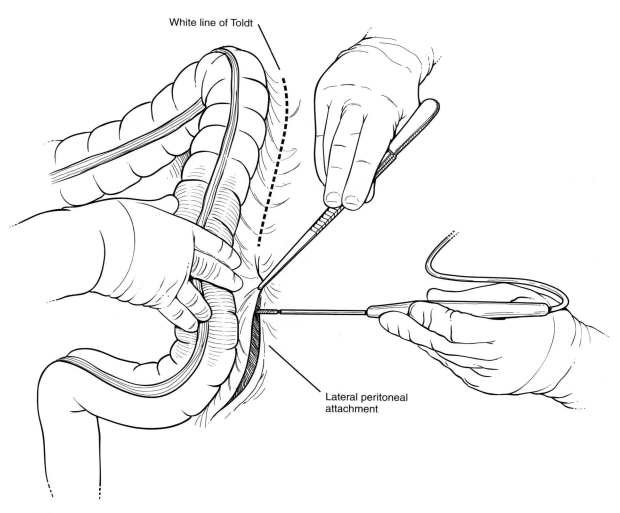

White line of Toldt

Lateral peritoneal attachment

FIGURE 60–2

- The sigmoid and descending colon is retracted medially, exposing the left ureter and gonadal vessel **(Figure 60-3).**

- Continuing cephalad along this retroperitoneal plane, divide the renocolic and splenocolic ligament to release the splenic flexure **(Figures 60-4 and 60-5).**

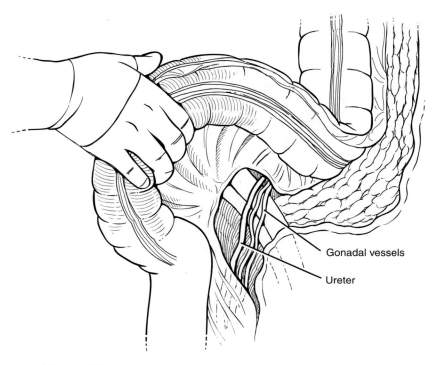

Gonadal vessels

Ureter

FIGURE 60–3

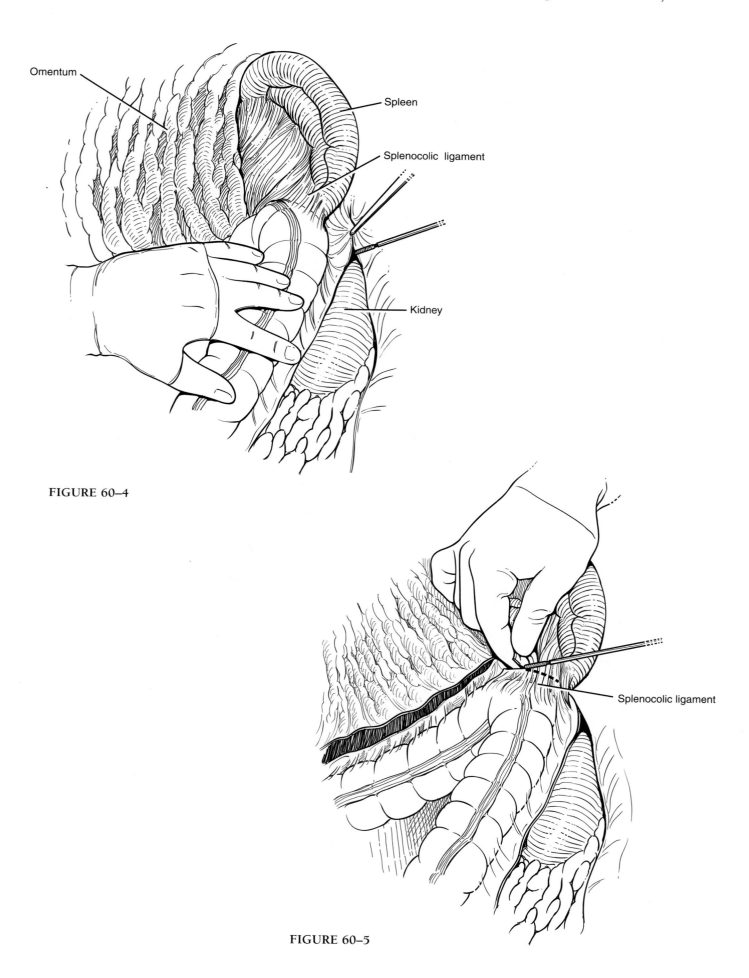

Omentum

Spleen

Splenocolic ligament

Kidney

FIGURE 60-4

Splenocolic ligament

FIGURE 60-5

◆ Dissecting from the left aspect of the omentum, mobilize the gastrocolic ligament off the transverse colon and splenic flexure **(Figure 60-6).**

◆ The least traumatic way of taking down the splenic flexure involves dividing these avascular ligaments from either side of the splenic flexure (see Figure 60-5) rather than pulling on the flexure with downward traction.

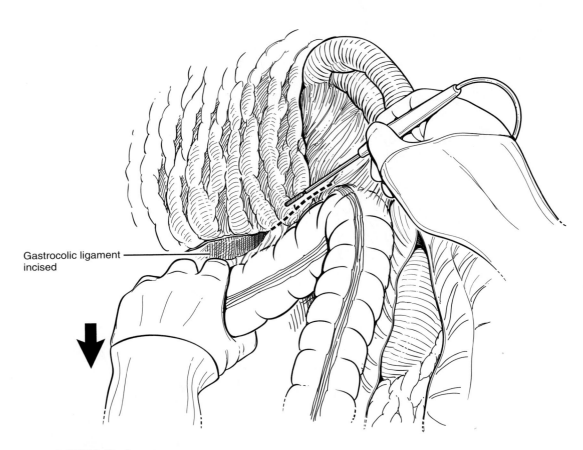

Gastrocolic ligament incised

FIGURE 60–6

◆ The blood supply to the left colon originates from the inferior mesenteric artery and mainly involves the left colic artery. The points of transection of the proximal and distal large bowel are decided upon based on the mesenteric blood supply. The colon is then divided with the gastrointestinal anastomosis (GIA) stapler at the proximal and distal resection margins **(Figure 60-7).** The left colic artery and proximal sigmoid arteries are ligated at their origins. Careful attention must be paid to the bowel ends to ensure a healthy blood supply and that the ends would reapproximate without tension.

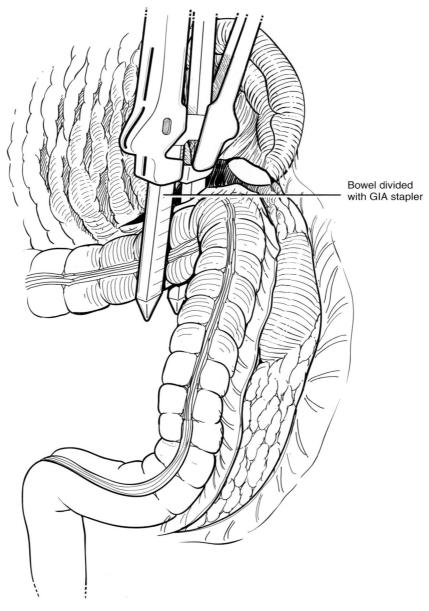

Bowel divided with GIA stapler

FIGURE 60–7

◆ The anastomosis joining the distal transverse and distal sigmoid colon can be hand-sewn **(Figures 60-8 through 60-11)** or stapled, as described previously. When performing an anastomosis using an end of bowel, such as an end-to-end anastomosis, at least a 1-cm edge of bowel must be cleared of fat, mesentery, and appendices epiploicae, exposing the serosa.

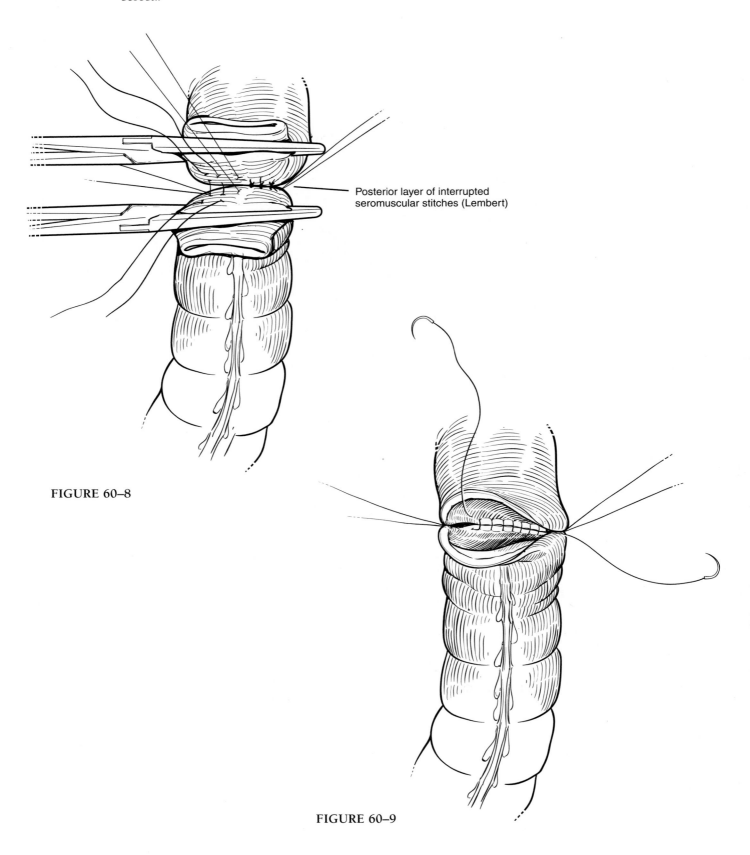

Posterior layer of interrupted
seromuscular stitches (Lembert)

FIGURE 60–8

FIGURE 60–9

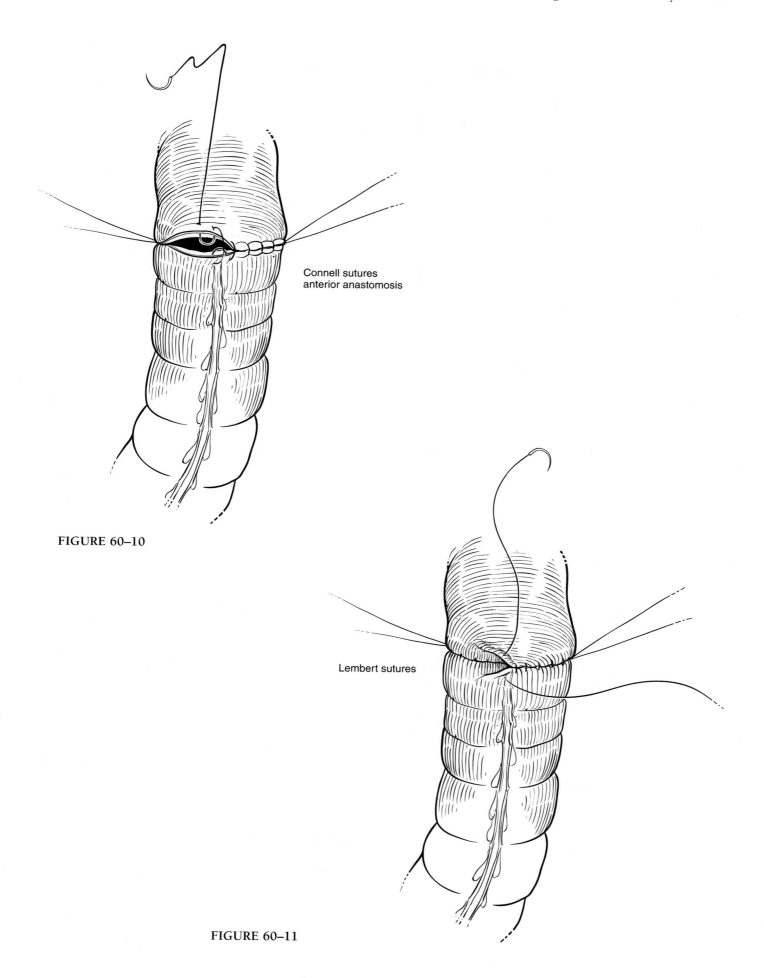

Connell sutures
anterior anastomosis

FIGURE 60–10

Lembert sutures

FIGURE 60–11

- The sigmoid colon may be resected if the tumor is located in the distal descending colon or sigmoid colon. As the retroperitoneum is exposed, the left ureter should be identified, typically anterior to the external iliac vessels. The limits of resection are determined: proximal sigmoid tumors will involve sacrifice of branches of the left colic artery, and distal sigmoid tumors will involve sacrifice of branches of the superior rectal artery and transecting the colon to the level of the sacral promontory. The splenic flexure may have to be mobilized to create a tension-free anastomosis.

- Hand-sewn end-to-end (see Figures 60-8 through 60-11) anastomosis: After noncrushing bowel clamps are applied proximal to the bowel ends, the staple lines are cut using electrocautery or Metzenbaum scissors. In a standard two-layer anastomosis, the posterior (outer) layer of the transverse colon and proximal rectum are reapproximated with 3-0 silk interrupted (Lembert) sutures. Two continuous absorbable sutures are used in the posterior inner row (see Figure 60-9), and each is brought anteriorly, where the transition to Connell sutures is made (see Figure 60-10).

- Finally, the anterior (outer) layer is completed with interrupted Lembert sutures (see Figure 60-11). The mesenteric defect can be reapproximated with a continuous absorbable stitch, with care to ensure that the underlying vessels supplying the bowel are not compromised.

3. CLOSING

- The abdominal cavity is irrigated with copious warm saline. The omentum can be overlaid on top of the newly formed anastomosis. After ensuring hemostasis, sponge counts, and instrument counts, close the abdomen using a no. 1 polydioxanone (PDS) suture. The subcutaneous tissue is irrigated again, and the skin is closed with skin clips.

STEP 4: POSTOPERATIVE CARE

- Ambulation and incentive spirometry on postoperative day 1 is important for the prevention of postoperative atelectasis. Oral intake of clear liquids can begin after removal of the nasogastric tube. The Foley catheter is left in place for a few days because of the high incidence of urinary retention in male patients.

STEP 5: PEARLS AND PITFALLS

- Injury to the spleen: Omental adhesions between the omentum and splenic capsule can cause inadvertent avulsion or injury to the splenic capsule if traction on the omentum is applied.

- Injury to the left ureter: After division of the renocolic ligament, the left ureter is visualized in the left retroperitoneum. The entire length of the ureter can be traced down to the pelvis if necessary.

SELECTED REFERENCES

1. Wille-Jørgensen P, Rasmussen MS, Andersen BR, Borly L: Heparins and mechanical methods for thrombo-prophylaxis in colorectal surgery. Cochrane Database Syst Rev 2004(4):CD001217.
2. Stahl TJ, Gregorcyk SG, Hyman NH, et al: Practice parameters for the prevention of venous thrombosis. Dis Colon Rectum 2006;49:1477-1483.

CHAPTER 61

LEFT AND SIGMOID COLECTOMY (LAPAROSCOPIC-ASSISTED)

Valerie P. Bauer

STEP 1: SURGICAL ANATOMY

♦ The descending colon is covered by peritoneum on the anterior and lateral surfaces and attaches to the retroperitoneum on the posterior side.

♦ Structures beneath the descending colon include the left kidney, the proximal ureter, and the inferior mesenteric vein.

♦ The splenic flexure is much higher than the hepatic flexure, a consideration to be noted when placing ports for laparoscopic dissection. Mobilization of the flexure requires division of the lienocolic ligament, a maneuver that must be carefully done to prevent splenic capsular tear.

♦ The main blood supply to the left colon includes the left colic artery and the superior sigmoid arteries. Collateral flow may be provided by the marginal arteries and the arc of Riolan, a meandering artery from the middle colic artery to the inferior mesenteric artery.

♦ The sigmoid colon is highly mobile, typically with a long mesentery and variable length. It is completely covered by peritoneum and is attached to the abdominal wall by the lateral peritoneal attachment called the "white line of Toldt," which extends upward to include attachment of the left colon, as well. Preservation of this attachment allows for countertraction during laparoscopic mobilization.

♦ The blood supply of the sigmoid colon includes the inferior mesenteric artery and its sigmoidal branches.

♦ The intersigmoid fossa is a recess at the base of the mesosigmoid that provides an anatomic landmark for locating the left ureter, which courses beneath the fossa and parallel just medial to the gonadal vein.

♦ The superior hypogastric plexus provides sympathetic innervation for erectile function and is situated at the bifurcation of the aorta in close proximity to the inferior mesenteric artery (IMA) pedicle. Care should be taken to avoid division of nerve fibers during high IMA division, which results in retrograde ejaculation in male patients.

STEP 2: PREOPERATIVE CONSIDERATIONS

♦ Preoperative considerations for laparoscopic left and sigmoid colectomy are similar to those outlined in Chapter 59.

♦ Bowel continuity may or may not be restored depending on the clinical circumstances.

♦ If an ostomy is planned, the patient should be marked preoperatively for either an end sigmoid colostomy or loop ileostomy and educated concerning the new ostomy.

♦ Indications for laparoscopic left and sigmoid colectomy include:
  ♦ Benign polyps or lesions not amenable to endoscopic resection
  ♦ Malignant lesions located in the splenic flexure, descending colon, and sigmoid colon
  ♦ Diverticulitis of the sigmoid colon
    ♦ Complicated as defined by history of perforation and abscess formation, stricture, and fistula
    ♦ In immunocompromised patients (steroid-dependent and transplant patients)
    ♦ In select few who had multiple episodes of recurrent simple disease
  ♦ Crohn's disease
  ♦ Sigmoid volvulus

♦ The hand-assisted technique is particularly beneficial in difficult cases, such as complicated diverticulitis and Crohn's disease, allowing for improved ease of dissection under operative conditions that are normally challenging even in the open setting.

♦ Informed consent addresses complications as outlined in Chapter 59, but should include possibility of damage to nerves, creating sexual dysfunction such as retrograde ejaculation.

STEP 3: OPERATIVE STEPS

1. POSITIONING

♦ The patient is placed supine on the operating table on a deflated bean bag covered with two hospital sheets.

♦ After general endotracheal anesthesia is administered, a Foley catheter is placed along with sequential compression devices on the lower extremities.

- During the setup, the surgeon confirms with the anesthesia team that the proper preoperative prophylactic antibiotic is being administered before initiating the procedure based on measures defined by the Physician Quality Reporting Initiative.

- The patient is placed in low lithotomy position using Allen stirrups. A soft roll is placed under the pelvis to elevate and pad the hips.

- The arms are padded and tucked so that the top sheet comes over and underneath the bottom sheet. Care is taken to ensure that all intravenous (IV) lines are padded away from the skin to prevent pressure necrosis. The hands are placed in slightly flexed position with circular roll to prevent intraoperative movement.

- The bean bag is inflated with the sides and top corners turned up. Padding is placed between the patient's head and the walls of the bean bag. A blue towel is placed across the patient's chest on which heavy tape is used to encircle the patient on the operating table. Attention is paid to ensure that the tape is not restricting to respiration.

- Abdominal and pubic hair is clipped off as needed.

- A warmer is placed appropriately to ensure normothermia during the procedure.

- An orogastric tube is placed by the anesthesia team for the duration of the procedure, to be removed upon completion of the procedure.

- The surgeon stands to the right of the patient, with the assistant between the patient's legs or next to the surgeon on the right.

- Monitors are placed on the upper and lower left side of the patient.

- Digital rectal examination is performed, followed by rigid proctoscopy. This confirms a clean rectal vault and absence of unappreciated rectal pathologic findings.

- The abdomen is prepped and draped in standard fashion according to the surgeon's preference.

2. INCISION

- Using a marking pen, mark the midline from the pubic symphysis to the xiphoid process to facilitate midline entry if rapid conversion to an open procedure is needed.

- The laparoscopic instruments are positioned accordingly on the operative field to include a 30-degree laparoscope, two insufflation tubing devices attached to CO_2 tanks, electrocautery, suction, and consideration for harmonic scalpel or LigaSure device.

- Port placement
  - Hand-assisted laparoscopic technique
    - A vertical midline incision is made 1 cm less than the width of the hand. It is carried through the center of the umbilicus, which will make up for the difference in length.
    - The abdomen is entered sharply. The midline fascia is divided beyond the limit of the skin incision both proximally and distally. Visible adhesions are taken down in standard fashion.
    - The GelPort (Applied Medical) is used by placing the Alexis retractor into the wound and rotating the outer ring inward, thus tightening the fit. A 5-mm blunt-tipped port is placed through the GelPort, which is attached to the outer ring. Insufflation is initiated on high flow to 15 mm Hg.
    - The left hand is introduced through the GelPort and the laparoscope through the 5-mm port.
    - Surgeons with larger hands may consider placing the camera through a 12-mm port in the upper midline.
    - A 12-mm port is placed in the right lower quadrant.
    - The patient is placed in steep Trendelenburg position and airplaned to the left.
  - Conventional technique
    - The Veress needle or Hassan technique may be used to access the abdomen above the umbilicus. A 12-mm port is placed in the right lower quadrant and a 5-mm port is placed at the lower midline. A second 5-mm port may be placed in the right upper quadrant for traction.

- The liver is visualized and inspected along with the peritoneal cavity for evidence of metastatic disease. Laparoscopic intraoperative ultrasound may be performed at this time.

3. DISSECTION

♦ The small bowel is retracted out of the pelvis and to the upper right of the abdomen. The sigmoid is pulled upward, and the base of the mesentery is exposed.

♦ A medial to lateral approach is taken to identify the left ureter **(Figure 61-1)**. The base of the mesosigmoid is lightly scored, and the IMA pedicle is lifted up so that the fine areolar tissue beneath can be dissected away. The left ureter is identified and freed from the overlying mesentery. It is retracted laterally.

♦ For oncologic resection of curable disease, a high ligation of the IMA is performed by skeletonizing and ligating the artery at its base, proximal to the origin of the left colic artery, using a white-load endoscopic gastrointestinal anastomosis (GIA) stapling device. The position of the ureter is checked before ligation. High ligation for advanced cancer provides no survival advantage and should not be performed; this is true for benign disease, as well.

♦ The posterior attachment of the descending colon to the retroperitoneum is mobilized by dissecting the avascular fine areolar plane proximally.

♦ The inferior mesenteric vein is identified and ligated proximally at the base of the pancreas for oncologic resections, allowing a tension-free anastomosis **(Figure 61-2)**.

♦ The lateral peritoneal attachments of the sigmoid colon are taken down. For sigmoid colectomy, the base of the mesosigmoid is entered posteriorly at the sacral promontory, in the avascular areolar plane. This is taken down to a point 5 cm distal from oncologic abnormality and to the upper rectum (as evidenced by splaying of the taenia coli) for diverticular disease.

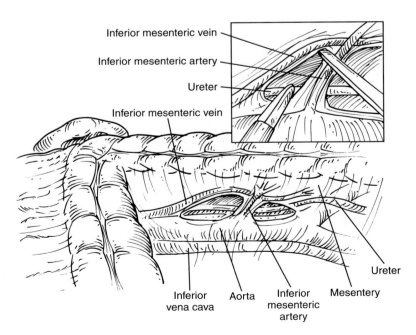

FIGURE 61–1

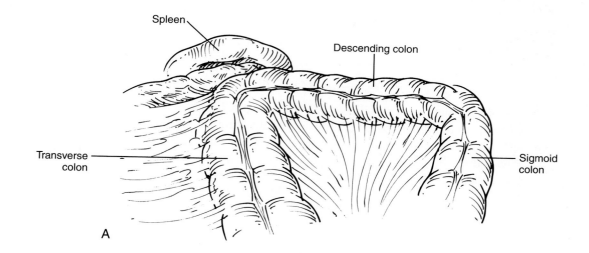

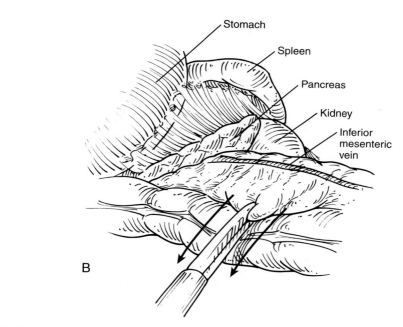

FIGURE 61–2

♦ A window is cleared between the bowel and mesentery. Use of the harmonic scalpel facilitates this without major blood loss. Mesentery may be divided using the harmonic scalpel
or an endoscopic GIA white vascular load stapler. The colon or upper rectum may be
divided using a reticulating endoscopic GIA blue load stapler **(Figure 61-3)**. Care should
be taken to ensure that the bowel is laid out like a "table," perpendicular to the staple line
to minimize an oblique division, undue thickness of the tissue, and inclusion of devascular-
ized segment in the anastomosis.

♦ The splenic flexure is mobilized for left colectomy and for creation of tension-free anastomosis in sigmoid colectomy **(Figure 61-4)**. In addition, if bowel continuity is not being
restored, mobilization will prevent tension on an end colostomy and subsequent retraction.
This is done by taking the lateral peritoneal attachment of the white line of Toldt down.
The gastrocolic ligament is divided at its colonic attachment in the distal transverse colon,
and the lesser sac is entered **(Figure 61-5)**. The lienorenal ligament is divided, and the retroperitoneal attachments are bluntly taken down.

♦ The proximal end of the anastomosis is determined according to the pattern of vascular
demarcation and location of the pathologic finding. In diverticular disease, an area free of
thickened colon is selected despite the possible presence of proximal diverticula.

♦ Pneumoperitoneum is reversed, and the mobilized segment is exteriorized.

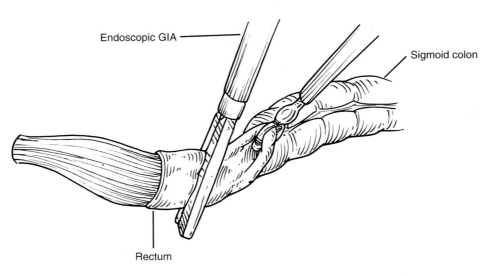

Endoscopic GIA

Sigmoid colon

Rectum

FIGURE 61–3

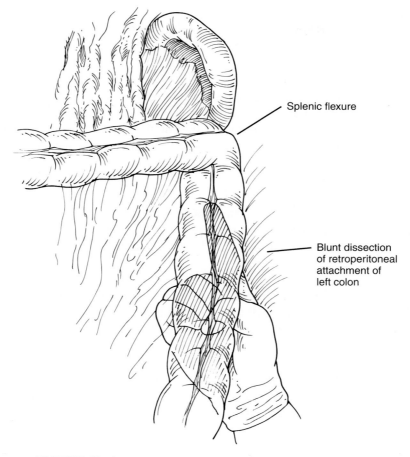

Splenic flexure

Blunt dissection
of retroperitoneal
attachment of
left colon

FIGURE 61–4

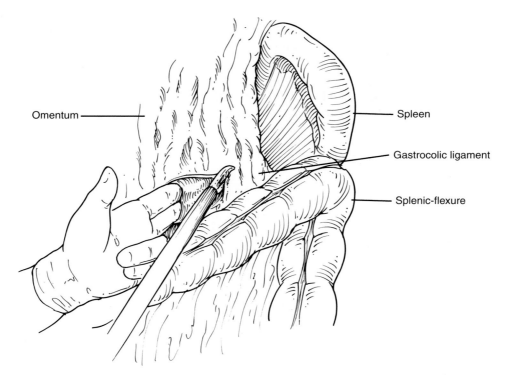

Omentum

Spleen

Gastrocolic ligament

Splenic-flexure

FIGURE 61–5

Primary Anastomosis

◆ The decision to restore bowel continuity depends on the primary diagnosis and clinical scenario.

◆ The mesentery to the proximal end of the anastomosis is clamped, divided, and ligated. An Ochsner bowel clamp is then placed across the bowel, and the specimen is divided and passed off the field. The proximal lumen of the colon is inspected for abnormalities and irrigated with saline. Care is taken to ensure full sterile technique is maintained without fecal spillage.

◆ A purse-string suture using 2-0 Prolene on an SH needle is taken circumferentially around the proximal end of the bowel. A 29-mm circular intraluminal stapler (ILS) is opened, and the anvil is placed in the lumen, synching the purse-string down **(Figure 61-6, A)**.

◆ The colon is replaced into the abdomen, and a pneumoperitoneum is recreated. An anvil grasper is used to pick up the anvil in the conventional laparoscopic technique. The left hand is used to guide the anvil to the pelvis in the hand-assisted technique.

◆ The perineal operator places the circular stapler into the rectum and is directed to the stapled end of the bowel. The main rod is deployed so that it exits either above or below the staple line **(Figure 61-6, B)**. The main rod and anvil are attached. The mesentery is checked for twists and for undue tension. The circular stapler is tightened and fired. The resulting rings are inspected for completion.

◆ A leak test is performed by introducing air into the rectum while occluding the proximal bowel. The anastomosis is submerged in saline and placed under intraluminal air tension. Presence of bubbles suggests an incomplete staple line and should be addressed accordingly.

◆ Loop ileostomy may be created to divert the fecal stream away from the distal anastomosis in the presence of unhealthy tissue or a tentative anastomosis.

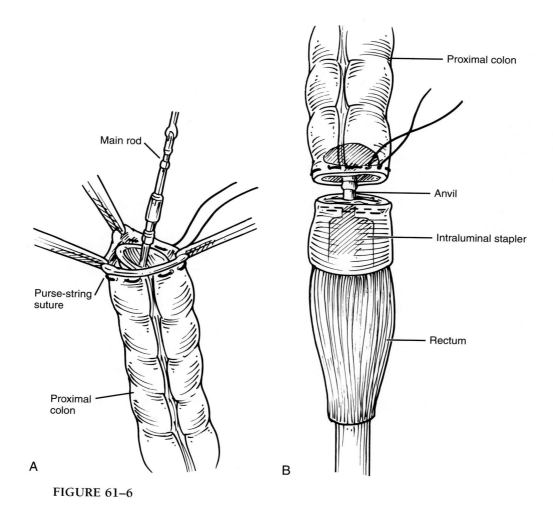

Main rod

Purse-string
suture

Proximal
colon

A

Proximal colon

Anvil

Intraluminal stapler

Rectum

B

FIGURE 61–6

Protecting Loop Ileostomy

- The following outlined steps may be done with the open abdomen using the Alexis wound retractor (Applied Medical) through the incision made to exteriorize the resected segment of colon.

- Umbilical tape is passed between the mesentery and distal ileum. A Vicryl stitch may be used to mark the up side of the ileostomy to avoid confusion in which side to mature.

- Two Ochsner clamps are placed on the anterior fascia of the rectus muscle, and an Allys clamp is placed on the skin between the two. The assistant maintains even traction so that all layers are parallel and aligned.

- An Ochsner clamp is placed on the skin over the ileostomy site and pulled up. A no. 10 blade knife is used to cut a circular disc.

- Electrocautery is used to cut through subcutaneous tissue down anterior rectus fascia, which is sharply divided. Muscle fibers are spread perpendicularly, and the peritoneum is cut longitudinally enough to snugly fit two fingers. Injury to the inferior epigastric vessels should be avoided.

- The ileostomy is wrapped in Seprafilm and brought out of the abdominal cavity through the ostomy site on traction using the umbilical tape for a length of at least 4 cm, taking care not to twist the mesentery. This will minimize adhesions and facilitate ease of takedown at a later time.

- The proximal limb is confirmed by visualizing the suture, and a transverse incision is made across the ileum using Bovie electrocautery.

- Vicryl sutures are placed through the mucosa at points equidistant from each other on the proximal limb, then through the seromuscular layer proximally at the skin level, and then to skin. The proximal limb is everted to form a spicket-like protuberance that falls into the ileostomy bag, diverting the sulcus away from the level of the skin. The distal limb is sutured to the inferior portion of the skin edge without eversion.

- The appliance is cut to fit circumferentially so that there are no gaps exposing the skin at the end of the procedure after skin is closed.

End Colostomy

- A left lower colostomy site is created in a similar fashion to the aforementioned technique for creation of a loop ileostomy.

- An Ochsner bowel clamp is passed through the aperture of the ostomy site and placed on the edge of the bowel to be exteriorized.

- The clamp is pulled through, taking care that there are no twists in the mesentery and no tension on the colostomy.

- The colostomy is matured in standard fashion after the abdomen is closed and the midline incision is protected.

4. CLOSING

- Surgical gloves are changed, and the Alexis wound retractor is removed, as are all other ports. Seprafilm is placed, and the anterior rectus fascia is reapproximated using 0 polydioxanone (PDS) in figure-of-eight interrupted sutures.

- The subcutaneous skin is irrigated with bacitracin antibiotic (50,000 U in 1 L saline).

- Staples are used to close the skin. A small umbilical bolster is created by placing a bacitracin-soaked cotton ball wrapped in Adaptic into the umbilical depression. This is left in place during the hospital stay and removed before discharge home.

- The orogastric tube is removed before extubation. A nasogastric tube should be placed if there is extensive lysis of adhesions or other indication for maintenance of a nasogastric tube postoperatively.

STEP 4: POSTOPERATIVE CARE

- The same principles of postoperative care followed for laparoscopic-assisted right colectomy apply to laparoscopic-assisted left and sigmoid colectomy, and can be referred to in Chapter 59.

STEP 5: PEARLS AND PITFALLS

- Division of the left colic artery may be necessary for adequate mobilization in creating a tension-free anastomosis. The ascending branch of the left colic artery should be preserved, allowing collateral flow from the middle colic artery back to the ascending left colic artery through the marginal arteries.

- Oncologic resection of the sigmoid colon mandates attention to preserve the meandering artery of Riolan during high ligation of the IMA for maintaining collateral blood flow to the proximal left colon.

- Consideration for placement of ureteral stents should be made for cases involving complicated diverticulitis or large bulky tumors. Although stents have not been shown to prevent injury, palpation of the stent may assist in timely recognition of ureteral location. In addition, injuries may be identified earlier during the intraoperative period by visualization of the stent, thus facilitating repair.

- The left ureter should be visualized and swept laterally before division of the IMA pedicle. Failure to do this may involve inclusion of the ureter with the pedicle, leading to one of the most common causes of ureteral injury during this procedure.

- High ligation of the IMA pedicle may injure the superior hypogatric (sympathetic) plexus because of entrapment and division of the nerves. This results in retrograde ejaculation. Care should be taken to identify the nerves and dissect them laterally before division of the pedicle.

- A lip of omentum may be mobilized to buttress the anastomosis, a consideration to make if the tissues are inflamed or friable.

- The inferior epigastric artery may be visualized and avoided before making the incision for an ostomy by transillumination of the anterior abdominal wall with the laparoscopic light.

- Tension on the ileostomy due to foreshortened mesentery or large abdominal pannus may be relieved by mobilization of the right colon.

SELECTED REFERENCES

1. Aalbers AG, Biere SS, van Berge Henegouwen MI, Bemelman WA: Hand-assisted or laparoscopic-assisted approach in colorectal surgery: A systematic review and meta-analysis. Surg Endosc 2008; 22:1769-1780.
2. Guidelines from the Joint Commission on Surgical Care Improvement Project Core Measurement Set. Available on the Internet: www.jointcommission.org/PerformanceMeasurement.
3. Zeng Q, Yu Z, You J, Zhang Q: Efficacy and safety of Seprafilm for preventing postoperative abdominal adhesion: Systematic review and meta-analysis. World J Surg 2007;31:2125-2131;2132 [discussion].

CHAPTER 62

TOTAL COLECTOMY

Valerie P. Bauer

STEP 1: SURGICAL ANATOMY

- A comprehensive understanding of the anatomy of the abdomen is critical before undertaking total abdominal colectomy **(Figure 62-1)**.

- The relationship of the colon to intraperitoneal and retroperitoneal attachments and structures should be fully understood.

- Particular attention should be paid to the location of the left ureter relative to the inferior mesenteric vascular pedicle. This is the most commonly injured area after vascular pedicle ligation.

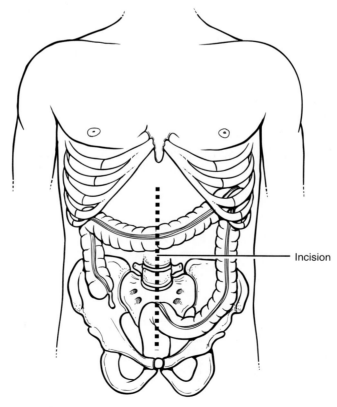

Incision

FIGURE 62–1

STEP 2: PREOPERATIVE CONSIDERATIONS

- Indications for total abdominal colectomy involve both emergent and elective scenarios for treatment of:
  - Ulcerative colitis
  - Crohn's disease of the large bowel with sparing of the distal sigmoid colon and rectum
  - Attenuated familial adenomatous polyposis
  - Synchronous multiple cancers
  - Perforated cecum due to distal colon cancer obstruction
  - Constipation

- Bowel continuity may or may not be restored depending on the clinical circumstance.

- If temporary or permanent ileostomy is planned, the patient should be marked preoperatively for either an end or loop ileostomy and educated concerning the new ostomy.

- Consideration for ureteral stenting should be made based on the extent of disease and prior abdominal operations.

- Aspirin, other blood thinners, and vitamin E should be stopped for 10 days before the procedure.

- Preoperative laboratory and cardiac evaluations should be obtained based on patient comorbidities.

- Patients taking steroids preoperatively should receive a stress dose of hydrocortisone 100 mg intravenously (IV) before the operation. This should be continued postoperatively and tapered accordingly.

- Consideration toward placing an epidural catheter preoperatively should be made for postoperative pain control and minimization of parenteral narcotic use and associated postoperative ileus.

- Bowel preparation should include mechanical bowel preparation of the surgeon's choice. Sodium phosphate bowel preparations should be used with caution because of acute phosphate nephropathy.

- Appropriate preoperative antibiotics are administered parenterally within 1 hour before cut time, according to the Surgical Care Improvement Project (SCIP) quality measures defined for elective colorectal operations. We use ertapenem (Invanz) 1 g IV without redosing, because it has 24-hour duration of action.

STEP 3: OPERATIVE STEPS

1. POSITIONING

- Proper positioning of the patient should be directed by the primary surgeon to ensure consistency and safety to the patient.

- The patient should be placed supine on the operating table. After administration of anesthesia, sequential compression devices should be placed on the legs and a Foley catheter inserted. The legs are placed in low lithotomy position with Allen stirrups. The boots are adjusted so that each leg rests in a flexed position without pressure on the popliteal fossa. Padding is used to shield the skin from all hard objects.

- Abdominal and pubic hair is clipped off.

- A Bair Hugger Warmer is placed across the patient's chest.

- An orogastric tube is placed, to be removed after surgery unless a nasogastric tube is indicated, as in cases of extensive lysis of adhesions.

- Rigid proctoscopy is performed to clean the rectum of residual stool and to confirm absence of pathologic findings in the rectum that may need to be addressed in the operating room.

- The abdomen and perineum are prepped in standard fashion according to the surgeon's preference. The scrotum should be positioned away from the perineum.

2. INCISION

♦ The pubic symphysis and manubrial notch are palpated and marked. A line is drawn down the entire midline in case the incision needs to be extended during the later part of the procedure **(Figure 62-2)**.

♦ A no. 10 blade knife is used to make an incision from a point 2 cm above the umbilicus down to the pubic symphysis.

♦ The abdomen is entered sharply. Care is taken to dissect around the bladder obliquely. The incision is extended through the pyramidalis muscle to the pubic symphysis.

♦ The abdomen is explored for additional pathologic abnormalities. The terminal ileum is identified and the entire small bowel is run proximally to the ligament of Treitz. The liver is palpated for the presence of masses.

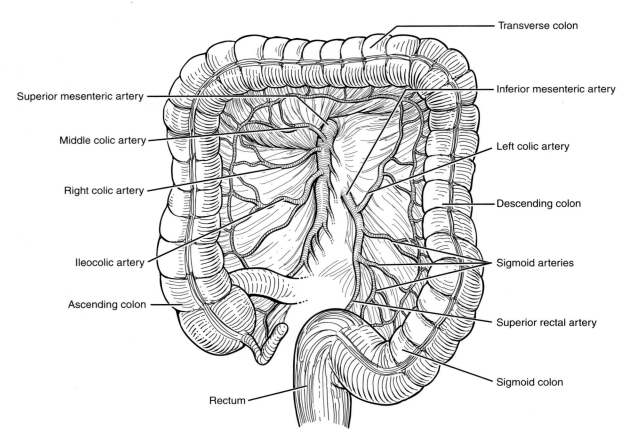

FIGURE 62–2

3. DISSECTION

◆ A Bookwalter retractor is set up. Laparotomy pads are placed along each side of the abdominal wall. Two ratcheted short Richardson retractors are positioned opposite each other in lower oblique fashion, taking care not to impinge on the femoral canal.

◆ The small bowel is packed upward using a moist blue towel with a radiopaque loop attached to it, and a wide Deaver ratcheted retractor is bent and placed to maintain exposure without compression of the aorta or inferior vena cava.

◆ In female patients, the uterus should be retracted by placing a figure-of-eight stitch with 2-0 Vicryl through the posterior wall of the uterus as a retraction stitch. A ratcheted bladder blade is then placed to retract the uterus and bladder.

◆ The surgeon on the right side of the patient pulls up on the sigmoid colon so that the lateral peritoneal attachment is on tension **(Figure 62-3).** Electrocautery is used to divide the attachment.

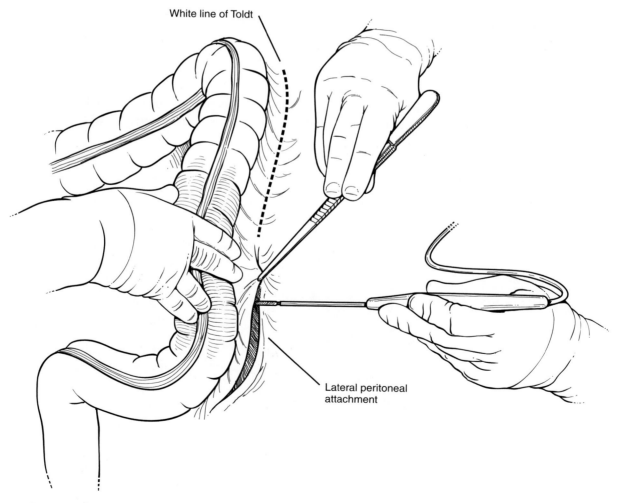

FIGURE 62–3

◆ The recess at the base of the mesosigmoid, called the intersigmoid fossa, is identified and delicately incised. The left ureter lies just deep to it and is identified and mobilized laterally. The ureter courses medially and parallel to the gonadal vessels, another important landmark to identify (**Figure 62-4**).

◆ The surgeon to the left of the patient isolates the inferior mesenteric pedicle. This is done by identifying the avascular window at the base of the mesosigmoid while tenting the mesentery up. The window is incised against the surgeon's finger from the right with electrocautery, and is extended proximally to the pelvic brim and distally down to the level of the sacral promontory bilaterally.

◆ The peritoneal covering of pedicle is cut, and excess mesenteric fat is thinned in preparation for ligation.

◆ Seurat clamps are used to divide the pedicle. A 2-0 Vicryl tie is used to ligate both the base and specimen side of the pedicle. If the artery feels calcified or has atherosclerotic plaque visibly extruding from the vessel after clamping, a 2-0 Vicryl stick tie should be placed to ensure hemostasis of the pedicle base (**Figure 62-5**).

◆ The rectosigmoid mesentery is sequentially clamped, divided, and ligated to the serosal edge of the colon. The surface is cleaned of excess mesenteric and epiploic fat in preparation for division.

◆ Before division, the left colon is mobilized as much as possible by being divided from its retroperitoneal lateral attachments upward toward the spleen (**Figure 62-6**).

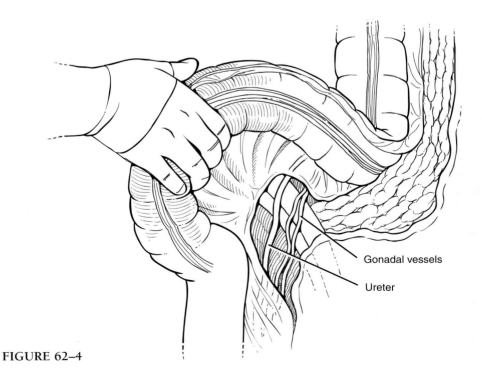

Gonadal vessels

Ureter

FIGURE 62–4

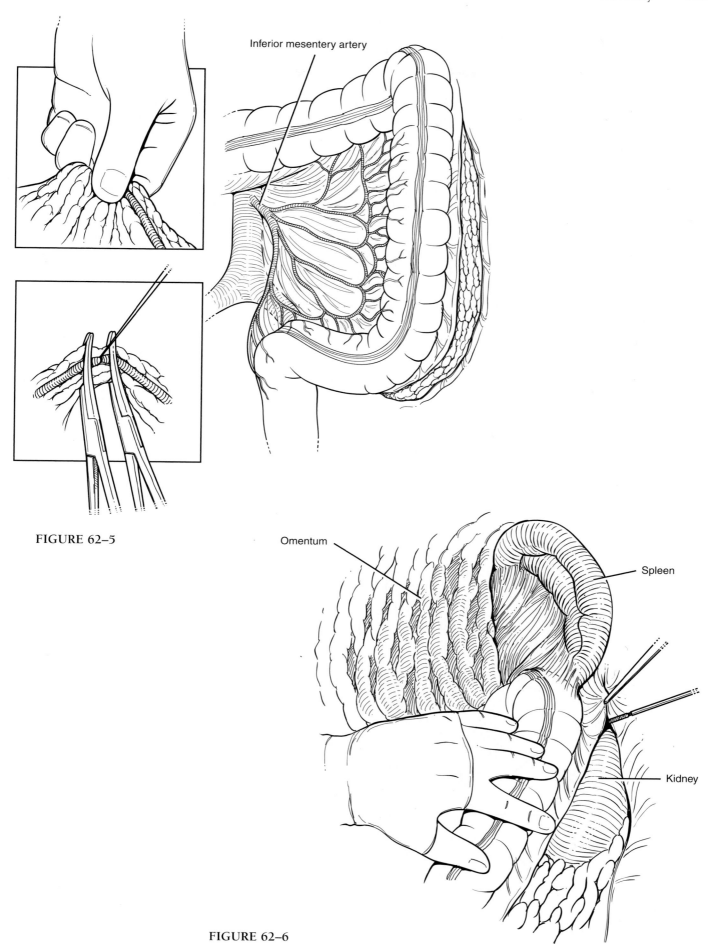

Inferior mesentery artery

FIGURE 62–5

Omentum

Spleen

Kidney

FIGURE 62–6

◆ Method of division of the rectosigmoid depends on whether intestinal continuity will be reestablished. Either a linear stapler or division between two Ochsner bowel clamps may be used to divide the bowel at the level of the sacral promontory **(Figure 62-7)**. The proximal rectosigmoid end is wrapped with a laparotomy pad and may be clamped if there is concern for fecal leakage through the staple line during mobilization. The distal stump is marked with a 2-0 Prolene suture for future recognition if reversal is a possibility.

◆ The Deaver blade is removed along with the blue towel. The transverse colon is pulled downward, and the lesser sac entered by incising the filmy attachment of the gastrocolic ligament to the colon **(Figure 62-8)**.

◆ The splenic flexure is mobilized by the surgeon standing on the patient's right side. The assistant may move to the position between the patient's legs for improved visualization. The splenocolic ligament is divided close to the bowel wall to avoid injury to the spleen **(Figure 62-9)**.

◆ Once the splenic flexure is down, the remainder of the gastrocolic ligament is detached from the transverse colon.

◆ Attention is then turned to the right colon. The small bowel may be loosely packed away, once again, depending on the surgeon's preference.

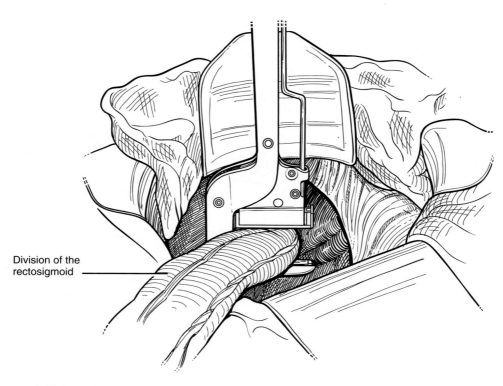

Division of the rectosigmoid

FIGURE 62–7

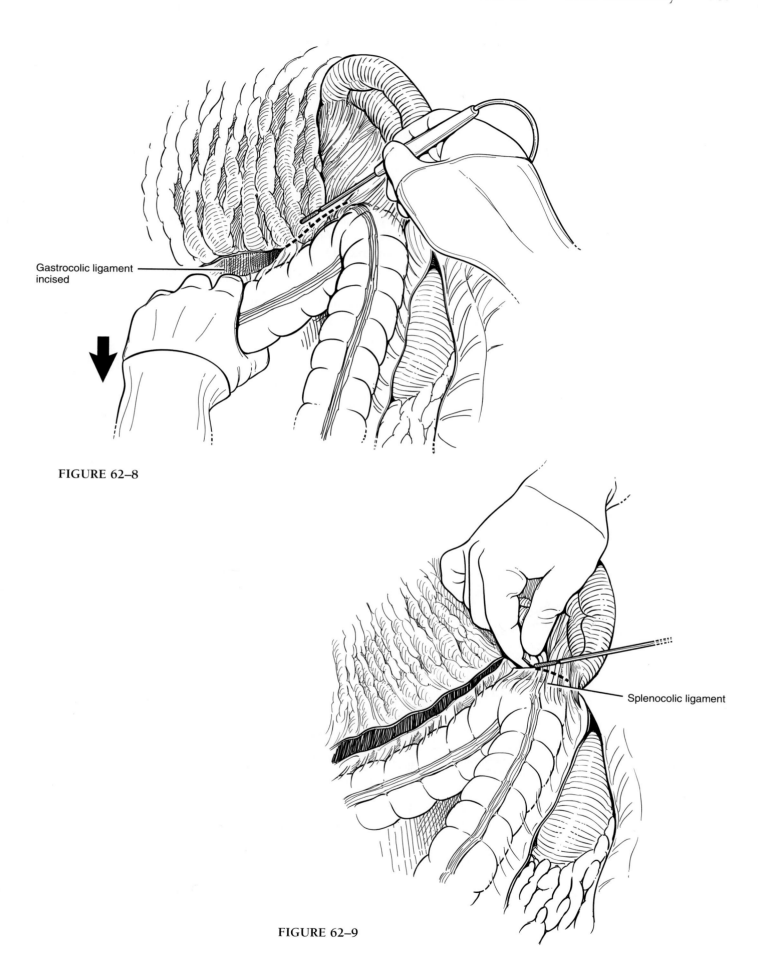

Gastrocolic ligament incised

FIGURE 62–8

Splenocolic ligament

FIGURE 62–9

◆ The cecum is retracted up away from the pelvic brim. The lateral peritoneal attachment is divided, and gentle blunt dissection is used to separate the ascending colon from the retroperitoneum. The duodenum is identified and dissected downward and away from colonic mesentery **(Figure 62-10)**.

◆ The phrenocolic and hepatocolic ligaments are clamped, divided, and ligated using 2-0 Vicryl suture.

◆ The ligament of Treves is identified and divided along with the parietal peritoneum of the terminal ileum. The ileocolic vascular pedicle is identified, clamped, divided, and ligated in similar fashion, as mentioned earlier **(Figure 62-11)**.

◆ The mesentery is scored to the point of ileal resection. The vascular arcades are clamped, divided, and ligated, and the ileum is divided between two Ochsner clamps.

◆ It is important to note that the method of pedicle ligation and mesenteric division will vary drastically for patients with ulcerative colitis. The possibility of having an ileal anal pouch in the future mandates that ileal length and vasculature be preserved. In this circumstance, the ileocolic artery is preserved, and the mesentery is divided close to the right colon **(Figure 62-12)**.

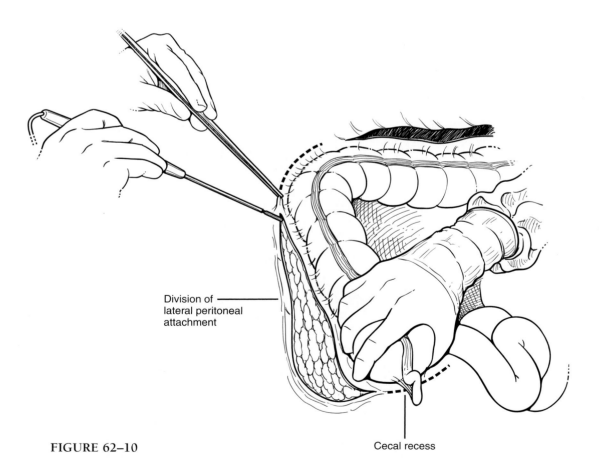

Division of lateral peritoneal attachment

Cecal recess

FIGURE 62–10

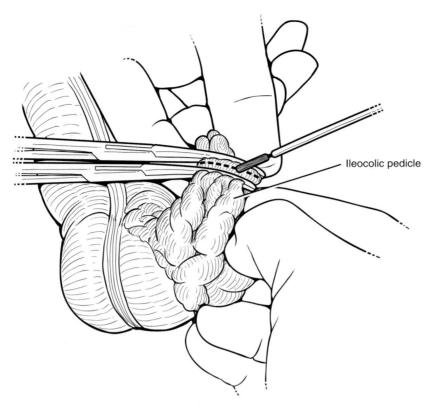

FIGURE 62–11

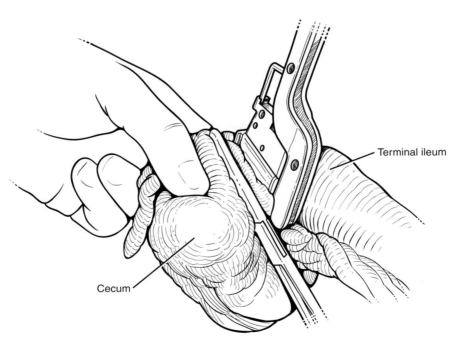

FIGURE 62–12

◆ The remaining vascular pedicles of the ascending, transverse, and descending colon are sequentially visualized, clamped, divided, and ligated. Remaining proximal to the vessels decreases the number of vessels that need to be divided.

◆ The specimen is removed from the table and opened off the field to confirm pathologic findings and rule out additional findings.

◆ All laparotomy pads are removed from the abdomen, and the Bookwalter retractor is taken down. If a retraction stitch was placed in the uterus, the stitch should be tied down to prevent bleeding from the myometrium.

◆ The abdomen is irrigated with warm sterile saline.

Brooke Ileostomy
◆ Two Ochsner clamps are placed on the anterior fascia of the rectus muscle, and an Allys clamp is placed on the skin between the two. The assistant maintains even traction so that all layers are parallel and aligned.

◆ An Ochsner clamp is placed on the skin over the ileostomy site and pulled up. A no. 10 blade knife is used to cut out a circular disc. The ileostomy is placed through the summit of the infraumbilical bulge through the split thickness of the rectus muscle. Electrocautery is used to cut through the subcutaneous tissue down to the anterior fascia of the rectus muscle, which is sharply divided. Muscle fibers are spread perpendicularly, and the peritoneum is cut longitudinally enough to snugly fit two fingers. Injury to the inferior epigastric vessels should be avoided.

◆ The ileostomy is brought out of the abdominal cavity for a length of approximately 5 cm, taking care not to twist the mesentery. If the ileostomy is temporary, it should be wrapped in a sheet of Seprafilm to prevent adhesions and facilitate takedown in the future.

◆ The abdomen is closed before the ileostomy is matured (see following section, Abdominal Closure), and the incision is protected with a clean, dry towel.

◆ Stitches using 2-0 chromic are placed through the mucosa at points equidistant from each other and through the seromuscular layer proximally at the skin level. The ileostomy is everted so that the end falls away from the mucocutaneous junction. The appliance is cut to fit circumferentially so that there are no gaps exposing the skin.

Ileorectal Anastomosis
◆ The decision to restore bowel continuity depends on the primary diagnosis and clinical scenario.

◆ Dissection for ileorectal anastomosis differs in sequence from the previously mentioned steps in that the operation begins with takedown of the right colon and proceeds clockwise to the final step of division of the sigmoid colon from the rectum.

◆ Preparation for open lumen of bowl mandates meticulous attention to detail to prevent fecal spillage into the abdominal cavity. A blue towel is folded and placed on the field, which will contain contaminated instruments: a metal pool sucker, Allys bowel clamps, and sponge stick. Moist laparotomy pads are packed around the rectum.

◆ A Glassman clamp is placed across the distal sigmoid colon, and a knife is used to detach the colon. Allys clamps are placed on the mesenteric and antimesenteric edges of the open lumen of bowel, and a sponge stick is used to blot and clean the edges.

◆ The terminal ileum is similarly divided off the Ochsner clamp and grasped with Allys clamps. Care is taken to place the Ochsner obliquely on the small bowel to match the size of the rectum. A Cheatle incision may be made on the antimesenteric border to enlarge the lumen.

◆ The antimesenteric and mesenteric borders of each lumen are lined up. Care is taken to ensure that the small bowel is not twisted around its mesentery.

◆ A double-armed 4-0 Maxon monofilament suture is used to create a single-layered running anastomosis.

◆ The integrity of the anastomosis may be checked using the proctoscope to insufflate through the rectum while submerged under saline. Presence of bubbles requires single interrupted sutures to repair the leak.

◆ The surgeons' gloves are changed before skin closure.

4. ABDOMINAL CLOSURE

◆ The omentum is moved to the side and placed in either paracolic gutter. One sheet of Seprafilm is cut in half and placed over the bowel under the incision. This minimizes adhesion formation and makes reentry easier for future operations.

◆ The abdomen is closed using no. 1 polydioxanone (PDS) running suture.

◆ The subcutaneous tissue is irrigated with bacitracin irrigation, and the skin is closed with staples.

◆ The umbilicus is reapproximated. A bacitracin-soaked cotton ball wrapped in Adaptic is packed into the umbilicus as a bolster.

STEP 4: POSTOPERATIVE CARE

◆ Adherence to a postoperative colorectal clinical pathway ensures standardization of care.

◆ Adequate pain control is achieved using patient-controlled analgesia or epidural catheter.

◆ Stress ulcer prophylaxis, such as famotidine (Pepcid) 20 mg IV every 12 hours, should be used if indicated.

◆ All patients should receive prophylaxis for deep venous thrombosis, consisting of sequential compression devices while in bed and heparin 5000 U subcutaneously every 8 hours or enoxaparin 40 mg subcutaneously within 24 hours of surgery. Dosing schedules should start on postoperative day 1 after results of morning laboratory tests are back to ensure that there is no significant drop in hemoglobin to suggest postoperative bleeding.

◆ Adequate intravenous fluid should be administered with monitoring of urine output via urimeter on the Foley bag.

◆ The diet may be limited to ice chips and sips of water in the postanesthesia care unit and on postoperative day 1. Return of bowel function is measured by the frequency and pitch of bowel sounds, lack of abdominal distention, and the patient's subjective will to eat. A clear liquid diet may be offered as sips of clear liquids without carbonation and without a straw to minimize accumulation of air in the intestine. This may be advanced ad lib as bowel function returns.

◆ Early ambulation is crucial for return of bowel function. Patients should be instructed to walk multiple times a day beginning on postoperative day 1, and should be encouraged to do so frequently.

◆ The umbilical bolster should be removed before the patient leaves the hospital. Skin staples are removed on postoperative day 10.

STEP 5: PEARLS AND PITFALLS

◆ Placement of deep ratcheted Richardson retractors may impinge on the femoral nerve against the psoas muscle, causing compression and femoral nerve neuropathy. The short ratcheted retractors should be used to avoid this, even in patients with thick body walls.

◆ The use of ertapenem 1 g IV for prophylaxis of surgical site infections after colon surgery has the advantage of once-a-day dosing so that therapeutic levels persist throughout the surgery without need for additional doses during long cases. Ertapenem is a broad-spectrum antibiotic covering enteric flora and has been approved by the SCIP as an acceptable prophylactic antibiotic for elective colorectal surgery.

- ◆ Visualizing the left ureter before dividing the inferior mesenteric artery will decrease the probability of inadvertent ureteral ligation. This step should be done every time after clamps are placed across the pedicle, before the artery is cut.

- ◆ In patients who may need future completion proctectomy, such as those with ulcerative colitis, care should be taken not to enter the avascular mesorectal plane after division of the mesosigmoid. This preserves the integrity of the tissue plane and improves the relative ease of future dissection.

- ◆ Every measure should be taken to preserve the ileal blood supply in patients with ulcerative colitis for potential future ileal pouch creation.

- ◆ Care should be taken not to twist the small bowel mesentery when bringing out an ileostomy or creating an ileorectal anastomosis. This can be done by identifying the superior mesenteric artery at the root and "shaking hands" with the mesentery to feel for twists.

- ◆ The use of Seprafilm underneath the incision minimizes abdominal adhesions and improves ease of entry on subsequent laparotomies. In addition, wrapping a temporary ileostomy with Seprafilm allows for easier takedown later.

SELECTED REFERENCES

1 Beck DE, Opelka FG: Perioperative steroid use in colorectal patients. Dis Colon Rectum 1996;39: 995-999.
2. Itani KMF, Wilson SE, Awad SS, et al: Ertapenem versus cefotetan prophylaxis in elective colorectal surgery. N Engl J Med 2006;355:2640-2651.
3. Zeng Q, Yu Z, You J, Zhang Q: Efficacy and safety of Seprafilm for preventing postoperative abdominal adhesion: Systematic review and meta-analysis. World J Surg 2007;31:2125-2131; 2132 [discussion].
4. Law WL, Bailey HR, Max E, et al: Single-layer continuous colon and rectal anastomosis using monofilament absorbable suture (Maxon): Study of 500 cases. Dis Colon Rectum 1999;42:736-740.
5. Max E, Sweeney WB, Bailey HR, et al: Results of 1,000 single-layer continuous polypropylene intestinal anastomoses. Am J Surg 1991;162:461-467.

CHAPTER 63

ILEOANAL ANASTOMOSIS (STRAIGHT AND J POUCH)

Valerie P. Bauer

STEP 1: SURGICAL ANATOMY

- A comprehensive understanding of the anatomy of the abdomen is critical before undertaking proctocolectomy.

- The relationship of the colon to intraperitoneal and retroperitoneal attachments and structures should be fully understood.

- The anatomy of the rectum and surrounding pelvic structures should also be appreciated. This includes understanding of the fascial relationship of the rectum to the anterior and posterior avascular planes of Denonvillier and Waldeyer; the sympathetic and parasympathetic innervation of the superior and inferior hypogastric nerve plexus and nervi erigentes; and arterial, venous, and lymphatic drainage of the rectum and anal canal.

- Particular attention should be paid to the location of the left ureter relative to the inferior mesenteric vascular pedicle. This is the most commonly injured area after inferior mesenteric artery (IMA) vascular pedicle ligation.

STEP 2: PREOPERATIVE CONSIDERATIONS

- Indications for proctocolectomy involve both emergent and elective scenarios for treatment of:
  - Ulcerative colitis
  - Crohn's disease of the large bowel and rectum
  - Familial adenomatosis coli
  - Synchronous multiple cancers

- Bowel continuity may or may not be restored depending on the clinical circumstance.

- Temporary loop ileostomy is used to protect the ileal pouch anal anastomosis (IPAA), and should be strongly considered in this operation. The patient should be marked preoperatively and educated concerning both the new ostomy and pouch.

- Consideration for ureteral stenting should be made based on the extent of disease and prior abdominal operations.

- Aspirin, other blood thinners, and vitamin E should be stopped for 10 days before the procedure.

- Preoperative laboratory and cardiac evaluations should be obtained based on the patient's comorbidities.

- Patients taking steroids preoperatively should receive a stress dose of hydrocortisone 100 mg intravenously (IV) before the operation. This should be continued postoperatively and tapered accordingly.

- Consideration toward placing an epidural catheter preoperatively should be made for postoperative pain control and minimization of parenteral narcotic use and associated postoperative ileus.

- Bowel preparation should include mechanical bowel preparation as per the surgeon's preference. Caution should be taken when using sodium phosphate preparation because of the risk of acute phosphate nephropathy.

- Appropriate antibiotics should be given parenterally within 1 hour of the incision.

1. POSITIONING

- Proper positioning of the patient should be directed by the primary surgeon to ensure consistency and safety to the patient.

- The patient should be placed supine on the operating table. A thromboembolism-deterrent (TED) hose and sequential compression devices should be placed on the legs, and a Foley catheter should be inserted.

- The legs are placed in low lithotomy position using Allen stirrups **(Figure 63-1)**. The boots are adjusted so that each leg rests in a flexed position without pressure on the popliteal fossa. Padding is used to shield the skin from all hard objects.

- Abdominal and pubic hair is clipped off.

- A warmer is placed appropriately on the patient to ensure normothermia during the procedure.

- An orogastric or nasogastric tube is placed after induction of anesthesia.

- A small roll is placed under the patient's lower back.

- Rigid proctoscopy is performed to clean the rectum of residual stool and to confirm absence of pathologic abnormalities in the rectum that may need to be addressed in the operating room.

- The premarked ileostomy site is scored using a needle to avoid losing the mark during the skin preparation.

- The abdomen and perineum are prepped. The scrotum should be positioned away from the perineum.

- Draping the patient:
  - The patient is draped in standard fashion according to the surgeon's preference.
  - An under buttocks drape should be included, because there will be work from the perineal side.

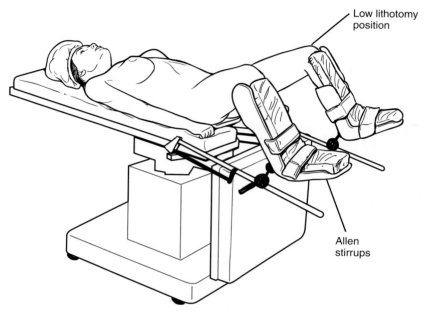

Low lithotomy
position

Allen
stirrups

FIGURE 63–1

STEP 3: OPERATIVE STEPS

1. INCISION

♦ A standard midline incision is made using a no. 10 blade knife from a point 2 cm above the umbilicus, through midline, and down to the pubic symphysis.

♦ The abdomen is entered sharply and dissection is carried around the bladder obliquely. The pubic symphysis is palpated, and the incision is extended through the pyramidalis muscle as the inferior boundary of the incision.

♦ The abdomen is explored for additional pathologic findings. The terminal ileum is identified, and the entire small bowel is run proximally to the ligament of Treitz. The liver is palpated for the presence of masses.

Exposure
♦ A Bookwalter retractor is set up so that the arm attaches to the right side of the table.

♦ Moist laparotomy pads are folded in half and placed along the length of each side of the abdominal wall. Two ratcheted Richardson retractors are positioned opposite each other in lower oblique fashion, taking care not to impinge on the femoral canal.

♦ The small bowel is packed upward using a moist blue towel with a radiopaque loop attached to it, and a wide Deaver ratcheted retractor is bent and placed to maintain exposure without compression of the aorta or inferior vena cava.

♦ In female patients, the uterus should be retracted by placing a figure-of-eight stitch with 2-0 Vicryl through the posterior wall of the uterus as a retraction stitch. A ratcheted bladder blade is then placed to retract the uterus and bladder.

2. DISSECTION

♦ Total abdominal colectomy is performed according to the steps outlined in Chapter 62. Please refer to that chapter for procedural details.

♦ The recess at the base of the mesosigmoid, called the intersigmoid fossa, is identified and delicately incised. The left ureter lies just deep to intersigmoid fossa and is identified and mobilized laterally. The ureter courses medially and parallel to the gonadal vessels, another important landmark to identify.

♦ The inferior mesenteric pedicle is isolated. This is done by identifying the avascular window at the base of the mesosigmoid while tenting the mesentery up. The window is incised and extended proximally to the pelvic brim and distally down to the level of the sacral promontory bilaterally.

- The pedicle is thinned, clamped, divided, and ligated in standard fashion. Identification of the left ureter should be made before this to ensure it has not been drawn up into the pedicle.

- The posterior avascular mesorectal plane is entered, and sharp dissection is carried down to the levator muscles. Care is taken to ensure that the superior and inferior hypogastric nerve plexus running deep to this fascial plane is not damaged (see comments in Pearls and Pitfalls section).

- Lateral dissection is then carried down in the appropriate avascular plane. Care is taken during division of the lateral rectal stalks. The pelvic plexus named nervi erigentes—affecting erectile function—as well as the middle rectal artery, are in close proximity to these stalks.

- Anterior dissection is carried between the anterior avascular plane of Denonvillier and the reproductive structures. This is done down to the levator ani muscles.

- The decision to staple or hand sew the ileal pouch anastomosis is determined by the clinical scenario. For example, patients with ulcerative colitis who do not have high-grade dysplasia may have a stapled anastomosis with mucosal surveillance on a regular basis. Patients at high risk for developing malignancy (presence of cancer or high-grade dysplasia) should have mucosectomy and hand-sewn ileal anal anastomosis.

- A stapled anastomosis may be placed as low to the dentate line as anatomically possible **(Figure 63-2)**. The posterior mesorectum tapers distally, so there should not be excess vascular tissue posteriorly, once the appropriate level of dissection has been reached.

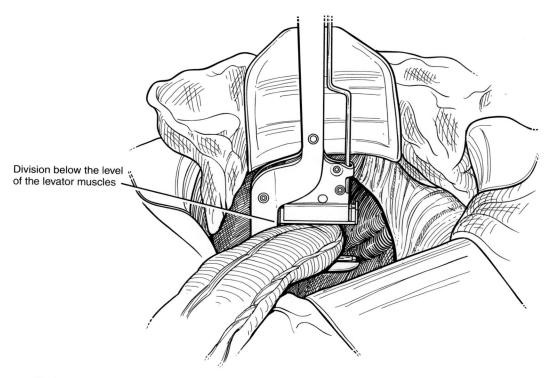

Division below the level
of the levator muscles

FIGURE 63–2

◆ The specimen is detached from the proximal small bowel using a 75-mm linear stapler **(Figure 63-3).**

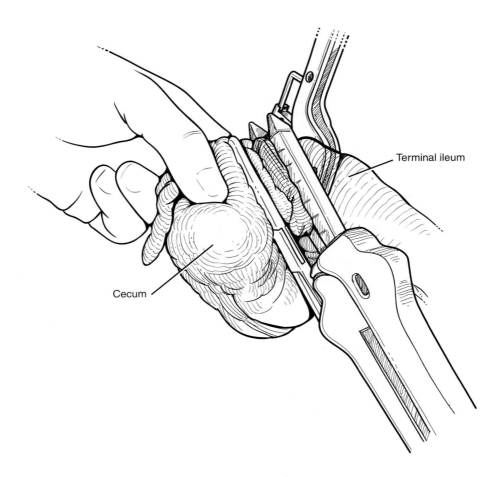

Terminal ileum

Cecum

FIGURE 63–3

Creation of the Ileal Pouch

◆ Attention to the method of pedicle ligation of the ileocolic artery is of paramount importance when performing proctocolectomy with the possibility of ileal pouch creation. The ileocolic artery should be preserved through its entire distance, taking care to hug the mesenteric border of the cecum and distal terminal ileum before division of the bowel.

◆ Adequate length of the mesentery will dictate reach to the pelvis. A good preliminary length is 1 to 2 cm distal to the pubic symphysis when measuring the apex of the pouch. Inadequate length may be regained by scoring the peritoneum or by distal ligation of the superior mesenteric artery (SMA), provided adequate collateral flow exists through the ileal branch **(Figures 63-4 and 63-5).**

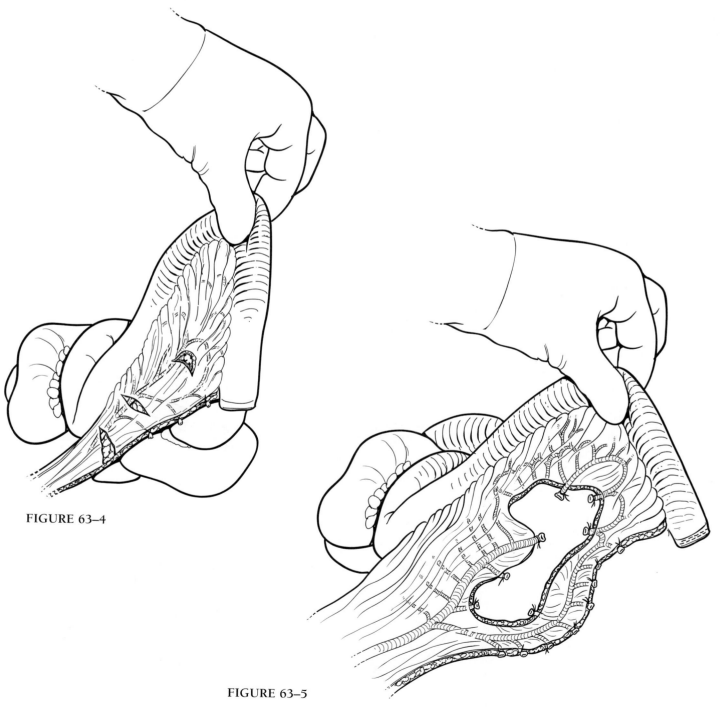

FIGURE 63–4

FIGURE 63–5

◆ The apex of the pedicle is identified, and the pouch is measured so that it is approximately 15 to 20 cm from the apex **(Figure 63-6)**.

◆ The apex of the pouch is entered using Bovie electocautery **(Figure 63-7)**.

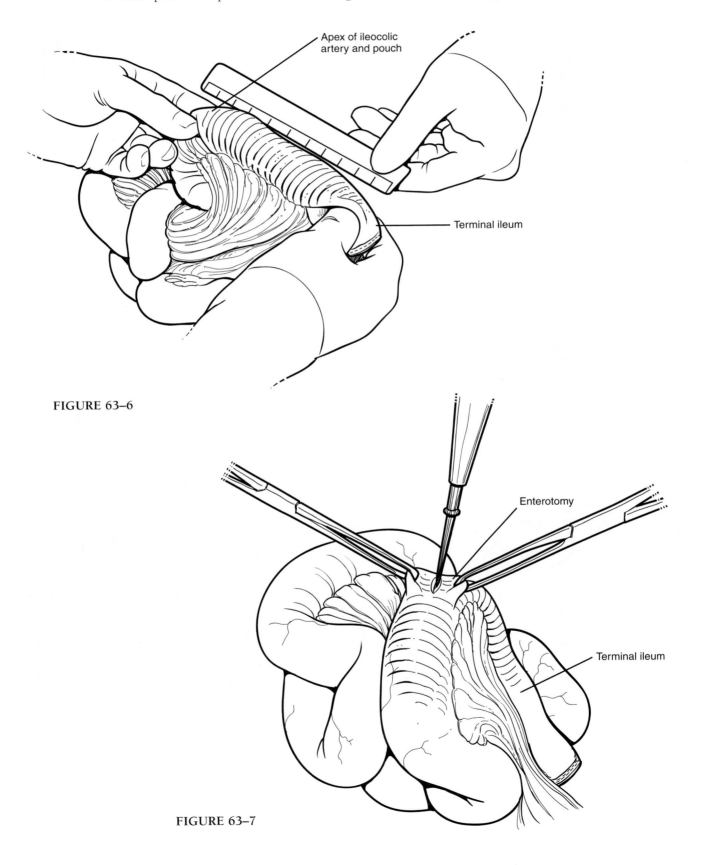

Apex of ileocolic artery and pouch

Terminal ileum

FIGURE 63–6

Enterotomy

Terminal ileum

FIGURE 63–7

◆ The mesentery is positioned anterior to the pouch, because this is the shortest distance to the pelvis with the least amount of tension on the pedicle.

◆ A 75-mm linear blue-load stapler is sequentially used to fire between the two limbs at the antimesenteric border, thus creating the pouch (**Figures 63-8 and 63-9**).

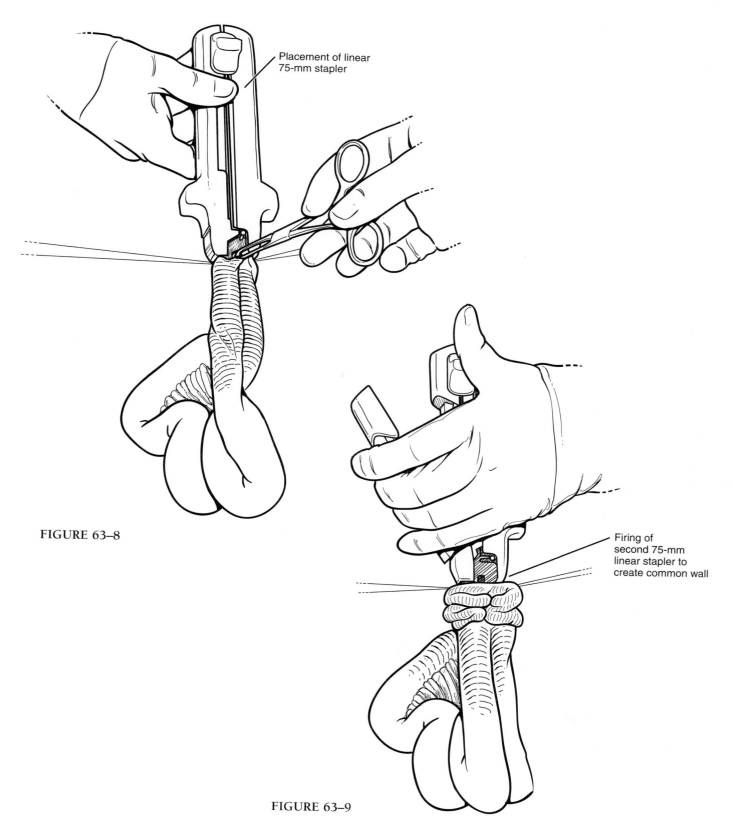

Placement of linear
75-mm stapler

FIGURE 63–8

Firing of
second 75-mm
linear stapler to
create common wall

FIGURE 63–9

Hand-Sewn Anastomosis

◆ The patient is positioned from low to high lithotomy **(Figure 63-10)**. The perineal operator places a Lone Star retractor in the anal canal. The dentate line is drawn down to the
anal verge by sequential placement of retractor hooks **(Figure 63-11)**. A Parks anal retractor may be placed to improve visualization of the anal canal. Mucosectomy is initiated first
by infiltrating 10 to 20 mL of 0.25% bupivacaine (Marcaine) with 1:200,000 epinephrine
circumferentially, raising the mucosa off the longitudinal muscle. The mucosa is circumferentially incised using electrocautery or sharp dissection. Metzenbaum scissors are used to
lift the mucosa off the muscle proximally. Once the mucosa falls back circumferentially, a
full-thickness incision is made laterally and carried circumferentially around the distal
rectum. Once the specimen is free, the ileal pouch is prepared for anastomosis.

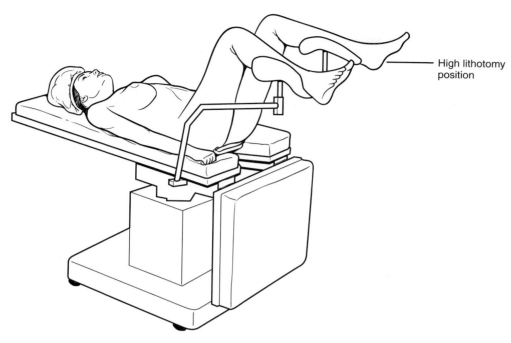

High lithotomy
position

FIGURE 63–10

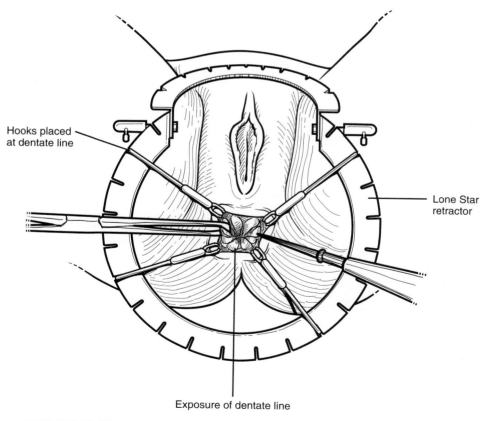

Hooks placed
at dentate line

Lone Star
retractor

Exposure of dentate line

FIGURE 63–11

◆ A full-thickness stitch using a long 2-0 Vicryl suture is taken at the antimesenteric edge of the pouch opening (posterior) and passed to the perineal operator through the anal canal **(Figure 63-12)**. Using the same suture, a full-thickness stitch is taken through the dentate line posteriorly. This process is repeated for both lateral sides, and finally the anterior side. The pouch is cinched down into the pelvis, and each suture is tied down **(Figure 63-13)**. Circumferential sutures are placed between each stitch in full-thickness fashion, taking care to incorporate an edge of pouch with the dentate line. The anastomosis and mesentery should be checked to ensure both are free from tension and there are no twists.

◆ The Lone Star retractor is removed, and the dentate is allowed to retract back into the anal canal. Proctoscopy is performed, and the anastomosis is checked for air leaks by insufflating while the proximal small bowel is clamped under saline.

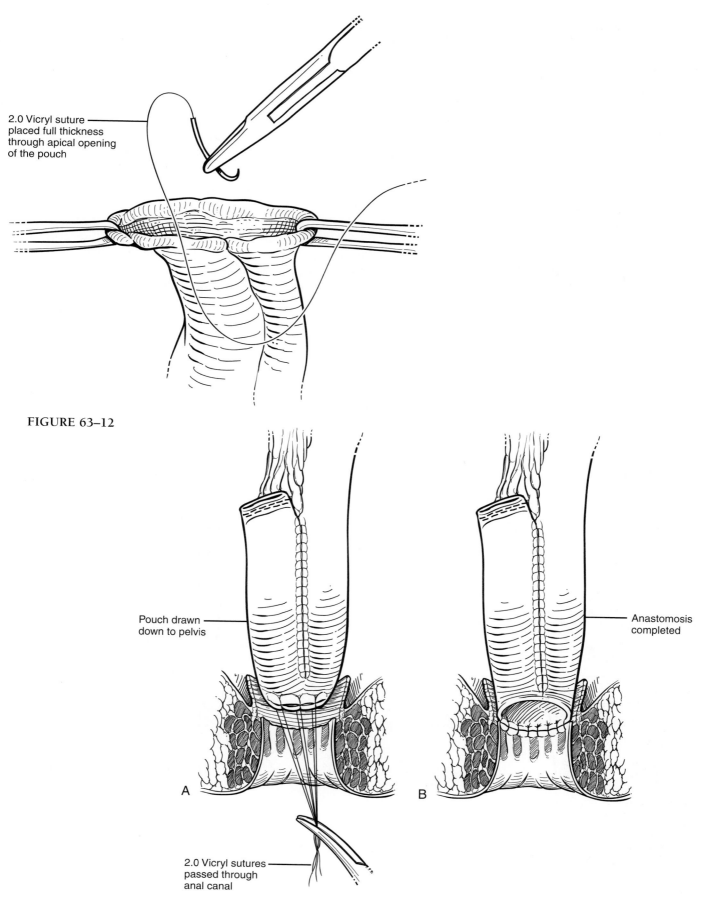

2.0 Vicryl suture
placed full thickness
through apical opening
of the pouch

FIGURE 63–12

Pouch drawn
down to pelvis

Anastomosis
completed

A   B

2.0 Vicryl sutures
passed through
anal canal

FIGURE 63–13

Stapled Anastomosis

◆ A purse-string suture using 2-0 Prolene on an SH needle is taken circumferentially around the proximal end of the bowel **(Figures 63-14 and 63-15).** A 29-mm circular intraluminal stapler (ILS) is opened, and the anvil is placed in the lumen of the pouch, cinching the purse-string down.

◆ The perineal operator places the circular stapler into the rectum and is directed to the stapled end of the bowel **(Figure 63-16).** The main rod is deployed so that it exits either above or below the staple line. The main rod and anvil are attached. The mesentery is checked for twists and for undue tension. The circular stapler is tightened and fired. The resulting rings are inspected for completion.

◆ A leak test is performed by introducing air into the pouch while occluding the proximal bowel. The anastomosis is submerged in saline and placed under intraluminal air tension. Presence of bubbles suggests an incomplete staple line and should be addressed accordingly.

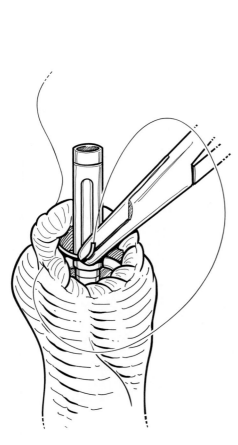

FIGURE 63–14

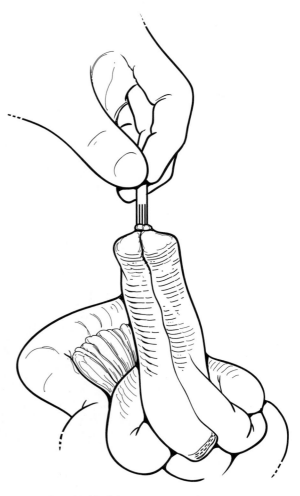

FIGURE 63–15

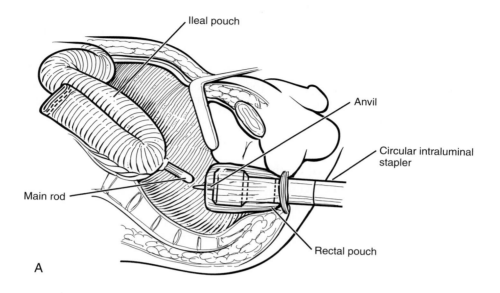

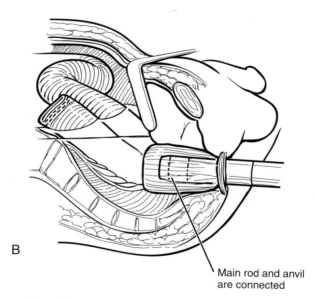

FIGURE 63–16

Brooke Ileostomy

◆ A protecting Brooke loop ileostomy may be created in the right lower quadrant through the rectus abdominis muscle to protect the pouch while it heals.

◆ Umbilical tape is passed between the mesentery and distal ileum. A Vicryl stitch may be used to mark the proximal limb of the ileostomy to avoid confusion about which side to mature.

◆ Two Ochsner clamps are placed on the anterior fascia of the rectus muscle, and an Allys clamp is placed on the skin between the two. The assistant maintains even traction so that all layers are parallel and aligned.

◆ An Ochsner clamp is placed on the skin over the ileostomy site and pulled up. A no. 10 blade knife is used to cut a circular disc.

◆ Electrocautery is used to cut through subcutaneous tissue down to the anterior rectus fascia, which is sharply divided. Muscle fibers are spread perpendicularly, and the peritoneum is cut longitudinally enough to snugly fit two fingers. Injury to the inferior epigastric vessels should be avoided.

◆ The ileostomy is wrapped in Seprafilm and brought out of the abdominal cavity through the ostomy site on traction using the umbilical tape for a length of at least 4 cm, taking care not to twist the mesentery. This will minimize adhesions and facilitate ease of takedown at a later time.

◆ The proximal limb is confirmed by visualizing the suture, and a transverse incision is made across the ileum using Bovie electrocautery.

◆ Vicryl sutures are placed through the mucosa at points equidistant from each other on the proximal limb, then through the seromuscular layer proximally at the skin level, and then to skin. The proximal limb is everted to form a spigot-like protuberance that falls into the ileostomy bag, diverting the sulcus away from the level of the skin. The distal limb is sutured to the inferior portion of the skin edge without eversion.

◆ The appliance is cut to fit circumferentially so that there are no gaps exposing the skin at the end of the procedure after skin is closed.

3. CLOSING

◆ A #10 closed suction Jackson-Pratt drain is placed in the pelvis.

◆ The omentum is moved to the side and placed in either paracolic gutter. Two Ochsner clamps are placed at the umbilicus opposite each other. One sheet of Seprafilm is cut in half and placed over the bowel under the incision. This minimizes adhesion formation and makes reentry easier for future operations.

♦ The abdomen is closed using no. 1 polydioxanone (PDS) running suture.

♦ The subcutaneous tissue is irrigated with bacitracin irrigation, and the skin closed with staples.

♦ The umbilicus is reapproximated. A bacitracin-soaked cotton ball wrapped in Adaptic is packed into the umbilicus as a bolster.

♦ A well-fitting ileostomy appliance is cut to size and placed so that skin is not visible around the wafer. This prevents early production of sulcus from draining into the healing mucocutaneous wound.

STEP 4: POSTOPERATIVE CARE

♦ Adherence to a postoperative colorectal clinical pathway ensures standardization of care.

♦ Adequate pain control is achieved using patient-controlled analgesia or epidural catheter.

♦ Consideration for stress ulcer prophylaxis should be given to patients with symptoms or history of peptic ulcer disease.

♦ All patients should receive prophylaxis for deep venous thrombosis, using sequential compression devices while in bed, and heparin 5000 U subcutaneously every 8 hours or enoxaparin 40 mg subcutaneously every morning, starting within 24 hours from surgery. Dosing schedules should start on postoperative day 1, after results of morning laboratory tests are back to ensure there is no significant drop in hemoglobin to suggest postoperative bleeding.

♦ Adequate intravenous fluid should be administered with monitoring of urine output via urimeter on the Foley bag. Adequate fluid resuscitation should be given based on the clinical assessment of intravascular volume status.

♦ The diet may be limited to ice chips and sips of water in the postanesthesia care unit and on postoperative day 1. Return of bowel function is measured by the frequency and pitch of bowel sounds, lack of abdominal distention, and the patient's subjective will to eat. A clear liquid diet may be offered as sips of clear fluids without carbonation and without a straw to minimize accumulation of air in the intestine. This may be advanced ad lib as bowel function returns.

♦ Early ambulation is crucial for return of bowel function. Patients should be instructed to walk multiple times a day beginning on postoperative day 1 and should be encouraged to do so frequently.

- The umbilical bolster should be removed before the patient leaves the hospital. Skin staples are removed in the office during the postoperative visit.

- The ostomy care nurse should be consulted, and adequate postoperative education and support should be given to the patient before discharge from the hospital.

- The closed-suction drain may be removed on postoperative day 3 or when the drainage has decreased to less than 50 mL/day.

STEP 5: PEARLS AND PITFALLS

- Damage to the superior hypogastric plexus during high ligation of the IMA or to the hypogastric nerves at the sacral promontory during mobilization of the upper mesorectum results in retrograde ejaculation.

- Damage to the inferior hypogastric pelvic plexus may also result in urinary dysfunction due to denervation and paralysis of the detrusor muscle.

- Damage to the nervi erigentes during lateral and anterior dissection in the pelvis results in erectile dysfunction.

- Shortened ileocolic mesentery may preclude pouch placement in the pelvis. The patient should be prepared to accept permanent ileostomy should this happen.

- Shortened small bowel mesentery or large body habitus may preclude formation of protecting loop ileostomy. The right colon may be mobilized to provide additional distance.

- Care should be taken not to twist the small bowel mesentery when bringing out an ileostomy or creating an ileoanal anastomosis. This can be done by identifying the SMA at the root and "shaking hands" with the mesentery to feel for twists.

- Strong consideration should be made in using a loop ileostomy to protect the pouch. Most patients with ulcerative colitis who are undergoing this procedure are malnourished, taking high-dose steroids, and at increased risk for impaired wound healing and anastomotic leak. The ileostomy may be reversed in 6 weeks after contrast study through the distal limb of the loop confirms anastomotic integrity.

- Patients taking high-dose steroids should follow an appropriate tapering of dosage after discharge from the hospital and should be cautioned on problems with wound healing.

SELECTED REFERENCES

1. Beck DE, Opelka FG: Perioperative steroid use in colorectal patients. Dis Colon Rectum 1996;39: 995-999.
2. FDA safety alert (12/11/2008): http://www.fda.gov/cder/drug/infopage/OSP_solution/default.htm
3. Zeng Q, Yu Z, You J, Zhang Q: Efficacy and safety of Seprafilm for preventing postoperative abdominal adhesion: Systematic review and meta-analysis. World J Surg 2007;31:2125-31;2132 [discussion].
4. Guidelines from the Joint Commission on Surgical Care Improvement Project Core Measurement Set. Available on the Internet: www.jointcommission.org/PerformanceMeasurement.

CHAPTER 64

LOW ANTERIOR RESECTION— TOTAL MESORECTAL EXCISION

Tien C. Ko

STEP 1: SURGICAL ANATOMY

- The mesorectum is covered by a visceral fascia and contains blood vessels, lymphatic channels, and lymph nodes.

- The pelvic sympathetic hypogastric nerves originate from the preaortic superior hypogastric plexus and travel laterally and caudally, parallel to the ureters.

- The pelvic parasympathetic sacral splanchnic nerves originate from S3 and S4 nerve roots and emerge from the sacral foramen to travel laterally and caudally on the pelvic side wall before joining the hypogastric nerve.

STEP 2: PREOPERATIVE CONSIDERATIONS

- Total mesorectal excision is indicated for all mid or low rectal cancers. Preoperative chemoradiation treatment is indicated for patients with T3, T4 lesions or tumors with enlarged pelvic lymph nodes found on pelvic computed tomography (CT) scan or endorectal ultrasound.

- Appropriate bowel preparation such as GoLYTELY or four bisacodyl (Dulcolax) tablets followed by HalfLytely should be administered the day before surgery. Preoperatively, a single dose of broad-spectrum antibiotic (such as ertapenem) is administered.

- After induction of general anesthesia, the patient is placed in a lithotomy position with the legs in padded stirrups at 30-degree abduction. A nasogastric tube is placed to prevent gastric distention, and a urinary catheter is placed to decompress the bladder.

- Intraoperative rigid proctoscopy is performed to determine the distal extent of the cancer.

STEP 3: OPERATIVE STEPS

1. INCISION

♦ A midline abdominal incision is made from the pubic symphysis to approximately 5 cm cranial to the umbilicus.

♦ The midline fascia is divided with electrocautery. The peritoneum is elevated with tissue forceps, and after ensuring that no bowel is entrapped by the graspers, the peritoneum is incised sharply with a scalpel.

2. DISSECTION

♦ Once the peritoneum has been entered, a systematic exploration is performed to search for metastatic diseases in the peritoneal cavity and the liver.

♦ A fixed retractor is placed to retract small bowel superiorly and laterally out of the operative field. Retraction of small bowel is aided by placing the patient in a Trendelenburg position.

♦ Mobilization of the sigmoid colon is achieved by using electrocautery to incise the lateral visceral fascia covering the mesosigmoid along the white line of Toldt, which can be easily visualized by retracting the sigmoid colon medially. Working through this avascular plane allows for easy identification of gonadal vessels and the left ureter as they course over the left iliac vessels into the pelvis **(Figure 64-1)**.

♦ The medial visceral fascia is incised with electrocautery, and the right ureter is visualized as it courses over the right iliac vessels **(Figure 64-2)**.

♦ The presacral space is entered by dividing the loose areolar tissue at the level of the sacral promontory. The presacral space is developed sharply with electrocautery caudally toward the levator ani muscle, under direct vision. A fiber-optic pelvic retractor is used for retraction of the bladder and the rectum to facilitate visualization in the pelvis. After the sharp posterior pelvic dissection is completed, the distal margin can be manually evaluated **(Figure 64-3)**.

♦ The mesorectum is mobilized laterally toward both the right and left pelvic side wall, preserving the hypogastric nerves on the sacrum. The mesorectum is divided laterally either with clamps and sutures or with a vessel sealer device, such as LigaSure.

♦ The rectum is mobilized ventrally by dividing the rectovaginal septum or the rectovesicle space. In males, the dissection plane is ventral to Denonvillier fascia, preserving the seminal vesicles.

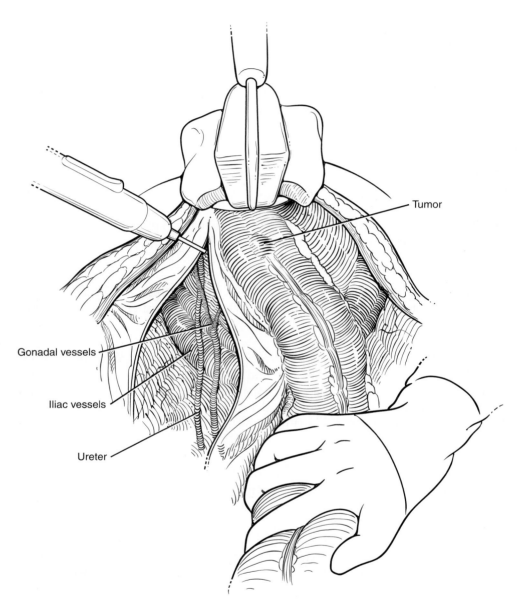

FIGURE 64–1

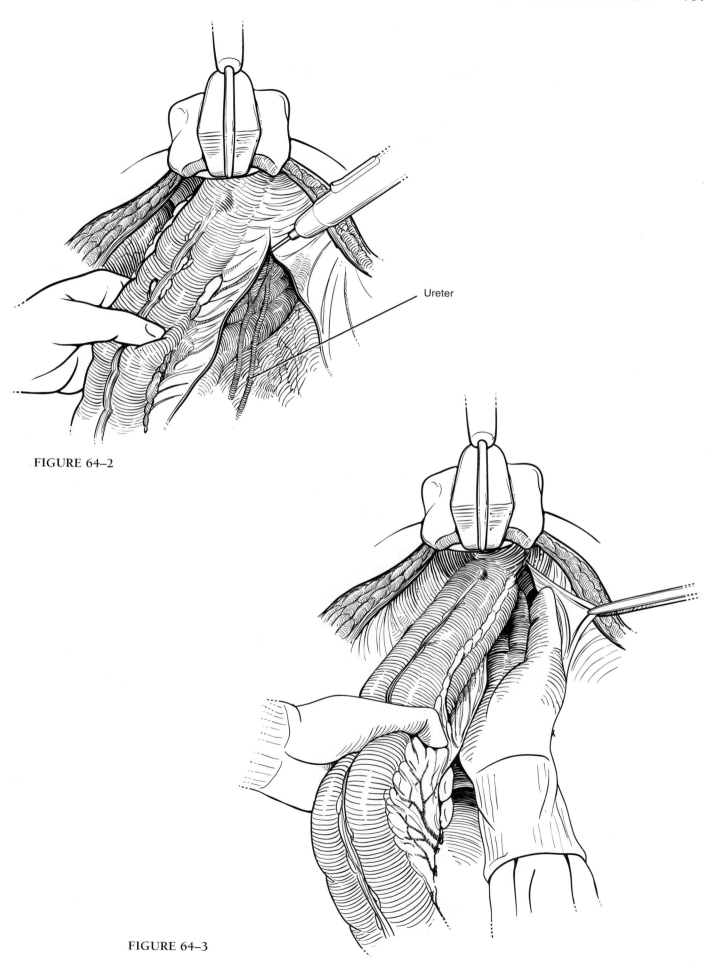

Ureter

FIGURE 64–2

FIGURE 64–3

◆ The distal rectum is closed with a linear stapler approximately 2 to 5 cm distal to the tumor **(Figure 64-4)**. The rectum is clamped just proximal to the staple line and divided with a scalpel. For low rectal tumors, a curved cutter stapler can help gain additional resection margin by avoiding the need for applying a clamp.

◆ The sigmoid colon is divided just distal to the first sigmoidal artery. The sigmoid colon is clamped proximally with a purse-string applicator and distally with a linear clamp if a stapled anastomosis is being performed **(Figure 64-5)** or with two linear clamps if a hand-sewn anastomosis is being performed. Transection is completed with a scalpel **(Figure 64-6)**. The mesosigmoid is divided with clamps and sutures or with a vessel sealer device.

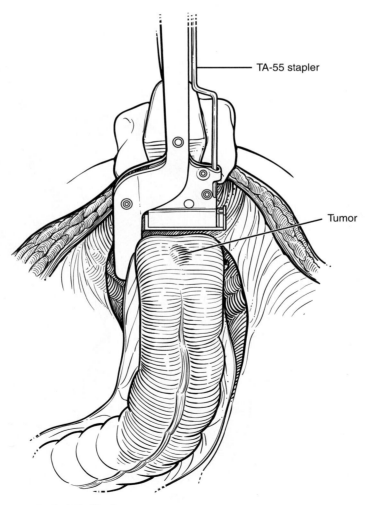

TA-55 stapler

Tumor

FIGURE 64–4

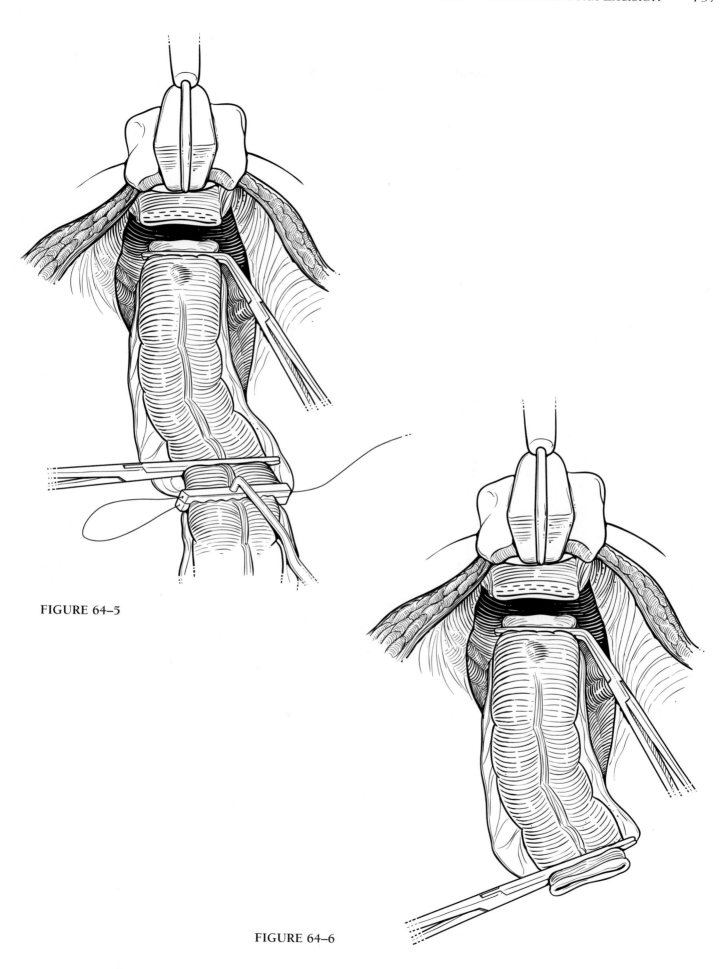

FIGURE 64–5

FIGURE 64–6

◆ A two-layer, hand-sewn colorectal anastomosis is performed by first placing a posterior layer of interrupted Lembert seromuscular sutures of 3-0 silk (**Figure 64-7**). Next, two running full-thickness sutures of 3-0 Monocryl are placed by beginning at the mid-point of the posterior layer (**Figure 64-8**). These sutures are continued anteriorly in a Connell fashion (**Figure 64-9**) and finished by tying to each other to complete the inner layer. Finally, an anterior layer of interrupted Lembert seromuscular sutures of 3-0 silk is placed (**Figure 64-10**).

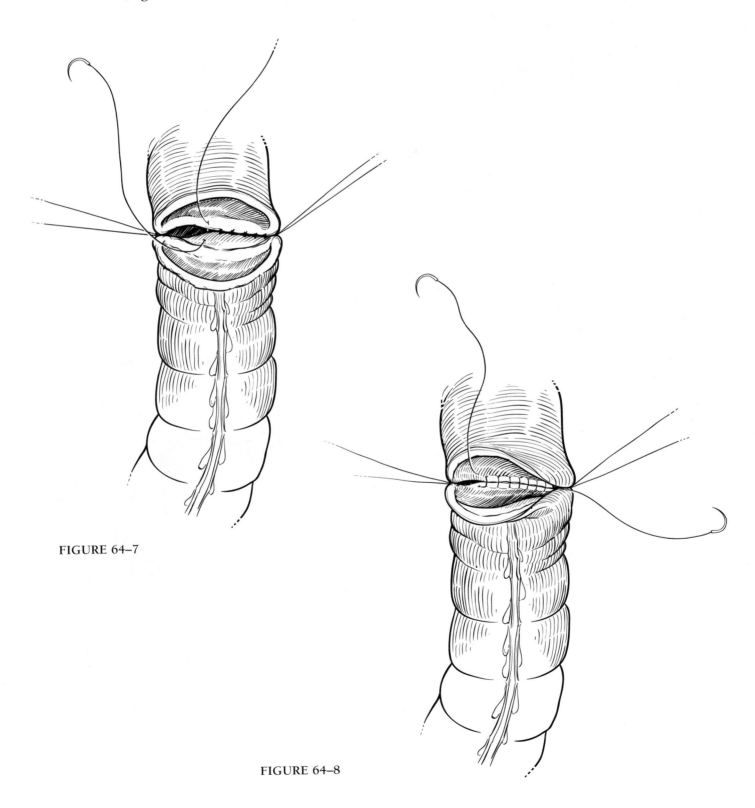

FIGURE 64–7

FIGURE 64–8

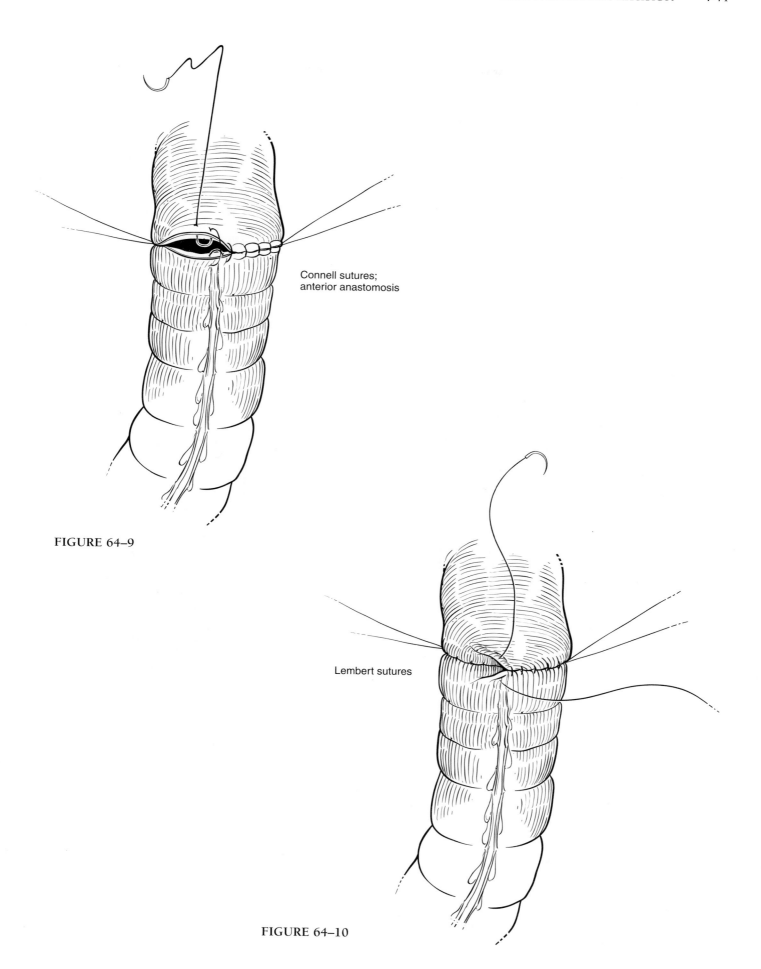

Connell sutures; anterior anastomosis

FIGURE 64–9

Lembert sutures

FIGURE 64–10

◆ Alternatively, a stapled colorectal anastomosis can be performed. After a purse-string applicator is used, the proximal sigmoid colon is dilated with increasing size of dilators, which also serves to determine the appropriate size of the stapler **(Figure 64-11).** Similarly, the distal rectum is sized with the dilators.

◆ The anvil of the circular stapler is inserted into the proximal sigmoid colon, and the purse-string is secured **(Figure 64-12).** The handle of the circular stapler is brought through the distal rectal staple line transanally (see Figure 64-12).

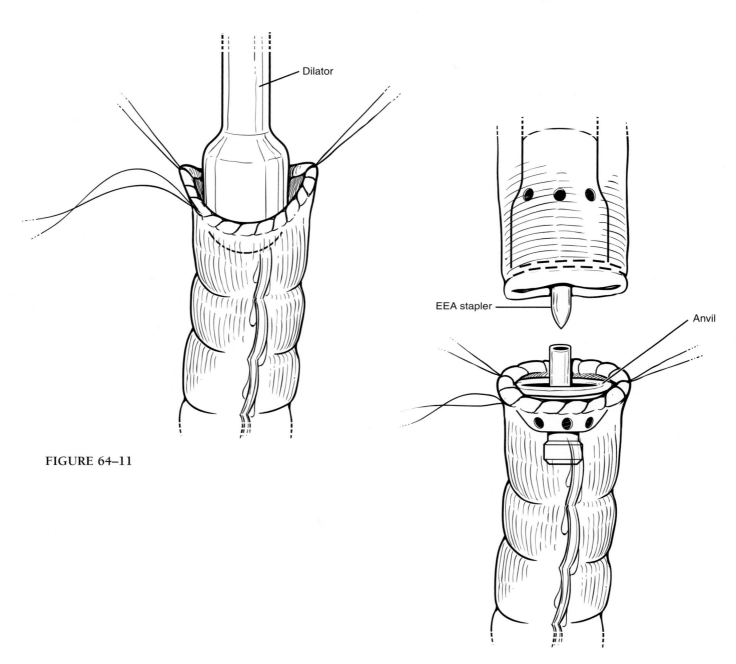

FIGURE 64–11

FIGURE 64–12

◆ The circular stapler is closed to appropriate tension and deployed (**Figure 64-13**). The circular stapler is opened partially and removed transanally (**Figure 64-14**). The stapler is then examined to ensure that there are an intact ring of sigmoid colon in the anvil and an intact ring of rectum in the stapler handle.

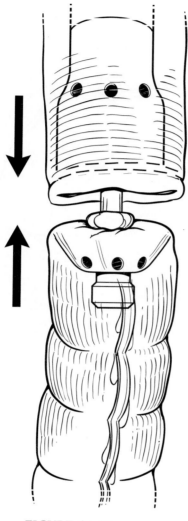

FIGURE 64–13

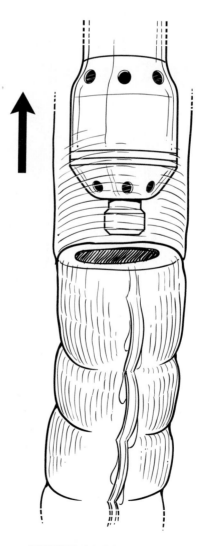

FIGURE 64–14

◆ The "bubble test" is performed to test the integrity of the colorectal anastomosis. The pelvis is filled with saline, and a rigid proctoscope is inserted into the rectum distal to the anastomosis. The lumen is gently distended by pumping air into the rectum, and absence of bubbles indicates an intact anastomotic line **(Figure 64-15)**.

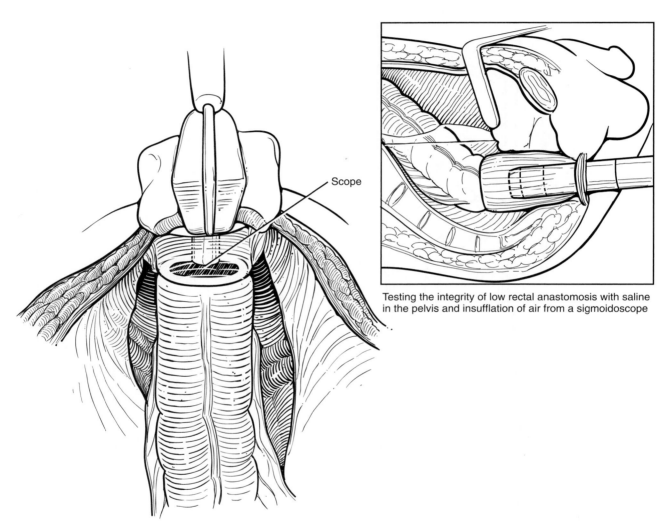

Scope

Testing the integrity of low rectal anastomosis with saline in the pelvis and insufflation of air from a sigmoidoscope

FIGURE 64–15

3. CLOSING

◆ The peritoneal cavity is irrigated with saline, and hemostasis is obtained. The midline fascia is closed in one layer with two running absorbable sutures of loop 0 polydioxanone (PDS) beginning at the cranial and caudal end of the incision. The skin is reapproximated with staples.

◆ No intraperitoneal drains are indicated.

◆ The nasogastric tube is removed before the patient emerges from anesthesia.

STEP 4: POSTOPERATIVE CARE

◆ Clear liquids are started on postoperative day 1, and diet is advanced as tolerated.

◆ Postoperative antibiotics are not necessary.

◆ The urinary catheter is left in place for 3 or 4 days to decrease the risk of urinary retention after pelvic dissection.

STEP 5: PEARLS AND PITFALLS

◆ The mesorectal dissection should be performed sharply under direct vision and not bluntly with the hand.

◆ The colorectal anastomosis must be tension free, and this may require division of the sigmoid artery at its origin and mobilization of the splenic flexure of the colon.

◆ In T3 and T4 rectal cancers, preservation of the pelvic autonomic nerves may not be possible.

◆ In most patients, the 29-mm circular stapler works well. Using the maximum-size circular stapler may create radial tension, leading to anastomotic leak.

◆ If the anastomosis fails the "bubble test," the anastomotic defect must be identified and repaired primarily. A protection loop ileostomy may be indicated for difficult or low anastomosis (<5 cm) and for patients who underwent preoperative chemoradiation treatment.

SELECTED REFERENCES

1. Havenga K, Grossmann I, DeRuiter M, Wiggers T: Definition of total mesorectal excision, including the perineal phase: Technical considerations. Dig Dis 2007;25:44-50.
2. Fry RD, Mahmoud N, Maron D, et al: Colon and rectum. In Townsend CM Jr, Sabiston DC (eds): Sabiston Textbook of Surgery, 18th ed. Philadelphia, Elsevier Saunders, 2008, pp 1348-1432.

CHAPTER 65

MILES ABDOMINOPERINEAL RESECTION WITH TOTAL MESORECTAL EXCISION

Tien C. Ko

STEP 1: SURGICAL ANATOMY

- For the total mesorectal excision, please see the discussion on pelvic autonomic nerves in Chapter 64.

- The seminal vesicles, prostate, and urethra are located ventral to Denonvillier's fascia cranially and the superficial transverse perineal muscle caudally.

STEP 2: PREOPERATIVE CONSIDERATIONS

- Miles abdominoperineal resection with total mesorectal excision is indicated for rectal cancer near the levator ani muscle or persistent or recurrent squamous cell cancer of the anus after chemoradiation treatment.

- Preoperative chemoradiation treatment is indicated for T3, T4 lesions or those tumors with enlarged pelvic lymph nodes on pelvic computed tomography (CT) scan or endorectal ultrasound.

- Appropriate bowel preparation such as GOLYTELY or four bisacodyl (Dulcolax) tablets followed by HalfLytely should be administered the day before surgery. Preoperatively, a single dose of broad-spectrum antibiotic (such as ertapenem) is administered.

- The permanent colostomy site is marked by an enterostomal nurse preoperatively to ensure the best placement of the colostomy.

◆ After induction of general anesthesia, the patient is placed in a lithotomy position with the legs in padded stirrups at 30-degree abduction. The coccyx is placed near the end of the table and elevated with a stack of towels **(Figure 65-1)**. A nasogastric tube is placed to prevent gastric distention, and a urinary catheter is placed to decompress the bladder. The rectum is irrigated with povidone-iodine (Betadine) solution until clear. The anus is closed with a 0 silk purse-string suture **(Figure 65-2)**.

STEP 3: OPERATIVE STEPS

1. INCISION

◆ A midline abdominal incision is made from the pubic symphysis to approximately 5 cm cranial to the umbilicus.

◆ The midline fascia is divided with electrocautery. The peritoneum is elevated with tissue forceps, and after ensuring that no bowel is entrapped by the graspers, the peritoneum is incised sharply with a scalpel.

◆ For the perineal dissection, an elliptical incision is made 2 cm away from the closed anus (see Figure 65-2).

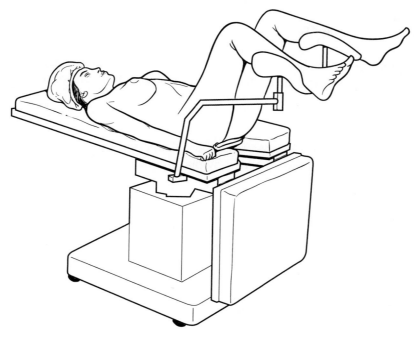

Patient lithotomy position

FIGURE 65–1

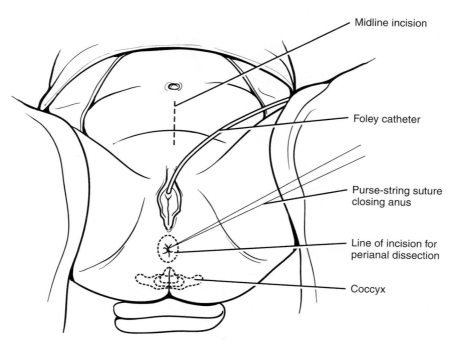

Midline incision

Foley catheter

Purse-string suture closing anus

Line of incision for perianal dissection

Coccyx

FIGURE 65–2

2. DISSECTION

◆ Once the peritoneum has been entered, a systematic exploration is performed to search for metastases in the peritoneal cavity, including the liver and the preaortic and iliac lymph nodes.

◆ A fixed retractor is placed to retract small bowel superiorly and laterally out of the operative field. Retraction of small bowel is aided by placing the patient in a Trendelenburg position.

◆ Mobilization of the sigmoid colon is achieved by using electrocautery to incise the lateral visceral fascia covering the mesosigmoid along the white line of Toldt, which can be easily visualized by retracting the sigmoid colon medially **(Figure 65-3)**. The left ureter is identified along its course over the left iliac vessels into the pelvis.

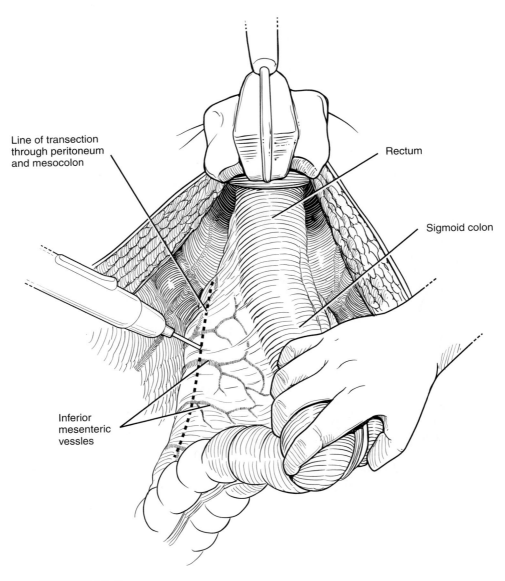

Line of transection through peritoneum and mesocolon

Rectum

Sigmoid colon

Inferior mesenteric vessles

FIGURE 65–3

◆ The medial visceral fascia is incised with electrocautery, and the right ureter is visualized as it courses over the right iliac vessels **(Figure 65-4)**. The line of proximal resection is also outlined but not carried out until the tumor is able to be fully mobilized.

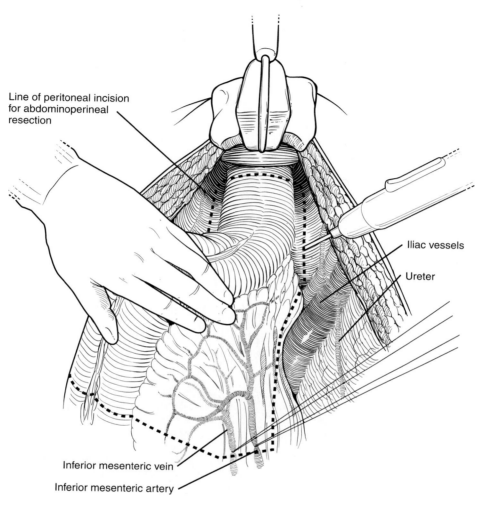

FIGURE 65–4

♦ The presacral space is entered by dividing the loose areolar tissue at the level of the sacral promontory. The presacral space is developed sharply with electrocautery caudally toward the levator ani muscle under direct vision. A fiber-optic pelvic retractor is used for retraction of the bladder and the rectum to facilitate visualization in the pelvis. Mobilization of the rectum continues caudally to the levator ani muscle. After the sharp posterior pelvic dissection is completed, the distal extent of dissection can be manually evaluated **(Figure 65-5)**. Care must be taken to avoid injuring the presacral plexus of veins during the posterior dissection.

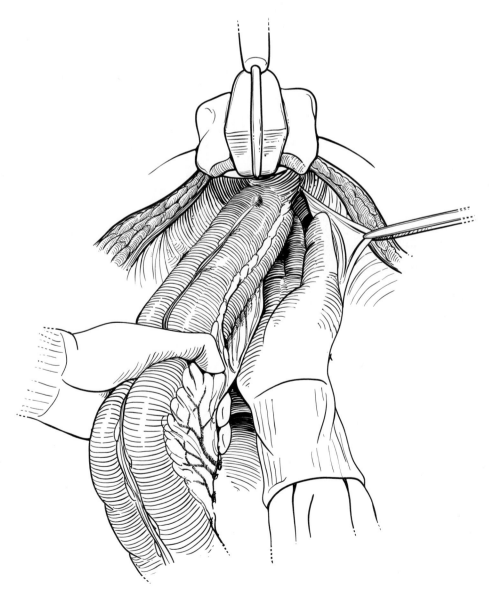

FIGURE 65–5

◆ The mesorectum is mobilized laterally toward the right and left pelvic side wall, preserving the hypogastric nerves on the sacrum. The lateral attachments to the pelvic wall containing the mesorectum are divided either with clamps and sutures (**Figure 65-6**) or with a vessel-sealer device, such as LigaSure.

◆ The rectum is mobilized ventrally by dividing the rectovaginal septum or the rectovesicle space. In males, the dissection plane is ventral to Denonvillier's fascia, preserving the seminal vesicles.

◆ Attention is directed toward the resection of proximal sigmoid colon. First, the inferior mesenteric artery is divided just distal to the origin of the left colic artery either with clamps and sutures or with a vessel-sealer device. Next, the proximal sigmoid colon is divided with a gastrointestinal anastomosis (GIA) stapler (**Figure 65-7**).

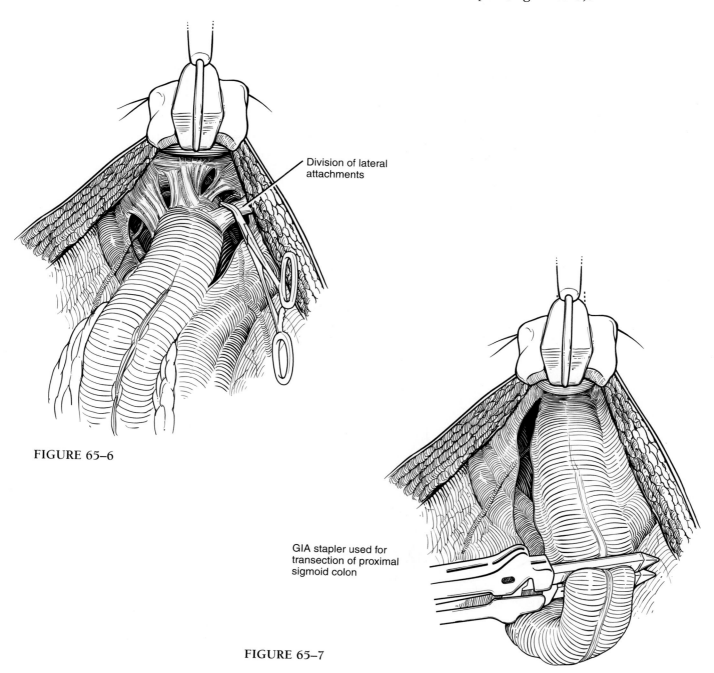

Division of lateral attachments

FIGURE 65–6

GIA stapler used for transection of proximal sigmoid colon

FIGURE 65–7

- A colostomy site is created in the left lower quadrant at either the premarked site or halfway between the umbilicus and the left anterior superior iliac spine. A 2 cm in diameter circle of skin is excised with a scalpel, and the subcutaneous tissue is divided with electrocautery. A cruciate incision is made in the anterior rectus abdominis fascia, and 2 cm of the rectus abdominis muscle is divided with electrocautery. The peritoneum is incised with electrocautery to complete the colostomy site, which should be approximately 2 fingerbreadths in diameter.

- The perineal dissection may be performed sequentially or simultaneously by a second team. After skin incision, the laterally ischiorectal space is entered. The skin and subcutaneous tissue is retracted with a self-retaining retractor to facilitate deep dissection **(Figures 65-8 and 65-9)**. Inferior hemorrhoidal vessels are secured with sutures and divided. The coccyx is identified posteriorly, and the anococcygeal ligament located posteriorly is divided. Laterally, the levator ani muscle is divided with electrocautery and the perineal fossa is entered.

- The distal stump of the transected sigmoid colon and the proximal rectum is delivered caudally through the opening of the levator ani muscle **(Figure 65-10)**. Ventral mobilization of the rectum is facilitated by the anterior retraction of the skin and subcutaneous tissue and the posterior retraction of the sigmoid colon and rectum. The superficial transverse perineal muscle is divided with electrocautery to completely mobilize the rectum. In males, the urethra courses ventrally to the superficial transverse perineal muscle and can be identified and protected by palpating the urinary catheter. The sigmoid colon and rectum are removed through the perineal wound.

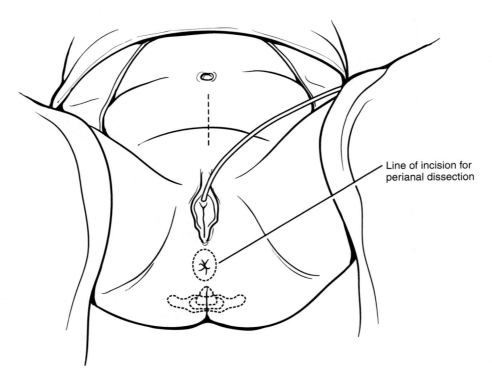

Line of incision for
perianal dissection

FIGURE 65–8

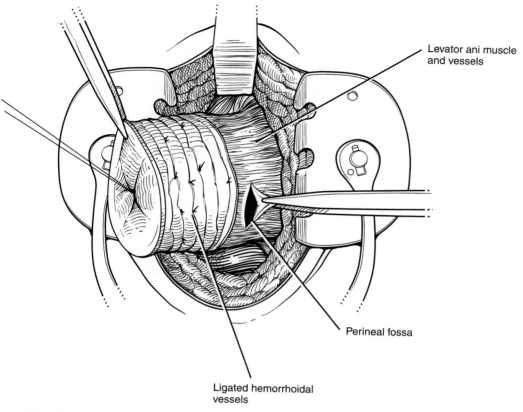

Levator ani muscle
and vessels

Perineal fossa

Ligated hemorrhoidal
vessels

FIGURE 65–9

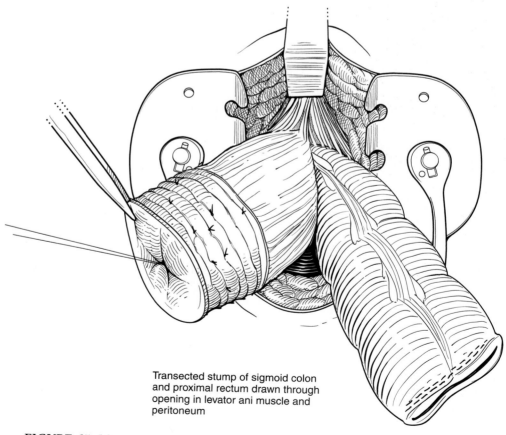

Transected stump of sigmoid colon
and proximal rectum drawn through
opening in levator ani muscle and
peritoneum

FIGURE 65–10

3. CLOSING

- The pelvis is irrigated with saline, and hemostasis is obtained. Two Silastic 10-mm drains are placed in the pelvis through stab incisions in the right and left gluteal regions, lateral to the perineal wound, and secured with sutures of 2-0 nylon. The levator ani muscle is reapproximated with a running suture of 2-0 Vicryl **(Figure 65-11)**.

- The subcutaneous tissue of the perineum is reapproximated with a running suture of 3-0 Vicryl. The skin is closed with interrupted vertical mattress sutures of 2-0 nylon **(Figure 65-12)**. The perineal incision is covered with povidone-iodine ointment and nonadhesive gauze.

- A pedicle of the greater omentum is mobilized from the transverse colon and placed into the pelvis to promote healing and prevent small bowel adhesions in the pelvis **(Figure 65-13)**. The proximal end of the resected colon is brought through the colostomy site, and the serosa of the colon is secured to the peritoneum with several interrupted sutures of 3-0 silk.

- The midline abdominal incision is closed by reapproximating the fascia in one layer with two running absorbable sutures of loop 0 polydioxanone (PDS), beginning at the cranial and caudal end of the incision. The skin is reapproximated with staples.

- The colostomy is matured by first removing the staple line with electrocautery. The full-thickness colonic mucosa is sutured to the dermis of the colostomy site circumferentially with interrupted sutures of 3-0 Monocryl. The colostomy is covered with a stoma appliance.

- The nasogastric tube is removed before the patient awakes from anesthesia.

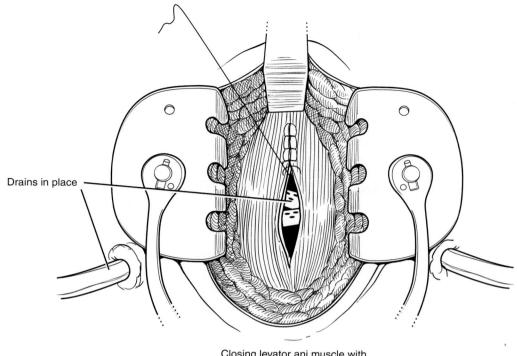

Drains in place

Closing levator ani muscle with
running sutures

FIGURE 65–11

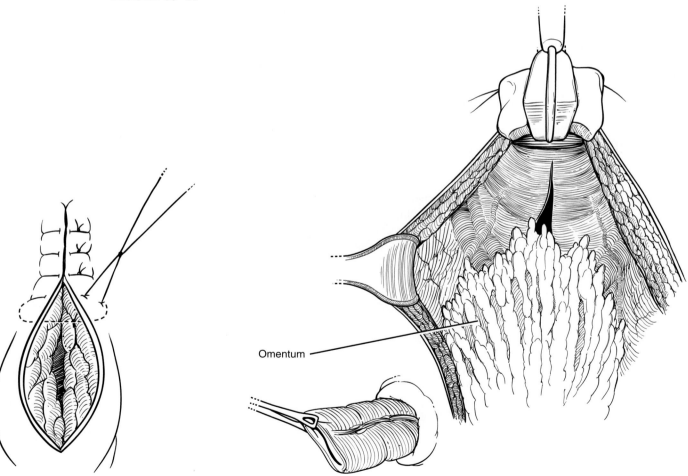

Omentum

FIGURE 65–12   **FIGURE 65–13**

STEP 4: POSTOPERATIVE CARE

- Clear liquids are started on postoperative day 1, and diet is advanced as tolerated.

- Postoperative antibiotics are not necessary.

- A urinary catheter is left in place for 3 to 5 days to decrease the risk of urinary retention after pelvic dissection.

STEP 5: PEARLS AND PITFALLS

- Obstructing rectal cancer may require a two-stage operation: a diverting descending colostomy, preoperative chemoradiation treatment, and a Miles abdominoperineal resection.

- Large anal or distal rectal lesions will require wider perineal resection and may require a rectus abdominis myocutaneous flap to close the perineal wound. Patients who received preoperative chemoradiation treatment should also be considered for perineal reconstruction with a myocutaneous flap. Alternatively, the perineal defect can be left open and covered with a wound V.A.C. to allow healing by secondary intention.

SELECTED REFERENCES

1. Havenga K, Grossmann I, DeRuiter M, Wiggers T: Definition of total mesorectal excision, including the perineal phase: Technical considerations. Dig Dis 2007;25:44-50.
2. Fry RD, Mahmoud N, Maron D, et al: Colon and rectum. In Townsend CM (ed): Sabiston Textbook of Surgery, 18th ed. Philadelphia, Elsevier Saunders, 2008, pp 1348-1432.

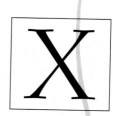

RECTUM

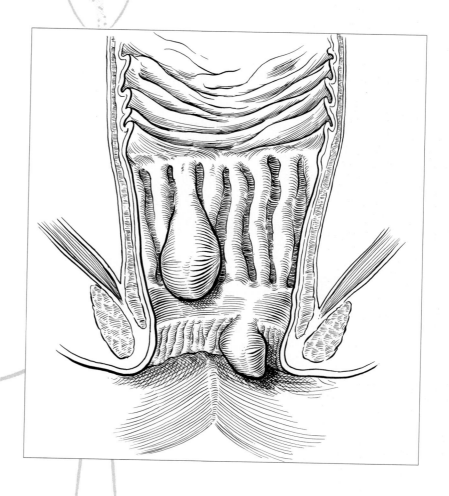

CHAPTER **66**

HEMORRHOIDECTOMY

Dennis C. Gore

STEP 1: SURGICAL ANATOMY

- ◆ Internal hemorrhoids arise proximal to the pectinate line and are insensate. These can be banded. External hemorrhoids arise distal to the pectinate line and are sensitive to touch. These are best treated with excision **(Figure 66-1)**.

- ◆ Indications are as follows:
  - ◆ Rectal bleeding attributed to the hemorrhoid
  - ◆ Persistent anal pain and pruritus

STEP 2: PREOPERATIVE CONSIDERATIONS

- ◆ A cleansing enema and oral mineral oil should be given several hours before the procedure.

- ◆ Ensure any bleeding tendencies are corrected.

- ◆ Anesthesia: spinal or general

- ◆ Position: prone; jackknife

- ◆ Operative preparation includes the following:
  - ◆ Before the hemorrhoidectomy, proctoscopy is advisable to exclude any rectal disease.
  - ◆ Ensure that genitals are not compressed by prone positioning.
  - ◆ Place a Foley catheter in the midgut.

STEP 3: OPERATIVE STEPS

1. INCISION

- ◆ Adherent tape is placed along the medial aspect of the buttocks then retracted laterally.

2. DISSECTION

◆ Place anal retractor opposite the hemorrhoid.

◆ Grasp hemorrhoid with Babcock clamp and retract.

◆ Place 2-0 Vicryl suture at the internal base of the hemorrhoid and ligate, thereby occluding venous backflow; leave a long segment of suture **(Figure 66-2)**.

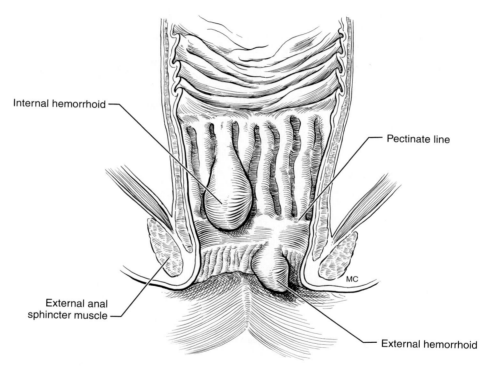

Internal hemorrhoid

Pectinate line

External anal sphincter muscle

MC

External hemorrhoid

FIGURE 66–1

◆ Use scalpel, Metzenbaum scissors, or electrocautery to excise the hemorrhoid, starting just external to the suture ligature **(Figure 66-3).**

◆ Use electrocautery or 4-0 Vicryl sutures to obtain hemostasis.

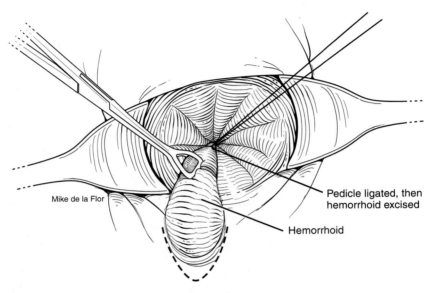

Mike de la Flor

Pedicle ligated, then hemorrhoid excised

Hemorrhoid

FIGURE 66–2

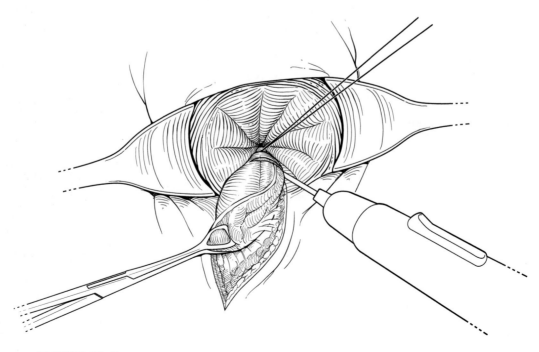

FIGURE 66–3

3. CLOSING

◆ With the remaining 2-0 Vicryl suture, reapproximate the wound edges in a running fashion, thus closing the hemorrhoidectomy wound. A running, locking suture can be used if needed for improved hemostasis (**Figures 66-4 and 66-5**).

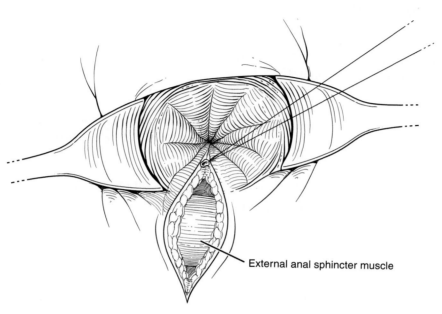

External anal sphincter muscle

FIGURE 66–4

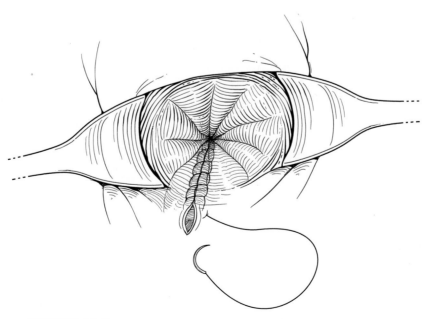

FIGURE 66–5

STEP 4: POSTOPERATIVE CARE

- ◆ Sitz baths

- ◆ Repeat oral mineral oil

STEP 5: PEARLS AND PITFALLS

- ◆ Excise no more than three hemorrhoids at one operative setting. Removal of excessive anal tissue may lead to stricture.

- ◆ Ensure in cases of rectal bleeding that other sources of gastrointestinal bleeding, such as colon cancer and diverticular disease, are excluded before the hemorrhoidectomy.

- ◆ Hepatic cirrhosis and other bleeding disorders should be addressed and thoroughly corrected, or the planned procedure should be aborted.

SELECTED REFERENCE

1. Zollinger R Jr, Zollinger R: Atlas of Surgical Operations, 5th ed. New York, Macmillan, 1983, p 416.

CHAPTER 67

DRAINAGE OF PERIRECTAL ABSCESS

Dennis C. Gore

STEP 1: SURGICAL ANATOMY

- ◆ See previous chapters for anatomy of the anus.

STEP 2: PREOPERATIVE CONSIDERATIONS

- ◆ Indication: abscesses requiring emergent drainage

- ◆ Position: prone, jackknife

- ◆ Anesthesia: spinal or general

- ◆ Operative preparation includes the following:
    - ◆ Administer antibiotics before procedure.
    - ◆ Ensure that genitals are not compressed by prone positioning.
    - ◆ Proctoscopy is advisable to exclude any rectal disease such as Crohn's disease.

STEP 3: OPERATIVE STEPS

1. INCISION

- ◆ Adherent tape is placed along the medial buttocks then retracted laterally.

◆ Use scalpel or electrocautery to incise over the most prominent point of the abscess **(Figure 67-1).**

2. DISSECTION

◆ Using manual inspection, ensure the abscess is completely drained.

◆ Irrigate abscess cavity copiously.

◆ Use electrocautery judiciously to ensure hemostasis.

◆ If hemostasis remains a concern, then the abscess cavity can be packed with moist gauze.

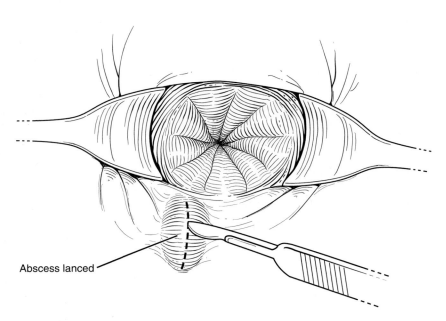

Abscess lanced

FIGURE 67–1

3. CLOSING

- None

STEP 4: POSTOPERATIVE CARE

- Mineral oil is given orally when feasible.

- Sitz bath

STEP 5: PEARLS AND PITFALLS

- Many abscesses are associated with anal fistulae. Fistulotomy may reduce abscess recurrence.

SELECTED REFERENCES

1. Zollinger RM Jr, Zollinger RM: Atlas of Surgical Operations. New York, Macmillan, 1983, p 418.
2. Schwartz SI, Shires GT, Spencer FC, et al: Principles of Surgery, 5th ed. New York, McGraw-Hill, 1989, p 1305.

CHAPTER 68

LATERAL SPHINCTEROTOMY

Dennis C. Gore

STEP 1: SURGICAL ANATOMY

- See previous chapters for anatomy of the anus.

STEP 2: PREOPERATIVE CONSIDERATIONS

- Indication: anal fissure

- Preoperative planning: a cleansing enema and oral mineral oil should be given several hours before procedure.

- Position: prone, jackknife

- Anesthesia: spinal or general

- Operative preparation includes the following:
  - Administer antibiotics before procedure.
  - Proctoscopy is advisable to exclude any rectal disease.
  - Ensure that genitals are not compressed by prone positioning.

STEP 3: OPERATIVE STEPS

1. INCISION

- Use two strips of strong adhesive tape placed 8 to 10 cm from midline, then retracted laterally and down and secured to the lower operating table. This tape placement allows retraction of the buttocks laterally.

2. DISSECTION

◆ Place anal retractor to expose lateral wall of anus **(Figure 68-1)**.

◆ Use scalpel or electrocautery to make a small incision from just distal to the anal verge laterally **(Figure 68-2)**.

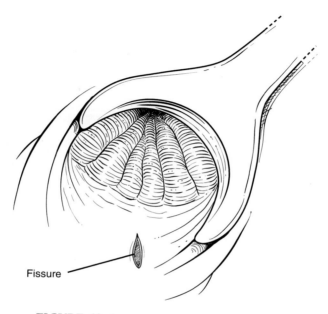

Fissure

FIGURE 68–1

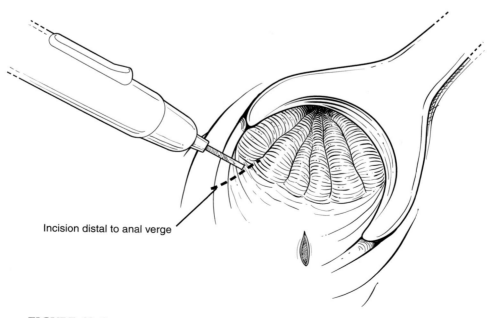

Incision distal to anal verge

FIGURE 68–2

◆ Insert either scalpel or electrocautery through incision and cut the external sphincter longitudinally **(Figure 68-3).**

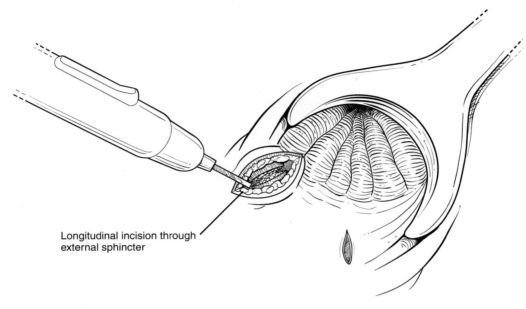

Longitudinal incision through
external sphincter

FIGURE 68–3

3. CLOSING

- 3-0 Vicryl interrupted suture (optional)

STEP 4: POSTOPERATIVE CARE

- Sitz bath

- Stool softeners

STEP 5: PEARLS AND PITFALLS

- Consider biopsy of fissure to exclude cancer or inflammatory bowel etiologies, especially if fissure is in a position other than posterior midline or if the patient is elderly.

SELECTED REFERENCE

1. Schwartz SI, Shires GT, Spencer FC, et al: Principles of Surgery, 5th ed. New York, McGraw-Hill, 1989, p 1303.

CHAPTER 69

PILONIDAL CYST CURETTAGE

Dennis C. Gore

STEP 1: SURGICAL ANATOMY

- **Figure 69-1** shows the posterior lower back with pilonidal cyst.

STEP 2: PREOPERATIVE CONSIDERATIONS

- Indication: pilonidal cyst

- Anesthesia: general, spinal, or extensive local

- Position: prone, jackknife

- Operative planning: Ensure genitals are not compressed by prone positioning.

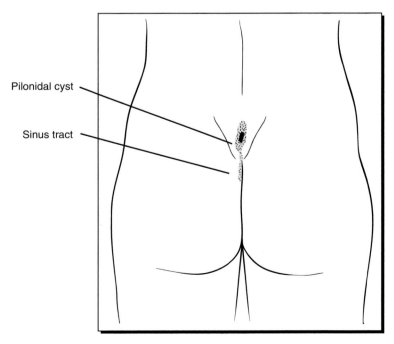

Pilonidal cyst

Sinus tract

FIGURE 69–1

STEP 3: OPERATIVE STEPS

1. INCISION

♦ Use two strips of strong adhesive tape placed 8 to 10 cm from midline retracted laterally, then down and secured to the lower operating table. This tape placement allows retraction of the buttocks laterally.

2. DISSECTION

♦ Place probe into the pilonidal opening and advance into sinus tracts **(Figure 69-2)**.

♦ With probe in place, use electrocautery to incise open sinus tracts **(Figure 69-3)**.

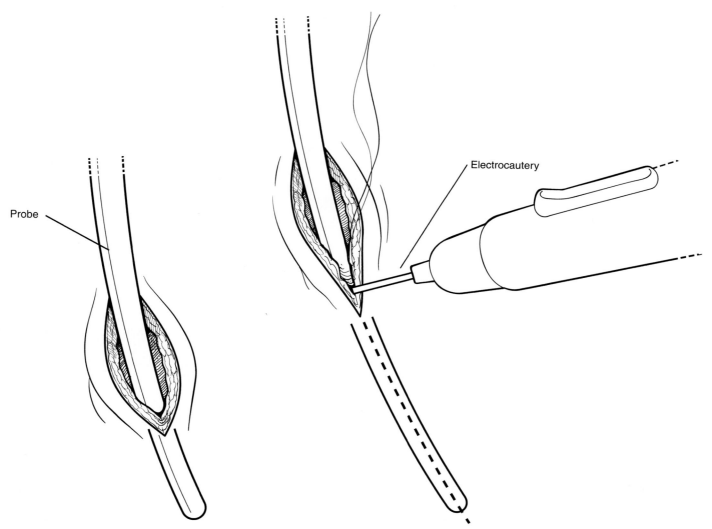

Probe

Electrocautery

FIGURE 69–2   **FIGURE 69–3**

◆ Use electrocautery or curettage to cauterize and remove inflammatory tissue and any foreign materials (usually hair) all along the pilonidal cyst and the accompanying sinus tracts **(Figure 69-4)**.

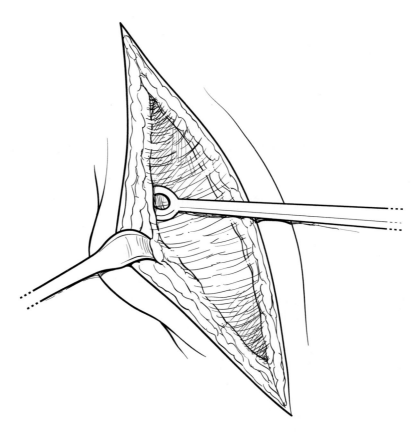

FIGURE 69–4

3. CLOSING

- None

STEP 4: POSTOPERATIVE CARE

- Wound dressing with moist gauze

STEP 5: PEARLS AND PITFALLS

- Pilonidal sinus tracts may extend into surrounding spaces at multiple finger-like projections.

- Search diligently for all tracts.

SELECTED REFERENCE

1. Zollinger RM Jr, Zollinger RM: Atlas of Surgical Operations, 5th ed. New York, Macmillan, 1983, p 422.

CHAPTER 70

INCISION OF FISTULA-IN-ANO

Dennis C. Gore

STEP 1: SURGICAL ANATOMY

See **Figure 70-1.**

- Indication: anal fistula

- Anus
  - Most anal fistulas originate from the crypts of Morgagni and extend with varying depth to the perianal opening.
  - Goodsall's rule describes the relationship of the external opening to the internal origin of the fistula.
    - If the external opening is anterior and 3 cm or less from the anus, then the fistula tract courses directly toward the anus (see Figure 70-1).
    - If the external opening is anterior and 3 cm or more from the anus, then the fistula tract may curve to enter at the posterior midline.
    - If the external opening is posterior to the anus, then the fistula tract will curve to enter at the posterior midline.

STEP 2: PREOPERATIVE CONSIDERATIONS

- Preoperative planning: A cleansing enema and oral mineral oil should be given several hours before the procedure.

- Position: prone, jackknife

- Anesthesia: general or spinal

- Operative position preparation includes the following:
  - Ensure that genitals are not compressed by prone positioning.
  - Proctoscopy is advisable to exclude rectal disease.
  - Administer antibiotics before the procedure.

Goodsall's Rule

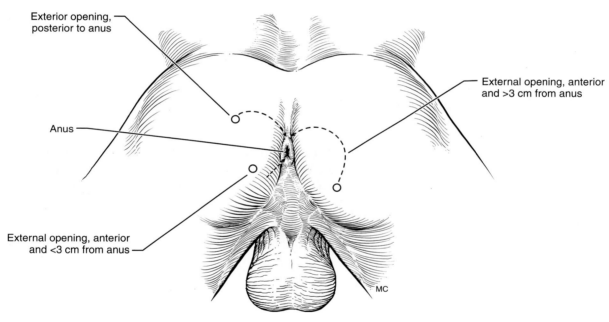

Exterior opening,
posterior to anus

External opening, anterior
and >3 cm from anus

Anus

External opening, anterior
and <3 cm from anus

MC

FIGURE 70–1

STEP 3: OPERATIVE STEPS

1. INCISION

♦ Adherent tape is placed along the medial aspect of the buttocks and retracted laterally.

2. DISSECTION

♦ Insert a probe through the external opening of the fistula and gently advance the probe to identify the fistulous tract **(Figure 70-2)**.

♦ With the probe in place, use a scalpel or electrocautery to incise skin overlying the fistulous tract **(Figure 70-3)**.

♦ Most anal fistulas arise from an anal crypt at the pectinate line; continue incision and exposure of fistulous tract to origin at anal crypt.

♦ Use electrocautery or curettage to cauterize and remove inflammatory tissue along the fistulous tract **(Figure 70-4)**.

♦ Many anal fistulas extend internally to circumscribe the external and very rarely the internal sphincters. To complete the fistulotomy, the sphincter muscle can be cut, but the sphincter muscle can be transected in only one place without precipitating incontinence.

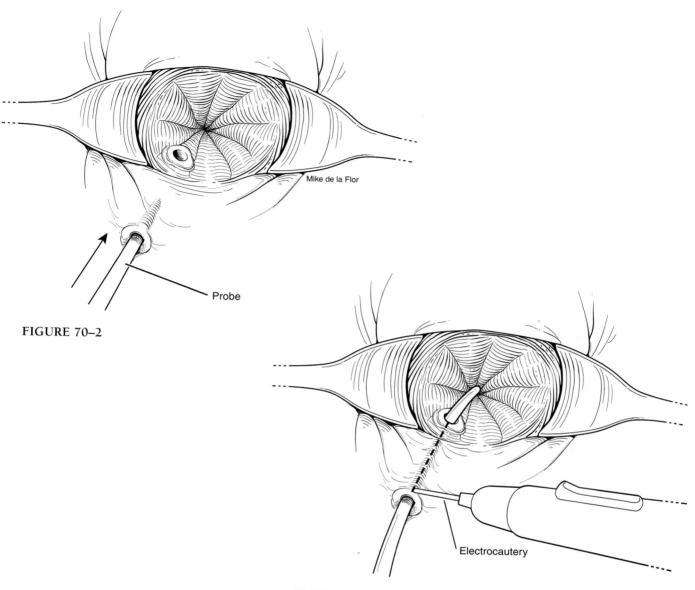

Mike de la Flor

Probe

FIGURE 70–2

Electrocautery

FIGURE 70–3

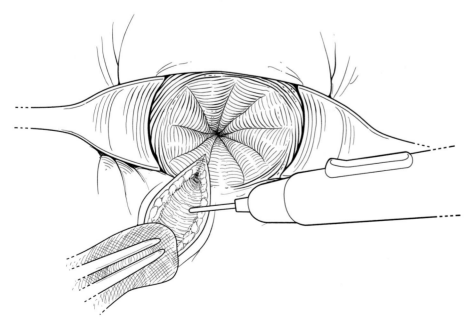

FIGURE 70–4

3. CLOSING

- For multiple, complex fistula-in-ano, place a 2-0 silk suture through those fistulous tracts that circumscribe an anal sphincter yet cannot be incised. Tie the ends of this suture together loosely to create a seton. With time the seton will incite sufficient granulation and fibrosis that the fistulous tract can be incised at a second operation or allowed to erode through the fistulous tract.

STEP 4: POSTOPERATIVE CARE

- Sitz baths

- Stool softeners

- Repeat doses of mineral oil given orally

STEP 5: PEARLS AND PITFALLS

- It is sometimes difficult to assert with confidence the path of the fistula-in-ano. Goodsall's rule relates that if the external opening is anterior to an imaginary line drawn across the midpoint of the anus and less than 3 cm from the anus, the fistula usually runs directly into the anal canal. If the external opening is anterior to but greater than 3 cm from the anus, then the fistulous tract may curve posteriorly to the posterior midline. If the external opening is posterior to this line, the tract will usually curve to the posterior midline.

SELECTED REFERENCE

1. Zollinger RM Jr, Zollinger RM: Atlas of Surgical Operations, 5th ed. New York, Macmillan, 1983, p 420.

HERNIAS

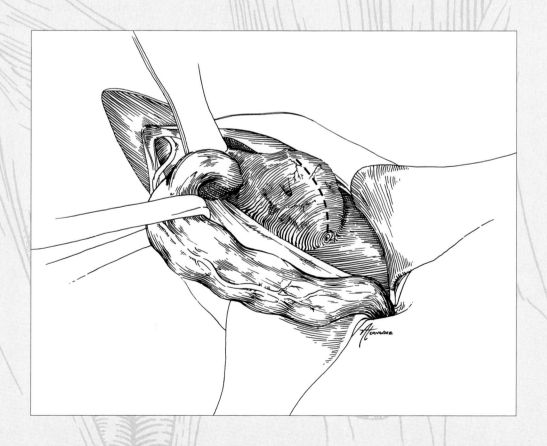

CHAPTER 71

Hernia Repair: General Principles—Tension-Free versus Tension

Thomas D. Kimbrough

STEP 1: SURGICAL ANATOMY

◆ Although the widespread adoption of mesh to repair hernias may lead the inexperienced and reckless to presume otherwise, a comprehensive understanding of the anatomy of the inguinal region is of paramount importance in inguinal hernia repairs.

◆ See **Figures 71-1 and 71-2** for surface and superficial anatomic structures. The typical location of each of the three inguinal hernia types is shown in Figure 71-2.

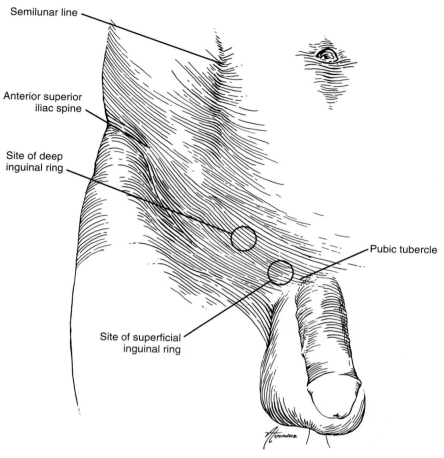

Semilunar line

Anterior superior iliac spine

Site of deep inguinal ring

Pubic tubercle

Site of superficial inguinal ring

FIGURE 71–1

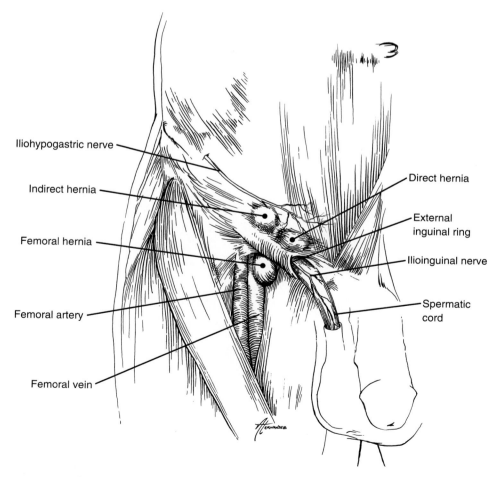

Iliohypogastric nerve

Indirect hernia

Femoral hernia

Femoral artery

Femoral vein

Direct hernia

External inguinal ring

Ilioinguinal nerve

Spermatic cord

FIGURE 71–2

◆ **Figure 71-3** is a parasagittal representation of the various layers at a point midway in the right inguinal canal.

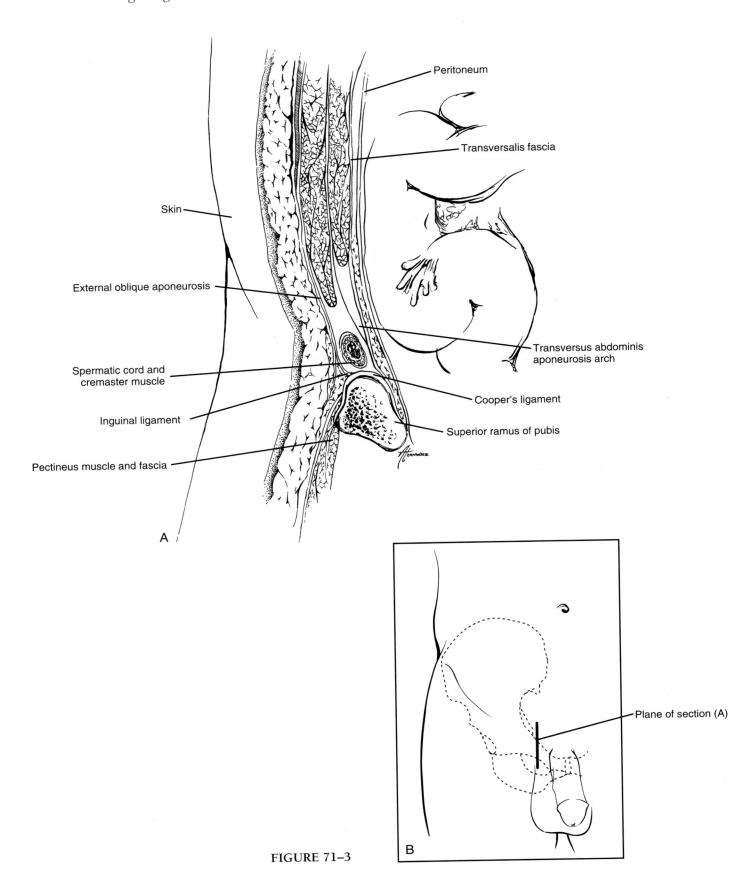

FIGURE 71–3

◆ **Figure 71-4** is a view from the inner surface of the abdominal wall—that is, from the preperitoneal space looking out.

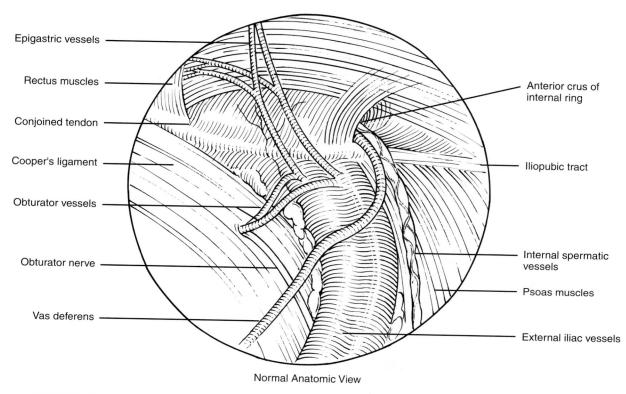

Epigastric vessels

Rectus muscles

Conjoined tendon

Cooper's ligament

Obturator vessels

Obturator nerve

Vas deferens

Anterior crus of internal ring

Iliopubic tract

Internal spermatic vessels

Psoas muscles

External iliac vessels

Normal Anatomic View

FIGURE 71–4

STEP 2: PREOPERATIVE CONSIDERATIONS

◆ The actual incidence of dangerous complications of untreated hernias is quite low, and the mortal risk from these complications, when they do occur, is similarly low.

◆ The few deaths that result from hernia repair are far more likely to be due to complications of comorbidities than operative complications, so any evaluation of a candidate for repair should include careful attention to other medical problems. Appropriate evaluation and referral for evaluation and treatment of other significant medical problems should take precedence over a recommendation for operative repair in elective cases.

◆ On the other hand, the probable natural course of an untreated inguinal hernia over time is an increase in size and symptoms, so it is not unreasonable to offer repair to a young individual with no other medical problems.

◆ The classic recommendation to evaluate and treat those conditions that might chronically increase intra-abdominal pressure, including chronic cough, constipation, and difficulty with urination, fits under the previous admonition to evaluate comorbidities and does not otherwise bear special consideration.

◆ In the final analysis, the recommendation for a hernia repair requires of the surgeon a careful balance and consideration of the natural history of untreated hernias, their symptoms and complications, the patient's age and comorbidities, and the presence of symptoms and their immediate and anticipated effect on quality of life.

TENSION VERSUS TENSION-FREE

◆ A basic precept of surgery is that wounds closed under tension are less likely to heal well than those closed with little or no tension.

◆ All of the classic tissue repairs require the approximation of tissues that do not exist in that state naturally and thereby to one degree or another create tension on wound closures.

◆ Recognition of this has led to the use of mesh to bridge hernia defects and reinforce what has been increasingly recognized as an often attenuated, hernia-prone portion of the abdominal wall, even in those areas away from the actual hernia defect at the time of operation.

◆ The purported advantages of the tension-free repairs obtained with mesh include the following:
  ◆ Mesh repairs have lower recurrence rates than tissue repairs.
  ◆ Postoperative pain is less, and recovery to full activity is faster.
  ◆ Long-term morbidity is the same as with tissue repairs.
  ◆ Although there are case reports of complications arising from the mesh itself, these are sufficiently rare to not preclude its use.

◆ The ideal material for tension-free repair has not been identified, and further research holds the promise of developing materials, whether chemical or biologic, that will decrease even further those problems associated with use of mesh.

◆ There are arguably some cases in which mesh should or cannot be used. For this reason, surgeons should be familiar with classic tissue repairs, although one has to recognize that the exposure of surgeons in training to these repairs will be quite limited in most cases.

STEP 3: OPERATIVE STEPS

1. INCISION

◆ The steps outlined here will be those used in the classic anterior approach to the inguinal canal, which is satisfactory for the performance of most mesh and tissue repairs.

◆ **Figure 71-5** illustrates two possible skin incisions for approaching the inguinal region. Incision A lies in the lower inguinal skin fold. Incision B directly exposes the external ring.

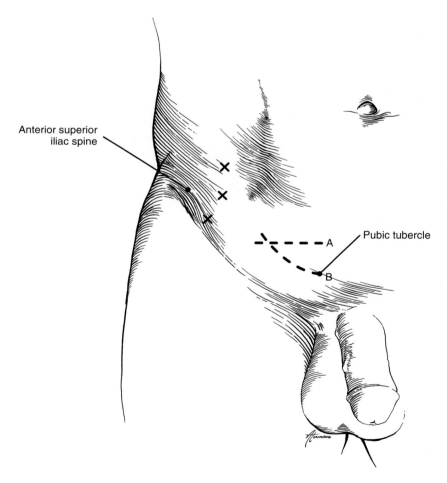

FIGURE 71–5

- Before the incision is made, 0.25% bupivacaine with epinephrine should be injected medial to the anterior superior iliac spine and deep to the external oblique aponeurosis. Approximate areas of injection are marked with an "X" on Figure 71-5. An additional 10 mL should be injected at the site of the incision.

- The skin incision should be carried through the superficial subcutaneous fat, Scarpa's fascia, and the deep subcutaneous fat until the easily recognized oblique fibers of the external oblique aponeurosis are identified.

2. DISSECTION

- The surgeon should then find the external inguinal ring, obtaining exposure as illustrated in **Figure 71-6.** Such exposure can be achieved with hand-held retractors or, as shown, with self-retaining ones.

- As shown in Figure 71-6, the aponeurosis of the external oblique should be divided in the line of its fibers through the external inguinal ring. Some advocate the use of a knife for the initial incision through the aponeurosis. I prefer scissors because they are less likely to injure underlying structures.

- Using a combination of blunt and sharp dissection, the external oblique aponeurosis should be freed superiorly and laterally from the underlying internal oblique muscle and fascia. Inferiorly and laterally, the cord structures should be swept off the undersurface of the external oblique aponeurosis down to the shelving edge of the inguinal ligament.

- The next step is longitudinal division of the fibers of the cremaster muscle that invests the structures of the spermatic cord as shown in **Figure 71-7.** Care should be taken to divide the cremaster away from the ilioinguinal nerve.

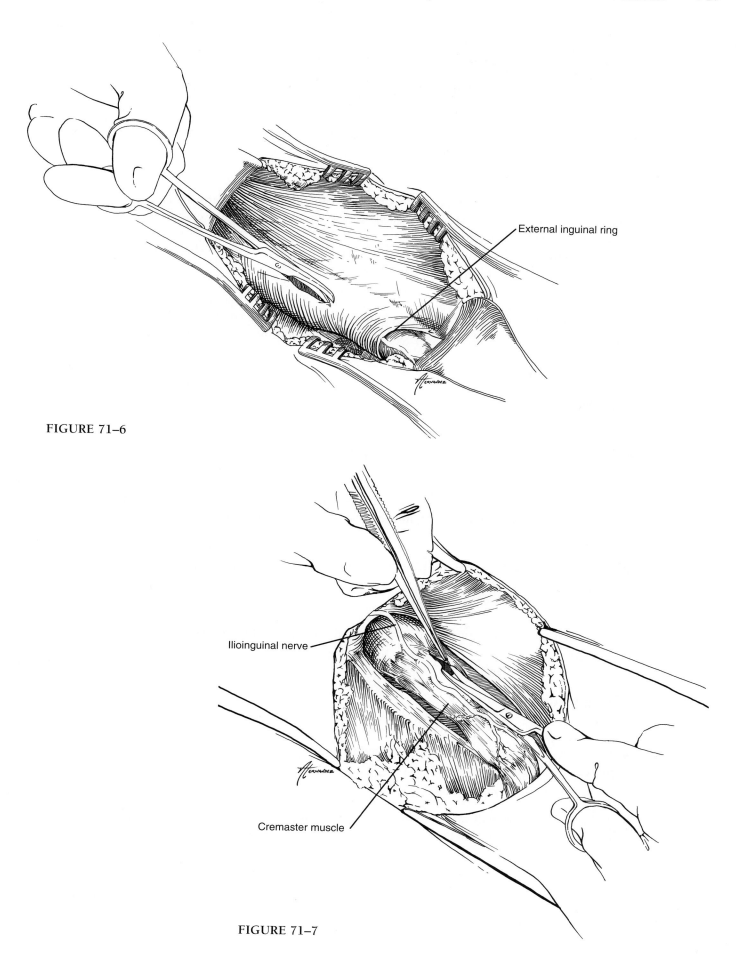

External inguinal ring

FIGURE 71–6

Ilioinguinal nerve

Cremaster muscle

FIGURE 71–7

- Superiorly, inferiorly, and posteriorly, the cremasteric fibers should be separated circumferentially from the structures of the spermatic cord. A Penrose drain can then be placed around the spermatic cord for traction as shown in **Figure 71-8.**

- In the case of an indirect hernia, this process will expose the hernia sac lying on the anterior superior part of the cord, as illustrated in Figure 71-8.

- The indirect hernia sac should then be separated carefully from the spermatic cord well up into the internal ring. Care should be taken to take down any soft tissue connections between the sac and the borders of the internal ring so that the sac can be restored to the preperitoneal space. Figure 71-8 illustrates the view on completion of this process. As shown, the inferior epigastric vessels can be seen medial to the sac and spermatic cord.

- **Figure 71-9** shows the appearance of a direct hernia. Once the spermatic cord is retracted with a Penrose drain, the direct sac can be easily dissected free of the cord and cremasteric fibers.

3. CLOSING

- Various options for repair of the hernia defect will be described in the following chapters.

- Once the repair is completed, the aponeurosis of the external oblique is reapproximated with a running absorbable suture, in the process recreating the external inguinal ring.

- Scarpa's fascia and superficial subcutaneous tissues are closed with interrupted absorbable suture.

- The skin is closed with running, subcuticular, absorbable suture reinforced with Steri-Strips.

STEP 4: POSTOPERATIVE CARE

- Most of these repairs are outpatient procedures, and patients can be discharged with a prescription for a mild analgesic agent.

- Activity instructions will vary with the type of repair and the opinion of the individual surgeon. In most cases, I advise patients to advance their level of activity as tolerated.

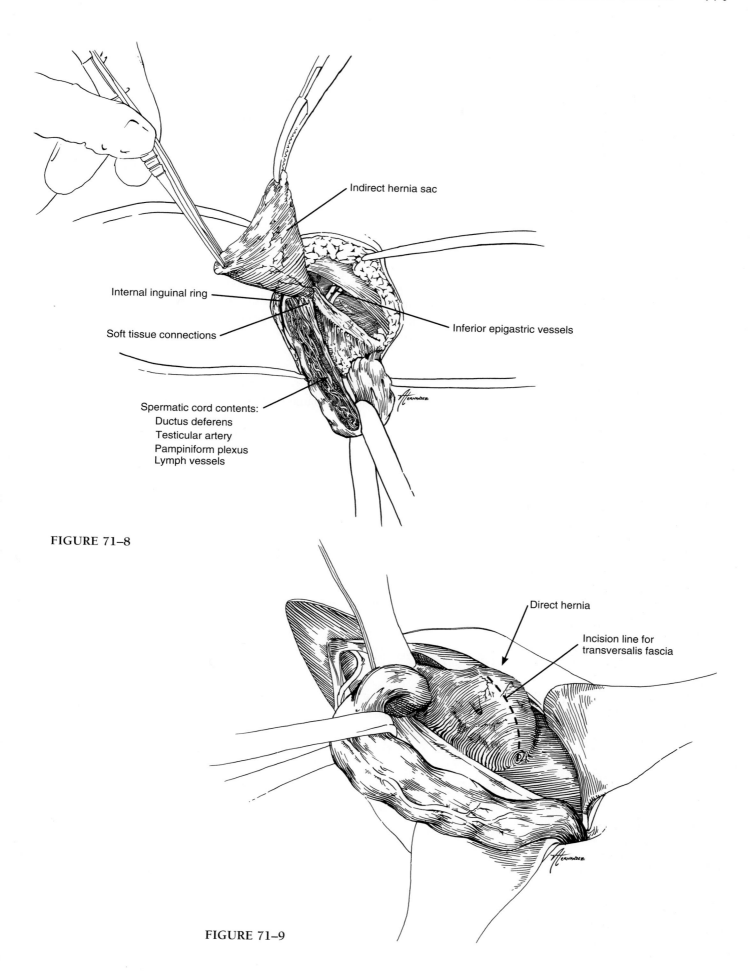

FIGURE 71–8

Indirect hernia sac

Internal inguinal ring

Soft tissue connections

Inferior epigastric vessels

Spermatic cord contents:
  Ductus deferens
  Testicular artery
  Pampiniform plexus
  Lymph vessels

Direct hernia

Incision line for transversalis fascia

FIGURE 71–9

STEP 5: PEARLS AND PITFALLS

- Although long-known as "intern cases," a careful review of the outcome literature on hernia repair shows conclusively that experience and knowledge produce better results.

- Superficial postoperative hematomas generally arise from a failure to secure the superficial epigastric veins that are encountered in exposing the external oblique aponeurosis. Although not always necessary, the safest course is to divide them between an appropriate suture ligature, such as 3-0 silk or Vicryl.

- In separating the structures of the spermatic cord from the investing cremasteric fibers, it is helpful to remember that the ductus deferens is usually the most posterior element that needs be mobilized and is easily identified by palpation. Although the genital branch of the genitofemoral nerve is posterior to the ductus deferens, I have not found it necessary to mobilize the nerve to obtain necessary exposure.

- Sharp dissection of an internal hernia sac off the spermatic cord with good exposure by traction and countertraction is less likely to lead to damage to the pampiniform venous plexus than blunt dissection.

SELECTED REFERENCES

1. Zinner MJ, Schwartz SI, Ellis H: Hernias. In Maingot R, Zinner M (eds): Maingot's Abdominal Operations, vol 1, 10th ed. Stamford, Conn, Appleton & Lang, 1997, pp 479-580.
2. Condon RE: The anatomy of the inguinal region and its relation to groin hernias. In Nyhus LM, Condon RE (eds): Hernia, 4th ed. Philadelphia, JB Lippincott, 1995, pp 16-72.

CHAPTER 72

MESH REPAIR

Thomas D. Kimbrough

STEP 1: SURGICAL ANATOMY

- See Chapter 71.

STEP 2: PREOPERATIVE CONSIDERATIONS

- There are several types of mesh repairs, and to date no studies have shown clear superiority of one over another.

- The Prolene Hernia System (PHS) repair, developed under the guidance of Dr. Arthur Gilbert, is illustrated here.

STEP 3: OPERATIVE STEPS

1. INCISION

- See Chapter 71.

2. DISSECTION

- The mesh used in the repair is illustrated in **Figure 72-1**. It comes in three sizes: extended, large, and medium.

- The technique of repair differs for indirect and direct hernias. The indirect repair will be described first. The initial operative steps for both indirect and direct hernias are outlined in Chapter 71.

- Mesh repair of an indirect hernia
  - After the hernia sac has been dissected free from all attachments to the spermatic cord and internal ring (as illustrated in Chapter 71), the next step is to return the sac to the preperitoneal space. It is not necessary to open the sac unless it contains irreducible contents, which require visual inspection. There is no advantage to resection and high ligation and that is not done. Associated cord lipomas, which are actually preperitoneal fat that has protruded through the internal ring, can be amputated or restored to their original location.
  - The preperitoneal space should be developed by bluntly pushing the peritoneal sac away from the transversalis or endoabdominal fascia. This can be facilitated by stuffing a gauze sponge through the internal ring and then withdrawing it.

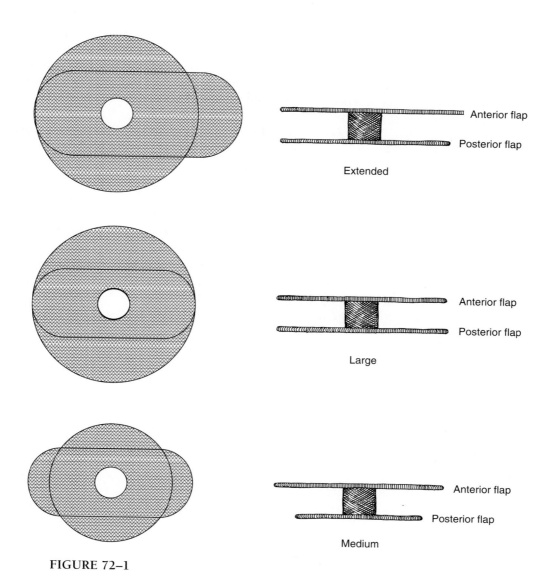

Extended

Anterior flap

Posterior flap

Large

Anterior flap

Posterior flap

Medium

Anterior flap

Posterior flap

FIGURE 72–1

- The PHS mesh is loaded onto an empty sponge forceps as illustrated in **Figure 72-2** and inserted through the internal ring. When the extended size is being used, the shorter of the two long anterior flaps should be positioned medially.
- The direction of insertion should be toward the umbilicus. The index finger of the opposing hand can be inserted through the ring into the preperitoneal space as a guide.
- The posterior flap of the mesh should be spread out in the preperitoneal space. This can be done with a finger or a pair of forceps, depending on the size of the internal ring. Medially and superiorly, the mesh should lie flat underneath the pubic tubercle and transversalis fascia. Inferiorly and laterally, the mesh will conform to the pelvic architecture and external iliac vessels.
- The anterior flap is then deployed in the floor of the inguinal canal. It is tacked into place in at least three locations with 2-0 Vicryl. Site *A* on **Figure 72-3** should be over the pubic tubercle with mesh overlap of at least 3 cm. Site *B* on Figure 72-3 should be a superficial site fixing the mesh to the fascia of the internal oblique only. Finally, as shown in Figure 72-3, a notch should be cut in the inferior part of the anterior mesh at the internal ring. The two flaps created should be wrapped around the spermatic cord at the internal ring and secured to each other and the shelving edge of the inguinal ligament with 2-0 Vicryl. The resulting opening through which the spermatic cord passes should be loose enough to allow easy introduction of a pair of forceps.
- The lateral flap is tucked under the uncut portion of the external oblique aponeurosis. Excess mesh on the anterior flap can be trimmed as desired.

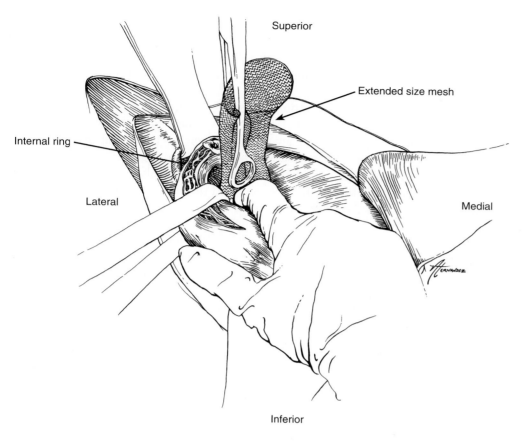

FIGURE 72–2

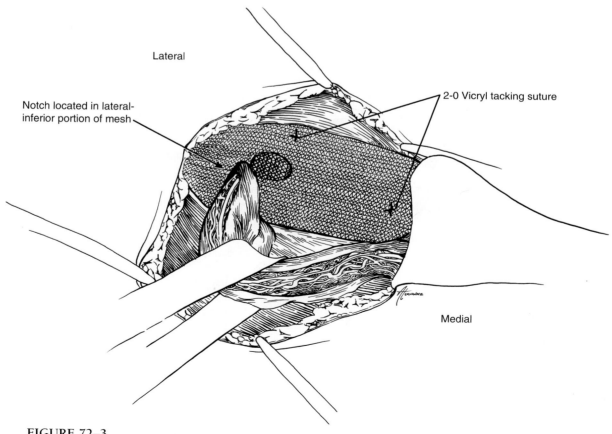

FIGURE 72–3

- Mesh repair of a direct hernia
    - In the PHS mesh repair of a direct hernia, the posterior flap of the mesh is deployed into the preperitoneal space through an incision in the attenuated transversalis fascia. If the hernia is a large direct hernia, you may desire to resect some of the attenuated transversalis fascia as shown in **Figure 72-4.**
    - As has always been the case, the spermatic cord should be inspected and explored to ensure there is not an indirect hernia also. The posterior flap of the mesh is deployed in the preperitoneal space as shown in **Figure 72-5.** Care must be taken to ensure that the mesh extends laterally to cover and protect for herniation through the internal ring. This is sometimes facilitated by dividing and ligating the inferior epigastric vessels.
    - In larger direct hernias, it is possible for the mesh to be extruded through the transversalis fascia before fibroblastic ingrowth and collagen deposition in the mesh interstices occurs. As a result, it is my practice to do the following: The connecting ring between the anterior and posterior flaps is left seated in the incision through the transversalis fascia after the posterior flap is deployed. The two sides of the cut portions of the transversalis fascia are affixed to each other and to the medial and lateral edges of the connecting ring, as shown in **Figure 72-6.** Should the incision through the transversalis be larger than the diameter of the connecting ring, additional sutures of 2-0 Vicryl are used to approximate the cut edges of the transversalis, again catching the underlying posterior mesh with each suture.

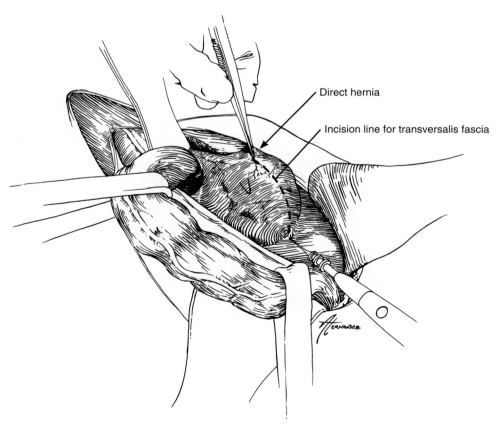

Direct hernia

Incision line for transversalis fascia

FIGURE 72–4

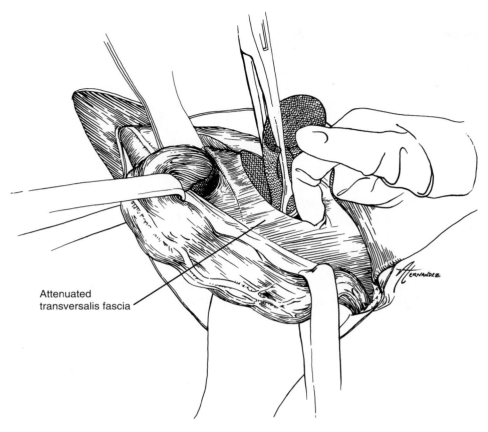

Attenuated
transversalis fascia

FIGURE 72–5

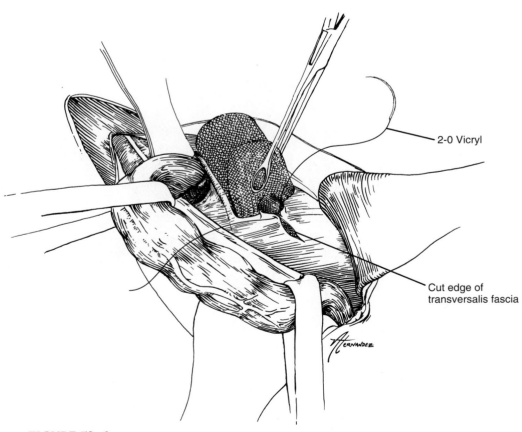

2-0 Vicryl

Cut edge of
transversalis fascia

FIGURE 72–6

◆ Deployment and fixation of the anterior flap is accomplished much the same as in repair of an indirect hernia with two exceptions (see Figure 72-6).

  ◆ The notch at the internal ring is cut in the lateral inferior part of the mesh because of the more medial placement of the connecting ring **(Figure 72-7)**.

  ◆ Most surgeons are more generous with tacking sutures because of the greater propensity for mesh extrusion early in the postoperative course.

3. CLOSING

◆ Closure is the same for either direct or indirect hernias with approximation of the external oblique aponeurosis over the completed repair with running 2-0 or 3-0 Vicryl. Care is taken to reconstruct the external ring.

◆ Scarpa's fascia and the superficial subcutaneous fat are closed with interrupted 3-0 Vicryl sutures to eliminate dead space and remove tension from the skin closure.

◆ The skin is closed with running subcuticular 4-0 Monocryl reinforced with Steri-Strips.

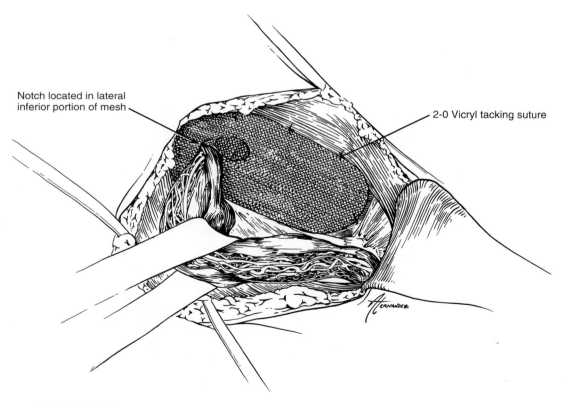

Notch located in lateral inferior portion of mesh

2-0 Vicryl tacking suture

FIGURE 72–7

STEP 4: POSTOPERATIVE CARE

- Wound care instructions are similar to those of any other abdominal operation. Patients are told that they can begin showering in 24 to 36 hours. Steri-Strips are left on until they fall off or need to be removed for other reasons.

- Patients are discharged on the day of surgery with prescriptions for oral pain medications.

- In general, patients are told that they may resume any and all activity in a stepwise progression as their own comfort dictates.

- The only exceptions are patients with large, blowout, direct hernias. In these cases, most patients limit activity for 3 to 4 weeks to help prevent mesh extrusion.

STEP 5: PEARLS AND PITFALLS

- I always use the extended size in adult males, preferring to trim any unnecessary mesh from the anterior flap rather than using too small a piece overall. In women, an extended or large size generally suffices. I have never used the medium size in an inguinal hernia repair.

- The anterior flap of the mesh is designed so that its long axis should parallel the long axis of the inguinal canal. Because the longitudinal orientation of the mesh is difficult to change once the posterior flap is deployed, correct orientation is best achieved by loading the mesh onto the sponge forceps such that the handles lie parallel to the long axis of the mesh and the inguinal canal at insertion.

- If, as is often the case, it is necessary to pull the anterior flaps out of the preperitoneal space after insertion on the sponge forceps, it is useful to place the index finger of the opposing hand in the connecting ring between the anterior and posterior flaps of the mesh. This will prevent accidental withdrawal of the posterior flap at the same time.

SELECTED REFERENCES

1. Zinner MJ, Schwartz SI, Ellis H: Hernias. In Maingot R, Zinner M (eds): Maingot's Abdominal Operations, vol 1, 10th ed. Stamford, Conn, Appleton & Lang, 1997, pp 479-580.
2. Condon RE: The anatomy of the inguinal region and its relation to groin hernias. In Nyhus LM, Condon RE (eds): Hernia, 4th ed. Philadelphia, JB Lippincott, 1995, pp 16-72.

CHAPTER 73

Inguinal Herniorrhaphy—Bassini

William J. Mileski

STEP 1: SURGICAL ANATOMY

- The anterior superior iliac spine and the ipsilateral pubic tubercle are identified and marked **(Figure 73-1)**.

STEP 2: PREOPERATIVE CONSIDERATIONS

- To avoid any confusion about the site of surgery, the site should be marked by the operating surgeon while the patient is awake in the preoperative area.

- Patient is positioned supine.

- Anesthesia may be general, regional, or local.

STEP 3: OPERATIVE STEPS

1. INCISION

- A near transverse incision is then made in the skin, paralleling Langer's lines, 1 to 2 inches inferior and medial to the iliac spine to a point 1 to 2 inches lateral and superior to the pubic tubercle (see Figure 73-1).

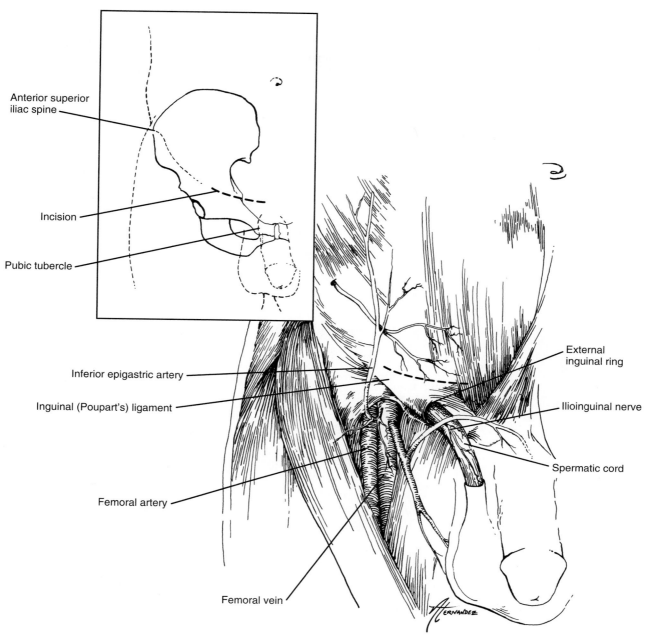

Anterior superior
iliac spine

Incision

Pubic tubercle

Inferior epigastric artery

Inguinal (Poupart's) ligament

Femoral artery

Femoral vein

External
inguinal ring

Ilioinguinal nerve

Spermatic cord

FIGURE 73–1

2. DISSECTION

◆ Subcutaneous fat is dissected, and the external oblique aponeurosis, inguinal ligament, and external inguinal ring are exposed **(Figure 73-2)**.

◆ The external oblique is incised from the external ring to a point lateral to the internal ring. Blunt dissection is used to separate the external oblique fascia from the underlying tissues, and the external oblique fascia is held with a self-retaining retractor **(Figure 73-3)**.

◆ The ilioinguinal nerve is dissected from the cord structures and cremaster and retracted to the inferior lateral aspect of the wound.

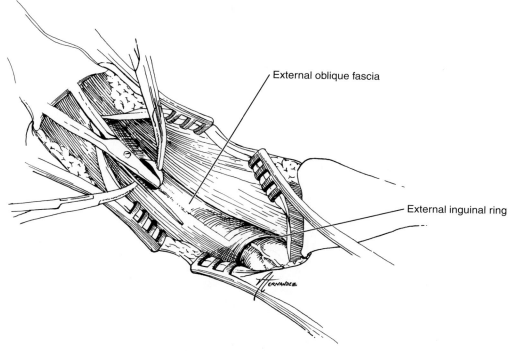

External oblique fascia

External inguinal ring

FIGURE 73–2

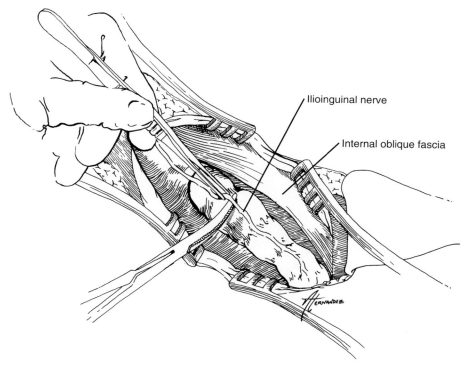

Ilioinguinal nerve

Internal oblique fascia

FIGURE 73–3

◆ The spermatic cord is then fully encircled at the pubis and retracted with a Penrose drain **(Figures 73-4 and 73-5)**. Cremasteric fibers are dissected from the cord structures, and if present the indirect hernia sac is identified; its contents are reduced; and the sac is ligated with a nonabsorbable suture, such as 2-0 silk **(Figure 73-6)**.

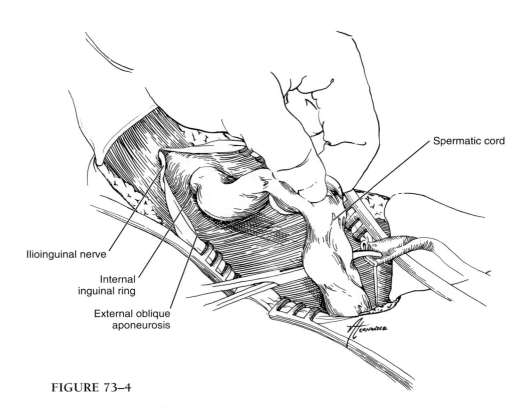

Spermatic cord

Ilioinguinal nerve

Internal
inguinal ring

External oblique
aponeurosis

FIGURE 73–4

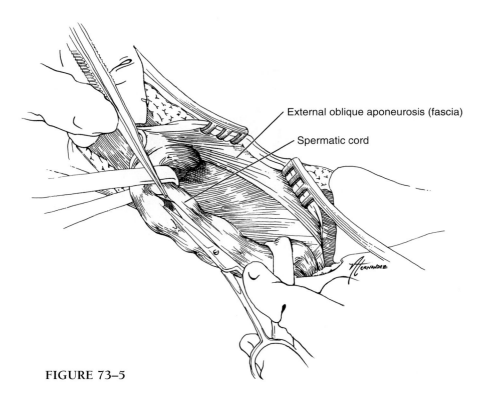

External oblique aponeurosis (fascia)

Spermatic cord

FIGURE 73–5

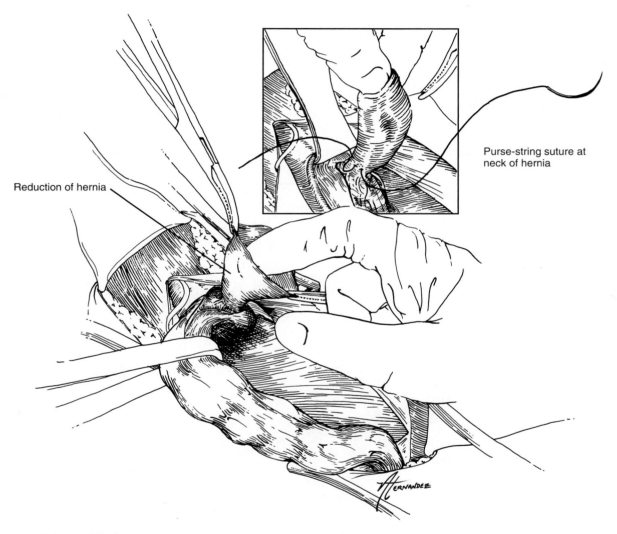

Reduction of hernia

Purse-string suture at
neck of hernia

FIGURE 73–6

◆ The repair of the inguinal floor can then be accomplished by approximating the reflex portion of the inguinal ligament to the inferior aspects of the transversalis fascia and the transversus abdominis muscles. In some patients this is clearly fused as a conjoint tendon; however most often the tissues of the transversalis and transversus abdominis are difficult to distinguish. This can be aided by retracting the internal oblique muscle with a rake or Senn retractor and grasping the transversalis fascia and transversus abdominis with several Allis clamps. Interrupted nonabsorbable sutures (0 silk or 0 Prolene) are then placed approximately 1 cm apart from the pubic tubercle to the internal ring. It is important to avoid injury to the femoral vessels as the sutures are placed near the internal inguinal ring. Two additional ligatures are placed lateral to the internal ring, leaving enough room for the spermatic cord without causing venous obstruction (**Figure 73-7**).

◆ The spermatic cord and ilioinguinal nerve are replaced, and the external oblique muscle is reapproximated using a running absorbable suture, such as 2-0 Vicryl (**Figure 73-8**).

3. CLOSING

◆ Skin is closed with a running subcuticular suture of 3-0 Monocryl (**Figure 73-9**).

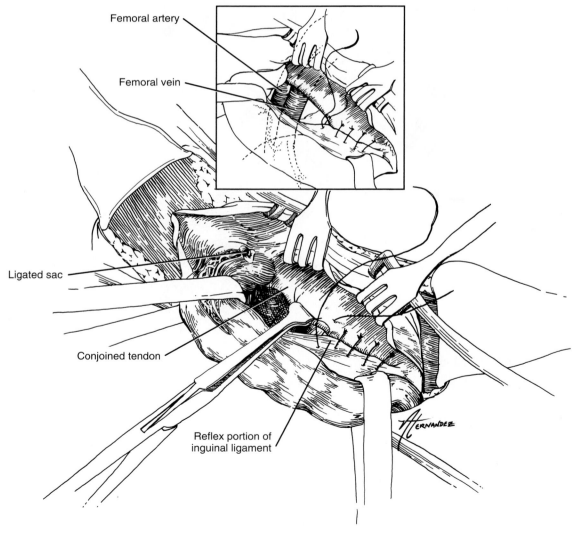

Femoral artery

Femoral vein

Ligated sac

Conjoined tendon

Reflex portion of inguinal ligament

FIGURE 73–7

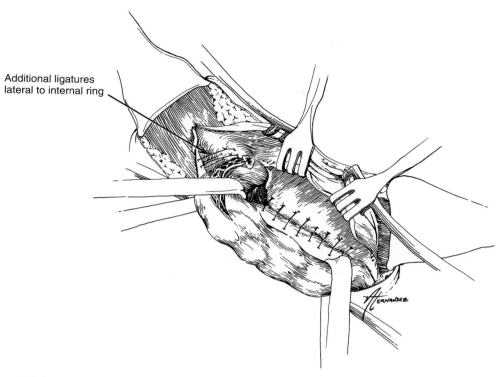

Additional ligatures
lateral to internal ring

FIGURE 73–8

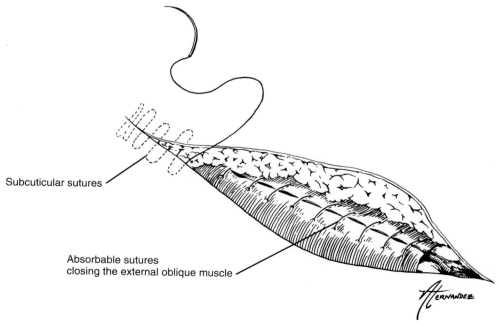

Subcuticular sutures

Absorbable sutures
closing the external oblique muscle

FIGURE 73–9

STEP 4: POSTOPERATIVE CARE

- The patient should be encouraged to participate in early ambulation and to void before discharge. No specific wound care is required; patients can shower on the first postoperative day. The patient should remain on stool softeners as long as postoperative analgesia requires the use of narcotics. The patient should be instructed to avoid heavy lifting (more than 8 pounds, or a gallon of liquid) for 4 to 6 weeks.

STEP 5: PEARLS AND PITFALLS

- Careful identification of the conjoint tendon and transversalis fascia are critical before approximation to the reflex portion of the inguinal ligament. Meticulous suture placement at 0.5 to 1.0 cm apart to distribute tension evenly helps ensure a sound repair.

SELECTED REFERENCES

1. Nyhus LM, Condon RE: Hernia, 3rd ed. Philadelphia, Lippincott, 1989.
2. Wantz GE, Henselmann C: Atlas of Hernia Surgery. New York, Raven Press, 1991.
3. Ponka JL: Hernias of the Abdominal Wall. Philadelphia, Saunders, 1980.
4. Wantz GE: The operation of Bassini as described by Attilio Catterina. Surg Gynecol Obstet 1989;168: 67-80.

CHAPTER 74

INGUINAL HERNIORRHAPHY (McVAY; COOPER'S LIGAMENT REPAIR)

Dennis C. Gore

STEP 1: SURGICAL ANATOMY

Important landmarks in the inguinal region include the ilioinguinal ligament, which runs from the anterior superior iliac crest to the symphysis pubis. The spermatic cord traverses anteriorly and medially relative to the ilioinguinal ligament, exiting the abdomen at the external ring. The femoral vessels traverse the ilioinguinal ligament posteriorly (**Figure 74-1**).

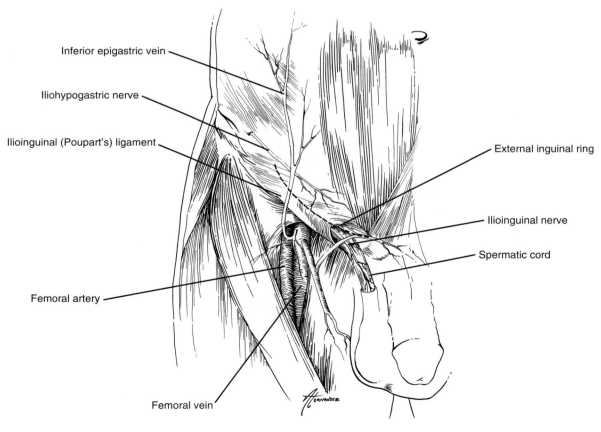

Inferior epigastric vein

Iliohypogastric nerve

Ilioinguinal (Poupart's) ligament

External inguinal ring

Ilioinguinal nerve

Spermatic cord

Femoral artery

Femoral vein

FIGURE 74–1

STEP 2: PREOPERATIVE CONSIDERATIONS

- Indications: inguinal hernia

- Anesthesia: general or spinal

- Position: supine

- Before the procedure, exclude and correct as feasible any conditions that may increase intra-abdominal pressure and thereby weaken the herniorrhaphy. For example, correction of prostatic hypertrophy, chronic cough, or constipation may aid in reducing hernia recurrence.

STEP 3: OPERATIVE STEPS

1. INCISION

- A skin incision is made 3 cm above and parallel to the ilioinguinal (Poupart's) ligament.

2. DISSECTION

- Use 3-0 Vicryl ligatures to secure hemostasis on the predominant veins that traverse the subcutaneous tissue along the incision.

- Use small Richardson retractors to bluntly dissect subcutaneous fat, exposing the external oblique aponeurosis.

- Manually identify the external ring.

- Make a small incision in the direction of the external oblique aponeurosis bands, and extend this incision to the external ring using scissors **(Figure 74-2)**.

- Dissect free the ilioinguinal nerve that commonly lies anterior to the spermatic cord. Retract the nerve away from the hernia/spermatic cord **(Figure 74-3)**.

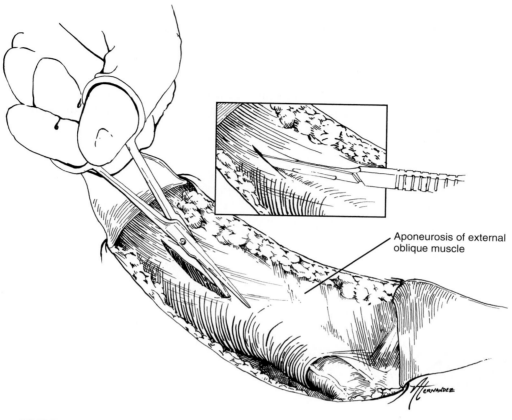

Aponeurosis of external
oblique muscle

FIGURE 74-2

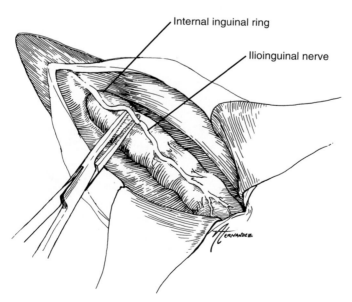

Internal inguinal ring

Ilioinguinal nerve

FIGURE 74-3

◆ Use manual dissection to free the spermatic cord from the underlying abdominal wall at the level of the prior external ring. Place a Penrose drain around the spermatic cord and retract the cord laterally (**Figure 74-4**).

◆ Use sharp dissection with forceps and retraction with hemostats to separate cremaster muscle, vas deferens, and spermatic vasculature away from any indirect hernia sac (**Figure 74-5**).

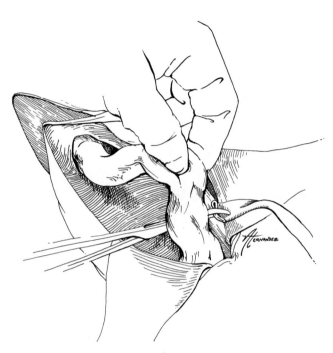

FIGURE 74–4

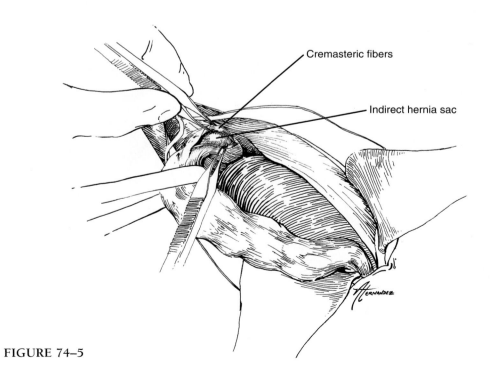

Cremasteric fibers

Indirect hernia sac

FIGURE 74–5

◆ Open the indirect hernia sac and reduce any contents back into the abdomen.

◆ Ligate the indirect hernia sac at the internal ring using 2-0 permanent braided suture **(Figure 74-6)**.

◆ Incise the anterior surface of the indirect hernia sac distally.

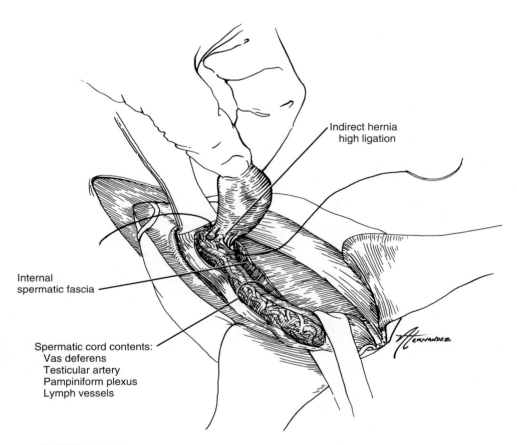

FIGURE 74–6

- Invert any direct hernia, place several 2-0 permanent braided sutures in a Lembert fashion to hold inversion of the direct hernia sac (**Figure 74-7**).

- Place two Richardson retractors cupping the external oblique aponeurosis and exposing the junction of the ilioinguinal ligament and symphysis pubis.

- Manually or with forceps start at this medial portion of the ilioinguinal ligament and dissect along the ligament to expose the underlying Cooper's ligament. Extend exposure laterally to the lacunar ligament.

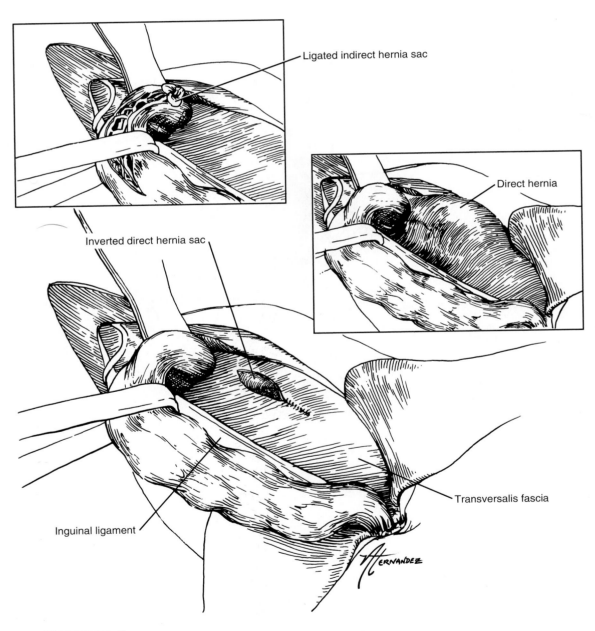

FIGURE 74-7

◆ Starting medially, use multiple 2-0 permanent braided sutures to approximate the transversalis fascia to Cooper's ligament **(Figure 74-8)**.

◆ After 3 to 5 interrupted sutures have secured the transversalis fascia to Cooper's ligament, place additional 2-0 sutures securing the transversalis fascia to the ilioinguinal ligament as this ligament passes anterior to the iliac vessels **(Figure 74-9)**.

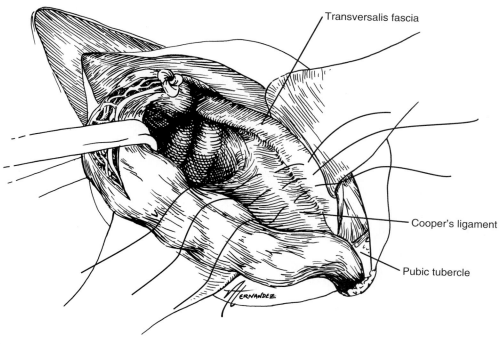

Transversalis fascia

Cooper's ligament

Pubic tubercle

FIGURE 74–8

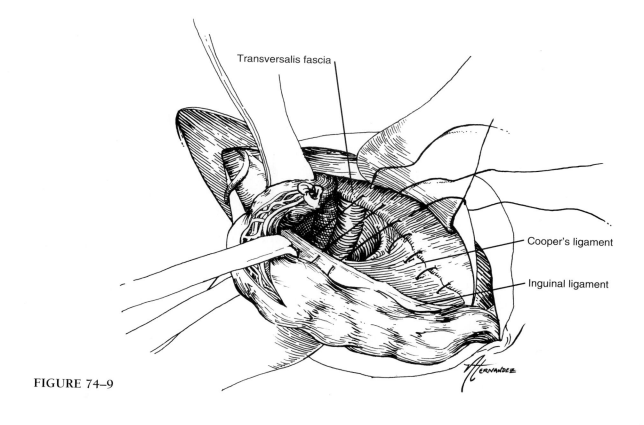

Transversalis fascia

Cooper's ligament

Inguinal ligament

FIGURE 74–9

◆ Place multiple small incisions through the fascia overlying the rectus abdominis muscle, thereby relaxing tension on the repair (**Figure 74-10**).

◆ Remove the Penrose drain and replace the spermatic cord and ilioinguinal nerve over the pelvic floor.

◆ Reapproximate the aponeurosis of the external oblique muscle using a running 3-0 Vicryl suture (**Figure 74-11**).

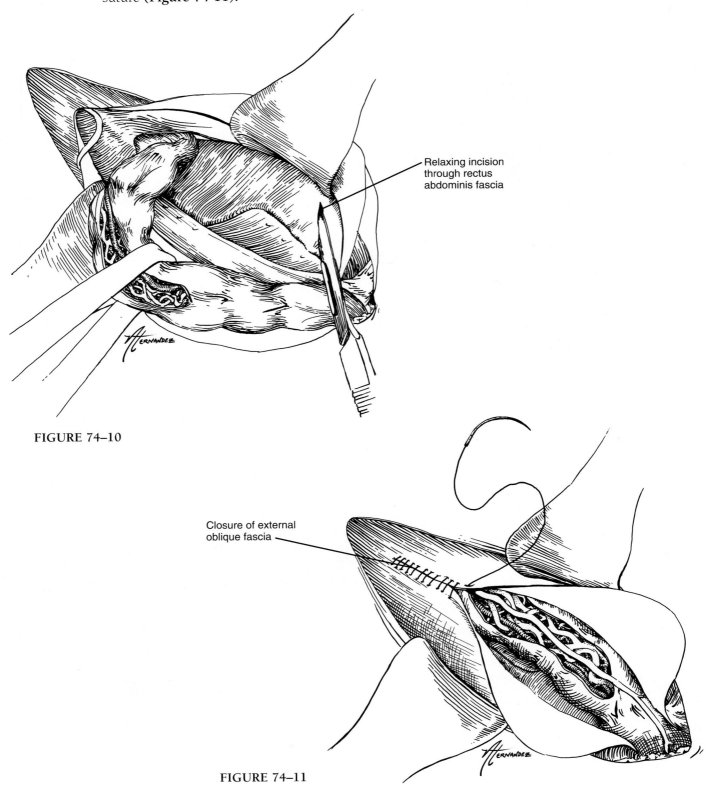

Relaxing incision through rectus abdominis fascia

FIGURE 74–10

Closure of external oblique fascia

FIGURE 74–11

3. CLOSING

- Close skin with staples or 3-0 or 4-0 permanent monofilament suture (Prolene).

STEP 4: POSTOPERATIVE CARE

- Instruct the patient to refrain from heavy lifting or aggressive activity for 3 to 4 weeks.

STEP 5: PEARLS AND PITFALLS

- For large indirect hernia sacs, simply incising along the anterior surface precludes the need for removal of the indirect hernia sac, thereby greatly reducing the incidence of subsequent hydrocele formation yet minimizing any bleeding associated with complete removal of the sac.

- Place sutures at unequal depth and distance when approximating the transversalis fascia or external oblique aponeurosis to reduce any sheer effect and thereby strengthen the closure.

SELECTED REFERENCE

1. Zollinger RM Jr, Zollinger RM: Atlas of Surgical Operations, 5th ed. New York, Macmillan, 1983, p 402.

CHAPTER 75

INGUINAL HERNIORRHAPHY— SHOULDICE

Michael D. Trahan

STEP 1: SURGICAL ANATOMY

- A thorough knowledge and understanding of the anatomy of the inguinal canal and pre-peritoneal space is critical to success in the tissue repair of the inguinal hernia.

- The site of incision and surface landmarks important to consider are demonstrated in **Figure 75-1.**

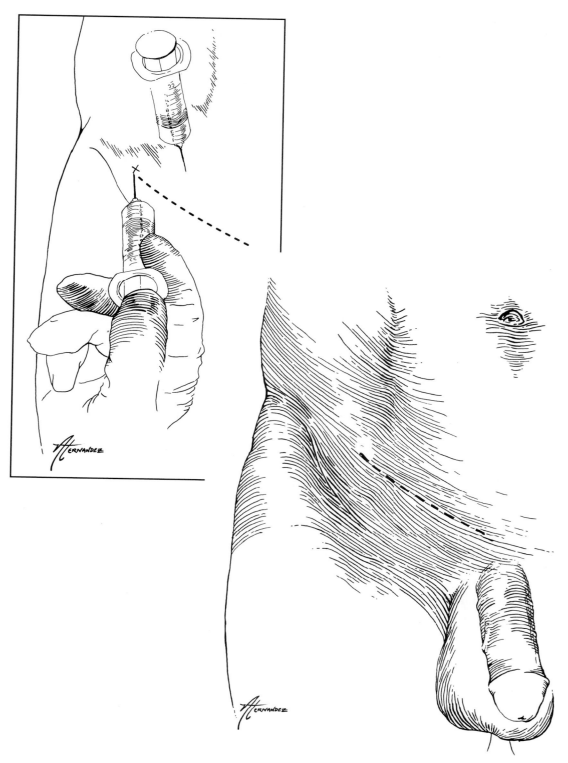

FIGURE 75–1

- The important structures of the male inguinal canal are illustrated in **Figure 75-2.**

- It is important to note that these structures may be significantly distorted by large or long-standing hernias, or both.

STEP 2: PREOPERATIVE CONSIDERATIONS

- Repair of an inguinal hernia should be considered for the patient with symptoms from the hernia that interfere with daily activities and for those hernias at risk for incarceration or strangulation.

- An effort should be made to diagnose and treat conditions that result in Valsalva, such as constipation, urinary straining, and chronic cough, before hernia repair.

- The Shouldice hernia repair has the lowest recurrence risk of all of the tissue repairs.

ANESTHESIA

- The choice of anesthesia should be tailored to the individual patient after evaluation by the anesthesiologist.

- This repair can be performed with general, regional (spinal), or local anesthesia.

- Five to 10 mL of a long-acting local anesthetic, such as bupivacaine, should be injected just medial to the anterior superior iliac spine and deep to the external oblique muscle.

- Ten milliliters of the local anesthetic is injected subcutaneously at the site of the incision.

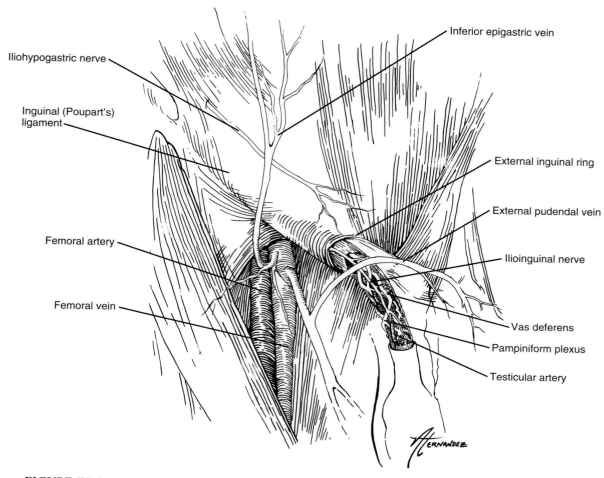

Iliohypogastric nerve

Inguinal (Poupart's) ligament

Femoral artery

Femoral vein

Inferior epigastric vein

External inguinal ring

External pudendal vein

Ilioinguinal nerve

Vas deferens

Pampiniform plexus

Testicular artery

FIGURE 75–2

STEP 3: OPERATIVE STEPS

1. INCISION

◆ Shaving should be avoided. If hair removal is necessary, it should be removed with an electric clipper.

◆ A linear incision is made over the external inguinal ring parallel to the course of the inguinal ligament.

◆ The subcutaneous fat and Scarpa's fascia are divided sharply to expose the external abdominal oblique aponeurosis and spermatic cord **(Figure 75-3)**.

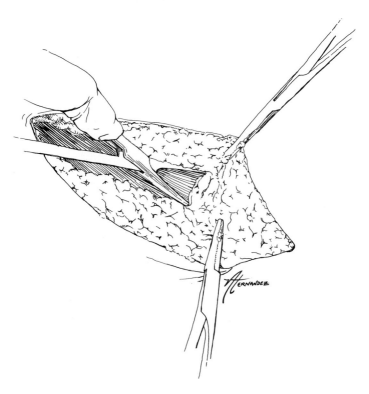

FIGURE 75–3

2. DISSECTION

◆ The external oblique aponeurosis is incised obliquely along the lines of its fibers, down through the external inguinal ring (**Figure 75-4**).

◆ The plane between the external and internal oblique muscle layers should be sharply dissected to the rectus sheath medially and the shelving edge of the inguinal ligament inferior laterally (**Figure 75-5**).

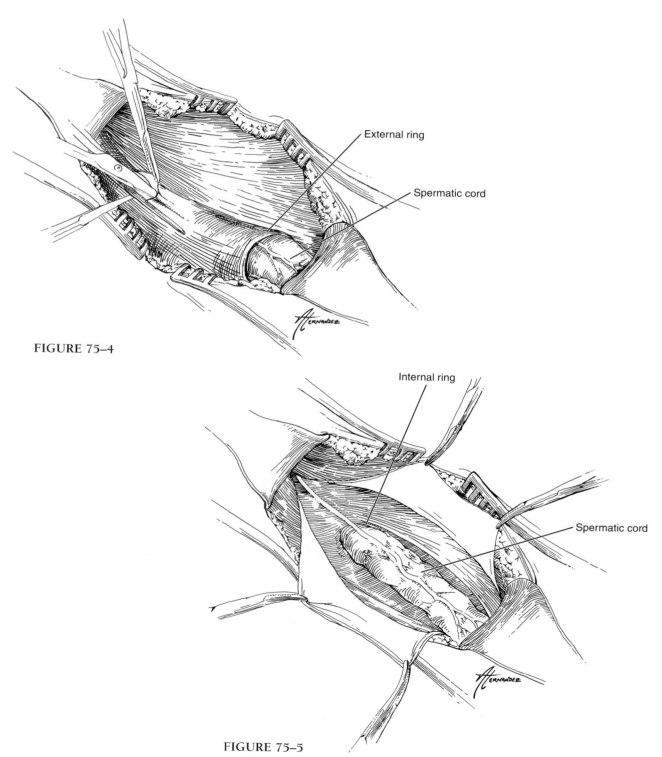

FIGURE 75–4

FIGURE 75–5

◆ The spermatic cord is mobilized from the floor of the inguinal canal and encircled with a Penrose drain **(Figure 75-6)**.

◆ The cremaster muscle is incised longitudinally to reveal the hernia sac and cord structures **(Figure 75-7)**.

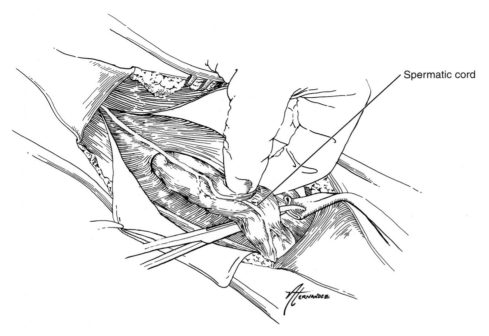

Spermatic cord

FIGURE 75–6

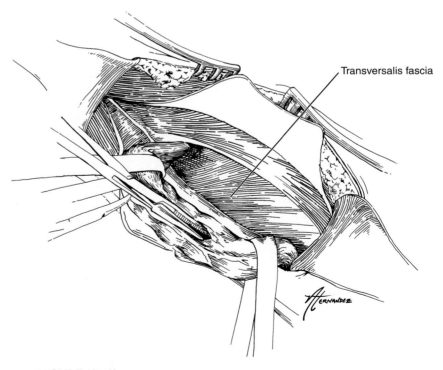

Transversalis fascia

FIGURE 75–7

◆ Dissection of the indirect sac and any cord lipomas from the cord structures should be complete up through the internal inguinal ring. Large sacs may be excised, whereas smaller sacs may be reduced through the ring **(Figure 75-8)**.

◆ The floor of the inguinal canal (transversalis fascia) is incised beginning near the pubic tubercle and proceeding laterally, with care taken to avoid the epigastric vessels as the internal ring is approached. The preperitoneal fat should protrude through the incision to ensure adequate opening of this layer **(Figure 75-9)**.

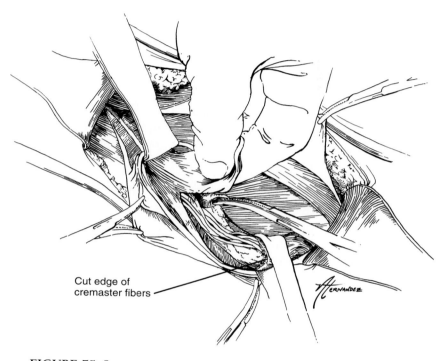

Cut edge of
cremaster fibers

FIGURE 75–8

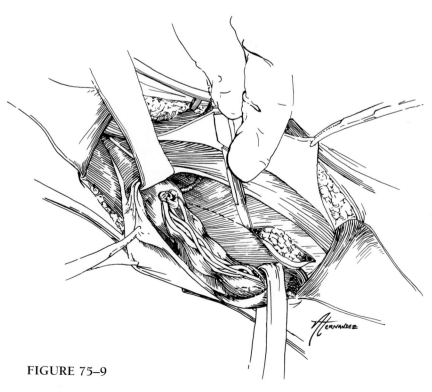

FIGURE 75–9

◆ The excess transversalis fascia of a large direct hernia may need to be trimmed.

◆ The preperitoneal fat should be swept off of the transversalis fascia to allow adequate mobilization of these flaps to complete the operation.

◆ Two nonabsorbable sutures such as 2-0 polypropylene are then used to perform the running four-layer closure.

◆ The first suture is started with a healthy bite of the pubic tubercle securing the lower layer of the transversalis fascia to the undersurface of the upper flap incorporating a bite of the rectus sheath. Small, closely spaced bites are used to close this layer progressing to the internal ring **(Figure 75-10)**.

◆ Without tying this suture, the second layer is started by approximating the upper flap of the transversalis to the shelving edge of the inguinal ligament, with care taken to not strangulate the cord. The second layer of the first suture ends at the pubic bone, where the suture is tied **(Figure 75-11)**.

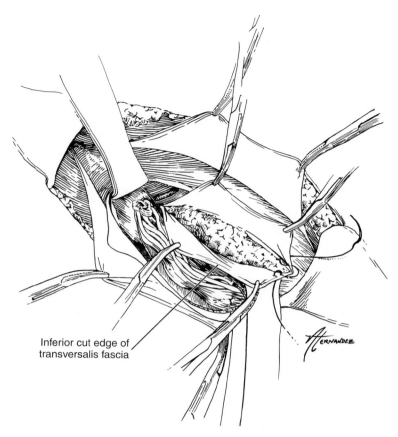

Inferior cut edge of
transversalis fascia

FIGURE 75–10

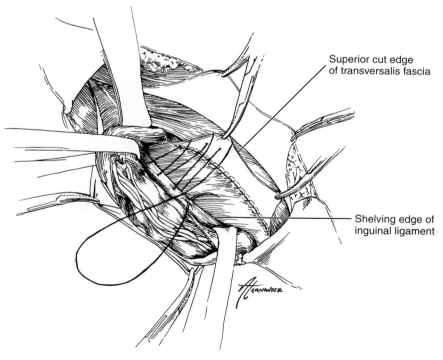

Superior cut edge
of transversalis fascia

Shelving edge of
inguinal ligament

FIGURE 75–11

◆ The second polypropylene suture is started laterally at the internal ring, and this third layer is used to oversew the second layer reinforcing the transversalis/internal oblique to inguinal ligament approximation **(Figure 75-12)**.

◆ After reaching the pubic tubercle again, in the final layer, the internal oblique muscle is sewn to the inguinal ligament. The suture is then tied at the inguinal ring **(Figure 75-13)**.

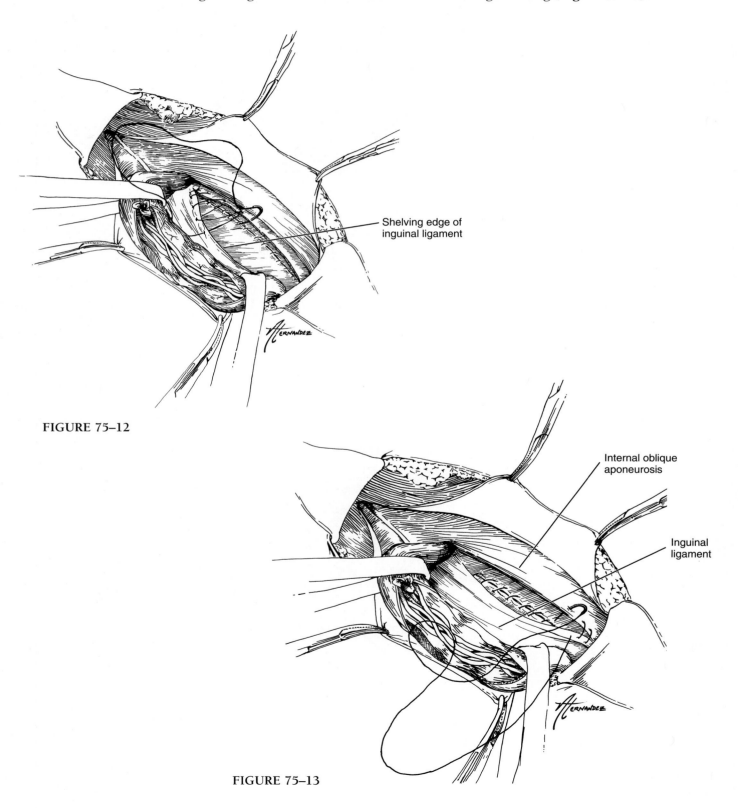

Shelving edge of inguinal ligament

FIGURE 75–12

Internal oblique aponeurosis

Inguinal ligament

FIGURE 75–13

3. CLOSING

◆ The spermatic cord is returned to its anatomic position, and the external oblique is closed with running 3-0 absorbable suture, such as Vicryl **(Figure 75-14)**.

◆ Scarpa's fascia is reapproximated with 3-0 Vicryl.

◆ Standard skin closure is the surgeon's choice of running subcuticular absorbable suture, such as 4-0 Monocryl or interrupted permanent suture, such as staples or 2-0 polypropylene **(Figure 75-15)**.

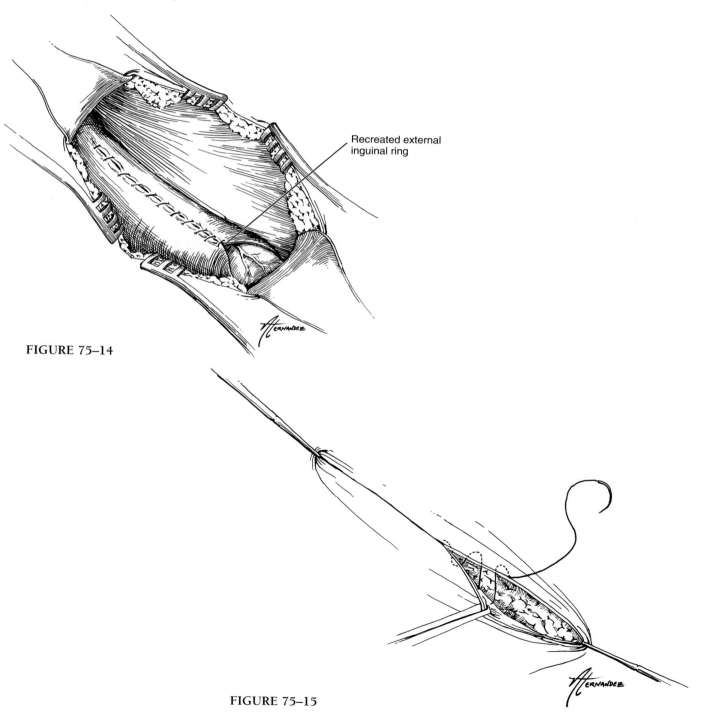

Recreated external inguinal ring

FIGURE 75–14

FIGURE 75–15

STEP 4: POSTOPERATIVE CARE

- ◆ Ice pack, oral hydrocodone or propoxyphene, and stool softeners are the standard post-operative orders.

- ◆ Activity and driving should be restricted until the patient is comfortable and no longer in need of pain medication.

- ◆ Severe pain and swelling of the testicle should be immediately evaluated for the possibility of ischemia.

STEP 5: PEARLS AND PITFALLS

- ◆ Hemostasis during sac dissection should be meticulous to avoid injury to the pampiniform plexus and the development of wound hematomas.

- ◆ Care must be taken to avoid crushing, burning, or entrapment of the cutaneous nerves in the inguinal canal to decrease the possibility of postoperative chronic pain syndromes.

- ◆ Patients should be thoroughly educated about the postoperative disability after a tension-producing repair of inguinal hernia.

SELECTED REFERENCES

1. Hay JM, Boudet MJ, Fingerhut A, et al: Shouldice inguinal hernia repair in the male adult: The gold standard? A multicenter controlled trial in 1578 patients. Ann Surg 1995;222:719-727.
2. Shouldice EE: The treatment of hernia. Ont Med Rev 1953;20:670-684.
3. Welsh DR, Alexander MA: The Shouldice repair. Surg Clin North Am 1993;73:451-469.

CHAPTER 76

SLIDING INGUINAL HERNIA

Thomas D. Kimbrough

STEP 1: SURGICAL ANATOMY

- A sliding inguinal hernia is defined as one in which a viscus or its attendant mesentery constitute a part of the wall of the hernia sac.

- Although sliding hernias have been reported in all three types of groin hernia, they are most common in the indirect location.

- Again, although a wide variety of organs have been reported, including female adnexa, appendix, ileum, ureter, and bladder, the sliding component most commonly is the cecum on the right side of the body and the sigmoid colon on the left.

- The part of the wall of the hernia sac involved is usually the posterior lateral region.

STEP 2: PREOPERATIVE CONSIDERATIONS

- Sliding hernias are rarely identified preoperatively, and in fact there is little reason to worry about doing so.

- Preoperative preparation should follow guidelines outlined in earlier chapters.

STEP 3: OPERATIVE STEPS

1. INCISION

- The standard incisions described in Chapter 71 are sufficient.

2. DISSECTION

◆ The most important step in dealing with a sliding hernia is its recognition. Failure to do so can result in unnecessary dissection leading to injury to the involved organ or its blood supply.

◆ It is important to differentiate between adhesions from abdominal organs to the inner surface of the hernia sac and true sliding hernias. Adhesions can be carefully lysed and the freed organ reduced back into the abdominal cavity.

◆ A right-sided sliding hernia is illustrated in **Figure 76-1.** Note the cecum forming part of the posterior lateral wall of the opened hernia sac.

3. CLOSURE

◆ Once any adhesions are taken down, the peritoneum is sewn shut, closing the hernia sac as shown in **Figure 76-2.** Care should be taken to avoid catching any part of the colon and its mesentery in the closure.

◆ Because a sliding hernia is a modification of an indirect hernia, once the sac is closed, it and the attached colon can be reduced back into the preperitoneal space in the fashion described in Chapter 71.

◆ Similarly, repair can then proceed by one of the techniques appropriate for an indirect hernia.

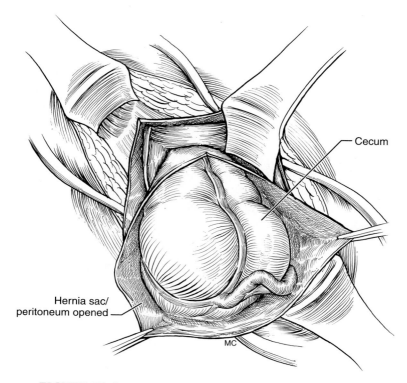

FIGURE 76–1

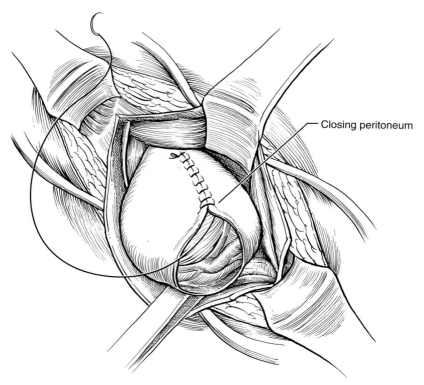

FIGURE 76–2

STEP 4: POSTOPERATIVE CARE

- There are no special considerations or steps necessary in postoperative care different from those mentioned in Chapter 71.

STEP 5: PEARLS AND PITFALLS

- Mentioned earlier but worth repeating, prompt recognition of the presence of a sliding hernia and avoidance of unnecessary and potentially damaging dissection is desirable.

- Because most of these are variants on the standard indirect hernia, any repair appropriate for a large version of that hernia will suffice here.

SELECTED REFERENCE

1. Nyhus LM, Condon RE (eds): Hernia, 4th ed. Philadelphia, JB Lippincott, 1995.

CHAPTER 77

INGUINAL HERNIAS IN INFANTS AND SMALL CHILDREN

Carlos A. Angel

INTRODUCTION

◆ The incidence of indirect inguinal hernias (which comprise 99% of the hernias found in small children) ranges from 1% to 5% of the population, with a male-to-female ratio of 8:1 to 10:1. Premature infants are at greater risk for developing inguinal hernias, with reported incidences ranging from 7% to 30% for boys and 2% for girls. The risk of incarceration is inversely proportional to the age of the patient and may exceed 60% in the first 6 months of life. Most neonatologists and pediatric surgeons recommend repair of inguinal hernias in premature babies before discharge from the hospital. The incidence of bilateral inguinal hernias in children and routine contralateral groin exploration at the time of repair are controversial topics. The possibility that bilateral inguinal hernias will be present at operation is greater in younger patients, but the risk of bilaterality subsequently decreases to 41% for children 2 to 16 years of age. Incidence of bilateral inguinal hernias seems to be greater in female patients in all age groups, with reported values ranging from 20% to 50%. Patients with ventriculoperitoneal (VP) shunts, peritoneal dialysis catheters, connective tissue disorders such as Ehlers-Danlos syndrome, and cystic fibrosis have a high enough incidence of bilaterality to justify routine contralateral exploration. Laparoscopic exploration of the contralateral inguinal ring by inserting a small 70-degree scope (or 120-degree, if available) through the hernia sac is a recent approach that is helpful in avoiding unnecessary and potentially morbid contralateral groin explorations. I continue to perform routine contralateral explorations in all premature infants with an inguinal hernia.

STEP 1: SURGICAL ANATOMY

◆ The processus vaginalis, which is a peritoneal diverticulum that extends in utero through the internal inguinal ring, is dragged along with testicular descent into the scrotum, where the portion surrounding the testicle will become the tunica vaginalis while the rest of the processus obliterates before the child's birth. Persistence of a patent processus vaginalis may lead to indirect inguinal hernias, hydroceles of the cord, or communicating hydroceles. Most inguinal hernias in children (99%) are indirect; that is, the sac originates lateral to the inferior epigastric vessels (although it may extend past them) and is close (on the anteromedial side) to the spermatic vessels and the vas deferens. All cord structures are enveloped by the deep spermatic fascia, which is very thin and translucent, and more superficially by the cremaster muscle, which originates from the internal oblique muscle.

STEP 2: PREOPERATIVE CONSIDERATIONS

♦ In most children, laboratory examinations or antibiotics are not indicated before hernia repair. The time at which ingesting clear fluids is stopped depends on the age of the patient and ranges from 3 to 6 hours before the procedure. Most anesthesiologists will administer an anxiolytic agent such as midazolam in the preoperative area to reduce separation anxiety and the fear that arises from an unfamiliar environment. Anesthetic technique varies depending on the level of comfort and experience of the anesthesiologist. In most patients, general endotracheal anesthesia will be preferred. In selected cases, such as very small infants with chronic pulmonary disease, in which endotracheal intubation can result in prolonged mechanical ventilatory support in the postoperative period, the procedure can be safely performed with the infant under a regional anesthetic such as a caudal block. Preoperative planning should include 23-hour postoperative observation and monitoring in all patients who were born prematurely within the previous 4 to 6 months.

STEP 3: OPERATIVE STEPS

1. INCISION

♦ The patient is placed on the operating table in the supine position. After anesthesia is induced, the lower abdomen, both groins, penis, and scrotum are prepped with a topical antiseptic solution and draped in a sterile fashion. A small (3- to 4- cm) incision is made along the lower abdominal crease **(Figure 77-1)**. The subcutaneous fat is grasped between mosquito hemostats and divided with electrocautery at very low settings. Two crossing veins can be either pushed off the midline, cauterized, or tied. Division of the subcutaneous fat stops when Scarpa's fascia becomes evident. Scarpa's fascia has a pearly, shiny appearance. Scarpa's fascia is opened with scissors, and blunt dissection is used, starting on the lateral aspect of the incision and working medially to expose the external oblique aponeurosis and the external inguinal ring. The external oblique aponeurosis is opened sharply, and this incision is extended until opening the external inguinal ring **(Figure 77-2)**. Care must be taken to avoid injury of the ilioinguinal nerve. The spermatic cord is grasped gently, avoiding any manipulation of the vas deferens. At this stage of the operation, bringing the testicle into the operative field should be avoided.

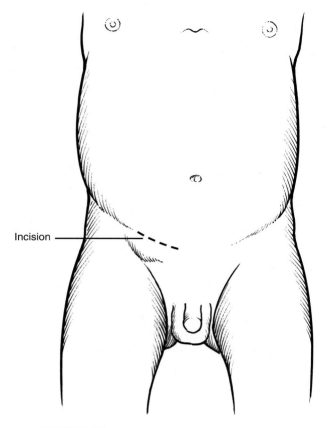

Incision

FIGURE 77–1

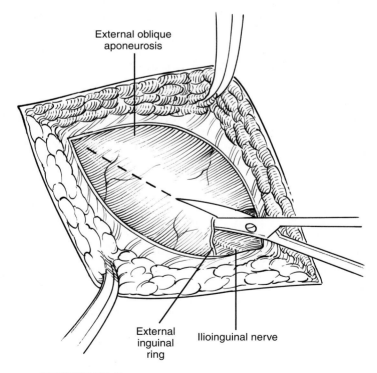

External oblique
aponeurosis

External
inguinal
ring

Ilioinguinal nerve

FIGURE 77–2

2. DISSECTION

◆ The cremasteric fibers that surround the spermatic cord are bluntly separated. Be aware that use of electrocautery in the vicinity of the spermatic vessels or the vas deferens is very hazardous, because transmitted heat or electrical current may damage these structures and may even result in testicular loss. The hernia sac will be found on the anteromedial aspect of the spermatic cord **(Figure 77-3)**. Gentle blunt dissection is used to separate the hernia sac from the spermatic vessels and the vas deferens, avoiding direct manipulation of the latter **(Figure 77-4)**. These structures must be positively identified before proceeding with the rest of the operation. Once the hernia sac has been separated from the vas deferens and the spermatic vessels, the hernia sac is divided between hemostats in its midcourse after it is ensured that there are no other tissues inside the sac and that there are no sliding components making part of the wall of the sac. I find it helpful to place the cord structures within a vessel loop for gentle traction to avoid injuries. The operation proceeds with dissection of the proximal portion of the hernia sac up to the level of the internal inguinal ring, where it is suture ligated with nonabsorbable suture and excised **(Figure 77-5)**.

If you wish to perform a diagnostic laparoscopy, a short 5-mm trocar is introduced through the sac and secured with a 3-0 Vicryl tie. Pneumoperitoneum is created with a maximum pressure of 4-8 mm Hg. The patient is placed in the Trendelenburg position, and the table is tilted toward the surgeon. A 120° telescope is introduced to inspect the contralateral inguinal ring. After this is done, the trocar is removed, the pneumoperitoneum evacuated, and the ligation of the sac completed.

In most cases, high ligation of the hernia sac is sufficient treatment for an inguinal hernia in a child. The distal portion of the sac is opened widely; no attempts are made to remove the sac because this may result in devascularization of the testicle. In patients in whom the floor of the inguinal canal is weak, repair may be performed using the Bassini technique by approximating the internal oblique muscle to the shelving edge of the inguinal ligament with two to three interrupted stitches. The most medial stitch approximates the internal oblique muscle (or the conjoint tendon when present) to the pubic spine. If a hydrocele is present, the tunica vaginalis is opened and the fluid is evacuated. The testicle can be brought back down into the scrotum by gentle caudad traction of the scrotal skin, which will pull the testicle down along with the gubernaculum testis.

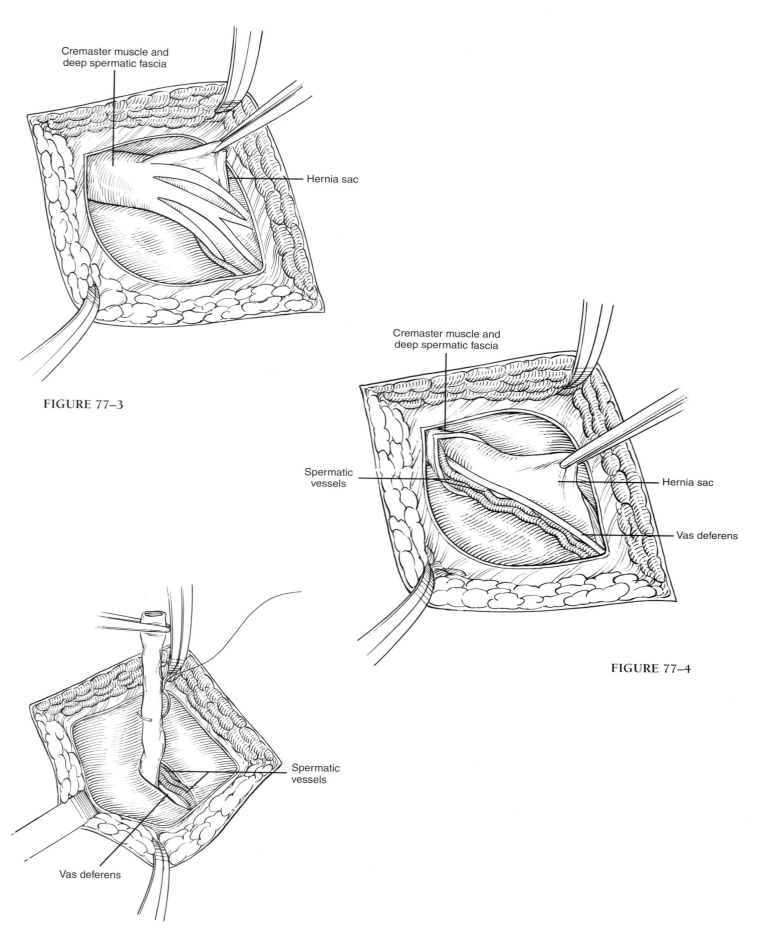

Cremaster muscle and
deep spermatic fascia

Hernia sac

FIGURE 77–3

Cremaster muscle and
deep spermatic fascia

Spermatic
vessels

Hernia sac

Vas deferens

FIGURE 77–4

Spermatic
vessels

Vas deferens

FIGURE 77–5

3. CLOSING

◆ The external oblique aponeurosis is closed with interrupted fine absorbable suture, making sure that the external inguinal ring does not constrict the cord structures **(Figure 77-6)**. Scarpa's fascia is closed with interrupted fine absorbable suture, and the skin is closed with a running fine absorbable monofilament subcuticular suture. The skin is dressed with adhesive strips.

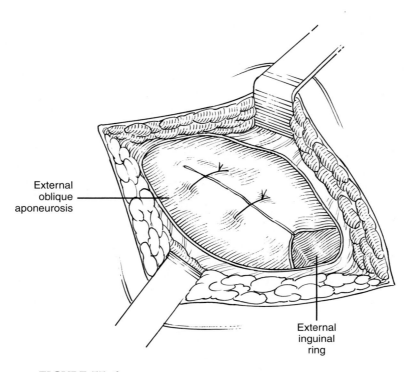

External oblique aponeurosis

External inguinal ring

FIGURE 77–6

STEP 4: POSTOPERATIVE CARE

- Most patients will have either a caudal block, an ilioinguinal block, or subcutaneous infiltration of the incision with local anesthetic in the operating room for postoperative pain control. An oral analgesic such as acetaminophen is prescribed to be given every 4 to 6 hours on the first postoperative day and then administered only as needed. Children are allowed to bathe normally 24 hours after the operation and can resume full activity after 2 weeks.

- Although rare, the most common complications are wound infections and hematomas. Injury to the vas deferens, epididymis, or spermatic vessels and hernia recurrence are reported in up to 1% of cases.

STEP 5: PEARLS AND PITFALLS

- Operating immediately after manual reduction of an incarcerated inguinal hernia in a child is technically difficult and fraught with complications, because the hernia sac is edematous and friable, and the structures of the cord are not easily identifiable. A period of 24 hours to allow some of the edema to subside is advisable.

- As a general rule, no structures should be divided until both the spermatic vessels and the vas deferens have been positively identified and placed within a vessel loop.

- Use of electrocautery in the vicinity of the spermatic cord is discouraged, because arcs of electrical current may result in thrombosis of the spermatic vessels and loss of the testicle.

SELECTED REFERENCES

1. Weber TR, Tracy TF, Keller MS: Groin hernias and hydroceles. In Ashcraft KW, Holcomb GW, Murphy JP (eds): Pediatric Surgery, 4th ed. Philadelphia, Elsevier Saunders, 2005, pp 697-705.
2. Engum SA, Grosfeld JL: Hernias in children. In Spitz L, Coran AG (eds): Operative Pediatric Surgery, 6th ed. London, Edward Arnold, 2006, pp 237-244.

CHAPTER 78

LAPAROSCOPIC INGUINAL HERNIA REPAIR

Michael D. Trahan

STEP 1: SURGICAL ANATOMY

- ◆ A thorough understanding of the preperitoneal space and important structures of the retroperitoneal space and inguinal canal is prerequisite to attempting laparoscopic inguinal hernia repair (**Figure 78-1**).

STEP 2: PREOPERATIVE CONSIDERATIONS

INDICATIONS

- ◆ A laparoscopic approach to inguinal hernias is indicated for any indirect, direct, or femoral hernia but is particularly suited to bilateral hernias and recurrences from anterior repairs.

- ◆ Larger hernias, especially with scrotal extension, can make the laparoscopic approach much more difficult.

PREPARATION

- ◆ A urinary catheter is inserted for bladder decompression.

- ◆ The patient is placed in the supine Trendelenburg position with the arms padded and tucked.

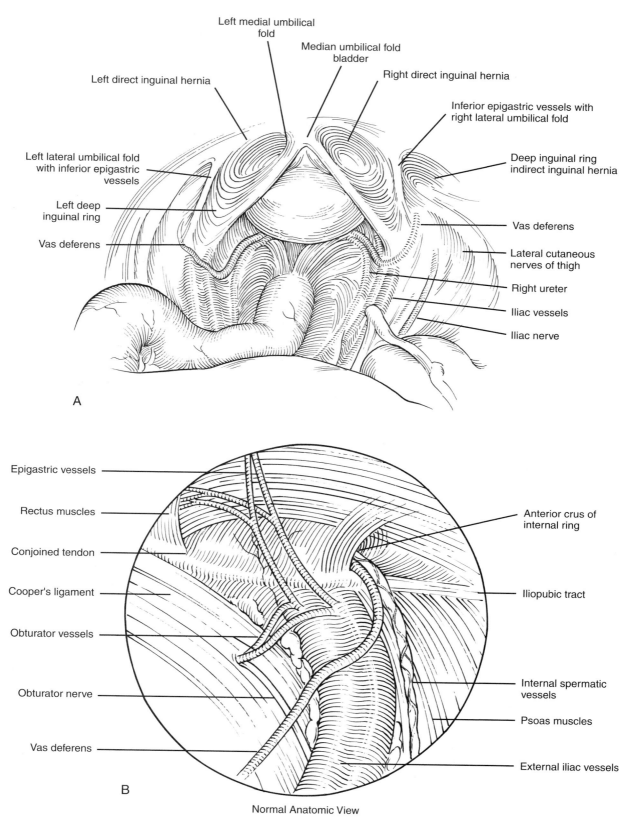

Left medial umbilical fold

Median umbilical fold
bladder

Left direct inguinal hernia

Right direct inguinal hernia

Inferior epigastric vessels with
right lateral umbilical fold

Left lateral umbilical fold
with inferior epigastric
vessels

Deep inguinal ring
indirect inguinal hernia

Left deep
inguinal ring

Vas deferens

Vas deferens

Lateral cutaneous
nerves of thigh

Right ureter

Iliac vessels

Iliac nerve

A

Epigastric vessels

Anterior crus of
internal ring

Rectus muscles

Conjoined tendon

Cooper's ligament

Iliopubic tract

Obturator vessels

Obturator nerve

Internal spermatic
vessels

Psoas muscles

Vas deferens

External iliac vessels

B

Normal Anatomic View

FIGURE 78–1

STEP 3: OPERATIVE STEPS

1. INCISION

- Three ports are used: one 10-mm port and two low-profile 5-mm ports **(Figure 78-2)**.

2. DISSECTION

- Transabdominal preperitoneal (TAPP) repair
  - An optically guided, bladeless 10-mm port is placed into the peritoneal cavity near the umbilicus. The two 5-mm ports are placed, guided by internal visualization to avoid the epigastric vessels.
  - The peritoneum is incised starting at the medial umbilical fold and proceeding laterally to or past the anterior superior iliac spine. The incision is made well away from the internal ring to provide ample tissue to cover the peritoneal defect at the end of the procedure **(Figure 78-3)**.
  - The peritoneum is peeled down and bluntly dissected from the underlying structures. An indirect hernia sac is gently pulled out of the internal ring and dissected free from the cord structures.

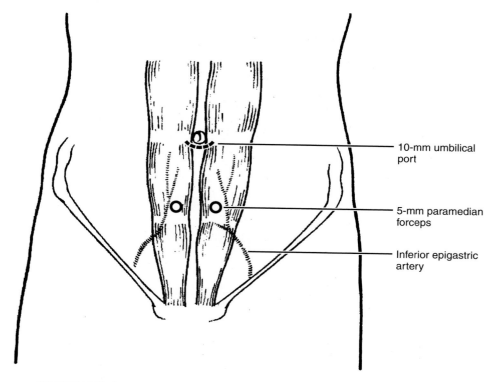

FIGURE 78–2

10-mm umbilical port

5-mm paramedian forceps

Inferior epigastric artery

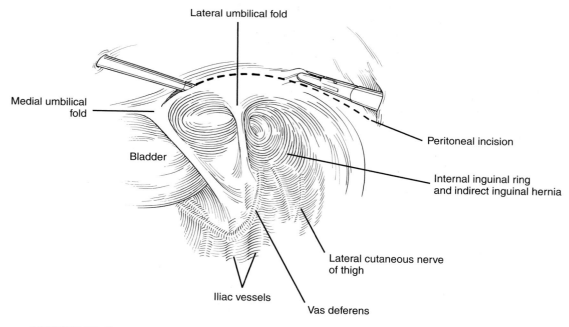

Lateral umbilical fold

Medial umbilical fold

Bladder

Peritoneal incision

Internal inguinal ring and indirect inguinal hernia

Lateral cutaneous nerve of thigh

Iliac vessels

Vas deferens

FIGURE 78–3

- The margins of a complete dissection are the midline medially, the iliac bone laterally, and Cooper's ligament inferiorly **(Figure 78-4, A-B).**
- The fatty contents of a direct hernia defect are reduced and trimmed away as necessary **(Figure 78-4, C).**

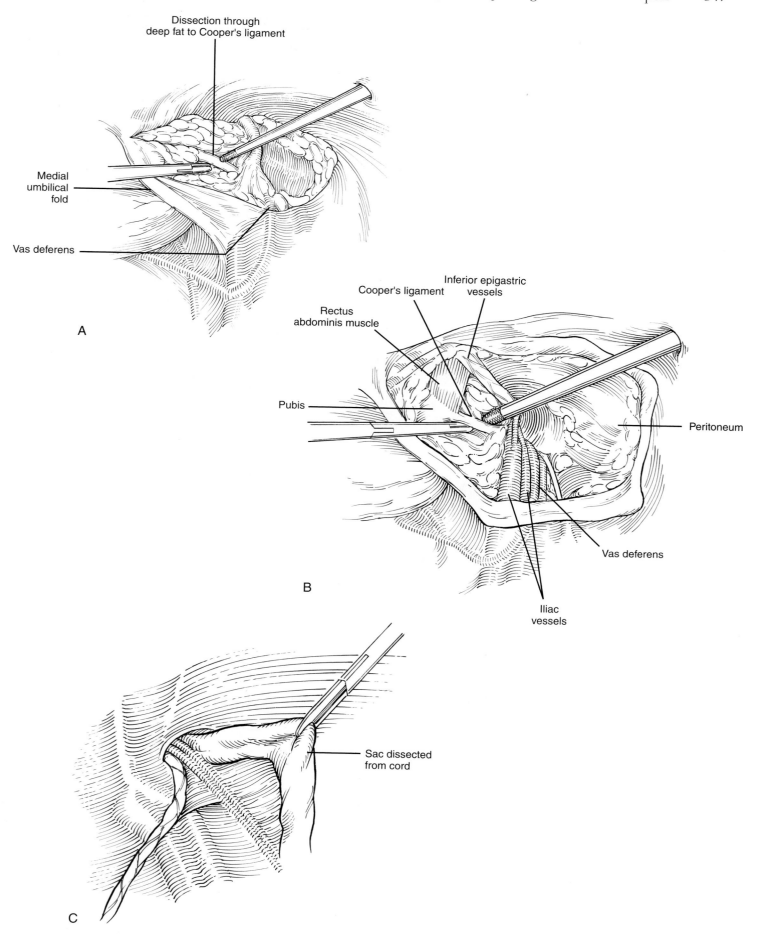

Dissection through
deep fat to Cooper's ligament

Medial
umbilical
fold

Vas deferens

A

Rectus
abdominis muscle

Cooper's ligament

Inferior epigastric
vessels

Pubis

Peritoneum

Vas deferens

Iliac
vessels

B

Sac dissected
from cord

C

FIGURE 78–4

◆ A sheet of polypropylene or polyester mesh is trimmed to shape, tightly rolled, inserted through the scope port, and spread out on the deperitonealized surface.

◆ The mesh should be anchored at the pubic bone, for a short distance along Cooper's ligament, and along the anterior abdominal wall, taking care to avoid the important neurovascular structures (**Figure 78-5**).

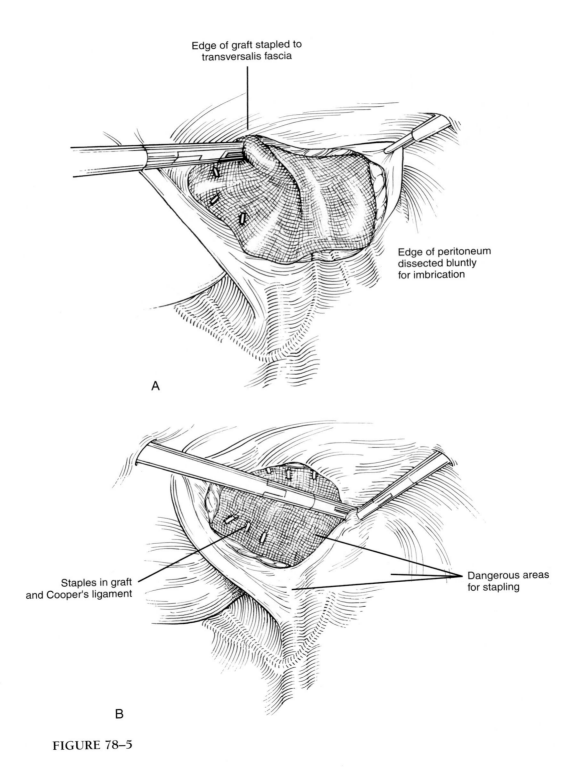

FIGURE 78–5

◆ The peritoneal flap is used to cover the mesh. The incision in the peritoneum is closed with clips or tacks **(Figure 78-6)**.

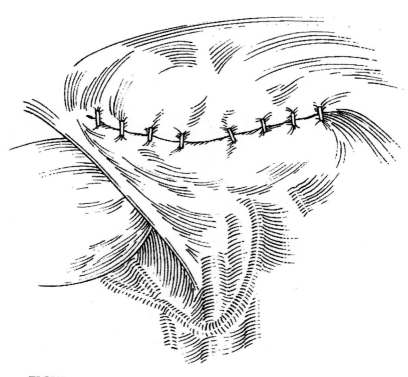

FIGURE 78–6

- Totally extraperitoneal (TEP) repair
  - The 10-mm port is first placed using an open approach. A small incision is made along the inferior edge of the umbilicus. The anterior rectus sheath is exposed and incised on either side of the midline. The rectus muscle is retracted laterally from the midline to expose the posterior rectus sheath.
  - The preperitoneal plane (between the rectus muscle and posterior rectus sheath) is bluntly dissected manually or, preferably, with a balloon dissector. This plane is developed down to the pubic bone **(Figure 78-7)**.

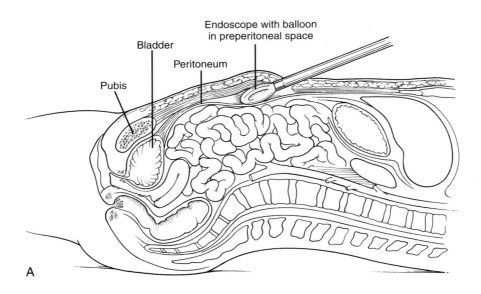

A

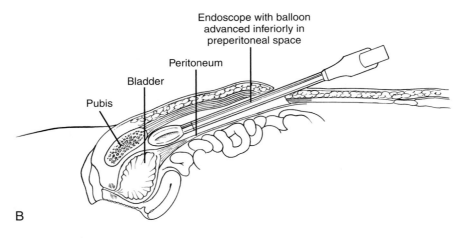

B

FIGURE 78–7

- The balloon dissector is inflated fully while the laparoscope is positioned to view internally. An interior view of the structures of the spermatic cord is usually observed at this point. A small indirect hernia sac may be reduced by inflation of the balloon **(Figure 78-8)**.
- The balloon is deflated and the balloon dissecting port is replaced with a working 10-mm port. CO_2 insufflation at 13 to 15 mm Hg is used to maintain the expansion of the preperitoneal space. The seal of the port to the anterior fascia can be provided by cinching the fascia with suture, placing a Hassan adapter, or using a balloon trocar (illustrated) **(Figure 78-9)**.
- The scope is inserted for placement of the two 5-mm ports and completion of the preperitoneal dissection. This dissection can usually be done bluntly without the need for the electrosurgical unit. However, care must be taken to avoid tearing the peritoneum, because this will lead to inflation of the peritoneal cavity and loss of adequate preperitoneal visualization. The structures entering the internal ring should be dissected until they are clearly seen (see Figure 78-1, B).

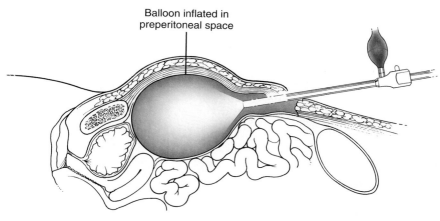

Balloon inflated in
preperitoneal space

FIGURE 78–8

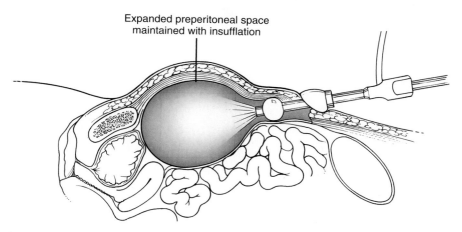

Expanded preperitoneal space
maintained with insufflation

FIGURE 78–9

◆ The fatty contents of a direct hernia defect should be reduced and usually excised **(Figure 78-10).**

◆ An indirect sac, if not reduced by the balloon inflation, is gently grasped and pulled out of the internal ring and carefully dissected it from the cord structures **(Figure 78-11).**

◆ The margins of dissection are the midline medially, the anterior superior iliac spine laterally, the transverse arch superiorly, and Cooper's ligament inferiorly. The polypropylene or polyester mesh is trimmed to shape, rolled tightly, inserted through the 10-mm port, and laid in place to cover the femoral and both inguinal potential orifices. A notch cut for the iliac vessels allows the mesh to lay with less buckling **(Figure 78-12).**

◆ The mesh can be anchored, if desired, to the pubis, Cooper's ligament, and the abdominal wall above the transverse arch avoiding the sites of neurovascular structures (see Figure 78-5).

◆ The insufflation is released (while the mesh is held in place if no anchoring is used), and the ports are removed.

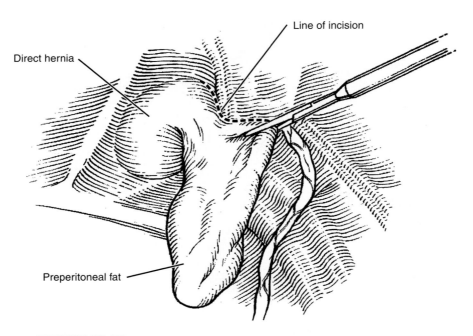

FIGURE 78–10

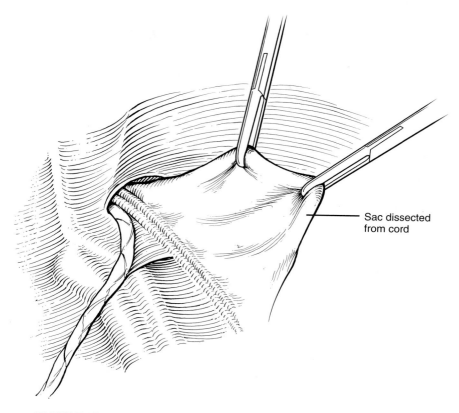

FIGURE 78–11

Sac dissected
from cord

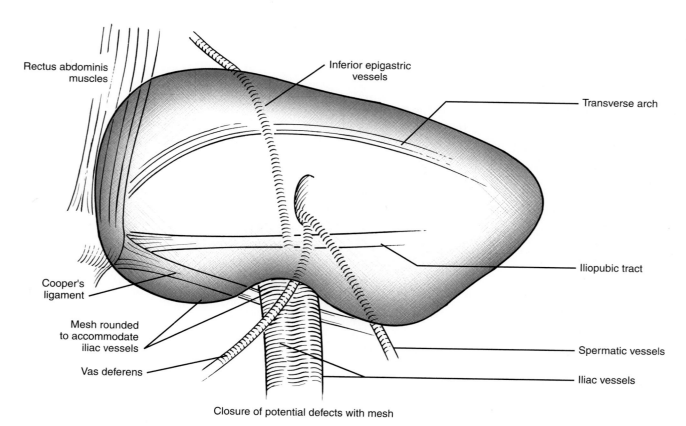

Rectus abdominis
muscles

Inferior epigastric
vessels

Transverse arch

Iliopubic tract

Cooper's
ligament

Mesh rounded
to accommodate
iliac vessels

Vas deferens

Spermatic vessels

Iliac vessels

Closure of potential defects with mesh

FIGURE 78–12

3. CLOSURE

♦ The anterior fascia is closed with absorbable suture. The skin incisions are closed with absorbable suture with a subcuticular technique.

♦ The incisions are dressed with tissue adhesive or tapes.

STEP 4: POSTOPERATIVE CARE

♦ These operations are usually performed in the outpatient setting.

♦ An oral narcotic such as hydrocodone is appropriate for pain management.

♦ Patients may return to regular activity as the surgical discomfort resolves.

STEP 5: PEARLS AND PITFALLS

♦ One must avoid fixation clips and tacks in the lower outer quadrant of the mesh. This is where the nerves and large vessels travel.

♦ If the peritoneal membrane is entered during a TEP, inflation of the preperitoneal space can be maintained by placing a Veress needle into the peritoneal cavity in the upper abdomen. Alternatively, the TEP procedure can be converted to a TAPP procedure.

♦ The inferior edge of the mesh should be tucked under the peritoneum as the pneumoperitoneum is released to avoid migration of the mesh.

SELECTED REFERENCES

1. McKernan JB, Laws HL: Laparoscopic repair of inguinal hernias using a totally extraperitoneal prosthetic approach. Surg Endosc 1993;7:26-28.
2. Stoppa RE, Warlaumont CR: The preperitoneal approach and prosthetic repair of groin hernia. In Nyhus LM, Condon RE (eds): Hernia, 3rd ed. Philadelphia, Lippincott, 1989, pp 199-225.
3. Liem MS, van Vroonhoven TJ: Laparoscopic inguinal hernia repair. Br J Surg 1996;83:1197-1204.

CHAPTER 79

FEMORAL HERNIA

Thomas D. Kimbrough

STEP 1: SURGICAL ANATOMY

♦ **Figure 79-1** shows, in a stylized fashion, the structures that pass underneath the inguinal ligament. Although large femoral hernias may extend laterally in the subcutaneous tissues of the thigh, most should be located medial to the palpated pulse of the femoral artery.

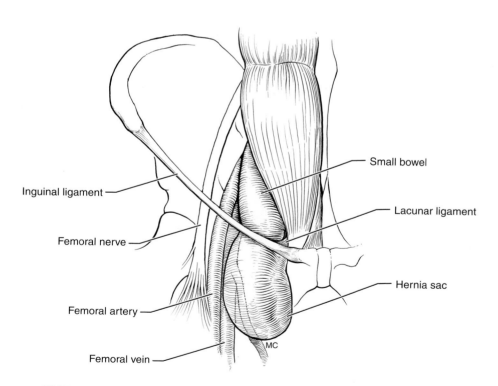

Inguinal ligament —

Femoral nerve —

Femoral artery —

Femoral vein —

MC

— Small bowel

— Lacunar ligament

— Hernia sac

FIGURE 79–1

- The hernia is protruding through the femoral canal, which remains only a potential space in most people. The space is bounded anteriorly by the inguinal ligament, posteriorly by the pubic ramus and pectineal ligament, laterally by the femoral vein and sheath, and medially by the lacunar portion of the inguinal ligament.

STEP 2: PREOPERATIVE CONSIDERATIONS

- The course of the inguinal ligament parallels a line drawn between the pubic tubercle and the anterior superior iliac spine. Any mass that lies beneath this line and medial to the femoral artery pulsation is a possible femoral hernia.

- As outlined later, some preoperative consideration regarding placement of the incision should take place.

STEP 3: OPERATIVE STEPS

1. INCISION

◆ The elective femoral hernia can be approached through a transverse incision, parallel to the inguinal ligament over the palpable mass in the medial thigh, just below the inguinal ligament.

◆ A standard incision should be considered for larger hernias, especially those that might require access to the preperitoneal space.

2. DISSECTION

◆ The exposed sac with surrounding structures is shown in **Figure 79-2.** In most cases, the sac can be reduced through the femoral canal back into the preperitoneal space and a repair effected.

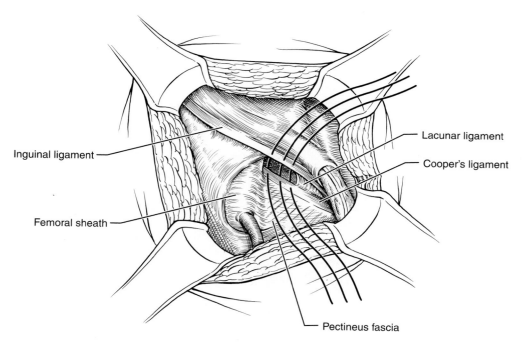

FIGURE 79–2

◆ The classic repair approximating the inguinal ligament to Cooper's ligament and the pectineus fascia with 2-0 monofilament polypropylene suture is shown in **Figure 79-3.**

◆ The relatively higher rate of recurrences associated with this and other tissue repairs has led most to use a tension-free mesh plug repair, as illustrated in **Figure 79-4.** A piece of polypropylene mesh approximately 2 inches long is rolled into a generous plug and inserted into the femoral canal. Suitable anchoring sutures are placed superiorly, medially, and inferiorly, as shown in Figure 79-4.

◆ In the case of emergency operations for strangulation or small bowel obstruction, careful consideration should be given to placement of the skin incision. In such cases, it may not be possible to reduce the hernia from below, and access to the preperitoneal space also through the floor of the inguinal canal may be necessary.

◆ **Figure 79-5** illustrates such an approach. After successful reduction, repair should include not only the mesh plug described but also a mesh repair of the inguinal floor, such as the Prolene Hernia System repair described in Chapter 72.

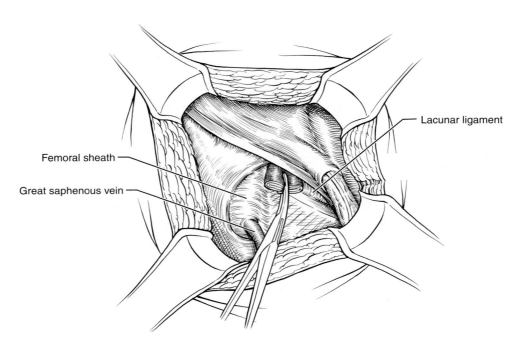

Lacunar ligament

Femoral sheath

Great saphenous vein

FIGURE 79–3

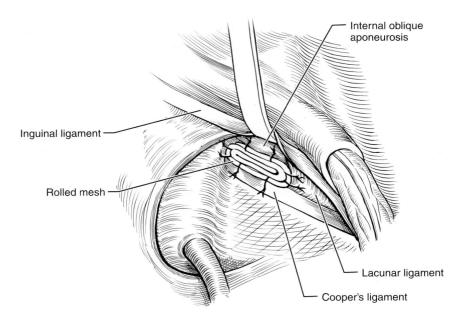

FIGURE 79–4

Internal oblique aponeurosis

Inguinal ligament

Rolled mesh

Lacunar ligament

Cooper's ligament

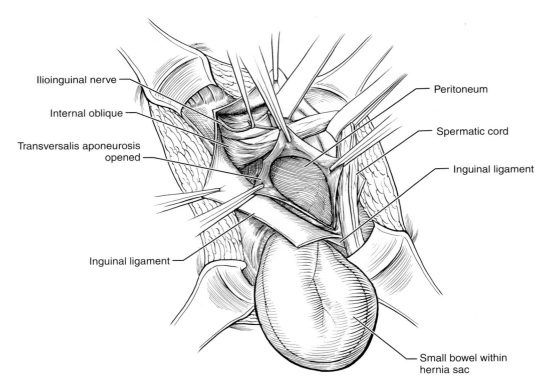

Ilioinguinal nerve

Internal oblique

Transversalis aponeurosis opened

Inguinal ligament

Peritoneum

Spermatic cord

Inguinal ligament

Small bowel within hernia sac

FIGURE 79–5

3. CLOSURE

◆ Closure is as described in Chapter 72.

STEP 4: POSTOPERATIVE CARE

◆ No instructions additional to those described earlier for mesh repairs of direct and indirect hernias are necessary.

STEP 5: PEARLS AND PITFALLS

◆ If in the approach to reduction of an incarcerated femoral hernia repair the sac cannot be reduced, the following is an option. Partial division of the lacunar ligament medially will enlarge the canal and usually allow reduction. If this is chosen, one should remember that if there is an aberrant course of the obturator artery, it can be lacerated during this maneuver. A far less desirable option is division of the overlying inguinal ligament.

◆ In any elderly patient with a bowel obstruction, especially women, the possibility of an incarcerated femoral hernia should be considered and looked for on physical examination. It is not only embarrassing for the surgeon to find such a hernia after a large midline laparotomy, but it is potentially quite harmful to the patient to experience the invasion of the abdominal cavity when an inguinal exploration would most likely have sufficiently solved the problem.

SELECTED REFERENCE

1. Nyhus LM, Condon RE (eds): Hernia, 4th ed. Philadelphia, JB Lippincott, 1995.

CHAPTER 80

UMBILICAL HERNIA (CHILD AND ADULT)

Michael D. Trahan

STEP 1: SURGICAL ANATOMY

- Most umbilical hernias are congenital. Conditions that increase intra-abdominal pressure can lead to an acquired hernia later in life.

- The hernia contents protrude through a defect in the linea alba through which the fetal umbilical vessels passed.

- The linea alba is the result of the midline fusion of the external oblique, internal oblique, and transversus abdominis muscles.

STEP 2: PREOPERATIVE CONSIDERATIONS FOR A CHILD

- Umbilical hernias are common in children and usually (up to 80%) close sometime during the first 4 years of life. Unless the hernia is complicated, repair should be delayed until 4 years of age.

- General anesthesia is preferred.

STEP 2: PREOPERATIVE CONSIDERATIONS FOR AN ADULT

- Umbilical hernias should be repaired in adults unless there is a contraindication. Contraindications may include patients unfit for anesthesia and the presence of massive ascites.

Anesthesia

- General anesthesia is preferred.

- Spinal anesthesia or deep sedation with local anesthesia are possibilities for small fascial defects in cooperative patients.

STEP 3: OPERATIVE STEPS FOR A CHILD

1. INCISION

- A curvilinear incision is made at the inferior rim of the umbilicus **(Figure 80-1)**.

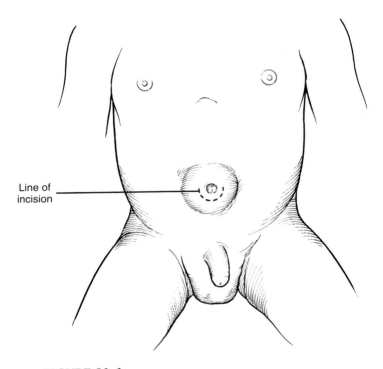

Line of incision

FIGURE 80–1

2. DISSECTION

♦ A combination of blunt and sharp dissection is used to expose the fascia of the abdominal wall and the hernia sac. The umbilical stalk is bluntly encircled with a right-angled hemostat **(Figure 80-2)**.

♦ The hernia contents, if present, are reduced, and the stalk is divided **(Figure 80-3)**.

♦ The excess sac is excised, and the fascia is approximated in the midline using 3-0 interrupted polypropylene suture.

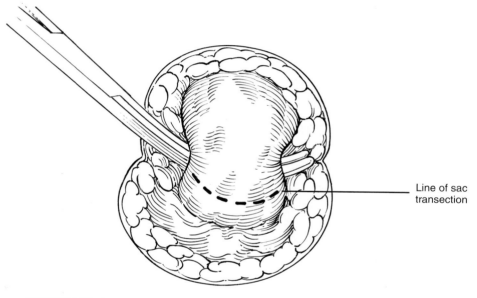

Line of sac transection

FIGURE 80–2

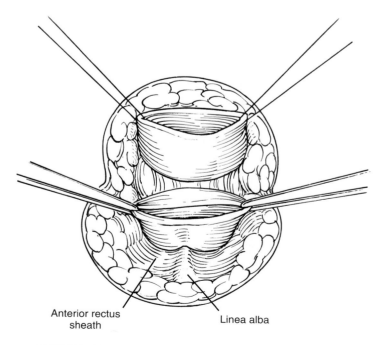

Anterior rectus sheath

Linea alba

FIGURE 80–3

3. CLOSING

♦ The dermis of the umbilicus is tacked down to the fascia using an absorbable 3-0 suture. The incision is closed with a running subcuticular absorbable 4-0 suture and dressed with tissue adhesive.

♦ A cotton ball or fluffed gauze is placed within the umbilicus, covered with gauze, and taped into place.

STEP 3: OPERATIVE STEPS FOR AN ADULT

1. INCISION

♦ For a small defect, an incision at the rim of the umbilicus may be used, but for larger hernias, a midline approach results in better exposure for placement of the mesh and a more acceptable postoperative cosmetic result **(Figures 80-4 and 80-5).**

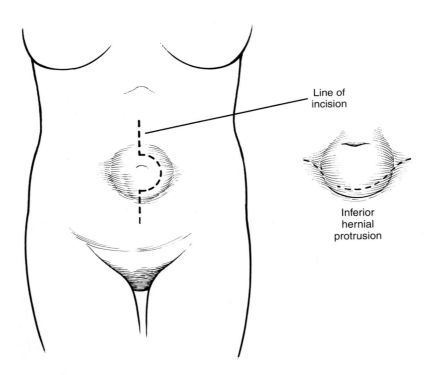

FIGURE 80–4

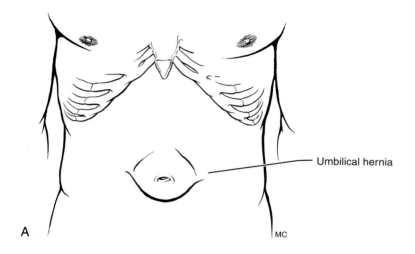

Umbilical hernia

A

MC

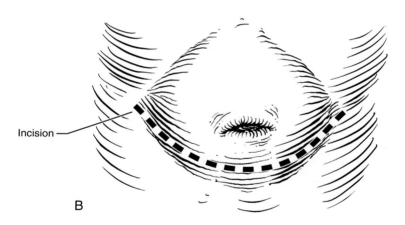

Incision

B

FIGURE 80–5

2. DISSECTION

♦ A combination of blunt and sharp dissection is used to expose the midline fascia and hernia sac. If possible, the hernia contents are reduced. If the contents are reducible or chronically incarcerated, an attempt is made to sharply dissect the sac from the overlying skin without opening the sac. For chronically incarcerated hernias, the midline fascia may need to be incised to completely reduce the contents **(Figure 80-6)**.

♦ For an acutely incarcerated hernia, the sac is opened so that its contents can be inspected for strangulation and ischemia **(Figure 80-7)**.

♦ The fascia may need to be carefully incised in the midline to release the incarcerated contents **(Figure 80-8)**.

♦ If determined to be nonviable, the hernia contents are excised. The healthy remaining intestine is repaired primarily **(Figure 80-9)**.

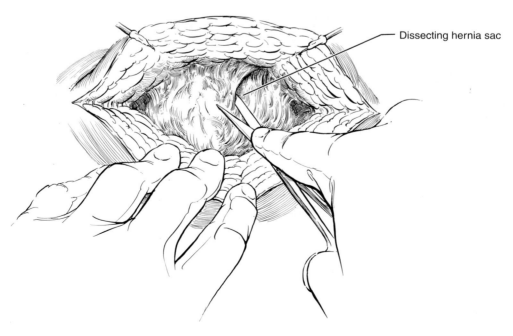

Dissecting hernia sac

FIGURE 80–6

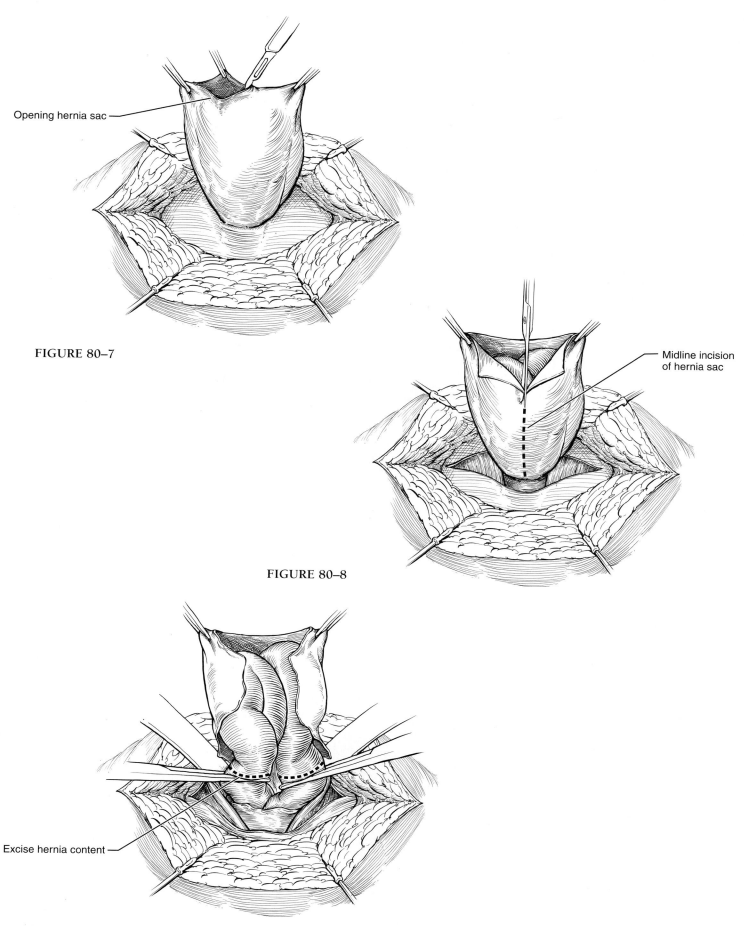

Opening hernia sac

FIGURE 80–7

Midline incision of hernia sac

FIGURE 80–8

Excise hernia content

FIGURE 80–9

◆ After complete reduction of the hernia contents, the sac is closed and the plane between the peritoneum and the posterior abdominal fascia is sharply dissected for a distance of 3 cm circumferentially if mesh is to be used. If this plane is not accessible, the mesh may be placed on the posterior rectus sheath, posterior to the rectus muscles **(Figure 80-10)**.

◆ Consideration may be given to primary midline approximation of smaller fascial defects using 2-0 interrupted nonabsorbable suture, especially if intestinal ischemia was encountered, but lower recurrence rates have been shown with mesh repairs.

◆ Polypropylene mesh is placed in the preperitoneal space with 3 cm of overlap with the fascia. The mesh is sutured circumferentially to the fascia without tension, and the edges of the fascia are sutured to the center of the mesh **(Figure 80-11)**.

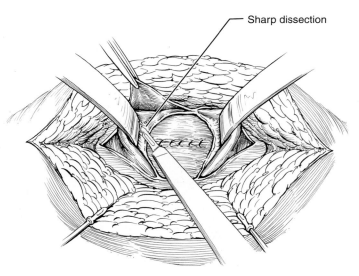

FIGURE 80–10

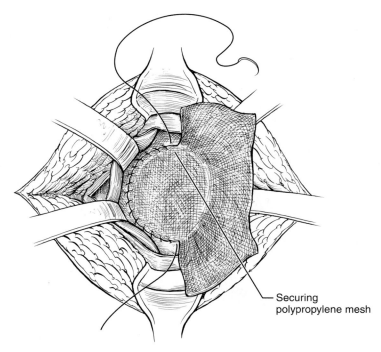

FIGURE 80–11

3. CLOSING

◆ A closed suction drain may be required to prevent postoperative seroma if the soft tissue space is excessive. The drain should exit the skin remote from the surgical wound. A two-layer closure using absorbable suture or skin staples completes the operation **(Figure 80-12).**

◆ To help prevent a wound seroma, a ball of cotton or gauze should be placed in the umbilicus and held in place with an abdominal binder.

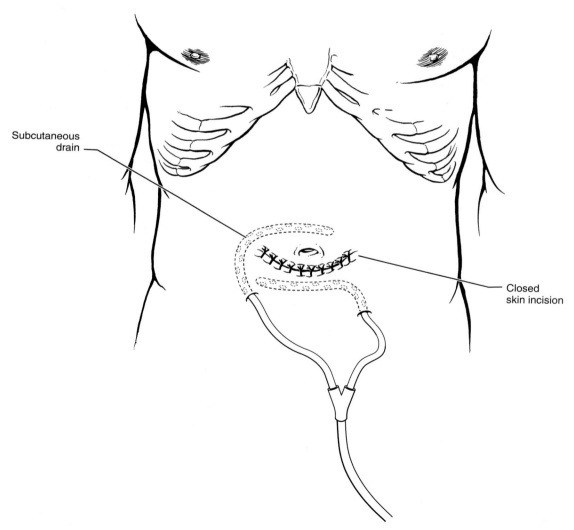

FIGURE 80–12

STEP 4: POSTOPERATIVE CONSIDERATIONS

- Drains usually may be safely removed once the output declines to less than 30 mL per day.

STEP 5: PEARLS AND PITFALLS

- In a contaminated field (e.g., resection of gangrenous intestine), an absorbable or biologic fascia substitute may be used with the expectation that a recurrence of the hernia is likely but may be repaired later after the eradication of the contamination.

- Polypropylene mesh should not be placed within the peritoneal cavity. If there is insufficient peritoneum to close in the midline, an expanded polytetrafluoroethylene mesh product may be placed, because formation of adhesions to this surface or erosion into adjacent viscera is unlikely.

SELECTED REFERENCES

1. Radhakrishnan J: Umbilical hernia. In Nyhus LM, Condon RE (eds): Hernia, 4th ed. Philadelphia, JB Lippincott, 1995.
2. Skinner MA, Grosfeld JL: Inguinal and umbilical hernia repair in infants and children. Surg Clin North Am 1993;73:439-449.

CHAPTER 81

INCISIONAL/VENTRAL HERNIA— MESH AND TISSUE FLAP

Thomas D. Kimbrough

STEP 1: SURGICAL ANATOMY

- ◆ A midline epigastric incisional hernia is represented in **Figure 81-1**.

- ◆ **Figure 81-2** is a cross-section of the hernia illustrating the relevant layers.

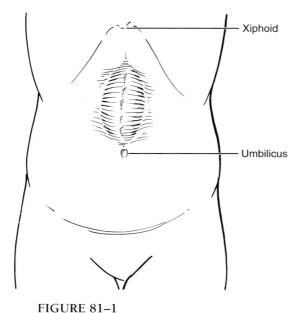

Xiphoid

Umbilicus

FIGURE 81–1

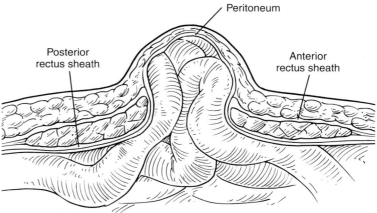

Peritoneum

Posterior rectus sheath

Anterior rectus sheath

FIGURE 81–2

873

STEP 2: PREOPERATIVE CONSIDERATIONS

◆ The most important preoperative consideration is whether the hernia should be repaired. Because the risk to the patient from the hernia decreases as its diameter increases, and the chance of recurrence and other surgical complications increases, the risk-to-benefit ratio should be carefully assessed.

◆ In the event repair is deemed desirable, many of these patients have significant comorbidities that must be addressed preoperatively and managed perioperatively. Neglect of these can lead to failure in spite of a technically superb surgical repair.

◆ There are many techniques for repair of incisional hernias, illustrating among other things that no one method has been judged superior. The technique illustrated here is but one of many acceptable available.

STEP 3: OPERATIVE STEPS

1. INCISION

◆ In the case of incisional hernias, the new incision is made by excising the old scar.

◆ In the case of a ventral hernia not related to a previous surgical procedure, the incision is best placed along the longer axis of the fascial defect.

◆ If the fascial defect is circular with no significant difference in the length of axes, transverse incisions leave better scars.

2. DISSECTION

◆ After the hernia sac is identified, its external peritoneal lining is dissected free from surrounding structures, including the innermost fascial layer of the abdominal wall.

◆ Although it is often necessary to open the peritoneum and even resect portions of it, preservation of enough of the peritoneum to close allows the imposition of a tissue layer between the mesh to be used and the contents of the intra-abdominal cavity. The end result is illustrated in **Figure 81-3**.

◆ **Figure 81-4** shows the next step, which is separation of the posterior rectus sheath from the overlying rectus abdominis muscle.

◆ Primarily the cut edges of the posterior sheath are then closed, even if under tension. This closure can be facilitated by application of the techniques of component separation.

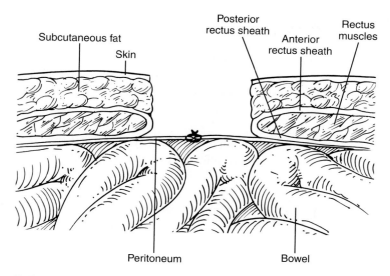

FIGURE 81–3

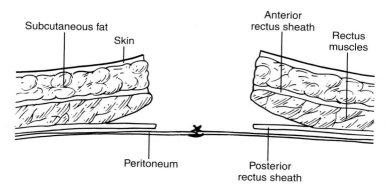

FIGURE 81–4

◆ A sheet of polypropylene mesh is then positioned on top of the posterior sheath and under the rectus muscle. There should be an overlap of 3 to 5 cm on all sides. Some choose to tack the mesh in place with mattress sutures through the rectus muscle and anterior sheath. I have found it sufficient to tack the mesh to the underlying posterior sheath with absorbable sutures. Either way the mesh should be tacked down as tautly as possible. The completion of these steps is illustrated in **Figure 81-5.**

◆ **Figure 81-6** shows the completed repair after primary closure of the anterior sheath. Again, fascial release techniques such as component separation can facilitate this process.

◆ It is, of course, not always possible to completely close the posterior and anterior fascial layers, even with releases. In that event, as much as possible is closed, even if under tension. Every effort is made to close some type of tissue layer between the abdominal contents and the mesh, and the mesh and the skin. As mentioned earlier, the peritoneum can be used in the first instance, and the subcutaneous tissues in the latter.

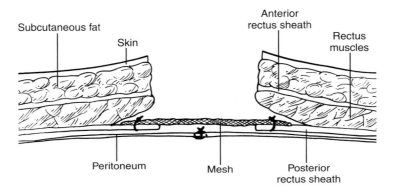

FIGURE 81–5

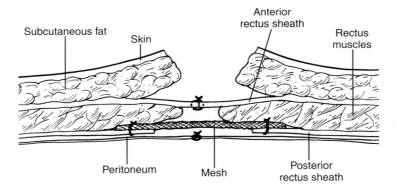

FIGURE 81–6

3. CLOSING

♦ Scrupulous attention should be paid to hemostasis, because postoperative hematomas are not uncommon and can create significant problems.

♦ Whether to use drains in any or all of the spaces created by the dissection is the choice of the individual surgeon. The drains are no substitute for good technique and offer a route for the introduction of bacteria.

STEP 4: POSTOPERATIVE CARE

♦ Most patients require a day or two in the hospital for adequate pain control.

♦ Patients are instructed to refrain from lifting or doing strenuous work for 4 to 6 weeks.

SELECTED REFERENCE

1. Zinner MJ, Schwartz SI, Ellis H: Hernias. In Maingot R, Zinner M (eds): Maingot's Abdominal Operations, vol 1, 10th ed. Stamford, Conn, Appleton & Lang, 1997, pp 479-580.

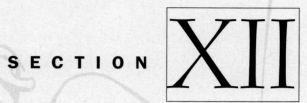

VASCULAR

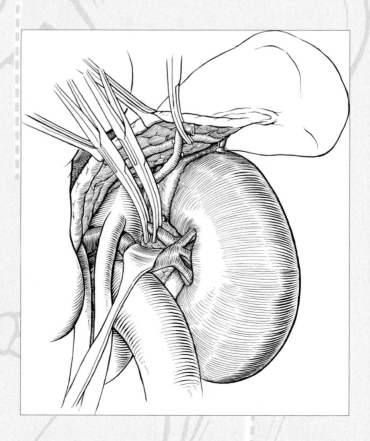

CHAPTER 82

RESECTION OF ABDOMINAL AORTIC ANEURYSM

Glenn C. Hunter

ELECTIVE ANEURYSM REPAIR

◆ Most patients with asymptomatic abdominal aortic aneurysms are operated on electively once the aneurysm exceeds 5.5 cm in diameter. If the aneurysm has ruptured, immediate operative repair is indicated. Some steps appropriate to emergency aneurysmectomy will be included in the discussion of elective aneurysm repair.

STEP 1: SURGICAL ANATOMY

◆ The aorta enters the abdomen between the crura of the diaphragm at the level of the 12th thoracic vertebra and bifurcates into the right and left common iliac arteries at the interspace between the fourth and fifth lumbar vertebrae. The aorta is crossed successively by the fourth portion of the duodenum, the left renal vein, and the root of the mesentery, and it is intimately related to the vena cava and iliac veins. The left common iliac vein runs posterior medial to the artery and is densely adherent to it (**Figure 82-1**).

◆ In most patients with abdominal aortic aneurysm, dilation begins distal to the origins of renal arteries and extends to the aortic bifurcation and iliac arteries. The elongation accompanying the aortic dilation results in tortuosity displacing the aorta off the vertebral column anteriorly or off to one side of the midline. The tortuosity may also involve the iliac arteries, resulting in their displacement into the pelvis.

◆ The inferior mesenteric vein is located in the mesentery anterior to the aneurysm. Care must be taken when ligating the inferior mesenteric vein to ensure that only the vein is ligated, because the collateral arterial supply to the colon often accompanies the vein in this location.

STEP 2: PREOPERATIVE CONSIDERATIONS

◆ A search for thoracic and iliac aneurysms and other associated anomalies, such as suprarenal extension, venous anomalies, horseshoe kidney, or aortocaval fistula, with computed tomography (CT) scanning, magnetic resonance imaging (MRI), or duplex ultrasound imaging should be made before repair of an abdominal aortic aneurysm. Assessment of cardiac, respiratory, and renal function should be undertaken and any abnormalities optimized before proceeding with aneurysm repair. A mechanical bowel preparation the night before surgery facilitates the operation. Prophylactic antibiotics are administered 1 hour before the incision.

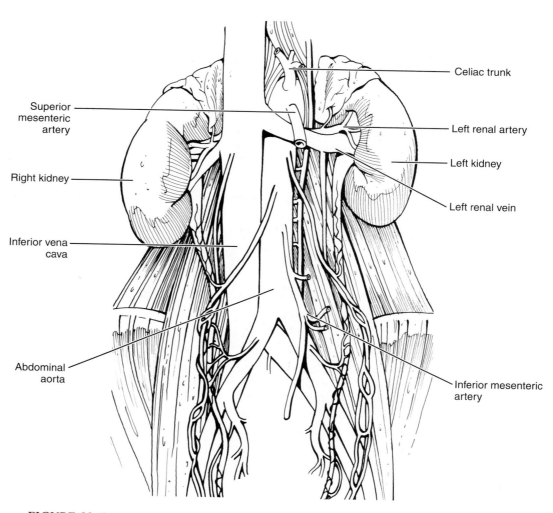

FIGURE 82–1

STEP 3: OPERATIVE STEPS

1. INCISION

◆ For elective aneurysm repair, the operative field is prepped from the nipples to the knees after induction of general anesthesia and placement of central venous and arterial monitoring lines. In the setting of a ruptured abdominal aortic aneurysm, the chest, abdomen, and groins should be prepared and draped before the induction of general anesthesia. Additional large-bore catheters are inserted peripherally and centrally, with the latter connected to a rapid infusion device capable of delivering large volumes of blood and blood products.

◆ Aortic aneurysm repair can be undertaken using either a transperitoneal or a retroperitoneal approach. With the transperitoneal approach, the patient is positioned supine on the operating table and in the right lateral decubitus position for retroperitoneal exposure of the aorta (**Figure 82-2**).

◆ A midline incision extending from the xiphoid process to the pubic symphysis or a transverse incision extending from flank to flank above or below the umbilicus provides excellent exposure of the entire intra-abdominal aorta.

◆ The retroperitoneal exposure is particularly helpful in patients with inflammatory aneurysms, horseshoe kidney, ostomies, or hostile abdomens. Although this approach allows exposure of the suprarenal aorta, exposure of the right iliac vessels may be limited and a counterincision required.

◆ The patient is placed in the right lateral decubitus position over a kidney rest, with the hips allowed to rotate to the supine position after induction of anesthesia and placement of monitoring lines.

◆ An oblique incision extending from the lateral border of the rectus sheath 2 cm below the umbilicus over the tip of the 12th rib is made. Dissection is continued through the external oblique, internal oblique, and transverse abdominis muscles. The retroperitoneal space is entered by incising the most lateral aspect of the posterior rectus sheath. Dissection is continued toward the midline anterior or posterior to the left kidney. The retroperitoneal structures are retracted to the right of the midline, and repair of the aneurysm is undertaken in the usual fashion.

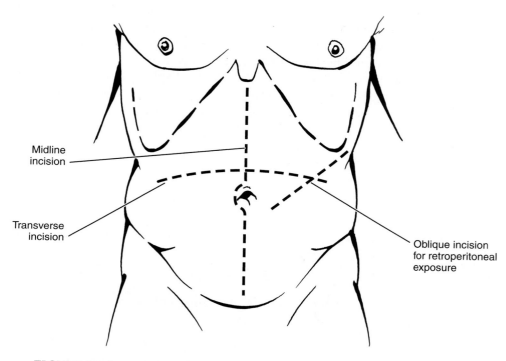

Midline
incision

Transverse
incision

Oblique incision
for retroperitoneal
exposure

FIGURE 82–2

2. DISSECTION

◆ The abdomen is explored to determine the presence of any other pathology.

◆ The transverse colon and mesocolon are then lifted cephalad, and the small intestine is moved to the right side of the abdomen. The peritoneum over the aneurysm is incised from the level of the left renal vein into the pelvis, a self-retaining retractor such as the Omni-Tract retractor is placed, and the small bowel returned into the abdomen (**Figure 82-3**).

◆ Proximal control must be immediately obtained if the aneurysm is ruptured. This is best achieved by dividing the triangular ligament and retracting the left lobe of the liver cephalad and to the right. The lesser omentum is entered near the level of the esophagogastric junction. The aorta is palpated through the fibers of the diaphragm, and the median arcuate ligament is divided. The fibers of the diaphragm are bluntly separated, a large angled aortic clamp is maneuvered into position, and the aorta is occluded. It is unnecessary to dissect and encircle the aorta before clamping. Once the bleeding is controlled, the dissection can proceed as for elective aneurysm repair.

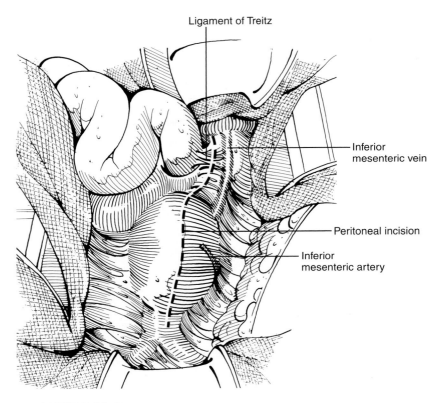

FIGURE 82–3

◆ The aorta is dissected between the aneurysm and the renal arteries; in 5% to 10% of patients, the suprarenal or pararenal aorta is involved. The surgeon should avoid injury to the left renal vein, which may be flattened over the proximal end of the aneurysm. Care should be taken to avoid injury to the iliac veins, which may be closely adherent to the arteriosclerotic arterial wall. This is best avoided by dissecting only the anterior and lateral surfaces of the common iliac arteries close to the arterial wall.

◆ The anterior and lateral surfaces of the aneurysm are more completely freed of overlying tissue, care being taken not to interrupt the collateral arterial supply to the descending and sigmoid colon as it descends in the arcade on the left side of the aneurysm. After the systemic administration of heparin (100 U/kg) and mannitol (12.5 to 25 g), the aorta and iliac vessels are occluded with vascular clamps. The clamps are placed on the iliac vessels first and then on the aorta to minimize the risk of distal embolization. When the aorta and iliac arteries are heavily calcified, occlusion of the aorta at the diaphragmatic hiatus and balloon catheter occlusion of the iliac arteries may be necessary. The anterior wall of the aneurysm is incised with a no. 11 blade or electrocautery, and the arteriotomy is continued to the right of the origin of the inferior mesenteric artery to avoid injury to the hypogastric autonomic plexus on the left **(Figure 82-4)**.

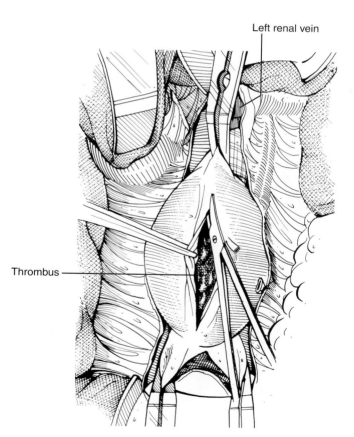

Left renal vein

Thrombus

FIGURE 82–4

◆ The laminated thrombus and the atherosclerotic debris are removed from within the aneurysmal sac, often by a sweep of the finger. Only adventitia and some media remain **(Figure 82-5).**

◆ Back-bleeding from lumbar and median sacral artery orifices is controlled with mattress sutures of 2-0 silk placed from within the opened aneurysm. Assessment of inferior mesenteric artery (IMA) backflow is then undertaken. If a large orifice with pulsatile back-bleeding is present, the vessel is ligated from within the aneurysm. If a large orifice with minimal back-bleeding is encountered, consideration should be given to reimplantation of the IMA **(Figure 82-6).**

◆ The aneurysm wall is cut transversely just distal to its beginning, except for the posterior third of the circumference if the neck is small. There is no objection to complete transection of the aorta unless the posterior aortic tissues are thin and friable, in which case it is helpful to have the retroaortic prevertebral fascia to aid in securing the posterior sutures. In most cases, the proximal anastomosis can be constructed using the Creech technique, in which the wall of the aneurysm is used to reinforce the suture line. A prosthetic graft of suitable diameter is selected, and the body of the graft is shortened to approximately 5 cm if a bifurcated graft is to be used. (The aortic portion of the graft is equal, under tension, to the length of the aortic aneurysm.) The iliac limbs of the graft are left long and appropriately trimmed just before completion of each anastomosis.

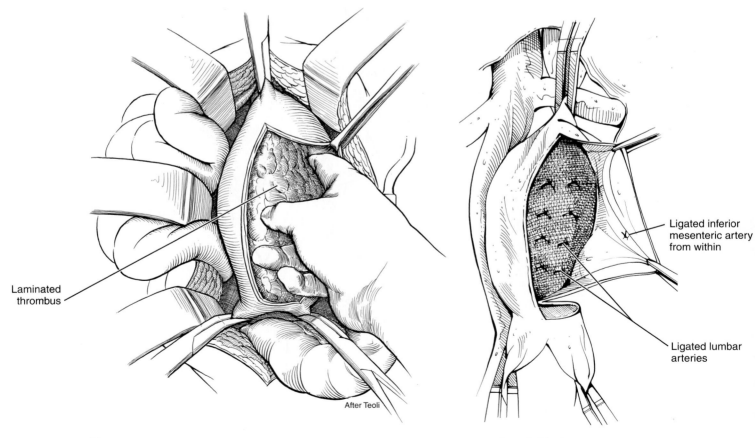

Laminated thrombus

After Teoli

Ligated inferior mesenteric artery from within

Ligated lumbar arteries

FIGURE 82–5   **FIGURE 82–6**

◆ Suturing the graft to the aorta is begun by passing the suture first through the graft and then through the aorta. Generous deep bites are taken through the aortic tissue to ensure a strong, blood-tight anastomosis. Several suturing techniques may be used. In this instance, a single 3-0 monofilament arterial suture is begun laterally at approximately the 3 o'clock position, sewing the posterior wall and continuing each end of the suture laterally and anteriorly where it is tied. Care must be taken to ensure that the suture is pulled tight before it is tied **(Figure 82-7, A)**.

◆ The graft should lie within the aortic lumen to allow better hemostasis and to prevent dissection beneath an atherosclerotic plaque at the suture line.

◆ The integrity of the aortic anastomosis is assessed by temporarily releasing the aortic clamp while the graft is occluded digitally or with a shod clamp. This is the time to be certain that the posterior suture line is secure, because it is difficult to expose this area later in the operation. A shod clamp is placed across the aortic tube graft or each limb of a bifurcated graft.

◆ Liquid blood, clots, and loose debris are aspirated from within the graft before proceeding with the distal aortic or iliac anastomosis. When a tube graft is used, the aorta above the bifurcation is partially divided transversely, leaving the posterior wall intact. The anastomosis is constructed using 3-0 polypropylene suture beginning at approximately the 3 o'clock position, taking deep bites of the posterior wall. Before placement of the final sutures, the graft and iliac arteries are flushed and the anastomosis completed **(Figure 82-7, B)**.

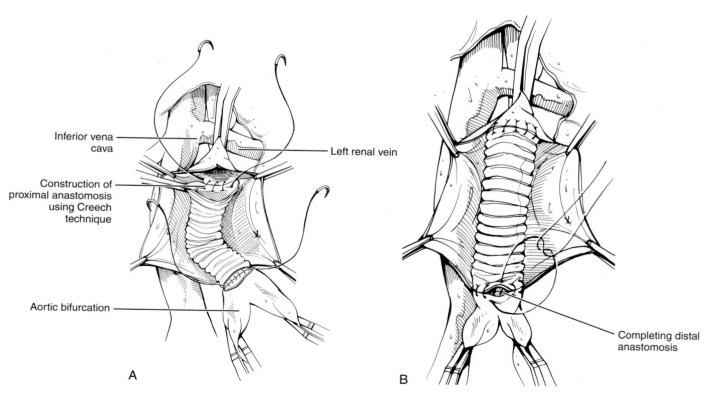

Inferior vena cava

Left renal vein

Construction of proximal anastomosis using Creech technique

Aortic bifurcation

Completing distal anastomosis

A   B

FIGURE 82–7

◆ When the distal anastomosis is to the iliac arteries, each iliac bifurcation is dissected, isolating the external and internal iliac arteries. The common iliac artery is divided 1 cm proximal to its bifurcation. If the common iliac artery is aneurysmal or otherwise unsuitable for anastomosis, the common iliac artery is oversewn or stapled and the external iliac or femoral arteries used for the distal anastomosis. The external iliac artery is allowed to back-bleed to ensure the absence of clot or debris and then flushed with heparinized saline. The limbs of the bifurcated graft are routed within the aneurysm bed to the iliac arteries.

◆ The proximal clamp on the right limb is removed with the distal end occluded digitally to assess the appropriate length of the graft so that it is long enough to allow for a tension-free anastomosis but not so long that kinking occurs.

◆ The distal anastomosis on the right is constructed first with a running 4-0 polypropylene suture. Before flow is reestablished, the iliac arteries are allowed to back-bleed, the iliac limb of the graft is flushed, and the remaining sutures are placed (**Figure 82-8**).

◆ The order of clamp removal is important in preventing of air or atheromatous debris material from passing into the legs. The clamps on the right internal iliac artery, the right limb of the graft, and the external iliac artery are removed in sequence and flow is reestablished.

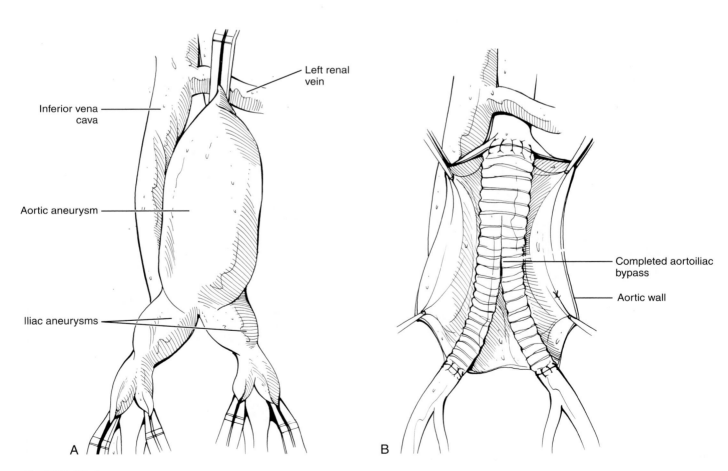

FIGURE 82–8

◆ The left limb of the graft is routed through the lumen of the left common iliac artery, and the anastomosis is completed in a similar fashion as on the right.

◆ After the aneurysmectomy is completed, hemostasis is secured and systemic heparin is reversed with protamine sulfate (1 mg/100 U heparin).

3. CLOSING

◆ The aneurysm wall is closed over the graft with 0 Vicryl suture **(Figure 82-9)**. To lessen the risk of an aortoduodenal fistula, omentum is placed adjacent to the anastomosis. The peritoneum is closed with absorbable suture, and the abdomen wall structures are reapproximated with a looped 1-0 running monofilament polydioxanone (PDS) or polypropylene suture.

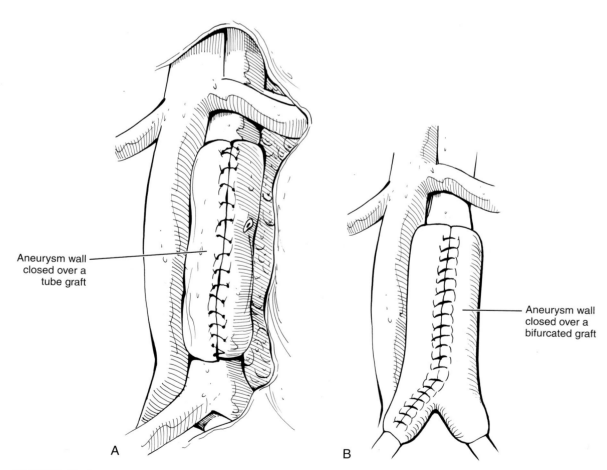

Aneurysm wall closed over a tube graft

Aneurysm wall closed over a bifurcated graft

A   B

FIGURE 82–9

STEP 4: POSTOPERATIVE CARE

◆ Careful control of fluid volume and heart rate are essential. Swan-Ganz catheter monitoring to assess cardiac output and fluid volume status is a useful adjunct. These patients often require large volumes of fluid within the first 24 to 48 hours postoperatively. Sufficient pain medication should be administered. Beta blockade begun preoperatively should be continued throughout the postoperative period. Inotropic agents should be used to ensure adequate cardiac output. Careful monitoring for evidence of mesenteric ischemia is especially important in patients with ruptured aneurysms.

STEP 5: PEARLS AND PITFALLS

JUXTARENAL ANEURYSM

◆ When the aneurysm involves the pararenal aorta, infrarenal clamping is unsafe. In this situation, supraceliac occlusion of the aorta and occlusion of the renal and superior mesentery arteries are necessary. The aorta and graft are appropriately beveled, and the patch of aorta with the visceral vessels is included in the repair. These maneuvers may require division of the left renal vein, which may be ligated or reapproximated at the completion of the aortic anastomosis.

HORSESHOE KIDNEY

◆ A horseshoe kidney occurs in 1 in 600 to 1800 individuals. The lower pole is most often fused. Each half of the kidney is usually supplied by a single renal artery. Vascular anomalies are often present, and great care should be taken to preserve the aberrant vessels.

HYPOGASTRIC ANEURYSM

◆ Although uncommon, hypogastric aneurysms usually occur deep inside the pelvis and are difficult to control with clamps. Endoluminal suture ligation of the orifice or preoperative coiling will control bleeding from the aneurysm.

AORTOCAVAL FISTULA

◆ Rarely, an undiagnosed communication between the aneurysm and the vena cava is encountered. This should be suspected if venous blood is seen flowing into the aneurysm after the thrombus has been removed from the aneurysm sac. Finger or sponge stick control of the venous bleeding and endoaneurysm repair of the communication with pledgeted monofilament sutures will usually suffice.

INFLAMMATORY ANEURYSM

◆ In approximately 5% of patients with abdominal aortic aneurysms, a dense fibrotic reaction involving the aortic wall and retroperitoneum is encountered. The inflammatory reaction may involve the duodenum, inferior vena cava, left renal vein, and ureters and is manifested as a thick white plaque overlying the aorta. Inflammatory aneurysm is an important cause of abdominal pain in patients with abdominal aortic aneurysms that must be distinguished from ruptured aneurysms on CT scans or MRI. These aneurysms are best repaired via the retroperitoneal approach mobilizing the aorta above the renal vein, taking care not to dissect the duodenum off the aneurysm wall. Venous anomalies such as left-sided or double inferior vena cava should be identified and preserved.

◆ No attempt should be made to dissect the aorta or iliac arteries circumferentially to minimize the risk of venous bleeding.

◆ Elective ligation and division of the left lumbar vein allows cephalad retraction of the renal vein, reduces the risk of bleeding, and improves exposure.

◆ Large lymphatic vessels and the cisterna chyli are often present at the level of the renal vein and should be suture ligated to prevent the rare occurrence of chylous ascites.

◆ Dissection of the left common iliac artery bifurcation should be undertaken by dividing the lateral peritoneal attachments of the descending colon, thus avoiding injury to the hypogastric nerves bilaterally. Routing the left limb of the graft through the lumen of the common iliac artery also minimizes the risk of this complication.

◆ If the renal vein is not present in its usual anterior location, a retroaortic renal vein should be suspected and care taken in placing the proximal clamp.

◆ Rectal bleeding in the early postoperative period should prompt careful sigmoidoscopy and prompt return to the operating room if significant ischemia is present or acidosis persists.

SELECTED REFERENCES

1. Standring S (ed): Gray's Anatomy: The Anatomical Basis of Clinical Practice, 39th ed. Philadelphia, Churchill Livingstone, 2005.
2. Lederle FA, Johnson GR, Wilson SE, et al: Prevalence and associations of abdominal aortic aneurysm detected through screening. Ann Intern Med 1997;126:441-449.
3. Sicard GA, Reilly JM, Rubin BG, et al: Transabdominal versus retroperitoneal incision for abdominal aortic surgery: report of a prospective randomized trial. J Vasc Surg 1995;21:174-181.

CHAPTER 83

AORTOFEMORAL BYPASS GRAFT FOR OCCLUSIVE DISEASE

Charlie C. Cheng and Michael B. Silva, Jr.

STEP 1: SURGICAL ANATOMY

SURGICAL ANATOMY OF THE FEMORAL REGION

- The inguinal ligament defines the transition from the external iliac to the common femoral artery. The common femoral artery and vein are encased in the femoral sheath in the proximal thigh bounded by the femoral triangle **(Figure 83-1)**. The lateral boundary of this triangle is formed by the sartorius muscle, the medial boundary by the adductor longus muscle, and the cephalad base by the inguinal ligament.

- Just proximal to the inguinal ligament, the external iliac artery has two branches: the inferior epigastric and the deep circumflex iliac arteries. Just distal to the inguinal ligament, the common femoral artery has three branches: the superficial epigastric, the superficial circumflex iliac, and the superficial external pudendal arteries.

- The common femoral artery divides into the superficial and the deep femoral arteries as it crosses the pectineus muscle. The superficial femoral artery traverses the thigh between the quadriceps and adductor muscles in the adductor, or Hunter's, canal. The origin of the deep femoral artery is 3 to 5 cm distal to the inguinal ligament. This artery is crossed by the lateral femoral circumflex vein (see Figure 83-1).

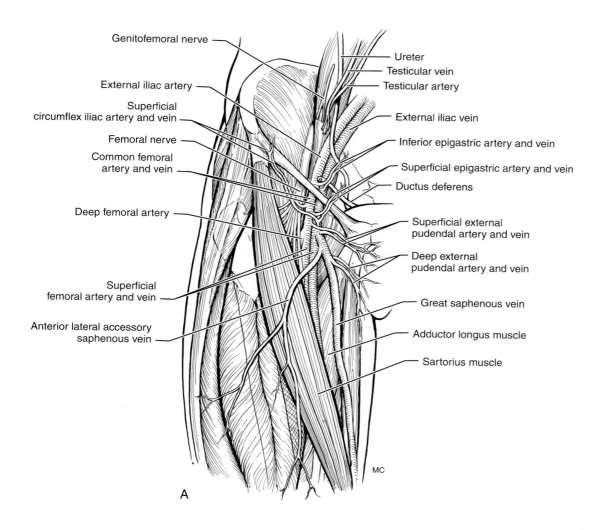

Genitofemoral nerve

External iliac artery

Superficial circumflex iliac artery and vein

Femoral nerve

Common femoral artery and vein

Deep femoral artery

Superficial femoral artery and vein

Anterior lateral accessory saphenous vein

Ureter

Testicular vein

Testicular artery

External iliac vein

Inferior epigastric artery and vein

Superficial epigastric artery and vein

Ductus deferens

Superficial external pudendal artery and vein

Deep external pudendal artery and vein

Great saphenous vein

Adductor longus muscle

Sartorius muscle

MC

A

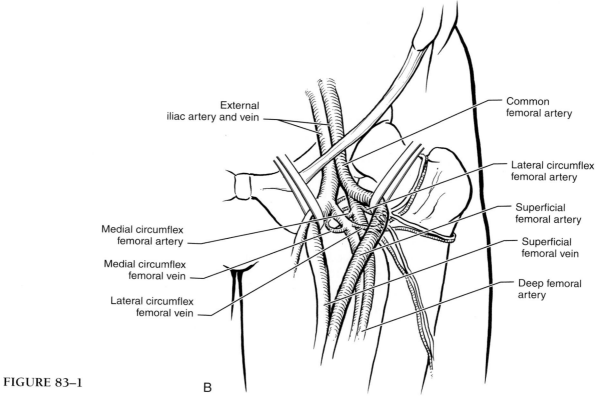

External iliac artery and vein

Medial circumflex femoral artery

Medial circumflex femoral vein

Lateral circumflex femoral vein

Common femoral artery

Lateral circumflex femoral artery

Superficial femoral artery

Superficial femoral vein

Deep femoral artery

FIGURE 83–1

B

SURGICAL ANATOMY OF THE ABDOMINAL AORTA

- The abdominal aorta has three large, unpaired midline branches that supply most organs: the celiac, superior mesenteric, and inferior mesenteric arteries **(Figure 83-2).** The celiac and superior mesenteric arteries arise at the level of the first lumbar vertebra. The inferior mesenteric artery arises at the third lumbar vertebra.

- The renal arteries arise at the level of the disc between the first two lumbar vertebrae from the lateral walls of the aorta (see Figure 83-2). The left-sided artery is usually slightly more cephalad than the right. The renal arteries lie posterior to the corresponding veins on each side. The left renal vein usually passes anterior to the aorta, whereas the right renal artery passes behind the inferior vena cava. A retroaortic left renal vein is a relatively common venous variant with an incidence of approximately 3%.

- The left renal vein serves as a landmark for cephalad dissection of the abdominal aorta. Beneath this vein, the origins of the right and left renal arteries can be located.

STEP 2: PREOPERATIVE CONSIDERATIONS

- Indications for aortobifemoral bypass are symptomatic atherosclerotic occlusive disease of the infrarenal aorta and both iliac systems, and peripheral atheromatous embolization (blue toe syndrome). Symptoms of occlusive disease include claudication, rest pain, and tissue loss. The presence of rest pain or tissue loss usually results from multilevel occlusive disease involving both the aortoiliac segment and the infrainguinal segment. Seventy-five percent to 80% of these patients can initially be managed with treatment of the inflow aortoiliac disease without treatment of the distal infrainguinal disease. This is usually adequate for patients with claudication or rest pain. However, in patients with tissue loss, the distal disease should also be treated to provide pulsatile flow to the foot. Embolization from atherosclerotic plaques in the aortoiliac system requires exclusion of the native aortoiliac arteries, even if the plaque lesions are not associated with hemodynamically significant stenoses.

- Up to 50% of patients with aortoiliac disease may have clinically evident coronary artery disease. The 30-day operative mortality for this bypass has decreased from 5% to 8% in the early 1970s to 2% in the past decade as a result of improved preoperative management of coronary artery disease. Patients should routinely be evaluated preoperatively for the presence of coronary artery disease and pulmonary, renal, and coagulation disorders.

- Preoperative imaging is needed in the evaluation of the entire abdominal aorta, the bilateral iliac arteries, and down to the origins of the deep femoral arteries. Arteriography has historically been the main imaging modality. Other contemporary alternatives include magnetic resonance imaging and computed tomography angiography. Complete bilateral lower extremity arteriography is also recommended.

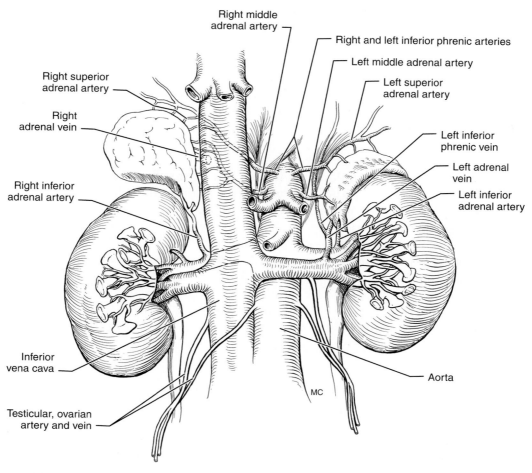

Right middle
adrenal artery

Right and left inferior phrenic arteries

Left middle adrenal artery

Right superior
adrenal artery

Left superior
adrenal artery

Right
adrenal vein

Left inferior
phrenic vein

Left adrenal
vein

Right inferior
adrenal artery

Left inferior
adrenal artery

Inferior
vena cava

Aorta

MC

Testicular, ovarian
artery and vein

FIGURE 83–2

STEP 3: OPERATIVE STEPS

1. INCISION

- The patient is placed supine, and the abdomen, groin, and thighs are prepared and draped. A narrow perineal towel is used, ensuring that it does not extend laterally to the groins. The perineum should remain excluded from the surgical field throughout the procedure. A povidone-iodine (Betadine)–impregnated self-adherent drape can be used to cover the abdomen, perineal towel, and groin areas to prevent the towel from becoming loose on the medial side of the femoral incisions.

- The groins are opened through vertical incisions directly over the femoral pulse, crossing the inguinal crease to expose the femoral arteries **(Figure 83-3).** The incision is made with one third of the incision above the inguinal ligament, and two thirds below it. If femoral pulse is not palpable, the vertical incision is made slightly medial to the midpoint of the inguinal ligament.

- The abdomen is opened through a full midline incision from the xiphoid process to the symphysis pubis. The peritoneal cavity is entered through the linea alba, and the abdominal aorta is exposed (see Figure 83-3). Alternatively, a retroperitoneal incision may be used. This may be the approach of choice in patients with a hostile abdomen from previous abdominal or aortic surgeries and poor pulmonary function. This incision is started from the lateral border of the rectus muscle, 2 cm below the level of the umbilicus, and is extended laterally to the tip of the 12th rib.

2. DISSECTION

- Femoral artery exposure
  - The groin incisions are deepened and extended proximally to the inguinal ligament. The fascia lata is opened along the medial margin of the sartorius muscle to expose the femoral sheath underneath. This sheath is opened to access the common femoral artery, and the artery is easily dissected free by separating the areolar tissue.
  - The common femoral artery branches into the superficial and deep (profunda) femoral arteries. The superficial femoral artery is exposed by dissecting distally from the common femoral artery on its anterior surface. The deep femoral artery often originates 3 to 5 cm distal to the inguinal ligament on the posterior lateral surface of the common femoral artery. The lateral femoral circumflex vein crosses anteriorly to the deep femoral artery, and caution should be used during dissection of this artery to avoid venous injury (see Figure 83-1).
  - The femoral arteries are examined for atherosclerotic occlusive disease and their suitability for distal anastomosis. The common, superficial, and deep femoral arteries are each encircled with tapes or vessel loops for control.

- Abdominal aorta exposure
  - Following the exploration of the abdomen for any incidental pathology, the transverse colon and the omentum are retracted upward toward the chest and protected from retraction injury. The small bowel is gathered and retracted to the patient's right side and wrapped in a moist laparotomy towel.

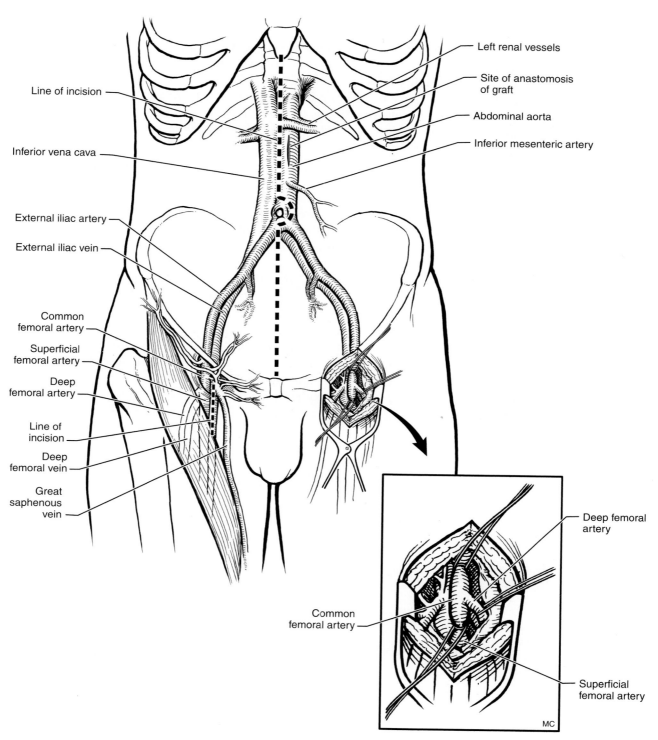

Line of incision

Inferior vena cava

External iliac artery

External iliac vein

Common
femoral artery

Superficial
femoral artery

Deep
femoral artery

Line of
incision

Deep
femoral vein

Great
saphenous
vein

Left renal vessels

Site of anastomosis
of graft

Abdominal aorta

Inferior mesenteric artery

Deep femoral
artery

Superficial
femoral artery

Common
femoral artery

MC

FIGURE 83–3

- The peritoneum is opened over the upper part of the aorta, and the ligament of Treitz is divided to mobilize the fourth portion of the duodenum and the first part of the jejunum. The patency of the celiac axis and the superior and inferior mesenteric arteries are confirmed by palpation.
- The aorta is exposed proximally to the left renal vein and distally to the inferior mesenteric artery using both sharp dissection and electrocautery of the small veins in the retroperitoneal tissue **(Figure 83-4).**
- The aorta is dissected free using blunt finger dissection or a curved instrument just below the left renal vein. The left renal vein is usually anterior to the aorta but can occasionally be retroaortic. Failure to accurately identify the left renal vein may result in iatrogenic injury during aortic cross-clamping.

- Aortofemoral bypass tunnel
  - The tunnel is used to connect the exposed aorta from the abdomen and the femoral arteries in the groins. It follows the course of the iliac and femoral arteries, lying anterior to the arteries and posterior to the ureter. This prevents compression of the ureter by the graft. The graft is protected in the retroperitoneal tissues.
  - Tunneling is started from the groin incision, with blunt finger dissection along the anterior surface of the common femoral artery. The inferior epigastric and deep circumflex iliac veins course anterior to the external iliac artery, and caution is used. These veins are routinely divided and ligated under direct vision to preclude inadvertent avulsion.
  - In the abdomen, tunneling is started on the anterior surface of the aortic bifurcation and continued onto the common iliac artery. The finger is passed blindly to meet with the finger advancing from the groin incision **(Figure 83-5).** The tunnel tract is maintained with passage of umbilical tape. The patient is systemically treated with anticoagulants, usually with unfractionated heparin, after the tunnel has been dissected and inspected for hemostasis.

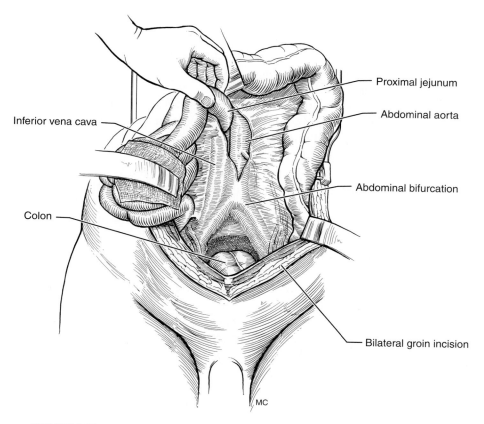

Proximal jejunum

Abdominal aorta

Inferior vena cava

Abdominal bifurcation

Colon

Bilateral groin incision

MC

FIGURE 83–4

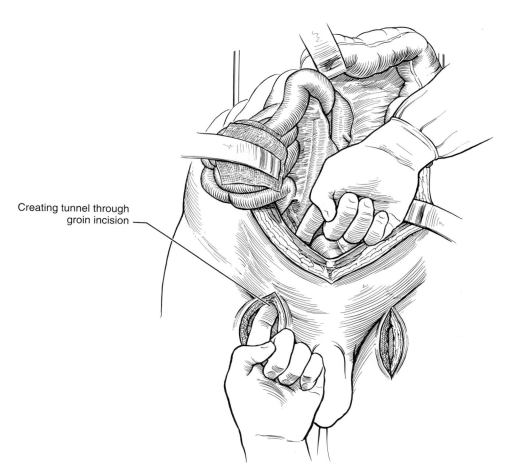

Creating tunnel through
groin incision

FIGURE 83–5

- Aortic anastomosis
  - The diameter of the aorta just below the left renal vein is assessed, and the size of the bifurcated prosthetic graft is chosen. The typical location of the proximal anastomosis is approximately 1 to 2 inches below the renal arteries. The aorta can be partially clamped or cross-clamped below the renal arteries.
  - The aortic limb of the aortic bifurcation graft is trimmed so that after the aortic anastomosis, the two limbs lie in a natural position through the tunnels in the pelvis and exit into the groin anterior to the femoral arteries. If the common trunk is too long, there is a risk of kinking of the two limbs, compromising flow.
  - The proximal aortic anastomosis can be performed in an end-to-end or end-to-side fashion. The end-to-end technique is used for patients who will not suffer circulatory compromise from interruption of prograde flow in the abdominal aorta. The end-to-side technique is used for patients who require prograde flow to perfuse an important hypogastric or inferior mesenteric artery.
  - For an end-to-side anastomosis, an arteriotomy is made on the aorta just below the renal vein, and the anastomosis is sutured with a running technique using a 3-0 nonabsorbable monofilament suture **(Figure 83-6)**. The suture can be tightened with a nerve hook.
  - For an end-to-end anastomosis, the aorta is divided sharply and the distal segment is oversewn with a heavy suture (3-0 nonabsorbable monofilament) using mattress stitches, followed by a second row using a running stitch over the cut edge. The graft is then anastomosed to the proximal aortic segment **(Figure 83-7)**.

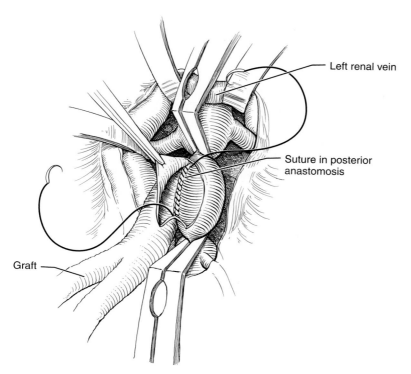

Left renal vein

Suture in posterior anastomosis

Graft

FIGURE 83–6

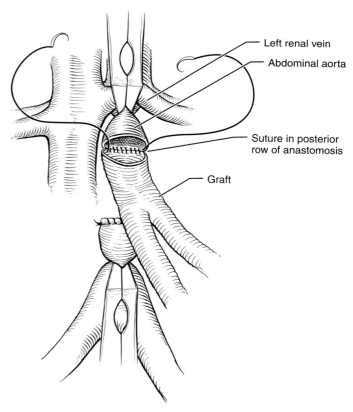

Left renal vein

Abdominal aorta

Suture in posterior row of anastomosis

Graft

FIGURE 83–7

- After the aortic anastomosis is completed, the clamp is released for several beats to flush clots, debris, and air. The limb to be used first is then flushed with heparinized saline. An aortic clamp is placed through the tunnel from the groin, and the limb is pulled out of the abdominal cavity **(Figure 83-8).**
- A plaque-free area in the distal common femoral artery is selected, and the artery is opened on the anterior surface. The length of the limb is trimmed, and the end of the graft is beveled. The anastomosis is performed with a 5-0 nonabsorbable monofilament suture, starting at the heel **(Figure 83-9).**
- Before the anastomosis is completed, the limb is flushed by removing the clamp from the limb, and the aortic clamp is released. The anastomosis is completed, and the flow is restored first to the common femoral artery and allowed to retrogradely fill the iliac artery in the pelvis so that debris is swept into this vessel rather than toward the feet. The superficial and deep femoral arteries are then reopened to restore flow to the lower extremity.
- The procedure is repeated for the other limb.

3. CLOSING

- The retroperitoneal tissue is closed over the graft to separate it from the viscera to prevent future adhesion or erosion of bowel. If this tissue is insufficient, the omentum can be used by bringing it around the left side of the colon and tacking it down on top of the graft. The bowel is returned to the abdominal cavity, and the nasogastric tube location is reconfirmed in the mid-portion of the stomach. The abdominal wall is closed using standard technique.

- The groin wound is closed in multiple layers with interrupted and/or running adsorbable 2-0 and/or 3-0 sutures using standard technique.

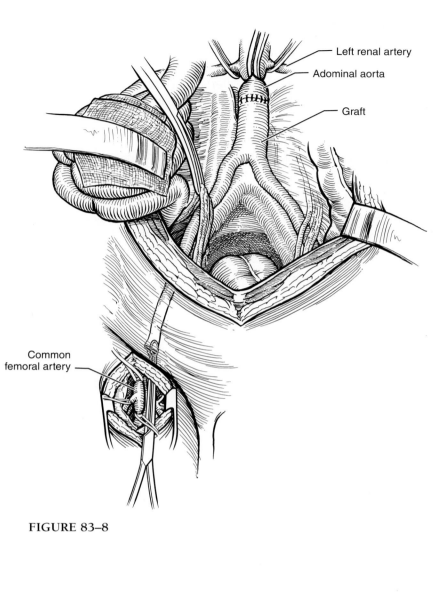

Left renal artery

Adominal aorta

Graft

Common
femoral artery

FIGURE 83–8

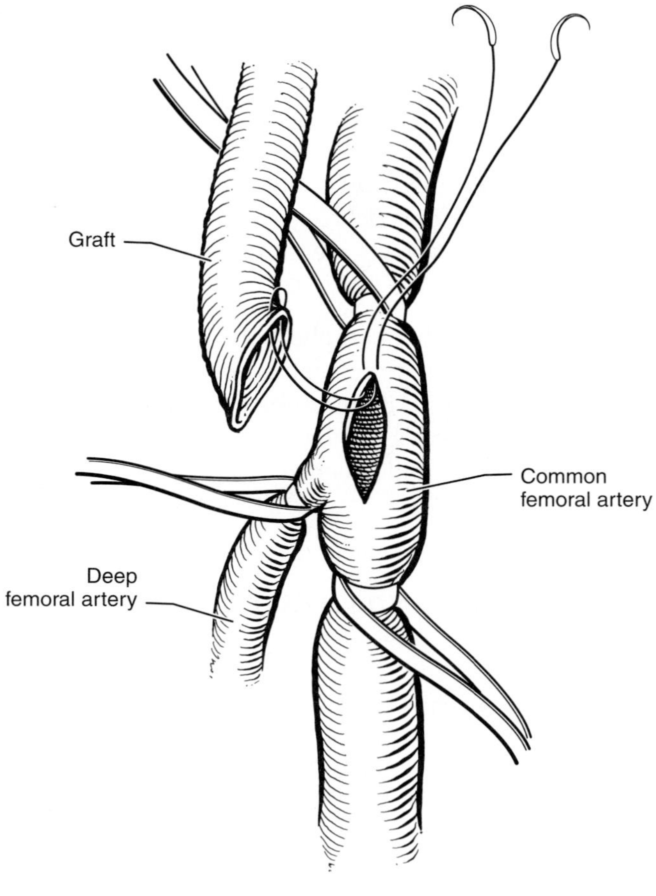

Graft

Common
femoral artery

Deep
femoral artery

FIGURE 83–9

STEP 4: POSTOPERATIVE CARE

- ◆ Patients are monitored in the intensive care unit immediately after surgery for several days and then transferred to the floor unit. Most patients are discharged on their seventh or eighth postoperative day.

- ◆ The nasogastric tube is removed with return of bowel function, usually on the third or fourth postoperative day.

- ◆ Patients are assisted by physical therapists for early mobilization with ambulation. Aggressive use of incentive spirometry is encouraged. Deep vein thrombosis prophylaxis is used.

- ◆ Patients are discharged when they have good pain control, exhibit return of bowel function, and are ambulatory.

- ◆ Surveillance of the bypass graft patency uses clinical cues, such as pulse examination, and objective criteria such as ankle-brachial indices (ABIs). Distal perfusion to the feet is verified in the operating room before closure of the wounds. Any unexpected findings require imaging and possible embolectomy. ABIs are followed in the postoperative period, at the first postdischarge clinic visit, and then at 6-month intervals.

- ◆ Initial graft patency rates are nearly 100%. The 5-year patency rates range from 80% to 90%. Long-term patency rate at 10 years is approximately 75%.

- ◆ Complications include pelvic ischemia caused by interruption of pelvic blood flow. Patients may develop colon ischemia, neurologic deficit from lumbar ischemia, and infarction of the pelvic musculature and skin.

- ◆ Embolization of large atheromatous debris may cause occlusion of major named vessels. Microscopic debris may cause injury ranging from minor focal toe ischemia to extensive tissue loss involving the major muscle groups of the buttocks, thigh, and leg.

- ◆ Other complications include lower extremity ischemia, male sexual dysfunction, and wound infection. Long-term complications include anastomotic pseudoaneurysms or stenoses. The most serious complication is aortic graft infection with development of aortoenteric fistula. Patients with this complication may present with acute gastrointestinal bleeding or chronic anemia.

STEP 5: PEARLS AND PITFALLS

- ◆ The lateral femoral circumflex vein is located between the origins of the superficial femoral and deep femoral arteries. Injury to this vein should be avoided during dissection of the deep femoral artery. When the vein is identified, it may be ligated to provide direct access to the deep femoral artery.

- The inferior epigastric and deep circumflex iliac arteries and veins can be found on the anterior surface of distal external iliac or proximal common femoral arteries beneath the inguinal ligament. Injury to these branches should be avoided during proximal dissection of the common femoral artery. Tunneling from the groin wound should be performed under direct visualization.

- In men, distal dissection should avoid the fibroareolar tissue on the anterior surface of the left common iliac artery. This tissue contains the autonomic nerves that control sexual function. Extended dissection can lead to nervous disruption and resultant retrograde ejaculation.

- The left renal vein anterior to the aorta can be divided to facilitate aortic exposure.

- A large pulsatile artery next to the inferior mesenteric artery on the left side of the aorta is likely a meandering mesenteric artery. This artery provides collateral circulation in the presence of mesenteric occlusive disease of the celiac or superior mesenteric artery, or both, and should not be divided.

- Interruption of pelvic blood flow should be avoided. The use of end-to-end or end-to-side aortic anastomosis is determined by preoperative arteriography of the abdominal aorta and bilateral iliac arteries. The end-to-end technique is used for patients who are not dependent on prograde flow in the abdominal aorta. The end-to-side technique is used for patients who require prograde flow to perfuse an important hypogastric or inferior mesenteric artery.

- The deep femoral artery can serve as the only outflow despite complete occlusion of the superficial femoral artery from atherosclerotic disease. The deep femoral artery is a low-resistance vessel that is usually free of atherosclerotic disease beyond its secondary branches.

- The common trunk of the bifurcated graft should be short, approximately 3 or 4 cm. This facilitates coverage of the graft with retroperitoneal tissue to separate the anastomosis from the overlying viscera. This also reduces the chance of kinking the graft limbs by decreasing the angle at the bifurcation.

- Proximal anastomosis on the aorta is performed just distal to the origins of the renal arteries. The infrarenal aorta can be affected by disease progression from atherosclerosis and later compromise graft patency.

SELECTED REFERENCES

1. Zarins C, Gewertz B: Atlas of Vascular Surgery, 2nd ed. Philadelphia, Churchill Livingstone, 2005.
2. Valentine RJ, Wind GG: Anatomic Exposures in Vascular Surgery, 2nd ed. Philadelphia, Lippincott Williams & Wilkins, 2003.
3. Moore WS: Vascular and Endovascular Surgery: A Comprehensive Review, 7th ed. Saint Louis, Saunders, 2006.
4. Zelenock GB, et al: Mastery of Vascular and Endovascular Surgery, 4th ed. Philadelphia, Lippincott Williams & Wilkins, 2005.

CHAPTER 84

Carotid Endarterectomy

Lois A. Killewich

STEP 1: SURGICAL ANATOMY

- The carotid sheath and its contents—including the extracranial carotid artery, the internal jugular vein, and the vagus nerve—are located in the anterior triangle of the neck, which is bounded by the mandible, the midline, and the strap muscles. Successful carotid endarterectomy requires a thorough understanding of the anatomy of the anterior triangle, in particular because a number of cranial nerves are located in the area and are easily injured if care is not taken to identify and preserve them.

- **Figure 84-1** demonstrates the structures found in the anterior triangle of the neck. The venous anatomy is variable. In the most commonly found situation, the anterior facial tributary crosses anterior to the carotid arteries at the level of the common carotid bifurcation and joins the internal jugular vein.

- The common carotid artery in the cervical region has no branches other than the external and internal carotid arteries. The internal carotid artery in this region also has no branches, except in rare situations. The persistent hypoglossal artery, a fetal structure that normally regresses before birth, is found in less than 0.1% of cases. The external carotid artery most commonly has three branches in the immediate region of the carotid bifurcation—the superior thyroid, lingual, and facial—although this anatomy can also be highly variable (see Figure 84-1, A and B).

906

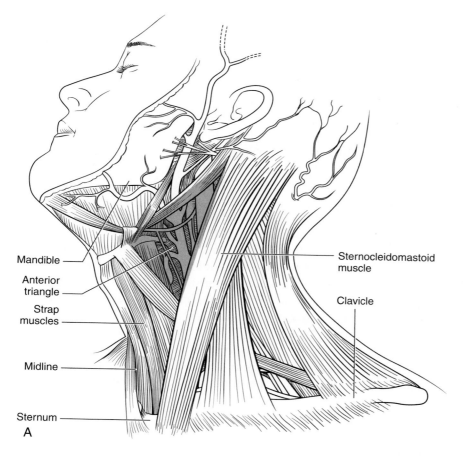

Mandible
Anterior triangle
Strap muscles
Midline
Sternum

Sternocleidomastoid muscle
Clavicle

A

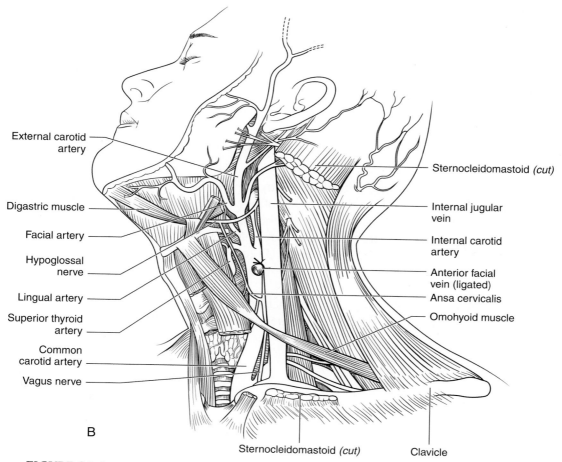

External carotid artery
Digastric muscle
Facial artery
Hypoglossal nerve
Lingual artery
Superior thyroid artery
Common carotid artery
Vagus nerve

Sternocleidomastoid (cut)
Internal jugular vein
Internal carotid artery
Anterior facial vein (ligated)
Ansa cervicalis
Omohyoid muscle

B

Sternocleidomastoid (cut)
Clavicle

FIGURE 84–1

STEP 2: PREOPERATIVE CONSIDERATIONS

◆ Standard indications for carotid endarterectomy include a stenosis of 50% or higher in a patient with a transient ischemic attack or stroke thought to originate from internal carotid artery plaque and 60% to 80% stenosis in an asymptomatic patient. Recurrent stenosis, stenosis secondary to radiation therapy, and high-risk patients with severe coronary artery or pulmonary disease are often treated with carotid stenting.

◆ Carotid endarterectomy can be safely performed with the patient under general, regional, or local anesthesia. Whichever technique is selected, a method must be used to ensure that the patient has adequate intracranial blood flow while flow through the operated internal carotid artery is interrupted. When local or regional anesthesia is used, the patient's neurologic status can be monitored by assessing contralateral motor function and, in some cases, speech. Many surgeons use a squeeze toy in the contralateral hand and instruct the patient to squeeze the toy to demonstrate that neurologic function is maintained when the carotid arteries are clamped. If general anesthesia is used, neurologic function can be monitored by measuring carotid back-pressure (the internal carotid artery pressure with the common and external carotid arteries; a mean arterial pressure of 25 to 40 mm Hg is sufficient), by using electroencephalographic or evoked potential monitoring, or by using routine carotid shunting.

◆ Patients should be administered 325 mg of aspirin by mouth daily, starting before the surgical procedure. In selected instances, clopidogrel (75 mg by mouth daily) may be used in addition to or in place of aspirin.

STEP 3: OPERATIVE STEPS

1. INCISION

◆ The head should be positioned with the neck hyperextended and rotated to the contralateral side. This can be facilitated by placement of a rolled sheet between the shoulder blades. The standard incision is placed along the medial border of the sternocleidomastoid muscle. The superior aspect should be extended posteriorly to the ear to ensure against division of the greater auricular nerve (**Figure 84-2, A**).

◆ For a more cosmetically pleasing result, the incision can be created in a mid-cervical skin crease, with an extension superiorly toward the ear (**Figure 84-2, B**).

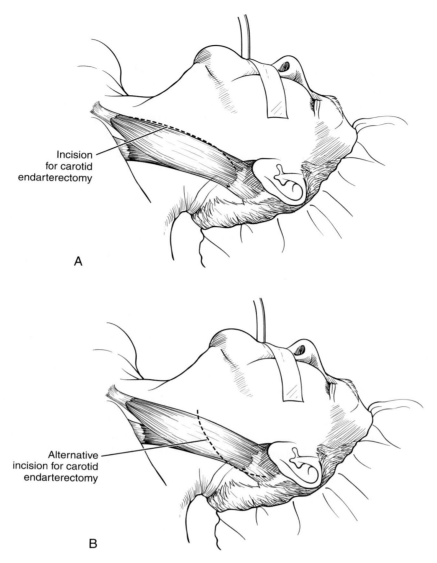

Incision
for carotid
endarterectomy

A

Alternative
incision for carotid
endarterectomy

B

FIGURE 84–2

2. DISSECTION

◆ After the incision is created, the platysma muscle is divided with electrocautery parallel to the skin incision. If the cervical skin crease incision is used, flaps must be created deep to the platysma muscle and extended superiorly toward the mandible and inferiorly toward the clavicle. This can be accomplished using a combination of electrocautery and blunt dissection, which enlarges the operative field to allow the dissection to be continued in standard fashion.

◆ The dissection is deepened along the medial border of the sternocleidomastoid muscle until the carotid sheath is identified (**Figure 84-3**). Small arteries and veins, which extend across the dissection line to supply the sternocleidomastoid muscle, are cauterized. The carotid sheath is opened using sharp dissection. (I prefer 7-inch Potts-Smith scissors, but either Metzenbaum or tenotomy scissors can also be used.)

◆ Once the sheath is opened, the dissection of the carotid arteries is completed using scissors (**Figure 84-4**). The common carotid artery is dissected first, followed by the external carotid artery and the superior thyroid artery. It is generally not necessary to continue the dissection of the external carotid artery beyond the second branch, which may be the lingual artery or a combined trunk of the lingual and facial arteries. Once this dissection is completed, anticoagulants are administered to the patient systemically, usually with unfractionated heparin at a dose of 100 units/kg body weight. The dissection of the internal carotid artery is completed while the heparin is circulating, which provides some measure of protection from embolization of plaque from the internal carotid artery during the dissection. When the dissection is completed, the arteries are controlled with vessel loops, sutures, or Rumel tourniquets.

3. DETERMINING THE NEED FOR INSERTION OF A SHUNT

◆ The dissected vessels are clamped so that the need for shunting can be determined. Except in the case of back-pressure monitoring, the internal carotid artery beyond the area of plaque is clamped first to prevent embolization into the intracranial circulation. I prefer a Gregory bulldog for clamping of the internal carotid artery; other choices include a Yasargil aneurysm clip or a small vascular clamp such as a Karchner. The common and external carotid arteries are also clamped with small vascular clamps; branches of the external carotid artery can be controlled with Yasargil clips, hemoclips, or Pott's knots.

◆ If back-pressure monitoring is used to determine the need for shunting, the internal carotid artery is not clamped. A 19-gauge butterfly needle or a small angiocatheter connected to pressure tubing is inserted into the artery distal to the plaque. It is imperative that this tubing be flushed thoroughly with heparinized saline before insertion to prevent introduction of air into the carotid, and hence intracranial, circulation. The back-pressure is then measured; I use a cutoff of 40 mm Hg mean arterial pressure to determine the need for insertion of a shunt.

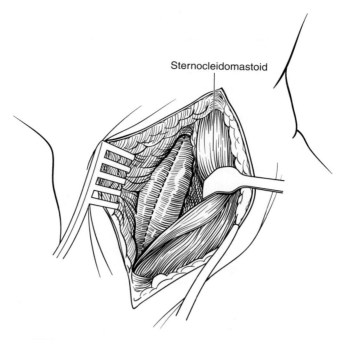

FIGURE 84–3

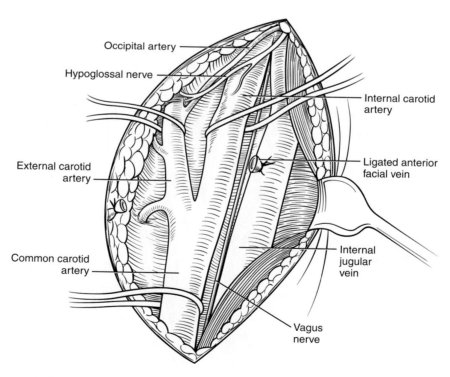

FIGURE 84–4

- Other methods for shunt determination include electroencephalogram, somatosensory evoked potentials, or awake patient monitoring. The electroencephalogram measures global hemispheric functioning, and evoked potentials measure peripheral nerve function. In general, a flattening of amplitude on the affected side indicates the need for a shunt. If the patient is awake and a shunt is required, the patient will lose function of the contralateral hand or foot, or both, and be unable to follow commands. It should be emphasized that these changes are almost immediate, so this assessment requires at most 3 minutes.

- Once the decision regarding shunting has been made, an arteriotomy is created on the distal anterior surface of the common carotid artery using a no. 11 blade and is extended through the region of plaque in the internal carotid artery using Potts scissors **(Figure 84-5)**.

- If a shunt is to be used, it should be flushed with heparinized saline and clamped in the midportion before insertion **(Figure 84-6, A)**. I insert the proximal end into the common carotid first, flush blood out the distal end, reclamp the mid-portion, insert the distal end into the internal carotid artery, check for bubbles, and then release the clamp **(Figure 84-6, B-C)**. Either specially designed shunt clamps or Rumel tourniquets can be used to fix the shunt in the arterial ends during endarterectomy. During the shunt insertion, the common and internal carotid arteries should be controlled with doubly looped vessel loops.

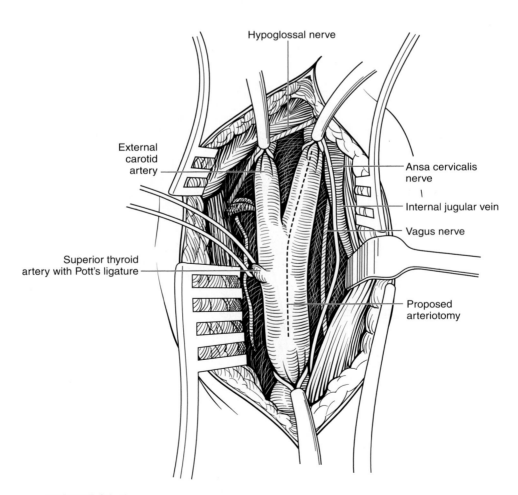

FIGURE 84–5

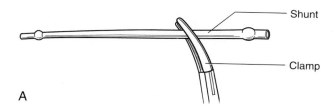

Shunt

Clamp

A

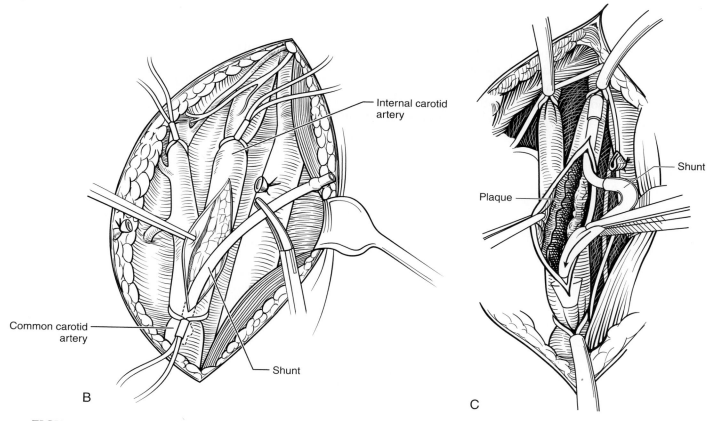

Internal carotid
artery

Common carotid
artery

Shunt

B

Plaque

Shunt

C

FIGURE 84–6

4. ENDARTERECTOMY

◆ The endarterectomy is performed using a Freer elevator **(Figure 84-7)**. This is inserted into the plane between the circular muscle fibers and the adventitia, beginning in the common carotid artery. The adventitia is pushed away from the muscle fibers extending distally. When the end of the plaque is reached, gentle pressure on the plaque pulling inferiorly and toward the contralateral side will usually separate it from the normal distal artery. Alternatively, a Beaver blade can be used to divide the plaque from the normal artery. The plaque can then be peeled off transversely. The remainder of the plaque is removed from the internal and common carotid arteries in a similar fashion.

◆ The plaque is removed from the external carotid artery using an eversion technique. The adventitia of the artery is everted by the surgical assistant, while the plaque and circular muscle fibers are dissected away circumferentially by the surgeon using the Freer elevator. The plaque is avulsed at its natural end.

◆ Once the specimen is removed, any remaining debris or circular smooth muscle fibers can be removed by scraping transversely with the Freer elevator or a Kittner sponge. If the edge of the distal endpoint has been lifted up, it should be tacked down with 7-0 Prolene as shown in **Figure 84-8.** The proximal endpoint does not need to be tacked because it will be pushed into the adventitia of the artery by the blood flow.

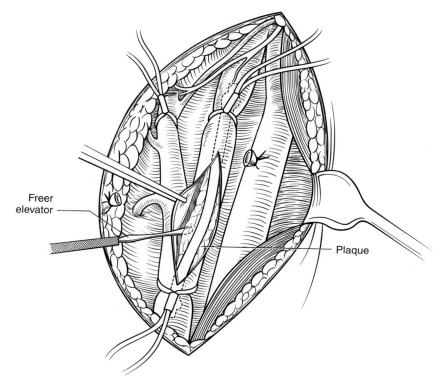

Freer
elevator

Plaque

FIGURE 84–7

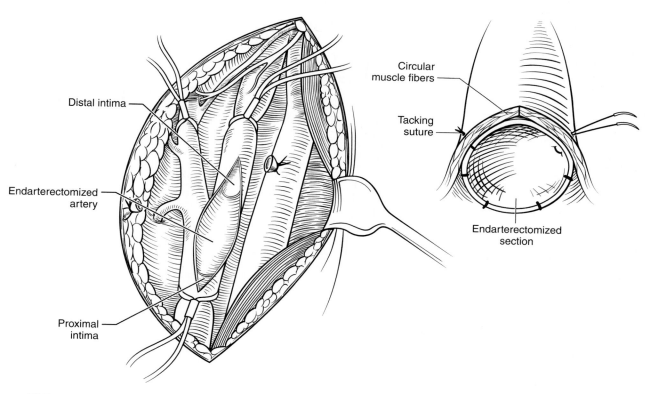

Distal intima

Endarterectomized
artery

Proximal
intima

Circular
muscle fibers

Tacking
suture

Endarterectomized
section

FIGURE 84–8

◆ It is the current standard of care to close the arteriotomy with a patch, as shown in **Figure 84-9.** Prosthetic patches are used most commonly, either Dacron or expanded polytetrafluoroethylene (ePTFE). Before the final closure, flushing should be performed with care taken to ensure that the internal carotid artery is flushed last. If a shunt has been used, this should be removed before flushing. Once flushing is completed, the inner surface of the endarterectomized vessel is irrigated copiously with heparinized saline, and the closure is completed. The internal carotid artery is then back-bled into the common carotid artery and gently clamped across its origin. (I use DeBakey pickups.) Flow is then restored through the common carotid artery into the external carotid artery, providing an additional means for flushing any remaining debris or air, or both, into the external carotid artery rather than the intracranial circulation. After 10 seconds, flow is restored through the internal carotid artery.

◆ It is possible to perform an intraoperative duplex ultrasound or angiogram to check the operative result, although this has not been my practice.

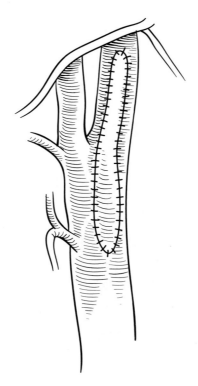

FIGURE 84–9

5. CLOSING

- The heparin can be reversed using protamine, if necessary. The platysma is closed with running 3-0 Vicryl. The skin is closed with 4-0 Monocryl and surgical glue. In some cases, I place a drain in the surgical site, bringing it out through a lateral skin stab incision. If a drain is used, it should be removed on the morning of the first postoperative day.

STEP 4: POSTOPERATIVE CARE

- Aspirin or clopidogrel, or both, should be continued daily throughout the postoperative period. Most surgeons would continue at least one of these medications for life.

- Drains should be removed on the first postoperative day.

- Hematoma in the neck can cause respiratory compromise. If a rapidly expanding hematoma or any evidence of respiratory compromise exists, the patient should be return emergently to the operating room for evacuation and control of the hemorrhage.

- Cranial nerves, which can be injured during the surgery, include the vagus, recurrent laryngeal, external branch of the superior laryngeal, hypoglossal, and marginal mandibular branch of the facial. Vagal and recurrent laryngeal injuries result in hoarseness secondary to vocal cord paresis or paralysis in the midline. A patient who is hoarse after carotid surgery should have a vocal cord assessment, in particular if contralateral carotid surgery is contemplated. Bilateral vocal cord paralysis requires emergent intubation or tracheostomy, or both. Injury to the external branch of the superior laryngeal nerve results in loss of the resonance and high tones in the voice. Hypoglossal nerve injury results in deviation of the tongue to the side of the injury; this can result in reduced ability to move food around in the mouth and drooling. Injury to the marginal mandibular nerve results in pulling of the inferior aspect of the mouth in a direction away from the injury. In general, hypoglossal and marginal mandibular nerve injuries are temporary.

- Patients, particularly those who undergo carotid endarterectomy under general anesthesia, can experience blood pressure instability after surgery. Most commonly, this is manifested as hypertension, which can be treated with intravenous medication such as nitroprusside. Hypotension, which is less common, can be treated with medication such as phenylephrine.

- The most feared complication after carotid endarterectomy is stroke, which can occur intraoperatively or postoperatively. Intraoperative strokes are usually treated with anticoagulant or antiplatelet therapy postoperatively. Postoperative strokes (in other words, the patient's neurologic examination is normal immediately after surgery, but changes within the first 12 to 24 hours) should be treated by emergent return to the operating room because of the possibility of carotid thrombosis. This can be treated with thrombectomy and possibly thrombolytic therapy.

STEP 5: PEARLS AND PITFALLS

- Injury to the marginal mandibular nerve can be avoided by not retracting the mandible too strongly.

- Division of an unusually large ansa cervicalis crossing anterior to the carotid bifurcation will usually result in hoarseness. Avoid cutting it if possible.

- Because of the risk of infection and carotid rupture, a tracheostomy adjacent to a fresh carotid endarterectomy is a disaster and should be avoided at all costs.

SELECTED REFERENCES

1. North American Symptomatic Carotid Endarterectomy Trial Collaborators: Benefit of carotid endarterectomy in symptomatic patients with high-grade carotid stenosis. N Engl J Med 1991;325:445-453.
2. North American Symptomatic Carotid Endarterectomy Trial Collaborators: Benefit of carotid endarterectomy in patients with symptomatic moderate or severe stenosis. N Engl J Med 1998;339:1415-1425.
3. Executive committee for Asymptomatic Carotid Atherosclerosis Study: Endarterectomy for asymptomatic carotid artery stenosis. JAMA 1995;273:1421-1428.
4. Ricotta JJ Jr, Malgor RD: A review of the trials comparing endarterectomy and carotid angioplasty and stenting. Perspect Vasc Surg Endovasc Ther 2008;20:299-308.

CHAPTER 85

FEMOROPOPLITEAL BYPASS (IN SITU)

Lori Cindrick Pounds

STEP 1: SURGICAL ANATOMY

◆ A comprehensive understanding of the anatomy of the leg is essential to performing the procedure and avoiding future complications. This anatomy includes the femoral triangle and the popliteal space below the knee. The saphenous vein can have many variations in its course in the thigh. Identifying the main branch and avoiding a flap are key points **(Figures 85-1 through 85-3)**.

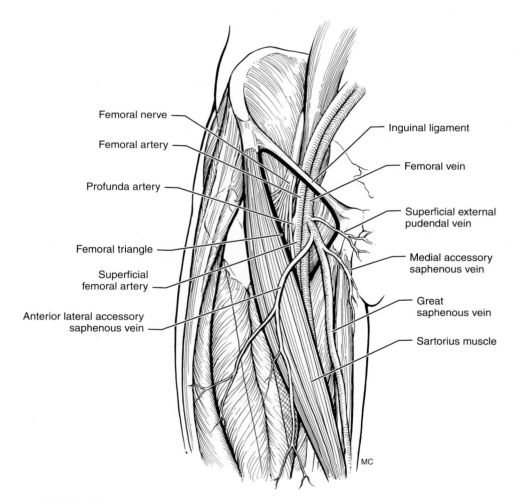

Femoral nerve
Femoral artery
Profunda artery
Femoral triangle
Superficial femoral artery
Anterior lateral accessory saphenous vein

Inguinal ligament
Femoral vein
Superficial external pudendal vein
Medial accessory saphenous vein
Great saphenous vein
Sartorius muscle

FIGURE 85–1

Posterior View

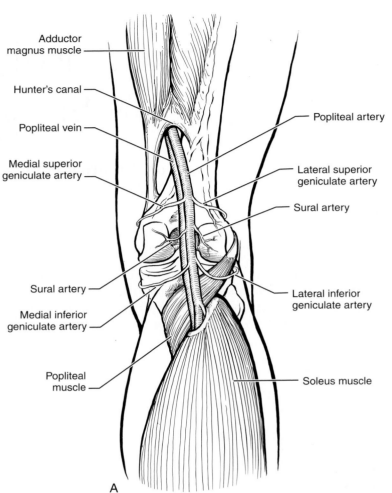

Adductor
magnus muscle

Hunter's canal

Popliteal vein

Medial superior
geniculate artery

Sural artery

Medial inferior
geniculate artery

Popliteal
muscle

Popliteal artery

Lateral superior
geniculate artery

Sural artery

Lateral inferior
geniculate artery

Soleus muscle

A

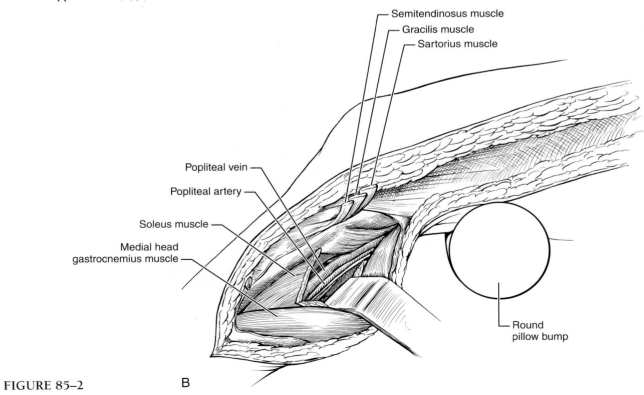

Semitendinosus muscle

Gracilis muscle

Sartorius muscle

Popliteal vein

Popliteal artery

Soleus muscle

Medial head
gastrocnemius muscle

Round
pillow bump

FIGURE 85–2

B

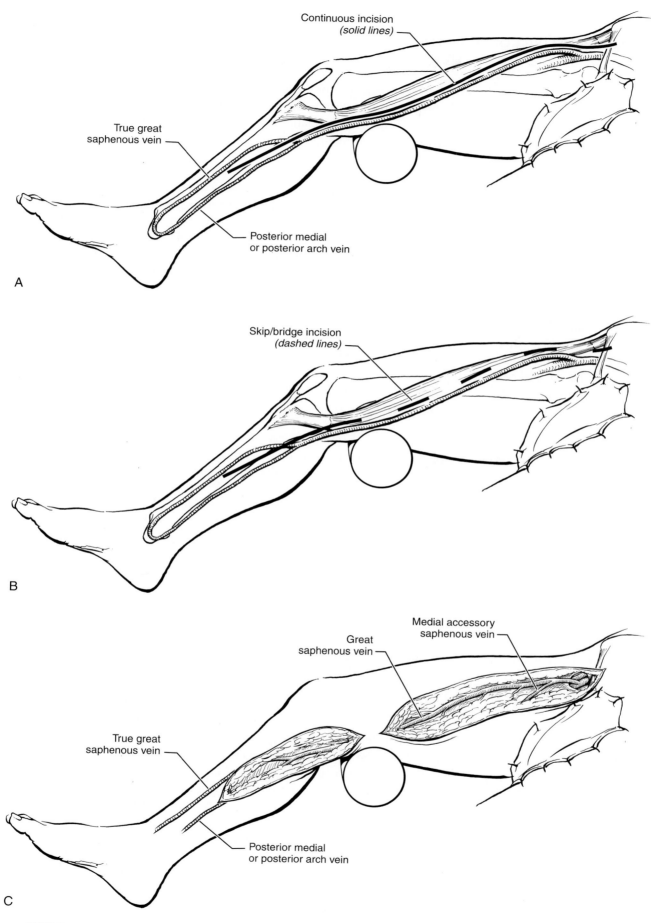

FIGURE 85–3

STEP 2: PREOPERATIVE CONSIDERATIONS

- The standard indication for reconstruction for occlusive disease is limb-threatening ischemia. This includes ischemic rest pain, ulceration, and gangrene. There are certain accepted indications for bypass in the setting of severe claudication that prohibit gainful employment or maintenance of the activities of daily living.

- The femoropopliteal in situ bypass is one of many open reconstructive options available to the surgeon. In general, when the vein is to be used for limb salvage, it is customary to use the below-knee popliteal segment. The above-knee segment may seem like an appropriate target, but it is known to have a high rate of progression of disease. The in situ technique offers the advantage of allowing the larger part of the saphenous to be placed on the larger common femoral artery and the smaller section of vein to be placed on the smaller outflow artery. The alternatives to this include a femoropopliteal bypass with vein that is reversed and buried in an anatomic tunnel that follows the native superficial femoral and popliteal arteries. A prosthetic infrageniculate (below the knee) graft is reserved for the individual who has exhausted all autogenous (vein) options in the lower and upper extremities—including the great and small (also known as the lesser or short) saphenous, as well as the basilic and cephalic veins. Last, with the endovascular revolution, many catheter-based options are available, including a percutaneous bypass with covered stent grafts, an atherectomy, or laser treatment, to name a few.

- Preoperative venous duplex (a grayscale B-mode ultrasound and doppler waveform analysis) of the superficial veins is very helpful to determine the quality of the vein and to help choose an operative plan. If the ultrasound can be arranged close to the bypass surgery date, it is helpful to have the technician mark the course of the vein. Many operative suites have an ultrasound available, and the vein can be marked before the leg is prepped. This may help reduce the risk of a flap formation.

STEP 3: OPERATIVE STEPS

- The patient is placed in a supine position. For occlusive disease, it is a good rule to prepare more than is needed. In general, both lower extremities should be draped in case further vein is needed to complete a procedure. The first incision is typically placed in the groin at the level of the inguinal ligament. The great saphenous vein is identified first at the fossa ovalis, below Scarpa's fascia. The femoral sheath is then opened longitudinally to identify the femoral vessels. The common femoral artery, superficial femoral artery (SFA), and profunda femoris artery (PFA) should be isolated. The saphenous vein can then be isolated either through a continuous incision that "unroofs" the entire vein or through a series of "skip" incisions, also known as bridge incisions. A continuous incision allows maximal visualization of all branches but can be associated with greater wound-healing and infection risks. The bridge technique can heal better but has limited viewing of the vein, which may result in either vein injury or inadequate ligation of all branches (see Figure 85-3). A third alternative is a hybrid between a traditional vein harvest and an in situ harvest—an endoscopic vein harvest. Some institutions may have a designated individual with extensive experience, such as a physician's assistant who harvests for coronary artery bypass grafting. This technique offers many advantages. There is one incision in the lower thigh that can be used to harvest the vein to the saphenofemoral junction. The vein can then be placed in the harvest tunnel—either reversed or nonreversed. This offers the advantage of an in situ technique, such as easy graft palpation or duplex surveillance. Additional benefits include fewer incisions at risk for wound dehiscence and graft exposure.

◆ Before the artery is clamped, the patient is given an unfractionated heparin bolus, typically between 5000 and 10,000 U. The artery is clamped proximally and distally, and an arteriotomy is made anteriorly. A standard spatulated end of the vein-to-side of artery anastomosis is created with Prolene suture, usually a 5-0 or 6-0 stitch **(Figure 85-4)**.

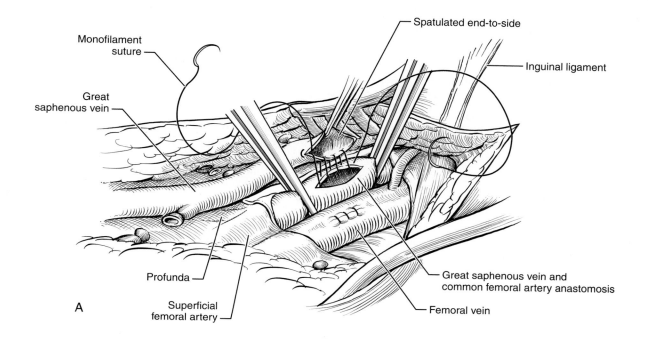

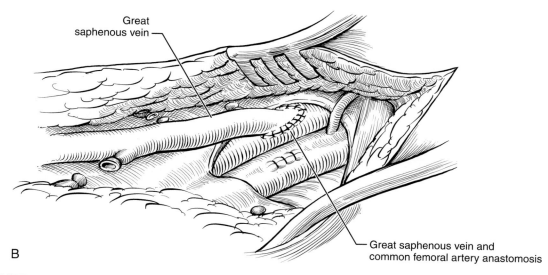

FIGURE 85–4

◆ The below-knee popliteal incision on the medial calf typically extends from the tibial tuberosity to the midcalf. A general rule for this exposure is to have a bump placed well above the knee so that the gastrocnemius and soleus muscles hang freely. The fascia is entered, and an avascular plane is developed by retracting the gastrocnemius and soleus muscles downward. The popliteal space is then entered, and the vein (anterior to the artery) is dissected free from the popliteal artery. The popliteal vein is commonly duplicated and that branch is lying posterior to the artery. It can be injured when trying to dissect bluntly with a right angle. It is best to use sharp dissection in this tight space, because it is much easier to repair a cut than an avulsed branch (see Figure 85-2).

◆ There are multiple methods for destruction of the valves. A hand-held valvulotome or scissors can be inserted through large side branches. There are also disposable products available **(Figure 85-5).** The proximal anastomosis should be created in a standard fashion (see Figure 85-4). The most proximal first and second valves are removed under direct vision before this anastomosis is started. It is important to remove the thin valve cusp flush with the vein wall. This will ensure that the cusp remnants do not become involved in the anastomosis, which would severely stenose or occlude the flow. Flow should then be established in the vein graft to identify whether any other valves are intact. There will be a decrease in pulsatility and flow detected by Doppler ultrasound where the valve is still intact.

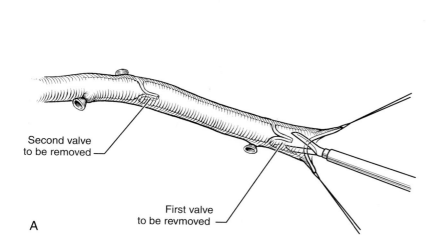

Second valve to be removed

First valve to be revmoved

A

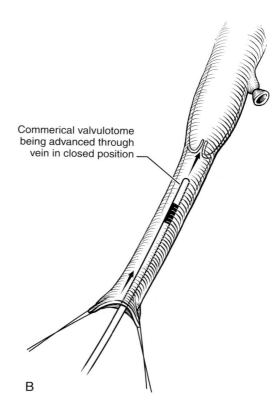

Commerical valvulotome being advanced through vein in closed position

B

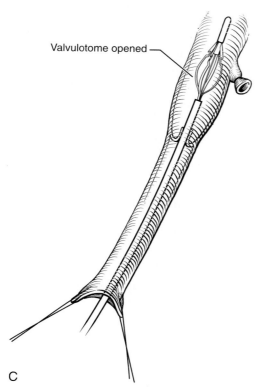

Valvulotome opened

C

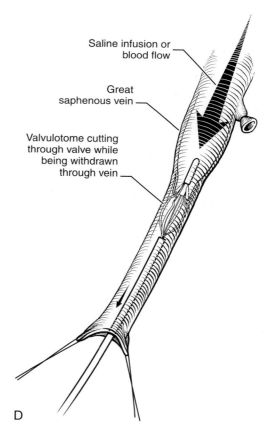

Saline infusion or blood flow

Great saphenous vein

Valvulotome cutting through valve while being withdrawn through vein

D

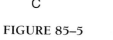

FIGURE 85–5

◆ Once adequate flow has been established in the vein, the distal anastomosis can be created in a similar fashion **(Figure 85-6)**. If the outflow artery is calcified, a tourniquet can be used to occlude the flow and avoid placing a clamp on the artery. Before the anastomosis is completed, it should be appropriately irrigated and flushed free of any potential debris or clot. A completion arteriogram can then be performed, ideally through a large preserved side branch with a radiopaque marking tape. This is essential if the entire vein had not been mobilized or if bridge incisions were used so that large branches can be ligated.

STEP 4: POSTOPERATIVE CARE

◆ Most patients undergoing surgery for peripheral arterial disease have multiple comorbidities including coronary artery disease. They can be monitored in an intensive care unit, step-down unit, or specialized floor bed depending on the protocols of the institution. Minimum requirements should include telemetry, and vital signs should be taken every 2 hours, including monitoring patency of the graft with Doppler ultrasonography. It is important to educate staff on the importance of using a quantitative measure such as a Doppler signal and not relying on an individual's experience at feeling pedal pulses.

◆ If medically stable, the patient should be moved to a floor bed as soon as possible. Rehabilitation therapy should begin immediately, even if it is as simple as sitting in a chair. Realistic expectations should be discussed with the family and staff about discharge planning. Many patients will need transition care either in a rehabilitation facility or by a skilled nurse facility (SNF) before they are independent and can go home by themselves or with a caregiver.

◆ Postoperatively, many surgeons prescribe a nonadjusted unfractionated heparin intravenous drip for 12 to 24 hours. It is common for the patient to take either an anticoagulant (warfarin) or a platelet inhibitor (aspirin or clopidrogel) after that. The decision on which to use needs to be individualized based on certain factors. In general, these include quality of the inflow, which should be adequate before attempting an infrainguinal procedure. The outflow artery may not always be ideal, and a substandard conduit such as ePTFE or a bad vein may convince the surgeon to use a stronger agent.

◆ After discharge, the patient should be seen in clinic and understand that he or she will have a relationship with the surgeon for the life of that graft. Routine graft surveillance with duplex scanning and ankle-brachial indices (ABIs) has been demonstrated to increase the primary patency of grafts (assisted primary patency). Protocols include a postprocedure baseline level and close follow-up (every 3 months for a year, then biannually). A drop in the ABI or a velocity elevation is suggestive of a stenosis in the graft and warrants an arteriogram and possible intervention.

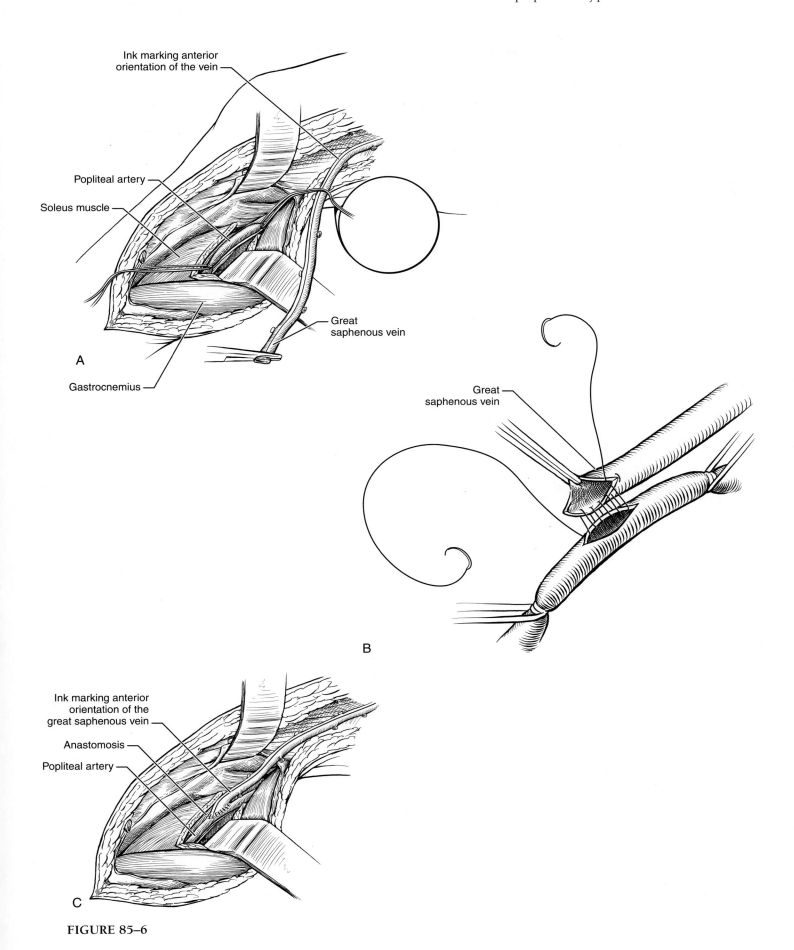

Ink marking anterior
orientation of the vein

Popliteal artery

Soleus muscle

Great
saphenous vein

A

Gastrocnemius

Great
saphenous vein

B

Ink marking anterior
orientation of the
great saphenous vein

Anastomosis

Popliteal artery

C

FIGURE 85–6

STEP 5: PEARLS AND PITFALLS

- ◆ The in situ bypass technique has been shown to be an excellent choice for infrainguinal reconstruction for occlusive disease. The location of the graft in the subcutaneous tissues makes it quite easy to feel and evaluate with duplex ultrasound. There are certain groups of patients with whom I am very cautious. The diabetic, end-stage renal patient is the classic individual to have a wound-healing issue. Because the graft is directly under the skin, any wound dehiscence will result in exposure of the adventitia and graft rupture if it is not dealt with expediently. One may consider leaving large skin bridges, or I find it preferable to place the graft in a more anatomic location adjacent to the artery and vein. Thus, when there are wound-healing issues, it is just a simple superficial or deep tissue infection and not an organ space (i.e., the graft) that is involved.

SELECTED REFERENCES

1. Ouriel K, Rutherford R (eds): Atlas of Vascular Surgery: Operative Procedures. Philadelphia, Saunders, 1998.
2. Norgren L, Hiatt WR, Dormandy JA, et al: Inter-Society Consensus for the Management of Peripheral Arterial Disease (TASC II). J Vasc Surg 2007;45:S5-S6.
3. Valentine RJ, Wind GG: Anatomic Exposures in Vascular Surgery, 2nd ed. Philadelphia, Lippincott Williams & Wilkins, 2003.
4. Rutherford RB: Atlas of Vascular Surgery: Basic Techniques and Exposures. Philadelphia, Saunders, 1993.

CHAPTER 86

FEMOROTIBIAL AND PERONEAL BYPASS

Lori Cindrick Pounds

STEP 1: SURGICAL ANATOMY

◆ A review of the proximal femoral and saphenous vein anatomy has been discussed at length in Chapter 85. The popliteal artery branches are commonly called the "trifurcation," denoting its division into three distinct arteries—(1) the anterior tibial artery (ATA), which crosses the interosseus membrane and runs in the anterior compartment until the ankle mortise; at that point it is called the dorsalis pedis artery (DPA). It has a large branch that also may be suitable to receive the bypass is the lateral tarsal artery; (2) the posterior tibial artery (PTA); and (3) the peroneal artery—which have a common trunk (tibioperoneal trunk) that courses in the deep posterior compartment. The PTA continues its course on to the foot at the medial malleous, where it divides into the medial and lateral plantar arteries. The peroneal artery does not cross the ankle joint, but gives out two consistent branches that collateralize to the DPA and PTA.

STEP 2: PREOPERATIVE CONSIDERATIONS

◆ The same standard indications for reconstruction are true for tibial bypass as are true for femoropopliteal reconstructions (see Chapter 85). They include limb-threatening ischemia (ischemic rest pain, ulceration, and gangrene). Typically the lower in the leg you have to go to find a suitable target, the greater the burden of disease. There are three basic sections of the arterial tree below the renal arteries: aortoiliac, femoropopliteal, and tibial (infrageniculate). When the disease is confined to one segment, then usually the patient will either be asymptomatic or have claudication. If two or more segments are involved, then the ischemia is more profound and the limb can be threatened. So if you are planning a femorotibial bypass, the occlusive lesions would be in two sections, the femoropopliteal and tibial distribution. It is generally a statement to the overall status of the patient as well, because these patients tend to have a heavier burden of atherosclerotic disease in other beds also (coronary and extracranial carotid arteries).

◆ Autogenous vein is clearly the best option for reconstruction below the knee. Similar considerations for vein assessment and procurement exist as for the femoropopliteal, but a longer section of quality vein is needed. At times, this can be hard to secure, and sections of different veins can be anastomosed to create a conduit. Always remember that the small saphenous, cephalic, and basilic veins are wonderful options. They can also be mapped with ultrasound before the surgery. Again, having to do this raises the degree of complexity and the possibility for adverse events.

◆ The decision to leave the vein in situ or bury it anatomically next to the native vessels is the choice of the surgeon. Each has been shown to be appropriate. A consideration would be the thin leg of a diabetic patient that has minimal subcutaneous tissue and is at risk for a wound dehiscence. This would leave the graft easily exposed and at risk for rupture.

STEP 3: OPERATIVE STEPS

◆ The patient is placed supine. For occlusive disease it is a good rule to prepare more than is needed. In general, both lower extremities should be draped in case further vein is needed to complete a procedure. The first incision is typically placed in the groin at the level of the inguinal ligament. The great saphenous vein is identified first at the fossa ovalis, below Scarpa's fascia. The femoral sheath is then opened longitudinally to identify the femoral vessels. The common femoral artery, superficial femoral artery (SFA), and profunda femoris artery (PFA) should be isolated. The saphenous vein can then be isolated either through a continuous incision that "unroofs" the entire vein or a series of "skip" incisions, also known as bridge incisions, or if available, endoscopic vein harvesting (please see Chapter 85 for more detail; see Figure 85-3).

◆ The target vessel has usually been identified on either a preoperative or intraoperative arteriogram. It is helpful to use a radiopaque ruler on the skin to show where the tibial vessel is good, otherwise you can reference a bony landmark (i.e., medial malleolus) and measure backward. The tibial arteries can be more difficult to isolate and work with than the popliteal artery. They are found deep in the muscular compartments of the leg and are generally smaller to sew to.

THE POSTERIOR TIBIAL ARTERY

◆ The PTA is approached through a medial calf incision (**Figure 86-1, A**) and is generally combined with the saphenous harvest incision (please see Chapter 85 for more details on a saphenous vein harvest). When the target is more proximal in the calf, say just past the tibioperoneal trunk, it can be easier to identify the popliteal artery and then divide more of the soleus muscle off the tibia. Immediately below will be the origin of the ATA and the tibioperoneal trunk. There is typically an extensive network of interconnected veins that will need to be ligated to allow full exposures. The origin of the PTA is approximately 2 to 3 cm below the ATA, if that is to be the target.

◆ In the mid to distal leg above the ankle, the PTA remains in the deep posterior compartment, and a thorough knowledge of the anatomy is helpful. The soleus is again removed from its tibial attachments and retracted toward the OR table (**Figure 86-1, B**). A plane can then be developed between the flexor digitorum longus and the soleus muscles. The artery will be surrounded again with a complex plexus of veins that need to be divided. In large muscular legs it can be helpful to use a Doppler pencil to guide the exposure.

◆ At the ankle, the PTA becomes much more superficial, allowing an easier dissection, but also raising the chances of wound complications. A reverse J-shaped incision is made at the ankle, and the flexor retinaculum is divided. The neurovascular bundle will be nestled in a groove between the tendons of the flexor hallucis longus and flexor digitorum longus muscles (**Figure 86-1, C**).

Posterior Tibial Artery Mid Calf

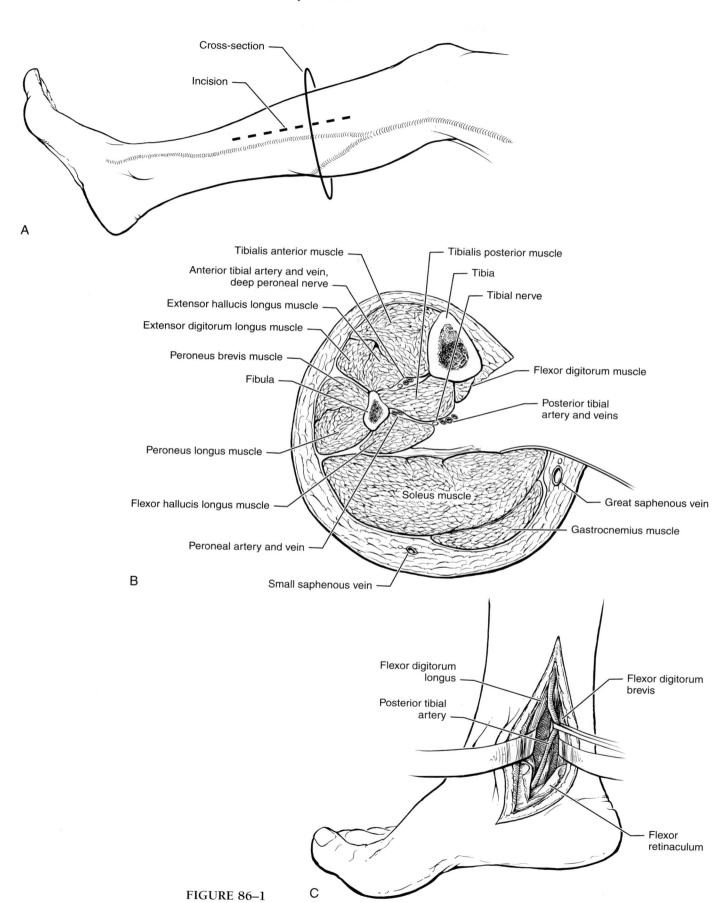

FIGURE 86–1

THE ANTERIOR TIBIAL ARTERY

- The ATA is isolated through an incision on the lateral calf between the tibia and fibula **(Figure 86-2, A)**. Sometimes in thin legs, you can appreciate the division between the anterior and lateral compartments of the leg and guide your incision more toward the anterior compartment. In the proximal leg, a plane can be developed between the tibialis anterior and **extensor digitorum longus** muscles **(Figure 86-2, B)**. The artery, vein, and nerve (deep peroneal) will be just anterior to the interosseus membrane. Once again there will be a rich network of surrounding veins.

- By the mid-portion of the leg, the **extensor hallucis longus** muscle originates and becomes more prominent, and the plane will be between it and the anterior tibialis muscle.

- In the distal third of the leg, the ATA courses much more anteriorly and is found between the tendon of the tibialis anterior muscle and the extensor hallucis longus muscles.

- The challenge with the ATA, however, is how to tunnel the vein graft. The two most popular options include an anatomic location with it going through the interosseus membrane in the popliteal space and then laterally in the anterior compartment. The other is to have the vein in a modified in situ position that courses from a medial to lateral position just below the skin. If the origin of the bypass is the femoral artery and it courses along the lateral knee, great care must be taken to account for the knee bending. If the origin of the bypass is the popliteal, then the options include laying it on top of the tibia or removing a section of the bone to allow it to sit better. Either way, if this approach is used, extra length of vein, which may not be available, is required.

Posterior Tibial Artery Mid Calf

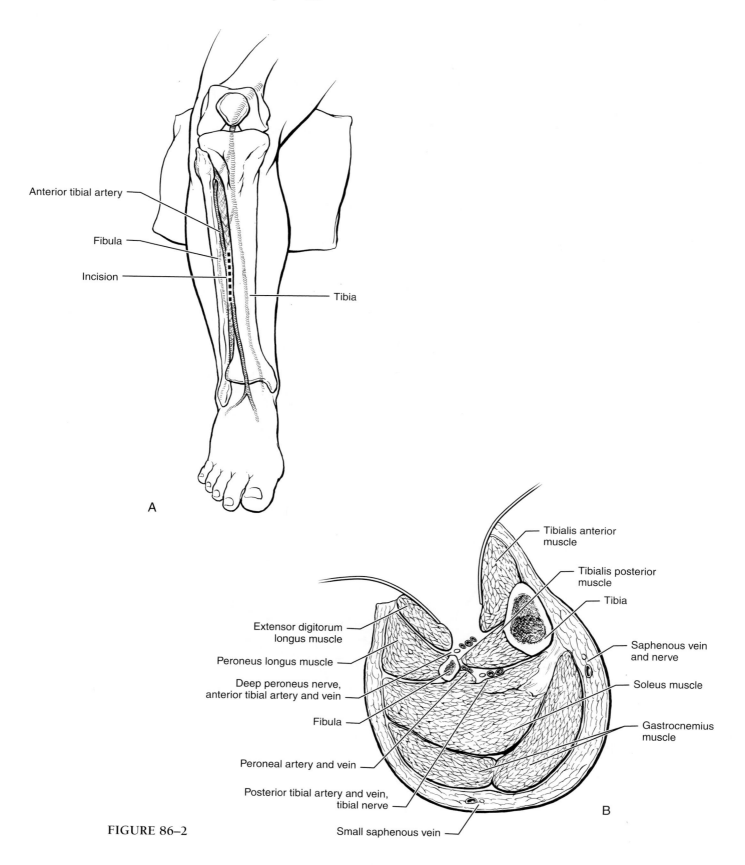

Anterior tibial artery

Fibula

Incision

Tibia

A

Tibialis anterior muscle

Tibialis posterior muscle

Tibia

Extensor digitorum longus muscle

Peroneus longus muscle

Deep peroneus nerve, anterior tibial artery and vein

Fibula

Saphenous vein and nerve

Soleus muscle

Gastrocnemius muscle

Peroneal artery and vein

Posterior tibial artery and vein, tibial nerve

Small saphenous vein

B

FIGURE 86–2

THE PERONEAL ARTERY

◆ The peroneal artery is the most difficult tibial artery to work with. It is always much deeper than expected. In a thin calf, the peroneal artery is generally approached medially. The same general dissection is used as for the PTA, but you must go deeper for the peroneal artery. The soleus is again divided and retracted posteriorly toward the OR table **(Figure 86-3)**. The PTA is left in its loose areolar tissue with the soleus muscle. The peroneal artery will be located on the anterior surface of the **flexor hallucis longus.** This makes sewing the distal anastomosis more challenging because seeing and sewing in a small deep space is more difficult.

Medial Approach Peroneal Artery

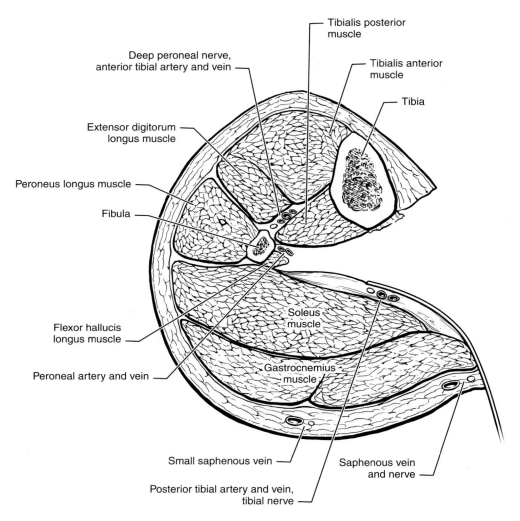

FIGURE 86–3

◆ If a leg is large or if the peroneal artery is best very distally in the leg, the artery can be approached laterally with removal of a section of the fibula (**Figure 86-4**).

Lateral Approach Peroneal Artery

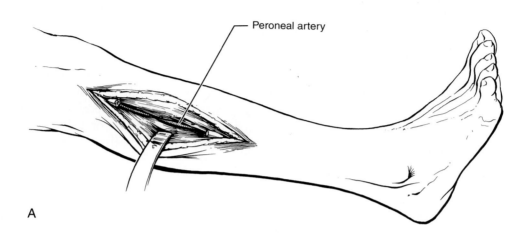

Peroneal artery

A

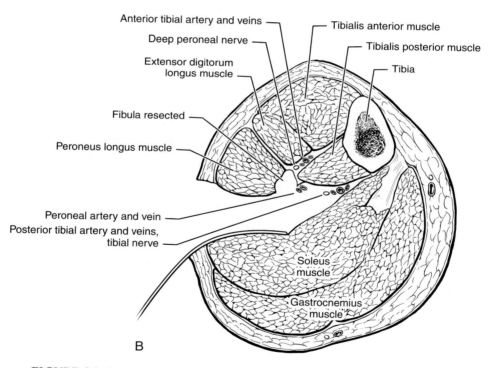

Anterior tibial artery and veins

Deep peroneal nerve

Extensor digitorum longus muscle

Fibula resected

Peroneus longus muscle

Tibialis anterior muscle

Tibialis posterior muscle

Tibia

Peroneal artery and vein

Posterior tibial artery and veins, tibial nerve

Soleus muscle

Gastrocnemius muscle

B

FIGURE 86–4

STEP 4: POSTOPERATIVE CARE

◆ Most patients undergoing surgery for peripheral arterial disease have multiple comorbidities including coronary artery disease. They can be monitored in an intensive care unit, step-down unit, or specialized floor bed depending on the protocols of the institution. Minimum requirements should include telemetry, and vital signs should be taken every 2 hours, including monitoring patency of the graft with Doppler ultrasonography. It is important to educate staff on the importance of using a quantitative measure, such as a Doppler signal, and not relying on an individual's experience at feeling pedal pulses.

◆ If medically stable, the patient should be moved to a floor bed as soon as possible. Rehabilitation therapy should begin immediately, even if it is as simple as sitting in a chair. Realistic expectations should be discussed with the family and staff about discharge planning. Many patients will need transition care either in a rehabilitation facility or a skilled nurse facility (SNF) before they are independent and can go home by themselves or with a caregiver.

◆ The need for postoperative modulation of the coagulation cascade is greater the longer the bypass is. Postoperatively, many surgeons prescribe a nonadjusted unfractionated heparin intravenous drip for 12 to 24 hours. It is common to prescribe either an anticoagulant (warfarin) or a platelet inhibitor (aspirin or clopidrogel) after that. The decision on which one to use needs to be individualized based on certain factors. In general, these include quality of the inflow, which should be adequate before attempting an infrainguinal procedure. The outflow artery may not always be ideal, or a bad vein may convince the surgeon to use a stronger agent. Most surgeons try to avoid prosthetic conduits (ePTFE) below the knee, but if it is used, warfarin is generally used.

◆ After discharge, the patient should be seen in the clinic and understand that he or she will have a relationship with the surgeon for the life of that graft. Routine graft surveillance with duplex scanning and ankle-brachial indices (ABIs) has been demonstrated to increase the primary patency of grafts (assisted primary patency). Protocols include a postprocedure baseline level and close follow-up (every 3 months for a year, then biannually). A drop in the ABI or a velocity elevation is suggestive of a stenosis in the graft and warrants an arteriogram and possible intervention.

STEP 5: PEARLS AND PITFALLS

◆ Femorotibial reconstruction is an excellent option for patients with advanced occlusive disease, most of which present with critical limb ischemia (rest pain or tissue loss). These individuals have a larger burden of disease and tend to have other serious comorbidities, such as cardiac disease and long-standing diabetes. They are more likely to have an adverse clinical event in the perioperative period. Great care must be taken to limit the risk of this, and such treatment as perioperative beta blockade is essential for this group.

◆ Just as in the in situ femoropopliteal reconstruction, the tibial bypass is also at risk for wound complication issues. Great care with tissue handling, keeping the graft as deep as possible, and avoiding a flap creation are essential to promote good wound healing.

SELECTED REFERENCES

1. Ouriel K, Rutherford R (eds): Atlas of Vascular Surgery: Operative Procedures. Philadelphia, Saunders, 1998.
2. Norgren L, Hiatt WR, Dormandy JA, et al: Inter-Society Consensus for the Management of Peripheral Arterial Disease (TASC II). J Vasc Surg 2007;45:S5-S6.
3. Valentine RJ, Wind GG: Anatomic Exposures in Vascular Surgery, 2nd ed. Philadelphia, Lippincott Williams & Wilkins, 2003.
4. Rutherford RB: Atlas of Vascular Surgery: Basic Techniques and Exposures. Philadelphia, Saunders, 1993.

CHAPTER 87

FASCIOTOMY—FOREARM AND LEG

William J. Mileski

STEP 1: SURGICAL ANATOMY FOR FOREARM

◆ The forearm is divided into multiple fascial compartments, each containing several muscles that are additionally enclosed within individual epimysial envelopes. Three forearm compartments are usually described: the volar, dorsal, and lateral (mobile wad) compartments.

◆ The interosseous membrane separates the volar and dorsal compartments from each other, and the posteriorly and radially located lateral compartment is demarcated by a connective tissue septum from the antebrachial fascia. In most cases of compartment syndrome, the volar muscles are the most severely affected, followed in severity by the muscles of the dorsal compartment and of the lateral compartment. Some communication exists among the three main compartments, and release of the volar compartment often relieves elevated tissue pressure in the dorsal compartment. Intraoperative pressure measurements and clinical findings may preclude the need for a separate dorsal fasciotomy to relieve this extensor compartment. The lateral compartment musculature is superficial and easily decompressed.

◆ Within the volar compartment, additional distinction can be made between the superficial and deep muscles. The superficial muscles include the pronator teres, palmaris longus, flexor digitorum superficialis, flexor carpi radialis, and flexor carpi ulnaris. The deep muscles include the flexor digitorum profundus, flexor pollicis longus, and pronator quadratus. The flexor digitorum profundus and flexor pollicis longus are particularly vulnerable in compartment syndrome, because they may be compressed against rigid bone and the unyielding interosseous membrane. Anatomic and clinical reports demonstrate that release of the superficial volar compartments may not be adequate to relieve deep pressures in these muscles.

◆ The dorsal compartment is also divided into superficial and deep muscles. The extensor digitorum, extensor carpi ulnaris, and extensor digiti minimi are the superficial group, which lie in a plane above the deeper abductor pollicis longus, extensor pollicis brevis, extensor pollicis longus, extensor indicis, and supinator (**Figure 87-1, A**).

Right Forearm
Lateral

Right Forearm
Medial

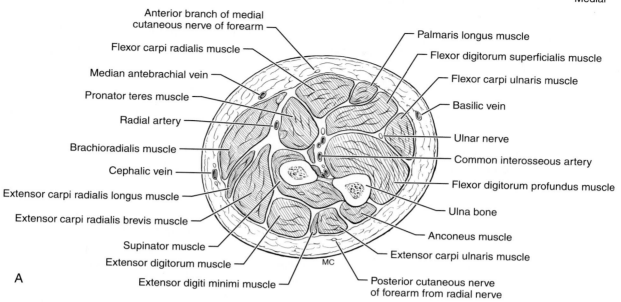

Anterior branch of medial cutaneous nerve of forearm

Flexor carpi radialis muscle

Median antebrachial vein

Pronator teres muscle

Radial artery

Brachioradialis muscle

Cephalic vein

Extensor carpi radialis longus muscle

Extensor carpi radialis brevis muscle

Supinator muscle

Extensor digitorum muscle

Extensor digiti minimi muscle

Palmaris longus muscle

Flexor digitorum superficialis muscle

Flexor carpi ulnaris muscle

Basilic vein

Ulnar nerve

Common interosseous artery

Flexor digitorum profundus muscle

Ulna bone

Anconeus muscle

Extensor carpi ulnaris muscle

Posterior cutaneous nerve of forearm from radial nerve

MC

A

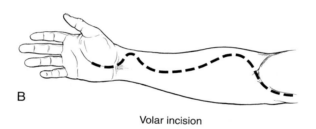

B

Volar incision

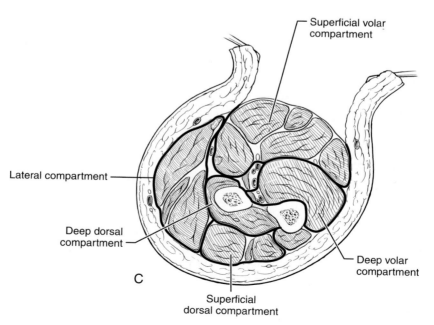

Superficial volar compartment

Lateral compartment

Deep dorsal compartment

Deep volar compartment

Superficial dorsal compartment

C

FIGURE 87–1

STEP 2: PREOPERATIVE CONSIDERATIONS FOR FOREARM

- Compartment syndrome is a surgical emergency that usually requires release of the superficial muscle compartments. In some clinical situations, it is imperative to also explore the deep muscle compartments.

- Forearm compartment syndrome requires immediate evaluation and treatment. The need for operation is established by careful review of the patient's history; the presence of physical signs and symptoms, such as pain with passive stretching, paresthesias, paresis, and palpably tense compartments; and, if needed, the measurement of elevated compartment pressures ($>$30 cm H_2O).

- The treatment of compartment syndrome requires expedient fasciotomy when nonoperative maneuvers such as cast removal are unsuccessful. If left untreated, elevated tissue pressure within the fascial confines decreases capillary blood perfusion below a level necessary for soft tissue viability. Most patients ultimately have minimal limb dysfunction when fasciotomy has been performed promptly and to an adequate depth. Postoperative loss of function may be caused by several factors, including damage from the initial injury, ischemia caused by elevated tissue pressure before fasciotomy, inadequate fasciotomy, and iatrogenic surgical injury.

- Mandatory exploration of deep muscle compartments is indicated in situations in which the deep muscles are preferentially injured, such as in cases of high-voltage electrical injury. The high electrical resistance of bone transmits a significant thermal injury to the adjacent muscles of the deep compartment. Other conditions that require exploration of the deep spaces include severe crush injuries; situations involving extended pressure, such as an unconscious patient lying on the limb; and when there is ongoing sepsis or suspicion of necrotic muscle, despite previous fasciotomy. If epimysiotomies of the deep muscles are not performed in these situations, necrosis and contracture may result.

- Limited incisions to minimize collateral morbidity from fasciotomy do not offer access to all components and increase the potential for missing an ischemic or necrotic muscle group.

STEP 3: OPERATIVE STEPS FOR FOREARM

1. INCISION

- A commonly used approach, begins 1 cm proximal and 2 cm lateral to the medial epicondyle. The incision is carried obliquely across the antecubital fossa and over the volar aspect of the mobile wad and is then curved medially to reach the midline of the forearm at the junction of its middle and distal thirds. The incision is continued straight distally to the proximal wrist crease ulnar to the tendon of the palmaris longus and is finally curved across to the midpalm (**Figure 87-1, B**).

2. DISSECTION

- The subcutaneous tissues are divided to expose the deep fascia, and individual muscles are mobilized for examination **(Figure 87-1, C)**.

- If the muscles of the dorsal compartment require release after the volar fasciotomy, a straight longitudinal incision is made below the lateral epicondyle toward the midline of the wrist.

- Other incisions described for the treatment of compartment syndrome criss-cross the forearm or gently sweep across it in various directions.

- Incisions that cross the forearm will transect more of the venous and lymphatic return than will a straight incision, and the resolution of forearm edema could be impaired. Such incisions may also prevent the future design of a radial forearm flap, because the vascular supply and outflow of the skin pedicle would be compromised.

3. CLOSING

◆ Dressings

◆ Cover the wound with saline-soaked gauze and a nonconstricting bandage.

STEP 1: SURGICAL ANATOMY FOR LEG

◆ The lower leg has four muscular compartments with dense investing fascia that contribute to the predisposition of this region to develop neurovascular compromise following injury generally referred to as compartment syndrome.

◆ The treatment of compartment syndrome requires incision of the investing fascia of all four compartments: anterior, lateral, superficial posterior, and deep posterior (**Figure 87-2, A**).

STEP 2: PREOPERATIVE CONSIDERATIONS FOR LEG

◆ Same as previously mentioned for the forearm procedure.

STEP 3: OPERATIVE STEPS FOR LEG

1. INCISION

◆ Medial and lateral skin incisions are carried from just proximal to the medial and lateral malleoli and carried cephalad to the level of the tibial plateau medially and the fibula head laterally, where care must be taken to avoid injury to the peroneal nerve (**Figure 87-2, B**).

2. DISSECTION

◆ Both the superficial and deep posterior compartments are released through the medial incision, and the anterior and lateral compartments are released through the lateral incision (**Figure 87-2, C**).

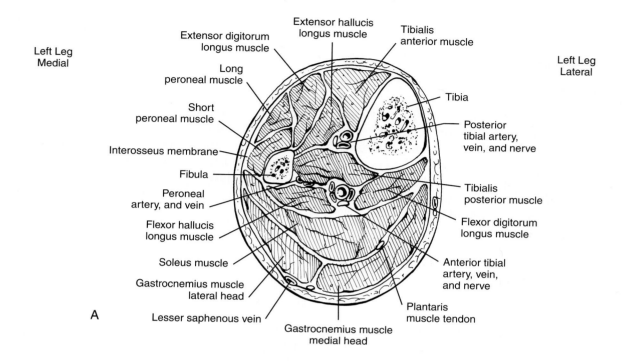

Extensor hallucis longus muscle

Extensor digitorum longus muscle

Tibialis anterior muscle

Left Leg Medial

Long peroneal muscle

Short peroneal muscle

Interosseus membrane

Fibula

Peroneal artery, and vein

Flexor hallucis longus muscle

Soleus muscle

Gastrocnemius muscle lateral head

Lesser saphenous vein

Gastrocnemius muscle medial head

Tibia

Posterior tibial artery, vein, and nerve

Tibialis posterior muscle

Flexor digitorum longus muscle

Anterior tibial artery, vein, and nerve

Plantaris muscle tendon

Left Leg Lateral

A

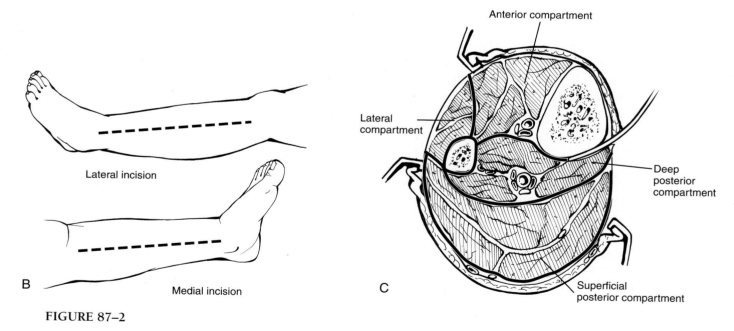

Lateral incision

Medial incision

B

Anterior compartment

Lateral compartment

Deep posterior compartment

Superficial posterior compartment

C

FIGURE 87–2

3. CLOSING

◆ Dressing of saline-soaked gauze and a nonconstricting bandage.

STEP 4: POSTOPERATIVE CARE

◆ Pain control is often a significant issue following fasciotomy and is best managed with a patient-controlled analgesia device. Wound care requires attention to aseptic technique and ensures adequate material: sterile gowns, gloves, and dressing supplies are at hand before dressing changes are begun to avoid contamination and serious morbidity associated with wound infection. Elevation of the extremity will help reduce edema and hasten the recovery and closure of the wound. The use of biologic dressings, either homograft or xenograft, may also help in wound care.

STEP 5: PEARLS AND PITFALLS

◆ Most cases of compartment syndrome are adequately treated by release of the superficial volar compartment, regardless of which surgical approach is chosen. Those clinical situations that mandate exploration of the deep volar or dorsal compartments, however, require a significant understanding of anatomy to follow a surgical approach that will minimize further injury. Clinical examples include high-voltage electrical injury, severe crush injuries, extended extrinsic forearm pressure (such as an unconscious patient lying on his or her forearm), and ongoing evidence of myonecrosis or sepsis despite previous superficial fasciotomy. In some cases, even after compartment fasciotomy, the epimysium of individual muscles must be incised to relieve persistently elevated tissue pressure. This can be achieved only with adequate visualization of the deep space.

SELECTED REFERENCES

1. Lagerstrom CF, Reed RL Jr, Rowlands BJ, Fischer RP: Early fasciotomy for acute clinically evident post-traumatic compartment syndrome. Am J Surg 1989;158:36-39.
2. Dente CJ, Feliciano DV, Rozycki GS, et al: A review of upper extremity fasciotomies in a level I trauma center. Am Surg 2004;70:1088-1093.

CHAPTER 88

RENAL REVASCULARIZATION

Glenn C. Hunter

Approximately 5% to 10% of patients with hypertension have renal artery stenosis (RAS) as the underlying cause. Atherosclerotic occlusive disease in individuals older than 65 years and fibromuscular dysplasia (FMD) in children and young adult females (20 to 40 years of age) are the most common etiologies. Atherosclerosis of the renal arteries is usually confined to the orifice and proximal third of the involved vessel (more commonly the left) and should be considered as an extension of aortic atherosclerosis. In 20% of patients with RAS, there is severe associated aortic aneurysmal or occlusive disease, which determines the extent and type of procedure to be performed. RAS may occur in isolation (anatomic stenosis) or in association with hypertensive ischemic nephropathy. FMD may be medial (85%), perimedial (10%), or intimal (5%) and usually involves the mid-portion of the main renal arteries and their segmental branches.

STEP 1: SURGICAL ANATOMY

◆ The renal arteries branch laterally from the aorta below the origin of the superior mesenteric artery. There is usually a single renal artery to each kidney. The right renal artery arises higher and is longer than the left renal artery. The right renal artery runs posterior to the inferior vena cava, right renal vein, head of the pancreas, and descending part of the duodenum to the renal hilum. The left renal artery passes posterior to the left renal vein, body of the pancreas, and splenic vein. Multiple renal arteries are present in up to 35% of patients and should be identified and evaluated before any surgical intervention.

STEP 2: PREOPERATIVE CONSIDERATIONS

◆ Medical history, physical examination, and assessment of renal and cardiac function should be performed in all patients. Features suggestive of RAS as the cause of hypertension include hypertension of abrupt onset, hypertension refractory to medical therapy (more than three drugs), unexplained azotemia or azotemia induced by angiotensin-converting enzyme (ACE) inhibitors, and hypertension in children and young adults.

◆ Screening and diagnostic studies: Duplex ultrasound is useful as a screening test for RAS and evaluation of kidney size. Interrogation of the renal arteries from their origin to the hilum can be achieved in 95% of cases. A peak systolic velocity of greater than 180 cm/sec and renal-to-aortic ratio ≥ 3.5 with distal turbulence is usually indicative of a hemodynamically significant stenosis ($>60\%$). Occlusion of the renal artery is usually identified by the absence of a Doppler signal.

- Computed tomography (CT) or digital angiography is used to delineate the stenosis before intervening. There is a high risk of contrast-induced nephrotoxicity, and care should be taken in performing these studies in patients with renal impairment. The administration of intravenous (IV) fluids (1.5 mL/kg/hr), limiting the dose of or diluting the contrast agent, and the administration of acetylcysteine 600 mg orally before and after the contrast procedure are among the measures used to reduce the risk of nephrotoxicity. Magnetic resonance angiography is an alternative method of assessing RAS in patients with a glomerular filtration rate $\geq$30 ml/min/1.73 m^2.

- Functional studies: A captopril renal scan may be helpful if there is unilateral stenosis and minimal parenchymal disease. The significance of unilateral RAS should be confirmed by plasma renin determinations. This may require admission to the hospital, withholding medications that interfere with renin release, and sodium restriction ($\leq$2 g Na$^+$/day) for approximately 2 weeks.

- Indications for the operative treatment of RAS include stenosis greater than 70% with poorly controlled hypertension, renal insufficiency, or recurrent bouts of congestive heart failure (CHF) with no attributable myocardial ischemia. Patients with branch vessel disease and FMD and selected patients with restenosis after angioplasty and stenting may be candidates for surgery.

STEP 3: OPERATIVE STEPS—AORTORENAL BYPASS

- The patient is admitted the day before the procedure for IV hydration, control of blood pressure, and a mechanical bowel preparation. Antihypertensive medications should be reduced to the minimum necessary to control the blood pressure. If the diastolic blood pressure is higher than 120 mm Hg, the patient should be admitted to the intensive care unit (ICU) and the blood pressure controlled with IV sodium nitroprusside or nicardipine.

1. INCISION

- A midline or transverse incision allows both access to the renal arteries and reconstruction of associated aortic disease if required. The abdomen is explored, the transverse colon and small bowel are lifted out of the abdomen, and a self-retaining retractor such as the Omni-Tract system is placed (**Figure 88-1, A**).

2. DISSECTION

- The peritoneum over the aorta is incised in the midline, and the dissection is carried down to the left renal vein superiorly and the aortic bifurcation inferiorly (**Figure 88-1, B**). The left renal vein is then mobilized and retracted cephalad or caudally depending on the location of the origin of the renal vessels. Retraction of the left renal vein is facilitated by ligation and division of the gonadal, adrenal, and lumbar veins.

- Both renal arteries are then dissected out 2 cm beyond the orificial stenotic lesion. An aortorenal bypass is the most common revascularization procedure performed but requires clamping of the aorta. This technique is applicable only to patients with large paired renal arteries with minimal aortic atherosclerosis or aneurysmal dilation.

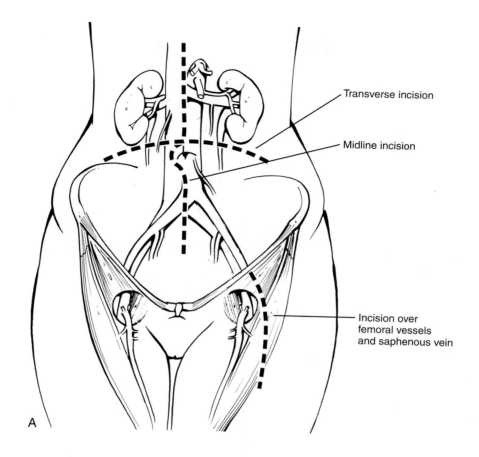

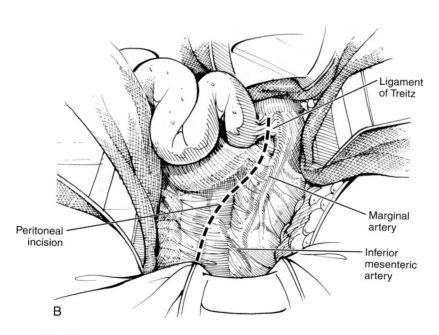

FIGURE 88–1

◆ The proximal right renal artery is exposed by retracting the left renal vein superiorly and the vena cava to the right. The distal portion of the renal artery is exposed by mobilizing the duodenum and hepatic flexure medially. If both renal arteries need to be exposed, the entire small bowel is mobilized from the ligament of Treitz to the mesentery of the cecum and along the right paracolic gutter to the foramen of Winslow. The peritoneal incision is extended along the inferior border of the pancreas, exposing the aorta above the origin of the superior mesenteric artery.

◆ Once the renal arteries have been isolated, a segment of the infrarenal aorta below the renal arteries is mobilized. After systemic heparinization (100 U/kg) and the administration of mannitol (12.5 to 25 g), the aorta is occluded below the renal arteries and above the bifurcation, and an ellipse approximately three times the diameter of the renal artery is excised from the anterior lateral aortic wall. Saphenous vein or a prosthetic Dacron or polytetrafluoroethylene (PTFE) graft 6 or 7 mm in diameter is beveled, and the aortic anastomosis is completed with 4-0 polypropylene suture (**Figure 88-2, A-C**).

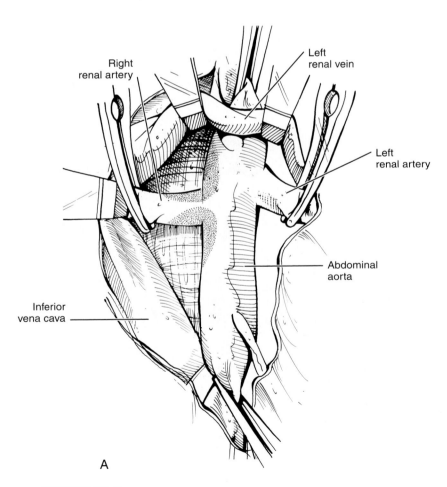

A

FIGURE 88–2

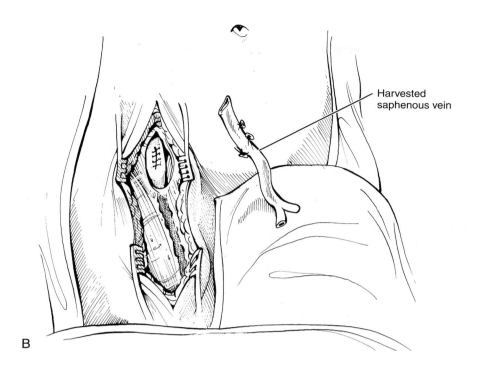

Harvested
saphenous vein

B

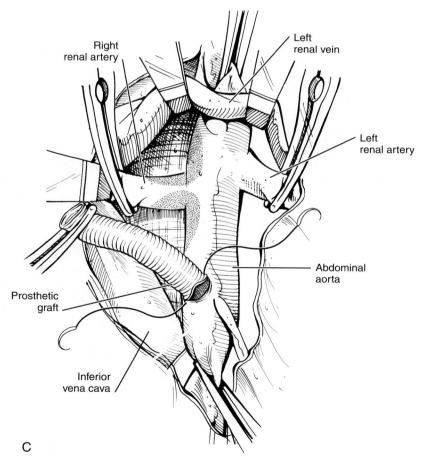

Right
renal artery

Left
renal vein

Left
renal artery

Abdominal
aorta

Prosthetic
graft

Inferior
vena cava

C

FIGURE 88–2, cont'd

◆ The renal artery is divided between clamps, and the proximal end of the artery is oversewn with 5-0 polypropylene suture. The saphenous vein or prosthetic graft is spatulated, and the distal anastomosis is constructed end-to-end with running (posterior wall) and interrupted 6-0 polypropylene suture **(Figure 88-2, D-E)**.

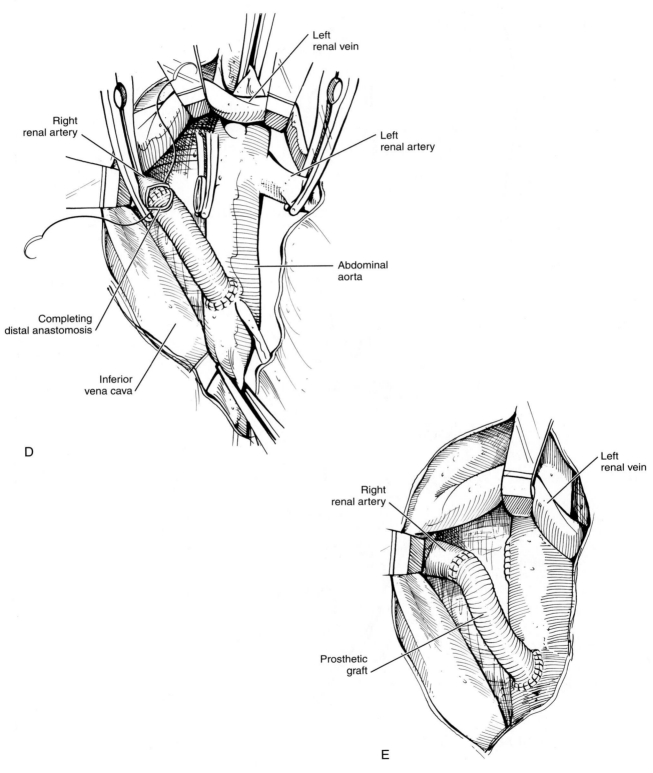

FIGURE 88–2, cont'd

- If bilateral renal revascularization is required, a 14 × 7 or 12 × 6 Dacron or PTFE bifurcated graft is used **(Figure 88-3).** Saphenous vein or hypogastric artery can be used as alternative conduits, especially in young adults and children with branch vessel disease. If the infrarenal aorta is severely diseased, the inflow of the bypass can originate from the supraceliac aorta or common iliac arteries.

- After the renal anastomosis is completed, heparin is reversed with protamine sulfate (1 mg/100 U heparin), and 40 mg furosemide is administered.

3. CLOSING

- The retroperitoneum is closed with 2-0 Vicryl, and the incision is closed with running looped monofilament 1-0 polydioxanone (PDS) or polypropylene suture.

- Dressings

- Cover the wound with saline-soaked gauze and a nonconstricting bandage.

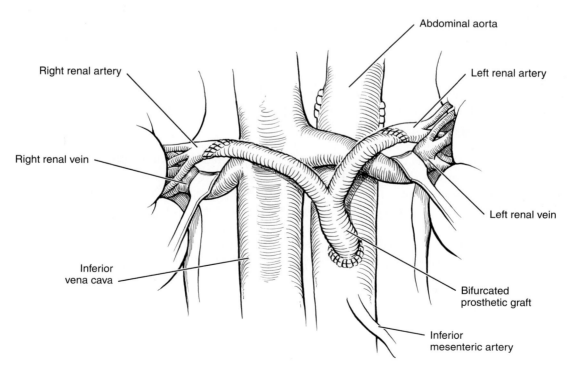

FIGURE 88–3

STEP 3: OPERATIVE STEPS—AORTORENAL ENDARTERECTOMY

Endarterectomy is used in selected patients with bilateral focal orificial atherosclerotic RAS.

1. INCISION

◆ The aorta is approached through a midline or transverse incision.

2. DISSECTION

◆ The aorta is mobilized from the level of the celiac artery to the inferior mesentery artery. This requires division of the diaphragmatic crural fibers, and the dense neural tissue that surrounds the origins of the celiac and superior mesenteric and renal arteries.

◆ This dissection should isolate a sufficient segment of aorta to allow safe placement of the proximal clamp above the renal or superior mesenteric arteries, if these vessels are so close that a clamp cannot be safely placed between them. The lumbar arteries are occluded with removable clips and clamps applied in sequence to the renal arteries, the superior mesenteric artery, and the infrarenal and suprarenal aorta.

◆ A longitudinal arteriotomy is made extending from the left side of the superior mesentery orifice to below the renal arteries **(Figure 88-4, A)**. The technique involves removal of the aortic intima in this section of the aorta. Once the aortic intima has been dissected proximally, each individual renal artery is approached. The aortic intima is grasped and gentle traction is applied, pulling to the opposite side. The renal ostial lesion is then dissected from the media by prolapsing the renal artery into the aorta **(Figure 88-4, B)**.

◆ Gentle advancement of the renal artery toward its orifice by the assistant facilitates feathering of the end point. The process is repeated on the contralateral side.

◆ The distal intima of the aorta is divided and secured with interrupted 6-0 polypropylene tacking sutures **(Figure 88-4, C)**. The arteries are flushed of atheromatous debris and air, and the arteriotomy is closed with running 4-0 polypropylene suture **(Figure 88-4, D)**. The adequacy of the renal endarterectomy is evaluated by intraoperative duplex ultrasound. If any residual plaque is detected, a transverse arteriotomy is made in the affected renal artery, the plaque is extracted, and the distal end point is secured with tacking sutures. The arteriotomy is closed with interrupted 7-0 polypropylene sutures.

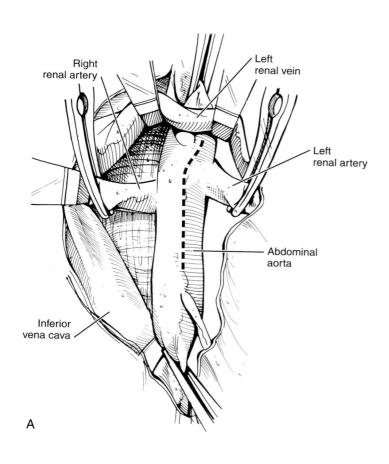

A

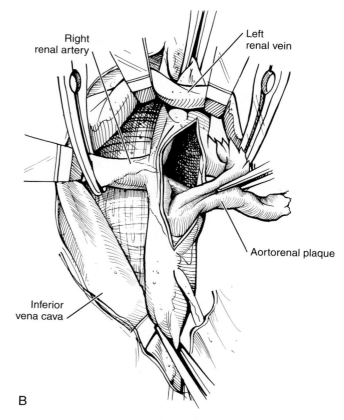

B

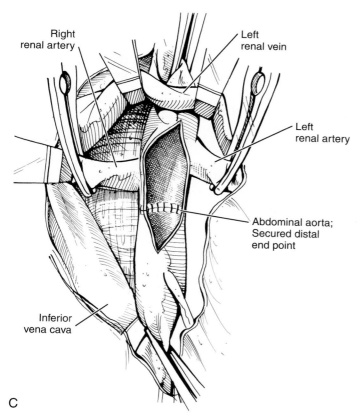

C

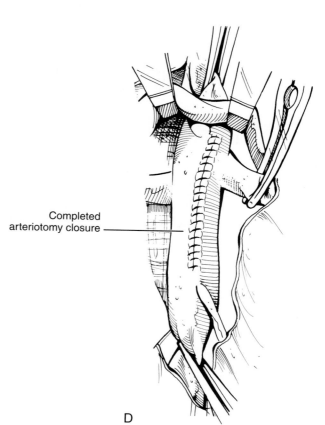

D

FIGURE 88–4

3. CLOSING

- The closure of the abdomen is similar for both aortorenal bypass and renal endarterectomy. The retroperitoneum is closed with 2-0 Vicryl, and the incision is closed with running looped monofilament 1-0 PDS or polypropylene suture.

STEP 3: OPERATIVE STEPS—SPLENORENAL BYPASS

- Both aortorenal bypass and renal endarterectomy may be contraindicated in elderly patients with severe aortoiliac occlusive or aneurysmal disease and multiple comorbidities. The presence of a dense fibrotic reaction from previous operations or renal angioplasty makes dissection difficult and increases the operative risk. The addition of an aortic bypass to renal revascularization, which may be indicated in younger patients, is associated with increased morbidity and mortality in older individuals. In these patients, alternative bypass procedures, such as splenorenal bypass for high-grade left RAS and hepatorenal bypass for disease on the right, should be considered. The more ischemic kidney is repaired first unless it is atretic.

- Careful angiographic assessment of the hepatic and splenic arteries with anterior posterior and lateral views is imperative before undertaking these alternative renal revascularization procedures, because extensive plaque may be present in the donor vessels, which may not be detected on standard anterior posterior angiographic views.

- For both splenorenal and hepatorenal bypass, the patient is positioned supine on the operating table with a sandbag elevating the affected side and prepped from nipple to knee.

1. INCISION

- The abdomen is entered via a left subcostal incision that can be extended medially and laterally if necessary. The splenocolic ligament, spleen, and pancreas are reflected medially, and a self-retaining retractor is placed (**Figure 88-5, A-B**).

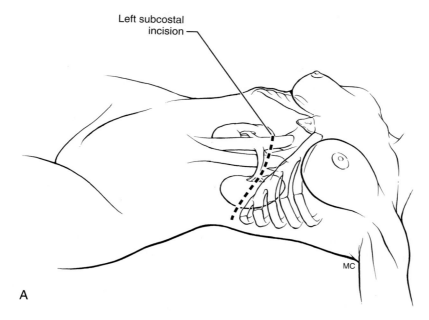

Left subcostal incision

MC

A

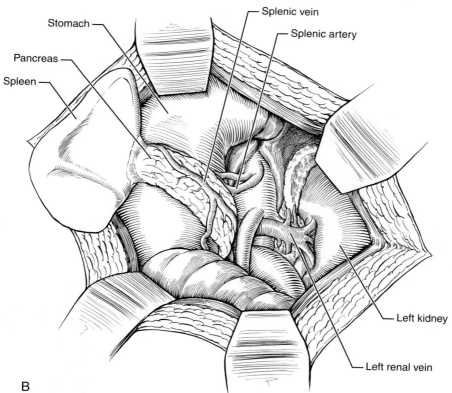

Stomach

Pancreas

Spleen

Splenic vein

Splenic artery

Left kidney

Left renal vein

B

FIGURE 88–5

2. DISSECTION

♦ The left renal vein is mobilized by dividing the lumbar and adrenal branches to expose the renal artery. The pancreas is retracted cephalad to expose the splenic artery and vein. The splenic arterial and venous branches to the pancreas are divided between 4-0 silk suture ligatures. A segment of splenic artery of sufficient length close to its origin (where its diameter is largest) is mobilized **(Figure 88-5, C-D).**

3. CLOSING

♦ After IV heparin is administered, the splenic artery is occluded and divided between clamps, and the distal end of the vessel is oversewn with 5-0 polypropylene suture. The renal artery is then mobilized, the proximal end is oversewn with 5-0 polypropylene suture, the vessels are spatulated, and an end-to-end anastomosis is constructed between the splenic and renal arteries using running (posterior wall) and interrupted 6-0 polypropylene suture **(Figure 88-5, E-G).** The patency of the anastomosis is evaluated with duplex ultrasound.

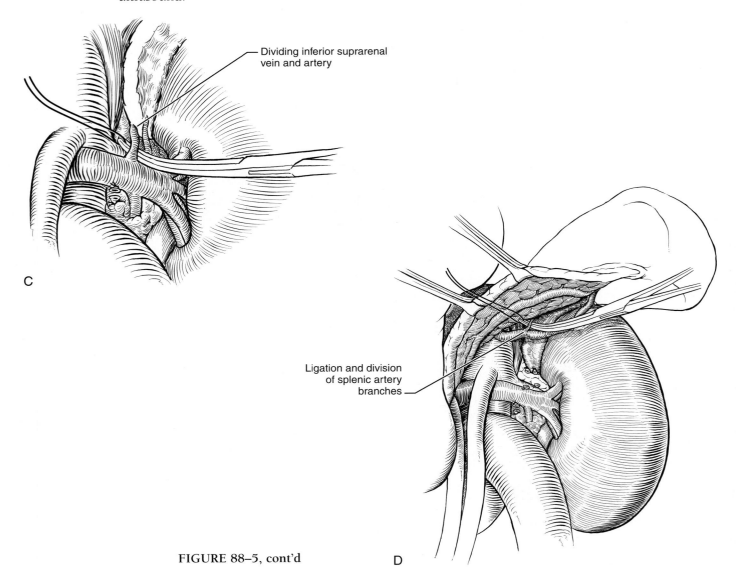

Dividing inferior suprarenal vein and artery

Ligation and division of splenic artery branches

FIGURE 88–5, cont'd   D

C

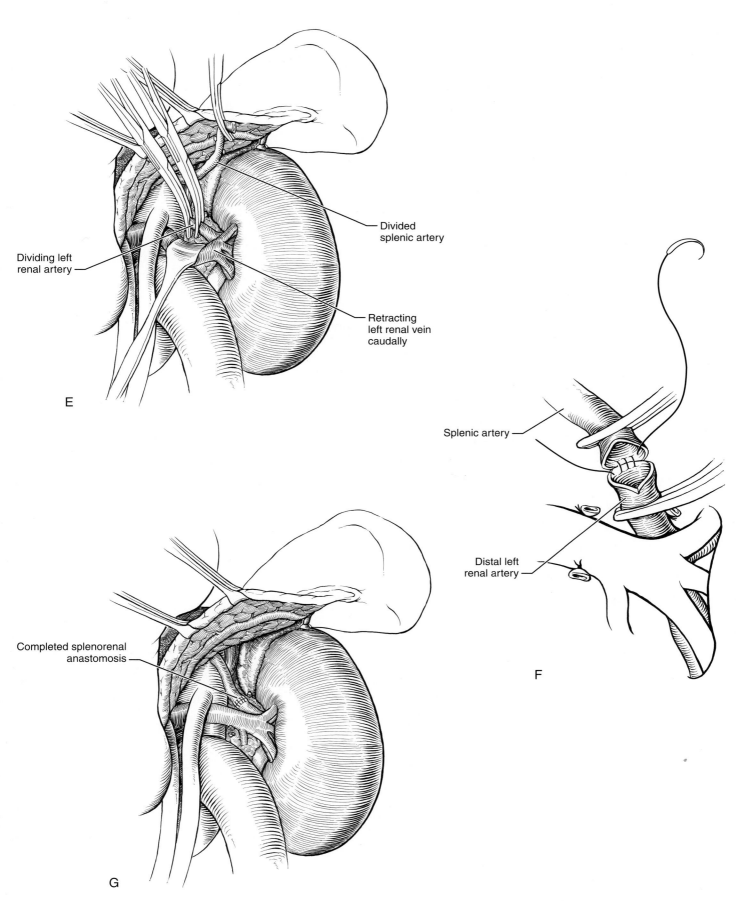

Divided
splenic artery

Dividing left
renal artery

Retracting
left renal vein
caudally

E

Splenic artery

Distal left
renal artery

F

Completed splenorenal
anastomosis

G

FIGURE 88–5, cont'd

STEP 3: OPERATIVE STEPS—HEPATORENAL BYPASS

♦ In patients with severe aortic atherosclerosis or aneurysmal degenerative disease and normal liver function with a high-grade right RAS, hepatorenal bypass should be considered.

1. INCISION

♦ The abdomen is entered via a right subcostal incision (**Figure 88-6, A**).

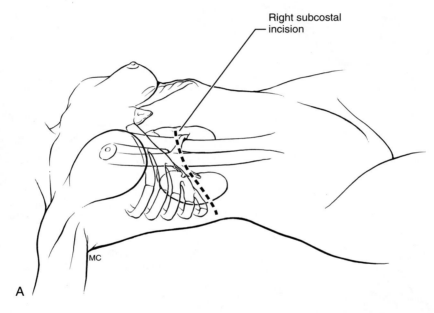

FIGURE 88–6

2. DISSECTION

◆ The hepatic flexure is mobilized, a Kocher maneuver is performed to mobilize the duodenum medially, and the Omni-Tract retractor is placed **(Figure 88-6, B)**.

◆ The hepatic artery is exposed between the portal vein and common bile duct **(Figure 88-6, C)**.

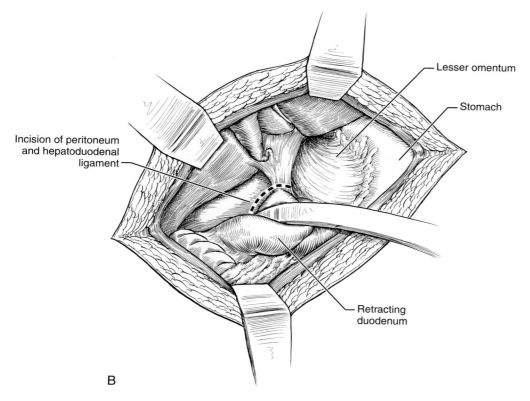

Lesser omentum

Stomach

Incision of peritoneum
and hepatoduodenal
ligament

Retracting
duodenum

B

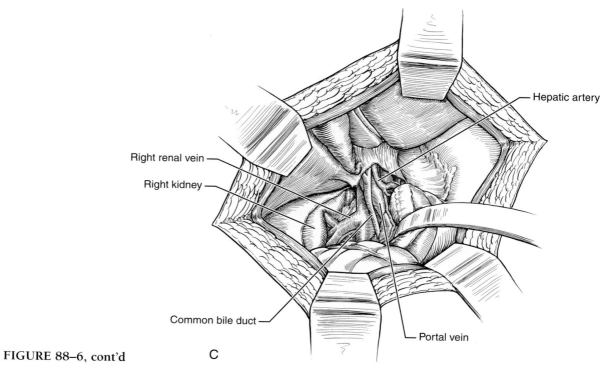

Hepatic artery

Right renal vein

Right kidney

Common bile duct

Portal vein

FIGURE 88–6, cont'd   C

- The right renal artery is exposed posterior to the vena cava by retracting the right renal vein cephalad and the vena cava to the left **(Figure 88-6, D)**.

- A 10-cm segment of saphenous vein is harvested and gently distended with a papaverine solution (see Figure 88-2, B). After systemic heparinization and the administration of mannitol, the hepatic artery is occluded between clamps and the saphenous vein graft is anastomosed end-to-side to the hepatic artery distal to the takeoff of the gastroduodenal artery with running 6-0 polypropylene suture **(Figure 88-6, E)**.

- The renal artery is similarly divided close to its origin from the aorta, and the proximal end is suture ligated with 5-0 polypropylene suture. An end-to-end spatulated anastomosis between the saphenous vein graft and the distal end of the renal artery is constructed with interrupted 6-0 polypropylene suture **(Figure 88-6, F-G)**. The patency of the anastomosis is evaluated with duplex ultrasound.

- After the renal anastomosis is completed, heparin is reversed with protamine sulfate (1 mg/100 U heparin), and 40 mg furosemide is administered intravenously.

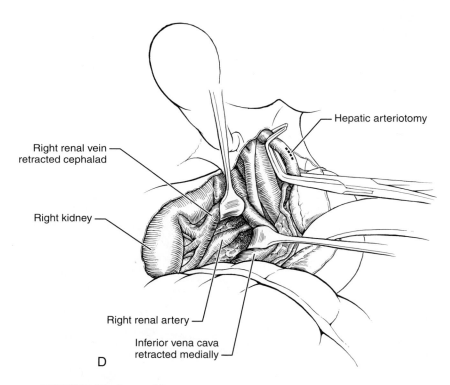

FIGURE 88–6, cont'd

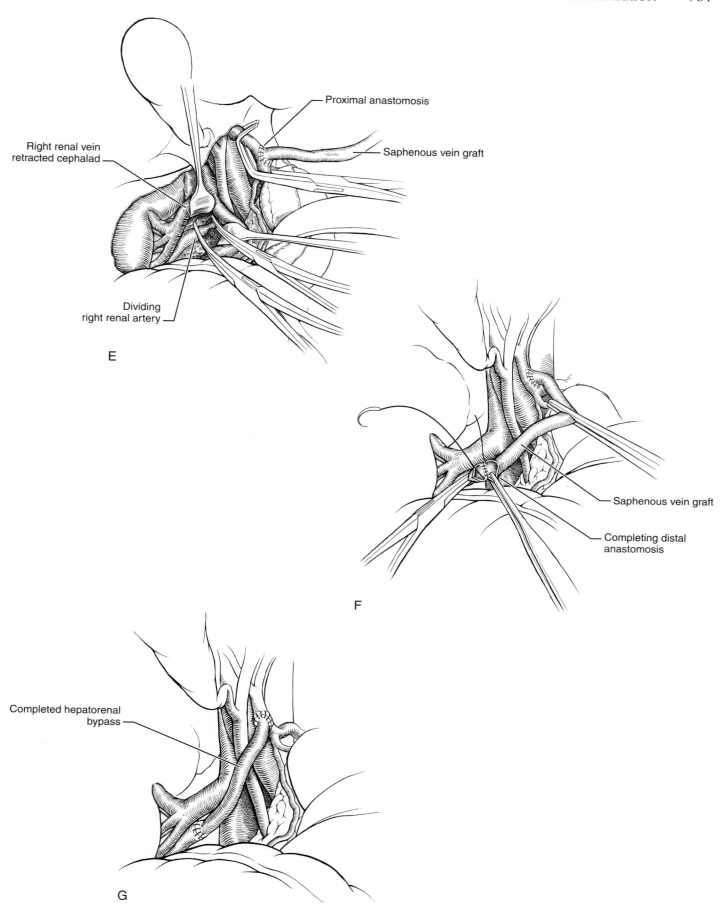

Proximal anastomosis

Saphenous vein graft

Right renal vein
retracted cephalad

Dividing
right renal artery

E

Saphenous vein graft

Completing distal
anastomosis

F

Completed hepatorenal
bypass

G

FIGURE 88–6, cont'd

3. CLOSING

- Both of the inner two layers of the right and left subcostal incisions are closed in a similar fashion with running absorbable suture (2-0 Vicryl), and the outer layers (external oblique and anterior rectus fascia) are closed with running monofilament (2-0 PDS or Maxon) suture.

STEP 4: POSTOPERATIVE CARE

- The patient is returned to the ICU with arterial line and Swan-Ganz pulmonary artery catheter in place. IV fluids are administered to control fluid volume and blood pressure. Nicardipine or sodium nitroprusside is used to control blood pressure. Beta blockade begun in the preoperative period is continued to control heart rate and blood pressure. Urine output is carefully monitored, and IV fluid administration is adjusted accordingly.

- There are often significant fluid shifts in the immediate postoperative period. A combination of fluid administration, vasopressors, and antihypertensive medications may be required to ensure adequate perfusion pressures and to prevent hypertensive crises.

STEP 5: PEARLS AND PITFALLS

- The renal artery should be carefully palpated to determine the distal extent of the plaque before an aortorenal bypass or endarterectomy is performed. This maneuver is especially important if endarterectomy is contemplated if difficulties with the end point are to be avoided.

- Each renal anastomosis should be completed in 15 to 20 minutes. If prolonged renal ischemic times are anticipated, cold electrolyte solution can be infused into the renal artery and the kidney packed in ice.

- Immediate evaluation of the patency of the repair with duplex ultrasound or renal isotope flow studies is indicated if anuria develops in the postoperative period. Prompt return to the operating room is indicated if the vessels are occluded.

- Atheroembolism is an uncommon but serious complication of renal revascularization. Careful preoperative assessment of the aorta to determine the presence and location of atheromatous debris or thrombus on a CT scan and the correct sequential application and removal of clamps is imperative if this complication is to be avoided. Oliguria or anuria that does not resolve, eosinophilia, and cholesterol crystalluria are clues to the diagnosis.

- In patients with oliguric acute renal failure dialysis, enteral or parenteral nutrition should be undertaken early to avoid the rapid loss of muscle mass encountered in these patients.

SELECTED REFERENCES

1. Hansen KJ, Tribble RW, Reavis SW, et al: Renal duplex sonography: Evaluation of clinical utility. J Vasc Surg 1990;12:227-236.
2. Wylie EJ, Perloff DL, Stoney RJ: Autogenous tissue revascularization techniques in surgery for renovascular hypertension. Ann Surg 1969;170:416-428.
3. Moncure AC, Brewster DC, Darling RC, et al: Use of the splenic and hepatic arteries for renal revascularization. J Vasc Surg 1986;3:196-203.
4. Benjamin ME, Dean RH: Techniques in renal artery reconstruction: Part I. Ann Vasc Surg 1996;10: 306-314.
5. Benjamin ME, Dean RH: Techniques in renal artery reconstruction: Part II. Ann Vasc Surg 1996;10: 409-414.

CHAPTER 89

MESENTERIC ISCHEMIA

Glenn C. Hunter

INTRODUCTION

- Despite recent advances in the diagnosis and treatment of mesenteric ischemia, the mortality rate remains between 59% and 93%. The low incidence of mesenteric ischemia, as well as the difficulties and delays encountered in establishing the diagnosis, contributes to the high morbidity and mortality rates. Acute mesenteric ischemia may either be caused by thromboembolic occlusive disease (80%) or result from nonocclusive ischemia (20%). The thromboembolic causes of mesenteric ischemia include mesenteric embolism (50%), thrombosis of a pre-existing atherosclerotic orificial stenosis (20%), and mesenteric venous thrombosis (10%). Nonocclusive mesenteric ischemia occurs in the absence of anatomic arterial or venous obstruction and is the result of hypoperfusion-induced vasoconstriction throughout the entire mesenteric circulation. Chronic mesenteric ischemia is due to atherosclerotic occlusive disease in most patients. Less common causes include aortic coarctation, aortic dissection, mid-aortic stenosis, vasculitides, fibromuscular dysplasia, neurofibromatosis, and celiac artery compression syndrome.

STEP 1: SURGICAL ANATOMY

- The blood supply to the abdominal viscera arises from the celiac, superior mesenteric, inferior mesenteric, and hypogastric arteries. The celiac artery arises from the aorta at the level of the T12 and L1 vertebral bodies and is 1.5 to 2.0 cm in length. The artery divides into the left gastric, splenic, and common hepatic arteries. At its origin, the artery is surrounded by the ganglia and fibers of the celiac autonomic nerve plexus.

- The superior mesenteric artery (SMA) arises 1 cm below the celiac trunk at the L1-L2 intervertebral disc. It lies posterior to the splenic vein and pancreas and is separated from the aorta by the left renal vein.

- The inferior mesenteric artery (IMA), the smaller of the three vessels, arises from the anterior lateral aspect of the aorta at the level of the third lumbar vertebra, approximately 3 to 4 cm above the aortic bifurcation.

- The abdominal viscera have a rich collateral blood supply formed by the interconnections between the three major vessels: the celiac artery and SMA communicate via the superior and inferior pancreaticoduodenal arteries and the SMA and IMA communicate via the arc of

Riolan (middle and left colic arteries). The marginal artery of Drummond formed by anastomoses between the main trunks and the arcades arising from the ileocolic, right colic, middle colic, left colic, and sigmoid arteries, augmented by the superior, middle, and inferior rectal arteries—branches of the hypogastric arteries.

STEP 2: PREOPERATIVE CONSIDERATIONS

EVALUATION

◆ The modes of presentation of patients with acute mesenteric ischemia are quite varied. The acute onset of severe abdominal pain, nausea, and vomiting in a patient with cardiac arrhythmias suggests mesenteric embolism. The exacerbation of symptoms in a patient with the symptom triad of abdominal pain, fear of eating, and severe weight loss is suggestive of thrombotic occlusion of a high-grade celiac artery or SMA stenosis. The symptom complex of diffuse abdominal pain, hypotension, and severe lactic acidosis in the setting of cardiogenic, septicemic, or hypovolemic shock is suggestive of nonocclusive mesenteric ischemia. The clinical presentation of mesenteric venous thrombosis is often more insidious and the physical findings more subtle than those of acute arterial ischemia. However, severe abdominal pain out of proportion to the physical findings is present in more than 80% of patients.

◆ A history of pre-existing congestive heart failure, use of digoxin or α-adrenergic agents, cardiac arrhythmias, valvular heart disease, recent myocardial infarction, cardiopulmonary bypass, hypercoagulable states, vasculitides, and malignancy should be elicited.

◆ In patients with chronic mesenteric ischemia, severe abdominal pain, fear of food, and weight loss in patients with atherosclerotic peripheral vascular disease (PVD) or underlying thrombotic or coagulation disorders should be elicited.

PHYSICAL EXAMINATION

◆ Careful assessment of the abdomen for the presence of distention, tenderness, signs of peritoneal irritation, bruits, and presence or absence of femoral pulses should be undertaken.

◆ In the early phases, signs of peritoneal irritation such as guarding and rebound tenderness are usually absent. As the bowel becomes more ischemic, abdominal distention, absent bowel sounds, excruciating tenderness, feculent vomiting, and occult bleeding become evident.

DIAGNOSTIC TESTS

◆ An electrocardiogram should be performed in all patients and an echocardiogram in selected patients with poor cardiac output. A complete blood count and routine laboratory chemistries for electrolytes, blood urea nitrogen, creatinine, troponin levels, liver function tests, and arterial blood gases should be performed. In patients with suspected hypercoagulable states, blood should be drawn for the prothrombotic work-up before the administration of heparin. Blood and blood products are typed and crossmatched.

◆ In patients suspected of having acute mesenteric ischemia, a plain abdominal radiograph may demonstrate "thumbprinting," ileus, or pneumatosis. A contrast-enhanced computed tomography (CT) scan with CT angiography provides the definitive diagnosis but does not allow treatment with intra-arterial vasodilators.

◆ Angiography with anterior posterior and lateral views of the aorta is indicated in patients with acute and chronic mesenteric ischemia and in whom diagnostic uncertainty exists. If nonocclusive mesenteric ischemia is present, the angiographic catheter is left in place for the infusion of vasodilators, such as papaverine, nitroglycerin, tolazoline, or verapamil. In patients with exacerbation or recent onset of symptoms (less than 3 hours) found to have a high-grade celiac artery or SMA stenosis, angioplasty and stenting should be considered.

◆ Resuscitation with intravenous fluid is begun while the investigation is ongoing. Broad-spectrum antibiotics are administered, and any potential underlying mechanism such as arrhythmias or congestive heart failure is corrected. A heparin infusion is begun to prevent extension of thrombus into the microvessels.

STEP 3: OPERATIVE STEPS

1. INCISION

◆ The abdomen is opened via an upper midline incision, and the extent of the ischemia is assessed **(Figure 89-1)**. Perfusion of the proximal 10 to 15 cm of jejunum is indicative of embolic occlusion, whereas bowel ischemia including this segment suggests arterial thrombosis. Both the small and large bowel appears dusky if nonocclusive mesenteric ischemia is present. Segmental ischemic changes with edema of the adjacent mesentery are indicative of mesenteric venous thrombosis. If the entire bowel is necrotic, the abdomen should be closed and comfort measures instituted.

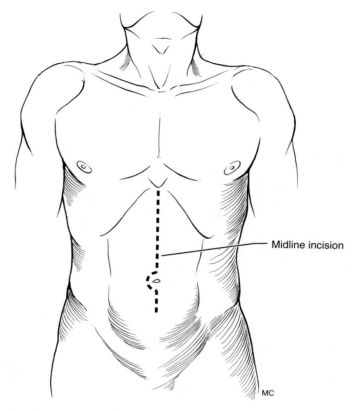

Midline incision

MC

FIGURE 89–1

2. DISSECTION

Mesenteric Embolism

◆ The transverse colon is elevated superiorly, and the fourth part of the duodenum is mobilized. The small bowel is retracted to the right, and a self-retaining retractor is placed. The SMA is isolated at the root of the mesentery and mobilized, taking care to preserve all its branches **(Figure 89-2)**.

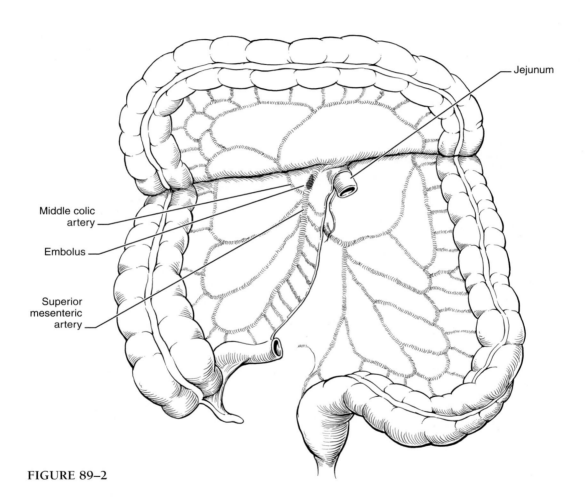

FIGURE 89–2

◆ An ACT is drawn and additional heparin is administered to ensure adequate heparinization (ACT >250). The SMA and its jejunal branches are occluded, and a transverse arteriotomy is made (**Figure 89-3, A**).

◆ A balloon catheter is then passed proximally toward the origin of the SMA, the embolus is extracted, and the proximal SMA is occluded once adequate inflow has been restored (**Figure 89-3, B**). The balloon catheter is also passed distally to ensure no thrombotic material remains (**Figure 89-3, C**). The clamps are temporarily removed, and the vessel is flushed proximally and distally.

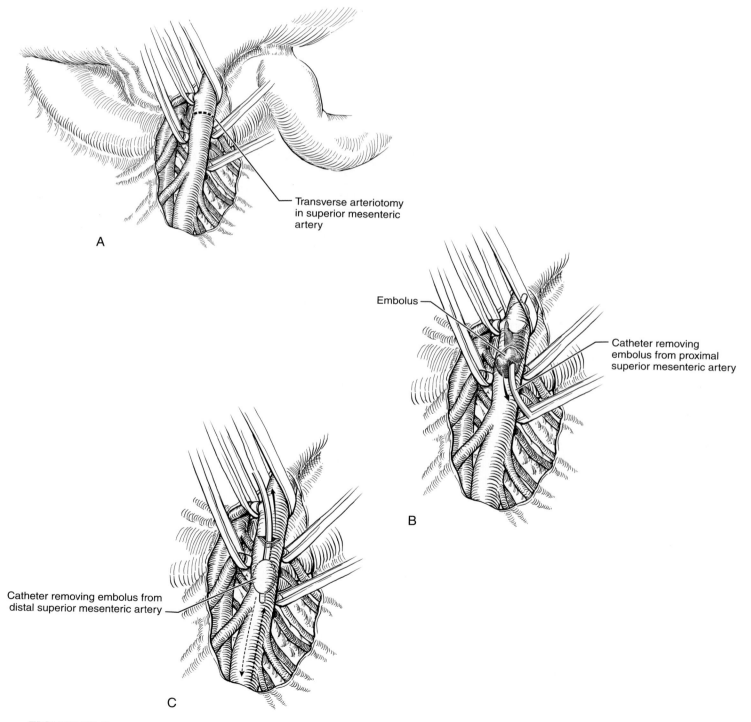

A — Transverse arteriotomy in superior mesenteric artery

Embolus — Catheter removing embolus from proximal superior mesenteric artery

B

Catheter removing embolus from distal superior mesenteric artery

C

FIGURE 89–3

◆ The lumen of the SMA is irrigated with heparinized saline, and the arteriotomy is approximated with interrupted 6-0 polypropylene suture **(Figure 89-3, D)**.

◆ The bowel is inspected, and mesenteric vessels are interrogated with Doppler ultrasound to ensure adequate perfusion. Nonviable segments of bowel should be resected.

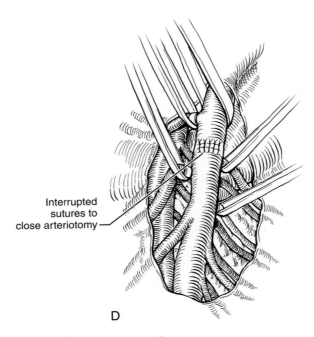

Interrupted
sutures to
close arteriotomy

D

FIGURE 89–3, cont'd

Mesenteric Thrombosis

♦ The proximal jejunum is usually ischemic because the stenosis involves the origin of the SMA, and thrombectomy alone will not suffice.

♦ The SMA is isolated as for SMA embolectomy.

♦ After systemic heparinization, the SMA is occluded and a longitudinal arteriotomy is made in the SMA below any palpable plaque.

♦ The thrombectomy catheter is then passed proximally and distally to remove any thrombus present. Antegrade blood flow is usually diminished or absent, but retrograde flow may be quite brisk because of well-established collaterals.

♦ Arterial inflow will be required from either the supraceliac, infrarenal aorta, or iliac arteries, which will be described subsequently.

Mesenteric Venous Thrombosis

♦ Mesenteric venous thrombosis may be primary or secondary to a number of conditions including cancer, hypercoagulable states, polycythemia, trauma, dehydration, and pancreatitis. Thrombus most often involves the superior mesenteric vein (70%) and inferior mesenteric vein (30%).

♦ At laparotomy, segmental small bowel congestion with edema of the mesentery is the usual finding. Segmental resection is usually the only treatment necessary. Long-term treatment with the anticoagulant warfarin (Coumadin) to prevent further thrombotic episodes is instituted postoperatively.

Chronic Mesenteric Ischemia

♦ Usually high-grade stenosis or occlusion of two of the three vessels (celiac artery and SMA) supplying the viscera is necessary to cause chronic mesenteric ischemia. Evidence of large collaterals on angiography suggests the diagnosis.

Retrograde Aortosuperior Mesenteric Bypass

♦ The SMA is exposed as described for mesenteric embolectomy, and a self-retaining retractor is placed.

♦ A segment of the abdominal aorta that is free of significant atherosclerosis (as determined on the CT scan) between the renal artery and IMA is isolated and mobilized.

♦ After systemic heparinization, the aorta is occluded between clamps, and an arteriotomy is made on its anterior lateral aspect.

◆ A harvested segment of saphenous or superficial femoral vein or 6- or 7-mm ringed polytet-rafluoroethylene (PTFE) or Dacron graft is fashioned and anastomosed end-to-side to the aorta with running 4-0 polypropylene suture **(Figure 89-4, A).** The graft is then routed in a gentle curve to the SMA. The SMA and its branches distal to the stenosis or occlusion are occluded with clamps and vessel loops, and a longitudinal arteriotomy is made beyond any palpable plaque.

◆ The graft is anastomosed end-to-side to the SMA with running 5-0 or 6-0 polypropylene suture, with care given to flush the artery and the graft before the anastomosis is completed **(Figure 89-4, B).**

◆ The entire bowel is then inspected, the mesenteric vessels are auscultated, and the anasto-moses are assessed with color flow Doppler ultrasound.

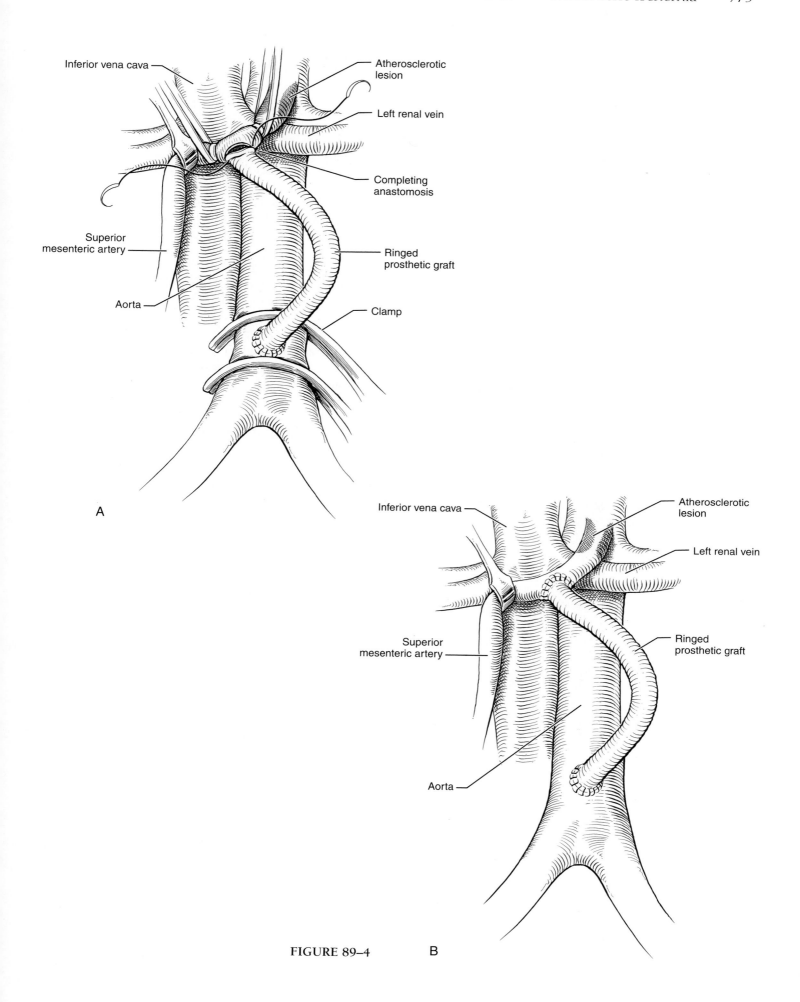

FIGURE 89–4

Antegrade Aortomesenteric Bypass

◆ When the infrarenal aorta is severely diseased, an antegrade mesenteric bypass originating from the supraceliac aorta should be considered.

◆ After the abdomen is explored, the left lobe of the liver is mobilized by dividing the triangular ligament, and the lesser sac is entered by dividing the gastrohepatic ligament.

◆ The stomach and esophagus are retracted to the left, with care given not to injure the vagus nerves. The left lobe of the liver is retracted to the right with a self-retaining retractor **(Figure 89-5, A)**.

◆ The diaphragmatic crura and median arcuate ligament are then divided in the midline, and the supraceliac aorta is mobilized for a distance of approximately 6 to 8 cm.

◆ The celiac artery and SMA are then identified and mobilized by dividing the autonomic neural fibers so that a segment of each artery uninvolved with atherosclerosis is identified. Heparin (100 U/kg) and mannitol (25 g) are administered.

◆ The celiac artery is then divided between clamps, and the proximal end is oversewn with 5-0 polypropylene suture **(Figure 89-5, B)**.

◆ The aorta is occluded between clamps, and an elliptical arteriotomy is made in the aorta **(Figure 89-5, C)**.

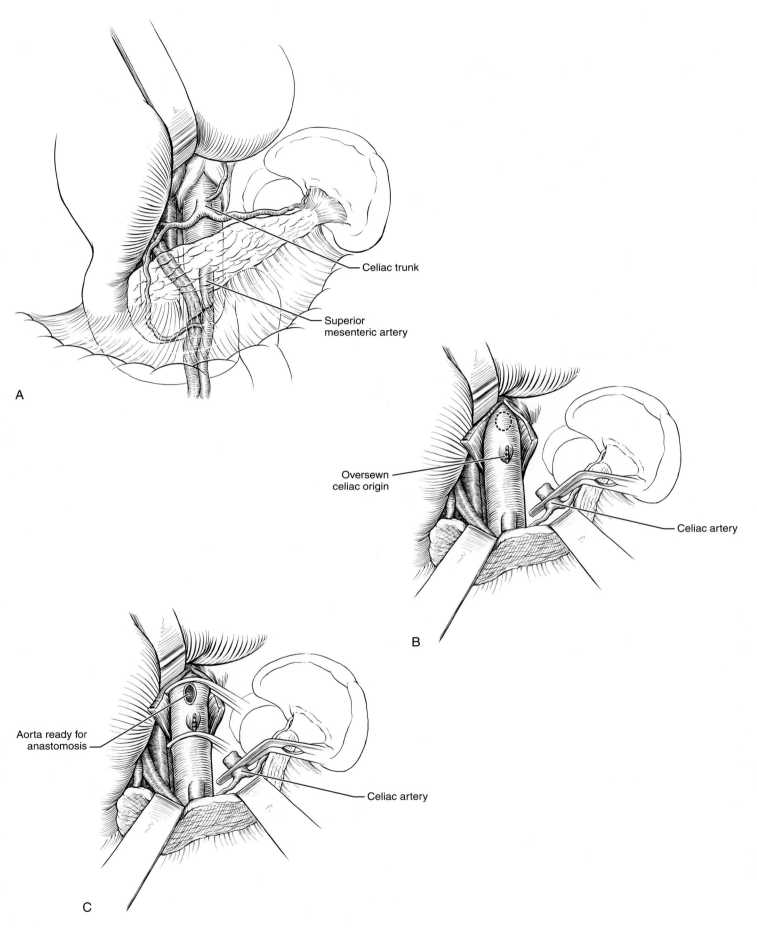

Celiac trunk

Superior
mesenteric artery

A

Oversewn
celiac origin

Celiac artery

B

Aorta ready for
anastomosis

Celiac artery

C

FIGURE 89–5

◆ A 14 × 7 bifurcated prosthetic graft is fashioned and anastomosed end-to-side to the aorta with running 3-0 Prolene suture. One limb of the graft is cut to an appropriate length, beveled, and anastomosed end-to-end to the distal celiac artery with 5-0 polypropylene suture **(Figure 89-5, D)**. The vessel and graft are flushed, the anastomosis is completed, and flow is reestablished.

◆ The second limb of the graft is routed behind the pancreas to the SMA. The SMA is occluded between clamps, and a longitudinal arteriotomy is made. The graft limb is distended with blood to its optimal length and is beveled, and the anastomosis is completed with 5-0 or 6-0 polypropylene suture **(Figure 89-5, E)**.

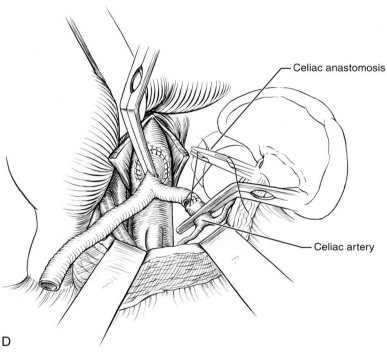

D

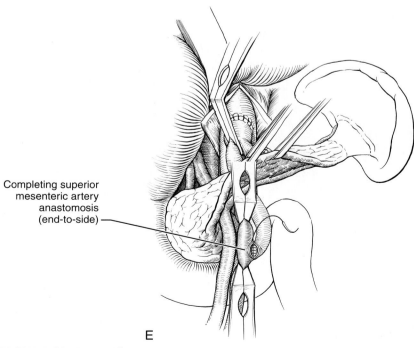

E

FIGURE 89–5, cont'd

Iliomesenteric Bypass

◆ When the supraceliac and infrarenal aorta are both severely involved with atherosclerosis or the patient is in poor general health, the common iliac artery can be used as the inflow vessel.

◆ The peritoneum over the common iliac artery is incised, and a segment of artery is mobilized, with care given not to injure the left common iliac vein.

◆ After systemic heparinization, the common iliac artery is occluded between clamps, and a longitudinal is arteriotomy made. A limb of a bifurcated prosthetic graft including cuff of the body or saphenous vein is fashioned and anastomosed end-to-side to the common iliac artery with 4-0 polypropylene suture (**Figure 89-6, A**).

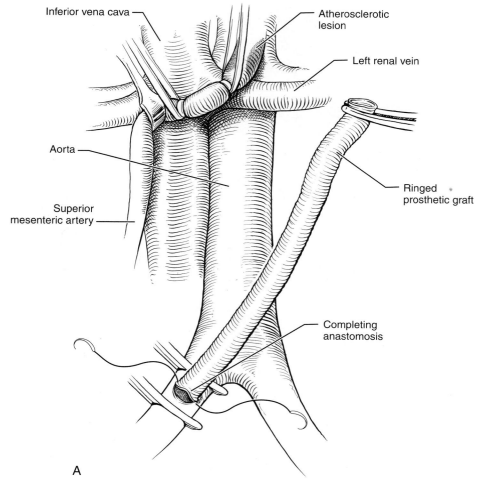

Inferior vena cava

Atherosclerotic lesion

Left renal vein

Aorta

Superior mesenteric artery

Ringed prosthetic graft

Completing anastomosis

A

FIGURE 89–6

- The limb of the graft is routed in a gentle curve to the SMA, and the anastomosis is constructed end-to-side to the SMA with running 5-0 polypropylene suture (**Figure 89-6, B-C**).

3. CLOSING

- Hemostasis is secured, and the blood supply to the viscera is carefully assessed by palpation and auscultation of the mesenteric vessels and interrogation of the anastomoses with color flow Doppler ultrasound.

- The abdomen is then closed with a looped 1-0 polydioxanone (PDS) suture.

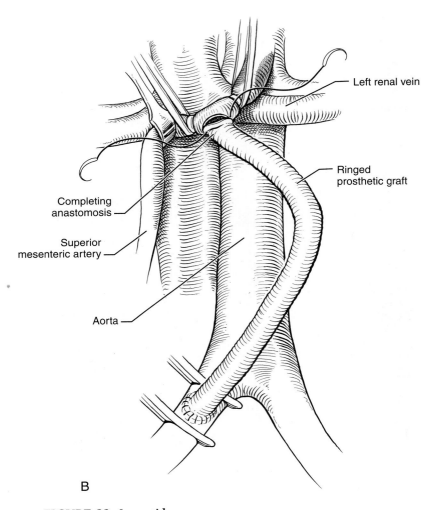

B

FIGURE 89–6, cont'd

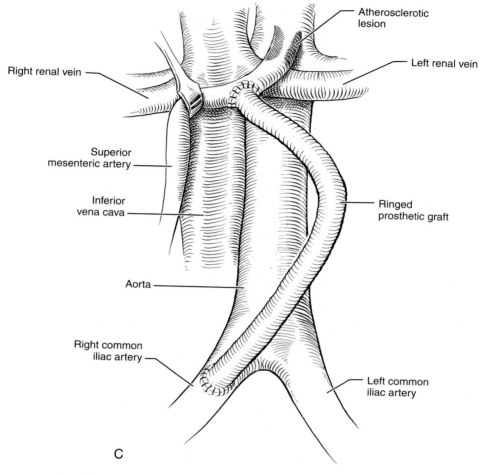

C

FIGURE 89–6, cont'd

STEP 4: POSTOPERATIVE CARE

- The patient is returned to the intensive care unit. Fluid volume, hematocrit, acid-base status, liver function tests, and clotting factors are carefully monitored and replaced. Persistent acidosis is usually indicative of ongoing bleeding or bowel or hepatic ischemia.

- Colonoscopy should be performed with care if colonic ischemia is suspected, because an intraluminal pressure greater than 30 mm Hg may further impair colonic blood flow. Prompt surgery is indicated if there is persistent acidosis, ongoing bleeding, or evidence of sepsis.

STEP 5: PEARLS AND PITFALLS

- Early diagnosis and treatment of mesenteric ischemia is essential if the survival rate is to be improved.

- A planned second-look operation to resect marginally viable segments of bowel is an integral part of the postoperative care of patients with mesenteric ischemia.

- Ongoing bleeding may be due to increased fibrinolysis, especially in patients undergoing antegrade mesenteric bypass with prolonged hepatic ischemia. After other causes of bleeding have been excluded, blood should be drawn for plasminogen levels, and an infusion of small amounts of epsilon aminocaproic acid should be considered.

- The choice of graft material is determined by the presence or absence of fecal contamination. Prosthetic grafts are preferred because they are less likely to kink. If there is gross contamination, an autogenous saphenous vein or superficial femoral vein graft should be used. These grafts should be carefully placed to avoid kinking and recurrent ischemia.

- Patients undergoing surgery for mesenteric ischemia may require large volumes of fluid intraoperatively and postoperatively and are prone to developing abdominal compartment syndrome. If there is significant bowel edema, the abdomen should not be closed primarily. Temporary abdominal content containment with plastic bags (Bogota bag) or polyglactin mesh or application of a wound vacuum-assisted closure (VAC) device and delayed primary closure should be done once the visceral edema has resolved.

- There is ongoing debate about the number of vessels to be revascularized. Patients with acute mesenteric ischemia are usually too critically ill to withstand total revascularization, and only the SMA should be revascularized. Revascularization of both the celiac artery and SMA should be considered in patients with chronic mesenteric ischemia.

SELECTED REFERENCES

1. Foley MI, Moneta GL, Abou-Zamzam AM, et al: Revascularization of the SMA alone for treatment of intestinal ischemia. J Vasc Surg 2000;32:37-47.
2. Morasch MD, Ebaugh JL, Chiou AG, et al: Mesenteric venous thrombosis: A changing clinical entity. J Vasc Surg 2001;34:680-684.
3. Wylie EJ, Stoney RJ, Ehrenfeld WK: Manual of Vascular Surgery. New York, Springer Verlag, 1980.

CHAPTER 90

HEMODIALYSIS ACCESS PROCEDURES

Kenneth J. Woodside

STEP 1: SURGICAL ANATOMY

- A comprehensive understanding of both the arterial inflow and venous outflow of the arm and forearm is critical to the successful placement and maintenance of hemodialysis access.

- **Figure 90-1** demonstrates typical target sites for arterial and venous anastomoses.

- **Figures 90-2 through 90-4** demonstrate key anatomic relationships underlying operative planning.

STEP 2: PREOPERATIVE CONSIDERATIONS

- Placement of new access should be initiated several months before the anticipated need for hemodialysis to allow time for fistula maturation and troubleshooting, as well as to avoid catheter placement and the associated risk of central vein stenosis.

- Physical examination for compressible veins in the forearm and arm should be performed, as well as Allen's test for palmar arch patency. Any history of congestive heart failure, diabetes, intravenous drug use, or chemotherapy should be elicited.

- In most patients, preoperative vein mapping should be obtained to maximize the creation of arteriovenous fistulae over graft placement. Target veins should have a diameter larger than 3 mm, although smaller distendable veins may be used.

- Access creation should occur in the nondominant forearm first, starting at the most distal site possible. Strategic placement of access is important to maximize the number of sites available over the life of the patient.

- In patients with more subcutaneous fat, consider vein transposition to make the vein closer to the skin surface and more accessible by the dialysis center.

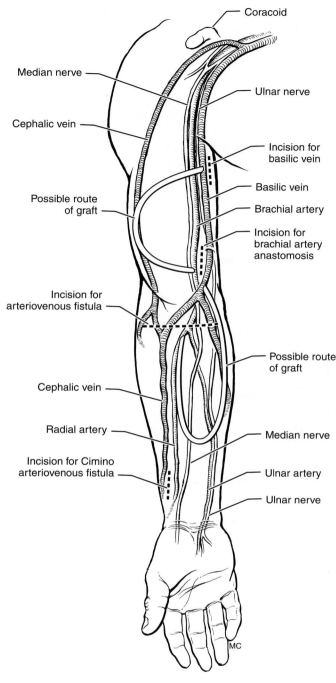

Coracoid

Median nerve

Cephalic vein

Possible route
of graft

Incision for
arteriovenous fistula

Cephalic vein

Radial artery

Incision for Cimino
arteriovenous fistula

Ulnar nerve

Incision for
basilic vein

Basilic vein

Brachial artery

Incision for
brachial artery
anastomosis

Possible route
of graft

Median nerve

Ulnar artery

Ulnar nerve

MC

FIGURE 90–1

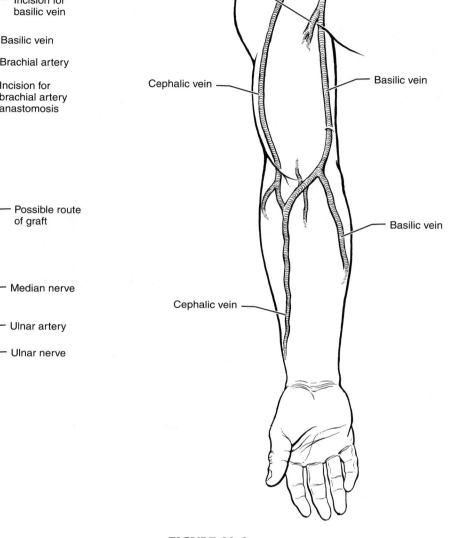

Brachial vein
(deep)

Cephalic vein

Basilic vein

Basilic vein

Cephalic vein

FIGURE 90–2

◆ Steal syndrome, in which too much blood is shunted away from the hand, is more likely to occur in patients with diabetes and in those with upper extremity atherosclerotic disease. In addition, placement of the access above the elbow or use of synthetic conduit increases the risk of steal symptoms.

◆ The axilla and shoulder must always be included in the surgical field. Fistulograms, shuntograms, and central venograms are often required, so a suitable vascular bed and arm board should be used. Preoperative antibiotics should be given at the appropriate time. Regional anesthesia may promote venous dilation and assist in successful fistula creation.

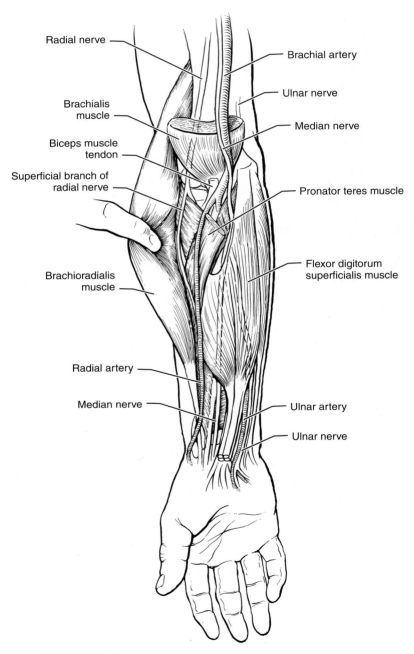

FIGURE 90–3

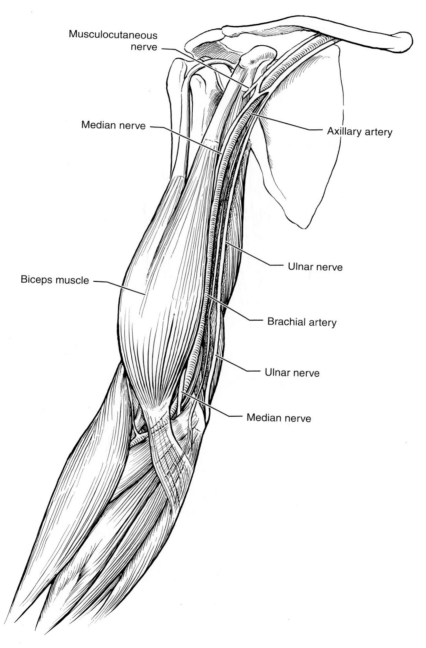

FIGURE 90–4

STEP 3: OPERATIVE STEPS—RADIOCEPHALIC ARTERIOVENOUS FISTULA

1. INCISION

♦ The patient is placed supine, with the arm placed on an arm board.

♦ The radial artery and the target cephalic vein are located. Intraoperative ultrasound can help the surgeon localize the vein and reassess patency of the vessel.

♦ A longitudinal incision is made between the target vein and the radial artery **(Figure 90-5)**.

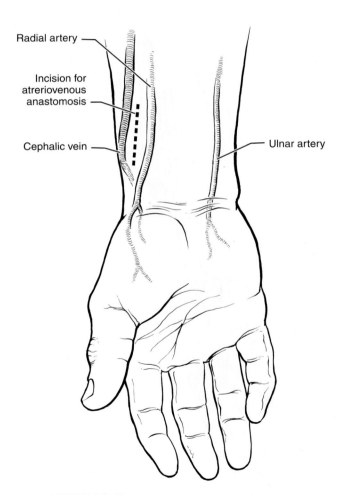

FIGURE 90–5

2. DISSECTION

♦ A small flap is made to allow mobilization of the cephalic vein. The vein is mobilized for a short distance and assessed for adequacy.

♦ The fascia over the radial artery is incised, and proximal and distal control of the vessel is obtained (**Figure 90-6**).

♦ The cephalic vein is divided as distally as possible, flushed with heparinized saline, and dilated manually.

♦ The patient is heparinized, and proximal and distal arterial clamps are placed.

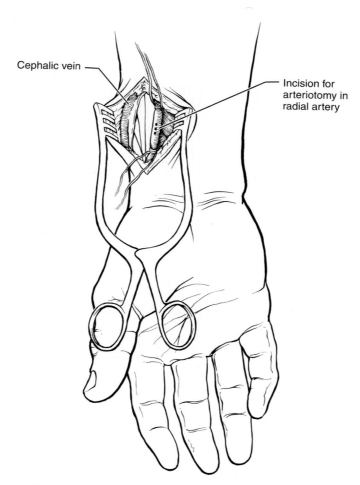

Cephalic vein

Incision for arteriotomy in radial artery

FIGURE 90–6

◆ An end-to-side anastomosis is performed with 6-0 Prolene suture **(Figure 90-7)**.

◆ The clamps are removed, with the distal arterial clamp removed last. The cephalic vein is palpated for a thrill. Revision may be necessary if a thrill is not readily palpable. If the fistula is pulsatile without a thrill, a distal obstruction may be present. If the obstruction is not from inadequate vein mobilization, a venogram may need to be performed.

3. CLOSURE

◆ The wound is closed in two layers with interrupted 3-0 Vicryl subcutaneous sutures and a running 4-0 Monocryl subcuticular layer.

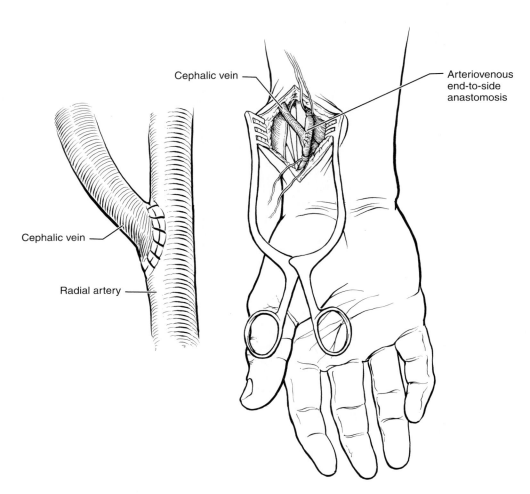

FIGURE 90–7

STEP 3: OPERATIVE STEPS—ANTECUBITAL ARTERIOVENOUS FISTULA

1. INCISION

◆ The patient is placed supine, with the arm placed on an arm board.

◆ Approximately 1 cm below the antecubital crease, a horizontal incision is made, with care taken to preserve the subcutaneous veins **(Figure 90-8).**

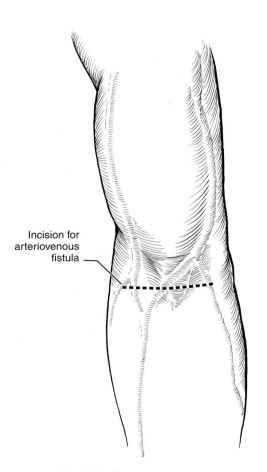

Incision for
arteriovenous
fistula

FIGURE 90–8

2. DISSECTION

♦ A suitable antecubital vein is identified and mobilized. The basilic, cephalic, or antecubital bridging veins are typically used. Strategically, flow through the cephalic vein will be easier to access at the dialysis center **(Figure 90-9)**.

♦ The brachial arterial pulse is identified just proximal to the elbow. The bicipital aponeurosis is divided, exposing the artery. Proximal and distal control is obtained. Communicating veins overlaying the artery may need to be divided to allow adequate control. Care must be taken to avoid damage to the nearby median nerve **(Figure 90-10)**.

♦ The vein is divided as distally as possible, flushed with heparinized saline, and dilated manually.

♦ The patient is heparinized, and proximal and distal arterial clamps are placed.

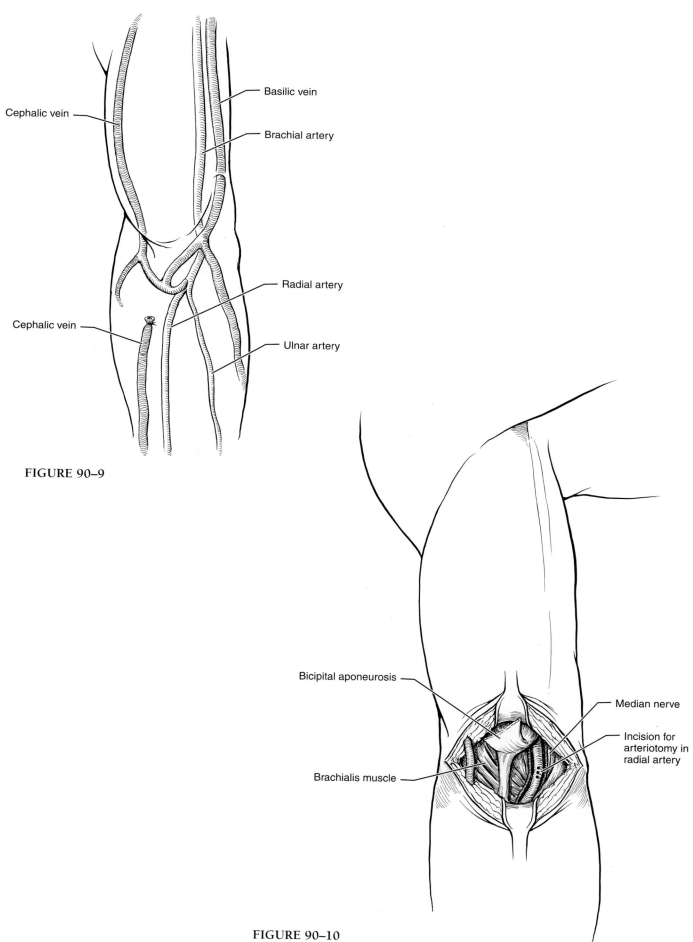

FIGURE 90-9

FIGURE 90-10

◆ An end-to-side anastomosis is performed with 6-0 Prolene suture **(Figure 90-11).**

◆ The clamps are removed, with the distal arterial clamp removed last. The proximal vein is palpated for a thrill. Revision may be necessary if a thrill is not readily palpable. If the fistula is pulsatile without a thrill, a distal obstruction may be present. If the obstruction is not from inadequate vein mobilization, a venogram may need to be performed.

3. CLOSURE

◆ The wound is closed in two layers with interrupted 3-0 Vicryl subcutaneous sutures and a running 4-0 Monocryl subcuticular layer.

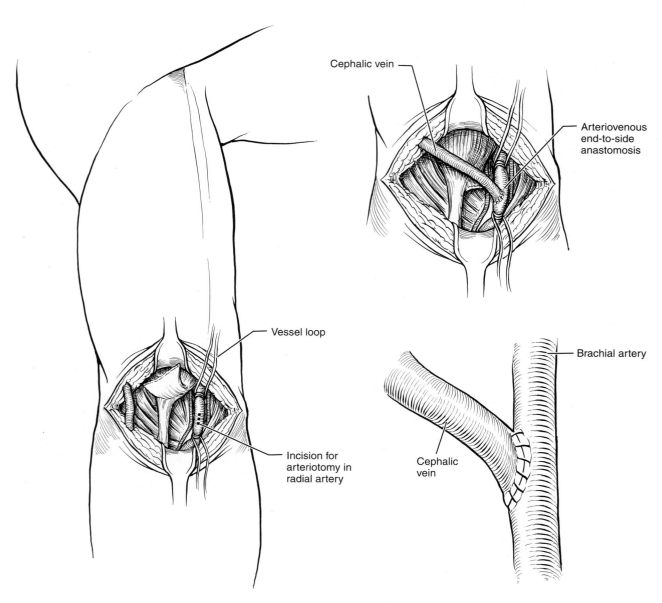

FIGURE 90–11

STEP 3: OPERATIVE STEPS—BRACHIOBASILIC UPPER ARM TRANSPOSITION

1. INCISION

◆ The patient is placed supine, with the arm placed on an arm board.

◆ Although any vein can be transposed, description of a brachiobasilic vein transposition is offered as an example of the surgical principles involved in creating such fistula. The exact incision and dissection should be tailored to the anatomic sites involved.

◆ A longitudinal incision is made along the biceps groove, starting just proximal to the elbow, with care taken to preserve the subcutaneous veins **(Figure 90-12)**.

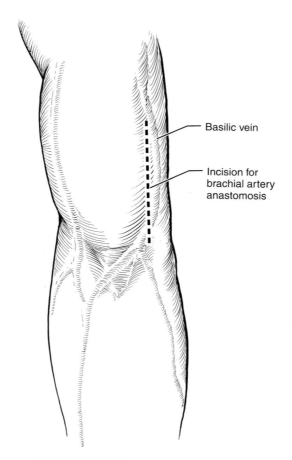

Basilic vein

Incision for brachial artery anastomosis

FIGURE 90–12

2. DISSECTION

◆ The basilic vein is identified, mobilized, and assessed for adequacy **(Figure 90-13)**.

◆ The deep fascia over the brachial sheath is divided, with care taken to preserve the median and ulnar nerves **(Figure 90-14)**.

◆ The brachial artery is identified and isolated. Communicating veins overlaying the artery may need to be divided to allow adequate control.

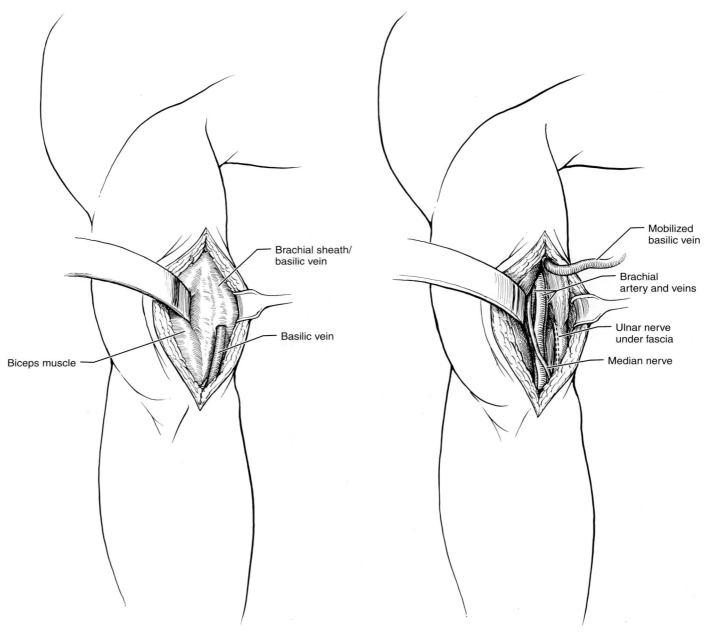

FIGURE 90–13   **FIGURE 90–14**

◆ The basilic vein is mobilized along its course as high as possible, with proximal extension of the incision as needed. Side branches are ligated with silk suture and divided. Some surgeons use skin bridges to minimize the size of the tissue flap. Sometimes, the basilic vein joins with the brachial vein early, preventing significant mobilization. If the vein is adequate distally, additional mobilization of the basilic vein below the elbow may offer additional length.

◆ The basilic vein is marked to prevent twisting. The vein is divided as distally as possible, flushed with heparinized saline, and dilated manually. The vein is tunneled through the subcutaneous tissue at a depth of approximately 4 mm (**Figure 90-15**).

◆ The patient is heparinized, and proximal and distal arterial clamps are placed.

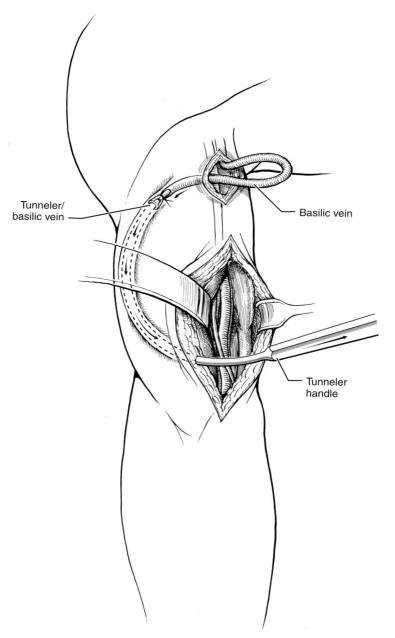

FIGURE 90–15

◆ An end-to-side anastomosis is performed with 6-0 Prolene suture (**Figure 90-16**).

◆ The clamps are removed, with the distal arterial clamp removed last. The proximal vein is palpated for a thrill. Revision may be necessary if a thrill is not readily palpable. If the vein twisted in the tunnel, the anastomosis may need to be taken down and the vein retunneled. If the fistula is pulsatile without a thrill, a distal obstruction may be present. A venogram can be performed to assess for stenotic lesions.

3. CLOSURE

◆ The wound is closed in two layers with interrupted 3-0 Vicryl subcutaneous sutures and a running 4-0 Monocryl subcuticular layer.

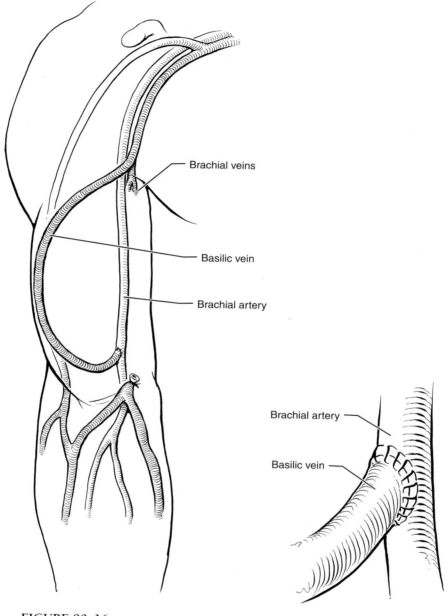

Brachial veins

Basilic vein

Brachial artery

Brachial artery

Basilic vein

FIGURE 90–16

STEP 3: OPERATIVE STEPS—ARTERIOVENOUS GRAFTS

1. APPROACH AND INCISION

◆ Although primary arteriovenous fistulae are preferred, some patients do not have adequate veins to allow fistula creation. In these cases, artificial conduit, most commonly standard wall 6-mm polytetrafluoroethylene (PTFE), is used. Occasionally, more distal PTFE grafts can bridge to later arteriovenous fistula creation by arterializing the downstream vein.

◆ Incisions are made according to the target vessels. Grafts may be placed in a looped, curved, or straight configuration, based on the availability of arterial inflow and venous outflow, as well as the anatomic position and future ease of access at the dialysis center. Again, the principle of distal placement is followed. Grafts that cross joints or have a sharp turn (e.g., a forearm hairpin turn) may require a short segment of ringed graft. Femoral grafts are avoided if possible, because they may interfere with future kidney transplant **(Figures 90-17 through 90-21)**.

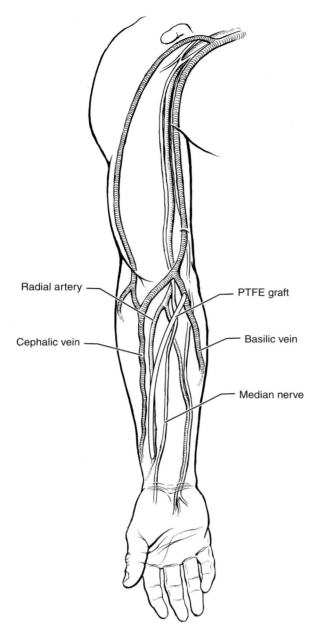

Radial artery

Cephalic vein

PTFE graft

Basilic vein

Median nerve

FIGURE 90–17

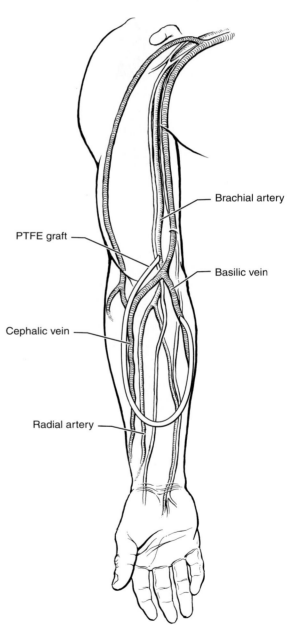

Brachial artery

PTFE graft

Basilic vein

Cephalic vein

Radial artery

FIGURE 90–18

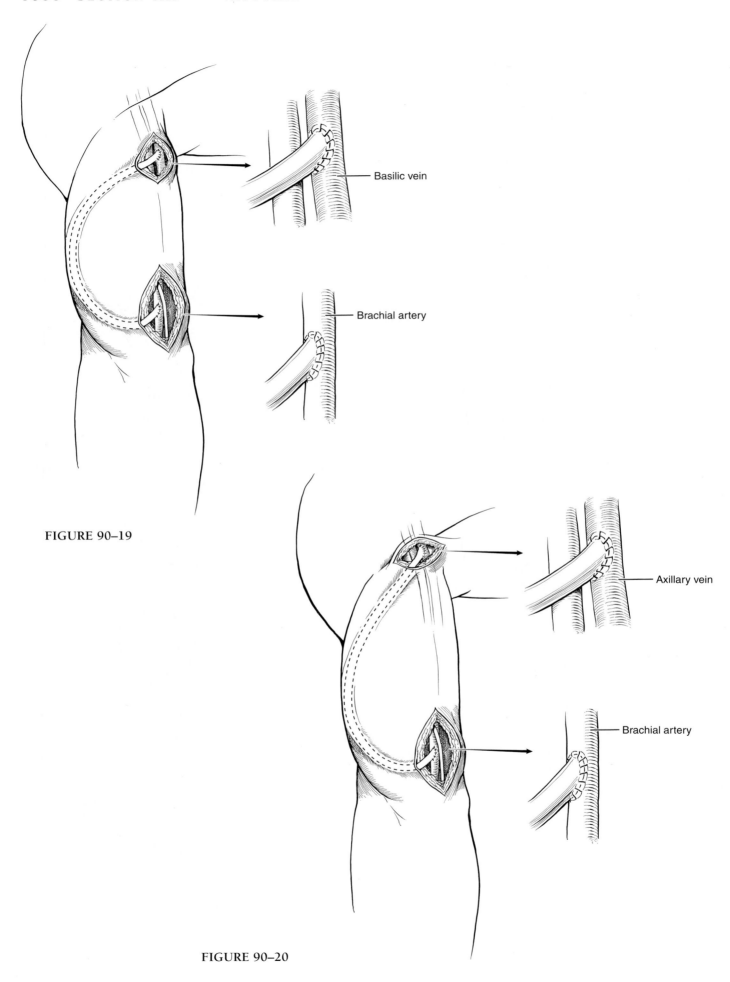

FIGURE 90–19

Basilic vein

Brachial artery

Axillary vein

Brachial artery

FIGURE 90–20

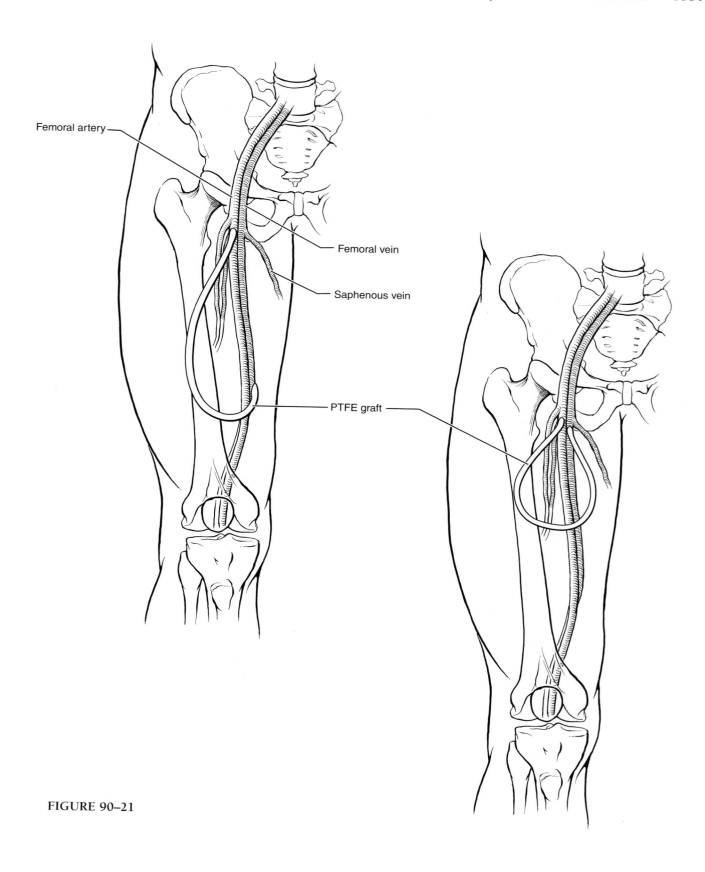

Femoral artery

Femoral vein

Saphenous vein

PTFE graft

FIGURE 90–21

2. DISSECTION

◆ Arterial inflow and venous outflow are isolated. Proximal and distal control of both vessels is obtained.

◆ The graft is tunneled, with care taken to keep the graft untwisted and to maintain a proper depth (approximately 4 mm). A counter-incision may be required, depending on the anatomic location **(Figure 90-22)**.

◆ Once the tunnel is completed, the patient is heparinized. A small hood is cut in each end of the graft, which is oriented according to the direction of flow. The vessels are clamped, and end-to-side anastomoses are performed to the target artery and vein with 6-0 Prolene suture. If the graft has a pre-existing (i.e., manufactured) venous hood, the venous anastomosis should be performed first to size the length of the graft appropriately.

◆ The clamps are removed, with the distal arterial clamp removed last. The graft is palpated for a thrill. Revision may be necessary if a thrill is not readily palpable. If the graft twisted in the tunnel, the anastomosis may need to be taken down and the vein retunneled. If the graft is pulsatile without a thrill, a distal obstruction may be present. A venogram can be performed to assess for stenotic lesions.

3. CLOSURE

◆ The wound is closed in two layers with interrupted 3-0 Vicryl subcutaneous sutures and a running 4-0 Monocryl subcuticular layer.

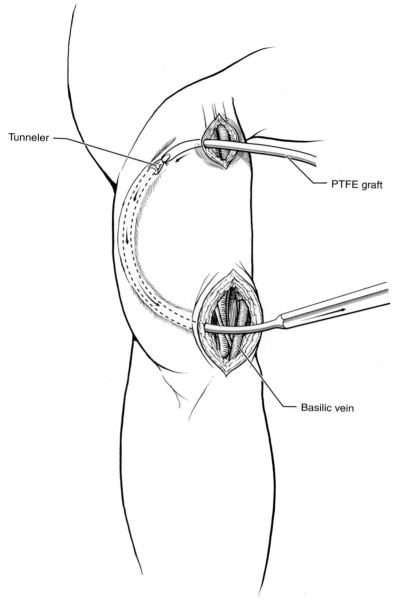

Tunneler

PTFE graft

Basilic vein

FIGURE 90–22

STEP 3: OPERATIVE STEPS—GRAFT REVISION: THROMBECTOMY

1. INCISION

- Most commonly, a small incision is made over the fistula or graft a few centimeters downstream from the arterial anastomosis.

2. OPERATIVE APPROACH

- Proximal and distal control of the fistula or graft is obtained. The patient is heparinized.

- A transverse incision is made in the conduit. A balloon thrombectomy catheter is passed up the venous limb first, and the clot is removed. The process is repeated for the arterial limb. There should be the return of strong, pulsatile flow on removal of the arterial clot **(Figure 90-23)**.

- A fistulogram or shuntogram is performed to assess for anatomic causes of the thrombosis. The central veins should be assessed as part of this venogram to evaluate for central stenoses. Peripheral or central stenoses may require balloon angioplasty or stenting.

- Short jump grafts or patch angioplasties are required for persistent anastomotic strictures **(Figure 90-24)**.

3. CLOSURE

- The wound is closed in two layers with interrupted 3-0 Vicryl subcutaneous sutures and a running 4-0 Monocryl subcuticular layer.

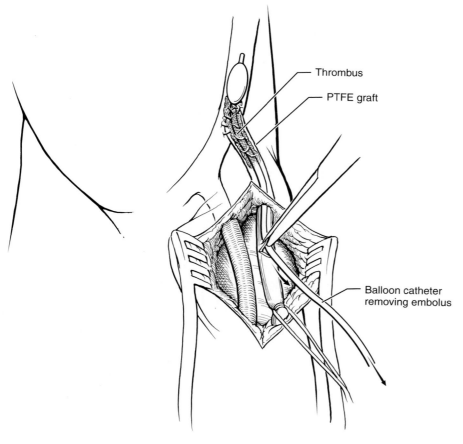

Thrombus

PTFE graft

Balloon catheter
removing embolus

FIGURE 90–23

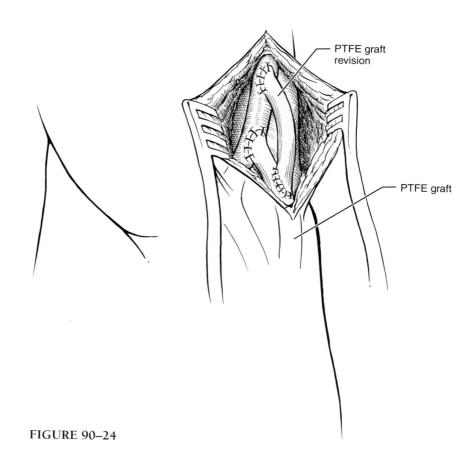

PTFE graft
revision

PTFE graft

FIGURE 90–24

STEP 4: POSTOPERATIVE CARE

- Patients should be examined again in the recovery room, and regularly until discharge, for a thrill and a bruit in the access.

- Fistulae require a minimum of 6 weeks to mature before cannulation. Most grafts require a minimum of 2 weeks before cannulation.

- Long-term catheters should be removed promptly once the fistula or graft has matured and has been used successfully for hemodialysis.

- Arm swelling that persists beyond the second postoperative week and does not respond to arm elevation should be investigated further with imaging.

- Fistulae often have venous side branches that prevent adequate maturation. If these are found, selective ligation of the branches can allow for maturation of the fistula. Imaging should be obtained of fistulae that do not mature by the sixth postoperative week.

- Mature fistulae (greater than 6 weeks after placement) are more likely to be usable if they meet the Rule of 6s criteria: flow greater than 600 mL/min, diameter larger than 6 mm, depth less than 6 mm, and discernable margins.

- Patients should be instructed in isometric hand exercises and in daily examination of the access for a thrill or signs of infection.

STEP 5: PEARLS AND PITFALLS

- Nondistendable veins are sclerotic and usually will not mature. Noncompressible veins are thrombosed. A history of intravenous drug use, chemotherapy, or multiple intravenous catheters at the site may indicate the presence of such veins.

- When a fistula or graft thromboses or has consistently high venous pressures, a fistulogram or shuntogram should be performed, which includes a central venogram. Because many of these patients have had multiple catheters, they are at risk for subclavian vein stenoses. If such a stenosis is found, it may be amenable to angioplasty and stenting. If the subclavian vein is actually occluded, the other arm should be assessed for access sites.

- Most of the arterial targets course near major nerves. Care should be taken to avoid traction injury or other damage to these nerves, especially in redo operations, where the anatomy may not be as well demarcated as usual.

- Steal syndrome, defined as ischemia of the hand, is more common with artificial conduit than autologous fistula, probably because the slower maturation of the fistula allows acclimation and collateralization to develop. Steal symptoms are also more common when the anastomosis is above the elbow or the patient is diabetic. These symptoms may occur sporadically, when the patient is on hemodialysis, or may be continuous. Any such symptoms require prompt evaluation. The access may need to be ligated or other procedures, such as a distal revascularization with interval ligation (DRIL), may be required to prevent hand loss and salvage the graft **(Figure 90-25)**.

◆ Potential future access sites should be preserved, with the patient counseled to avoid blood draws and catheters at those sites.

◆ Large aneurysmal dilations often indicate a downstream stenosis, especially if they occur away from cannulation sites, and should be investigated further.

◆ The patient's dialysis center should be sent a diagram of the access detailing the conduit, course, and anastomotic sites, as well as any findings of importance (e.g., angioplasty or stent sites).

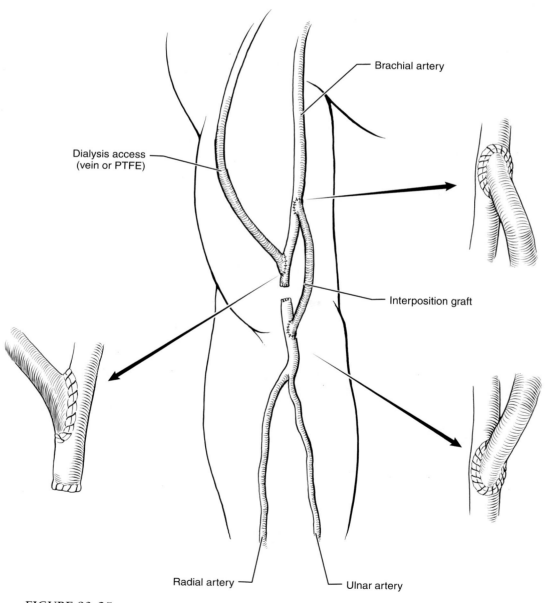

FIGURE 90–25

SELECTED REFERENCES

1. National Kidney Foundation: KDOQI clinical practice guidelines and clinical practice recommendations for 2006 updates: Hemodialysis adequacy, peritoneal dialysis adequacy, and vascular access. Am J Kidney Dis 2006:48: S1-S322.
2. Haisch CE, Parker FM, Brown PM Jr: Access and ports. In Townsend CM Jr (ed): Sabiston Textbook of Surgery: The Biological Basis of Modern Surgical Practice, 17th ed. Philadelphia, Elsevier Saunders, 2004, pp 2081-2094.
3. Bohannon WT, Silva MB: Venous transpositions in the creation of arteriovenous access. In Rutherford RB (ed): Vascular Surgery, 6th ed. Philadelphia, Elsevier Saunders, 2005, pp 1677-1684.
4. Lumsden AB, Bush RL, Lin PH, Peden EK: Management of thrombosed dialysis access. In Rutherford RB (ed): Vascular Surgery, 6th ed. Philadelphia: Elsevier Saunders, 2005, pp 1684-1692.
5. Knox RC, Berman SS, Hughes JD, et al: Distal revascularization-interval ligation: A durable and effective treatment for ischemic steal syndrome after hemodialysis access. J Vasc Surg 2002;36:250-255.

CHAPTER 91

INSERTION OF TENCKHOFF CATHETER

Kristene K. Gugliuzza

STEP 1: SURGICAL ANATOMY

◆ Place the uppermost trocar or the incision in a paramedian position. This allows for burial of the cuff of the catheter under the muscle and decreases the incidence of cuff erosion through the incision. Make the optimal placement by placing the catheter on the abdomen in a position where the end of the catheter or the bottom of the cuff is situated on the symphysis pubis and the first cuff lies over the rectus muscle. Place the incision where the first cuff lays on the abdomen. The exit site is usually lateral to the first trocar. Use this site for the second trocar (**Figure 91-1**).

◆ Achieve the optimal placement of the exit site with the aid of a home dialysis nurse. This provider can meet with the patient preoperatively to design the exit site that is most functional for the patient. Functionality is predicated by the handedness of the patient (usually more comfortable when the catheter is placed on the same side as the dominant hand) and body habitus (different placement for a patient with a large panniculus versus a thin patient; patient comfort in having the catheter below the belt line or above).

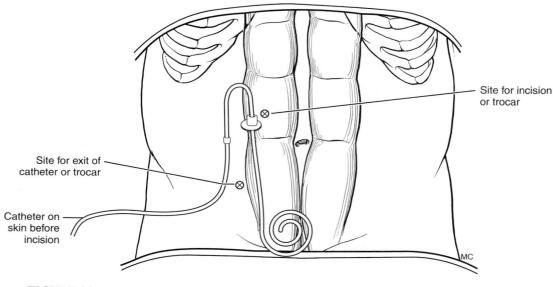

Site for incision or trocar

Site for exit of catheter or trocar

Catheter on skin before incision

FIGURE 91–1

STEP 2: PREOPERATIVE CONSIDERATIONS

- Twenty million Americans, one in nine adults, have chronic kidney disease (CKD), and 20 million more are at increased risk. The peritoneal dialysis (PD) catheter is one of the three options for treatment of stage 5 CKD (glomerular filtration rate [GFR] < 15 ml/min). The other options are hemodialysis and transplantation. Fifteen percent of the population dependent on dialysis chooses the option of PD.

- There are four methods to place a PD catheter. One is an emergent, temporary catheter at the bedside. Use this method only in a patient who requires immediate dialysis and cannot be moved from the intensive care unit (ICU). The second method is an open placement usually performed in the operating room with the patient under local or general anesthesia. The third and fourth methods are placed laparoscopically, either as an assist to open surgery or as the primary technique for placement of the catheter.

- Use the emergent and the laparoscopic-only procedures when there is no fear of adhesions that increase the risk of perforation of bowel through the blind insertion of the trocar or needle.

- The emergent placement of a PD catheter is similar to the procedure of diagnostic peritoneal lavage (DPL). The Seldinger technique (using a blunt-tipped flexible guidewire inside a finder needle to introduce a sheath or a catheter into the peritoneal space) is a safe method to place the catheter. You can accomplish this technique with an incision through the skin down to the peritoneum or as a puncture through the skin.

- It is helpful if the patient's bowel is deflated. Encourage the patient to ingest only liquids the day before the procedure.

STEP 3: OPERATIVE STEPS—OPEN PROCEDURE

- Patient positioning
  - Place the patient supine.
  - The surgical preparation should include the skin from the nipples to the symphysis pubis and laterally from the mid-anterior axillary line to the anterior axillary line.

1. INCISION

- To estimate the correct position of the incision for the first cuff of the catheter, lay the catheter on the abdomen with the bottom of the curl placed on the symphysis pubis. The first cuff will lay lateral to the umbilicus on the side of the exit site mark that has been placed preoperatively by the dialysis nurse. Make the incision approximately 1 cm above and below the area of the cuff (see Figure 91-1).

◆ If you are performing an open procedure without the aid of the laparoscope, carry the incision down through the skin and subcutaneous tissues to the muscle **(Figure 91-2)**. Incise the fascia of the muscle and split it down to the posterior fascia. Place a purse-string suture in the fascia with the diameter approximately the size of a dime and then make an incision in the middle of the circle **(Figure 91-3)**.

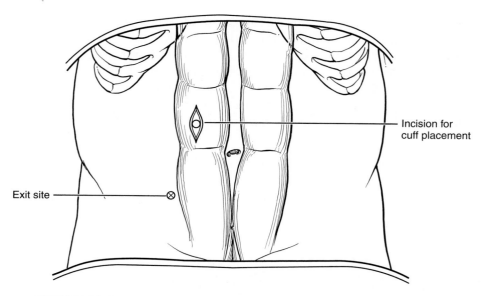

Incision for cuff placement

Exit site

FIGURE 91–2

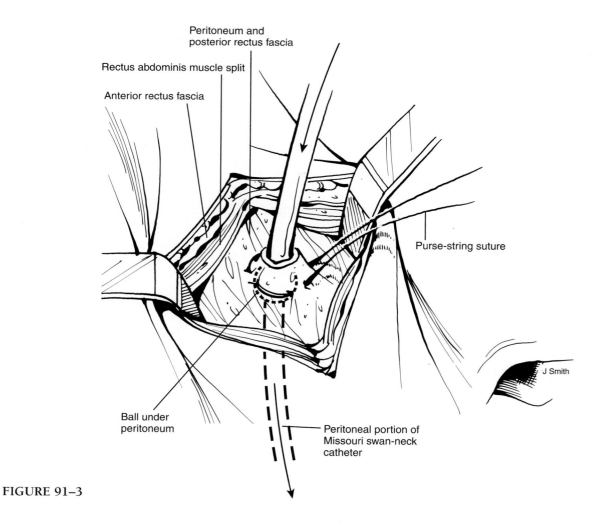

Peritoneum and posterior rectus fascia

Rectus abdominis muscle split

Anterior rectus fascia

Purse-string suture

Ball under peritoneum

Peritoneal portion of Missouri swan-neck catheter

J Smith

FIGURE 91–3

2. DISSECTION

◆ Place the catheter over a long metal guide or stylet that has been lubricated with water-soluble gel. Take care to look at the catheter because some have a white line that you must keep in the anterior or "up" position. With care, place the catheter and the guide through the hole into the peritoneal cavity. Guide the catheter along the posterior surface of the abdominal wall toward the iliac crest. Once there, aim the catheter toward the symphysis pubis. This allows for placement of the tip or bottom of the curl in the pelvis area close to the abdominal wall (Figure 91-4). After removing the stylet, test the function of the catheter by instilling a dilute heparinized saline through the end of the catheter. You should be able to instill, aspirate, and siphon the fluid easily through the catheter without force or interruption of flow. Usually, placing the patient in a reverse Trendelenburg position and administering approximately 100 mL of fluid aids in this maneuver.

◆ If there is difficulty in any of these three maneuvers, reposition the catheter.

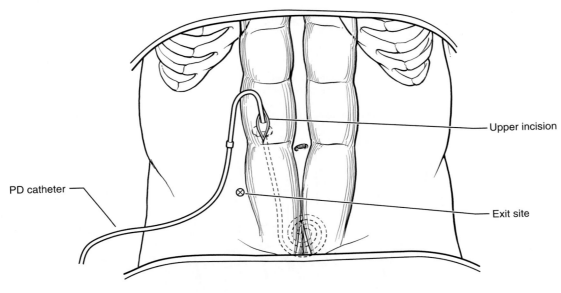

FIGURE 91-4

◆ After successfully testing the function of the catheter, tighten the purse-string around the catheter below the cuff (or between the intraperitoneal ball and the flat disc of the Missouri swan-neck catheter) and suture the cuff or disc to the posterior peritoneum in a whipstitch fashion. You must avoid puncturing the catheter with the needle **(Figure 91-5)**.

◆ Tunnel the end of the catheter through the rectus muscle and subcutaneous tissue to the exit site that was previously marked by the home dialysis nurse. The use of a sharp curved trocar is best to decrease the dead space around the catheter. To decrease the incidence of infection caused by an extruded cuff, make sure to have the second cuff of the catheter remain in the subcutaneous space and at least 1 cm from the exit site.

3. CLOSING

◆ Close the incisions in one or two layers, as per the tradition of the institution. Do not close the exit or place a suture around the catheter. Apply a simple clear air-permeable dressing over the exit site and the catheter to lessen the movement of the catheter.

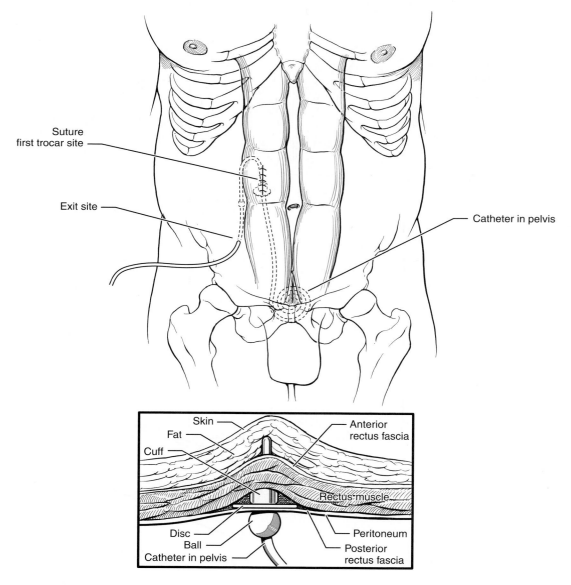

FIGURE 91–5

STEP 3: OPERATIVE STEPS—LAPAROSCOPIC OPTION

- ◆ When using the laparoscopic techniques, the surgeon must arrange the patient and the equipment in the most useful positions. Place the patient supine. Place the monitor at the foot of the bed, because the pelvis is the primary area of interest and is where the tip or the base of the curled catheter is going to lay **(Figure 91-6)**.

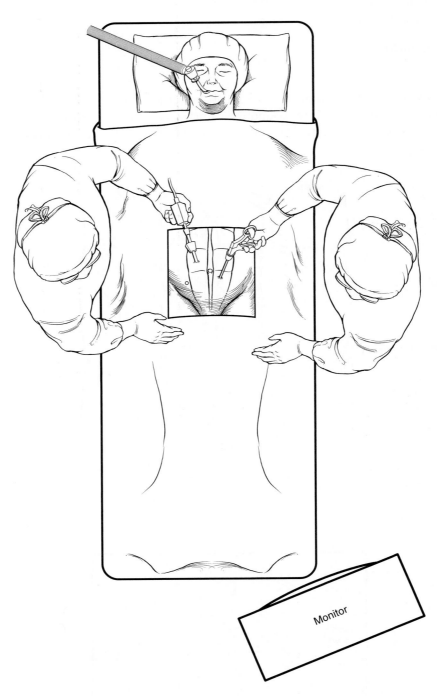

Monitor

FIGURE 91–6

1. INCISION

◆ When laparoscopic assistance or laparoscopic placement only is being used, the methods are similar to the open procedure. Place the 5-mm trocar in the most cephalad position blindly or open as described previously (see Figure 91-7, *1*). If placed open, the trocar can be easily placed through the hole in the posterior fascia and the purse-string tightened around the trocar **(Figure 91-7)**. Secure the string with a rubber-shod clamp. Insufflate the abdominal cavity with CO_2 to proper pressures (12 to 18 cm H_2O pressure). Place the 5-mm camera through this trocar. An exploration of the cavity will reveal adhesions to the abdominal wall that can be taken down with the placement of two trocars (5 mm). These can be placed under direct vision. Place the trocars tangentially to separate the outer and the inner holes, which allows for less leakage if the catheter is to be used quickly. One trocar is placed at the marked exit site (see Figure 91-7, *2*) and the other in the midline or contralateral aspect of the abdomen (see Figure 91-7, *3*).

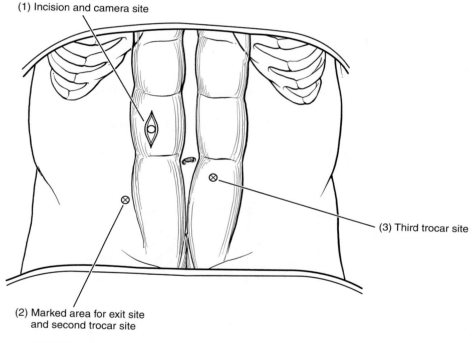

(1) Incision and camera site

(3) Third trocar site

(2) Marked area for exit site
and second trocar site

FIGURE 91–7

♦ When the pelvis and lower aspect of the peritoneal cavity is free from adhesions, move the camera to one of the other trocars. Remove the upper trocar and advance the catheter over the stylet through the purse-string into the cavity. To decrease the loss of intra-abdominal pressure, hold the purse-string tight around the catheter as it is advanced. Once the cuff is at the posterior fascia, hold the suture in place with a rubber-shod clamp.

2. DISSECTION

♦ Using the camera and a grasping instrument through the remaining trocar, place the end of the catheter (or the curl) in the pelvis above the bowel and omentum. Securing the catheter to the posterior abdominal wall is an advantage because it prevents catheter migration and enhances return of dialysate. Make a small incision in the skin in the midline and above the symphysis pubis. Using a laparoscopic suture passer, pass an absorbable suture (2-0 or larger) into the abdominal cavity under direct vision. Then guide the suture around the catheter, at the start of the curl if using a curled catheter, or at least 5 to 8 cm above the end of a straight catheter, and retrieve by the suture passer. Bring the suture to the outside and then tie it down securely.

3. CLOSING

♦ The completion of this procedure is identical to the open procedure described previously including testing for function of the catheter, securing the first cuff, bringing out the end of the catheter at the exit site, and closing the wounds **(Figure 91-8)**.

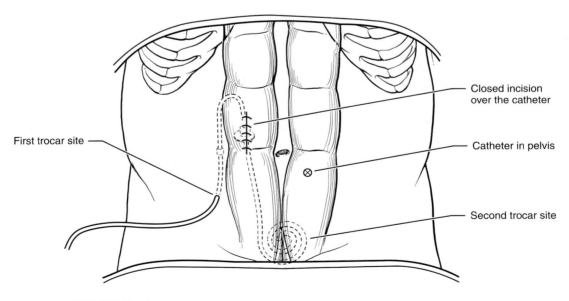

First trocar site

Closed incision over the catheter

Catheter in pelvis

Second trocar site

FIGURE 91–8

STEP 4: POSTOPERATIVE CARE

◆ Make sure that the patients are under the care of a home dialysis program. The standard of care is for the patient to see the dialysis nurses within 2 to 3 days. At that time, the nurses begin to set up the schedule for the home dialysis training. Each dialysis center individualizes the dressings for the exit site. The nurses have protocols that are followed rigorously.

◆ Tell the patient not to swim or take baths. Taking a shower is the primary option for bathing.

◆ Give instructions to the patients regarding signs of infection and contact numbers in case any redness, tenderness, swelling with pain, or discharge occurs at the sites of the incisions or exit site.

◆ Use of the dialysis catheter is also individualized. If the cuff is secured to the posterior fascia, the catheter can be used immediately with low volumes, increasing the volumes slowly over several days to the therapeutic levels. Usually, the wait is 2 weeks for healing of the incision sites and scarring of the outer cuff in the tunnel.

STEP 5: PEARLS AND PITFALLS

◆ Use the home dialysis nurses to help with the placement of the exit site. The patients have greater satisfaction when the exit site is in a convenient spot.

◆ If the catheter cuff is secured to the posterior fascia and the 5-mm trocars are placed tangentially through the abdominal wall, the likelihood of leaking is less and the catheter may be used sooner (if not immediately).

◆ The use of the laparoscope allows the surgeon to perform other procedures, if needed (e.g., lysis of adhesions, hernia repair, cholecystectomy, partial omentectomy).

◆ Securing the catheter to the anterior abdominal wall may prevent catheter migration and enhance return of dialysate.

◆ Take care not to puncture the catheter outside of the abdominal cavity, because it will not heal and you will have to place another one.

◆ Do not suture the catheter at the exit site. Place a clear, air-permeable dressing over the site and catheter. Then call your home dialysis nurses to come re-dress the site while the patient is in the postanesthesia care unit or the day surgery unit. The dialysis nurses are part of the team and they are diligent about reducing the risk of infection.

SELECTED REFERENCE

1. Tsimoyiannis EC, Siakas P, Glantzounis G, et al: Laparoscopic placement of the Tenckhoff catheter for peritoneal dialysis. Surg Laparosc Endosc Percutan Tech 2000;10:218-221.

CHAPTER 92

INSERTION OF PERITONEAL VENOUS SHUNTS

Kristene K. Gugliuzza

STEP 1: SURGICAL ANATOMY

- The target of the venous portion of the procedure is the internal jugular vein. The vein sits in the minor supraclavicular fossa between the sternal and clavicular heads of the sterno-cleidomastoid muscle and the clavicle and under the platysma muscle. It is encased in the fibrous carotid sheath, independent of and anterior lateral to the carotid artery. The phrenic nerve is posterior lateral; the ansa cervicalis crosses lateral to medial at the level of the carotid artery bifurcation and above the omohyoid muscle; and the vagus nerve is posterior medial. On the left, under the clavicle is the thoracic duct, which crosses from medial to lateral and enters the subclavian vein **(Figure 92-1)**.

- The target of the peritoneal portion of the procedure is the peritoneum, or the confluence of the posterior fascia of the abdominal musculature with the peritoneum.

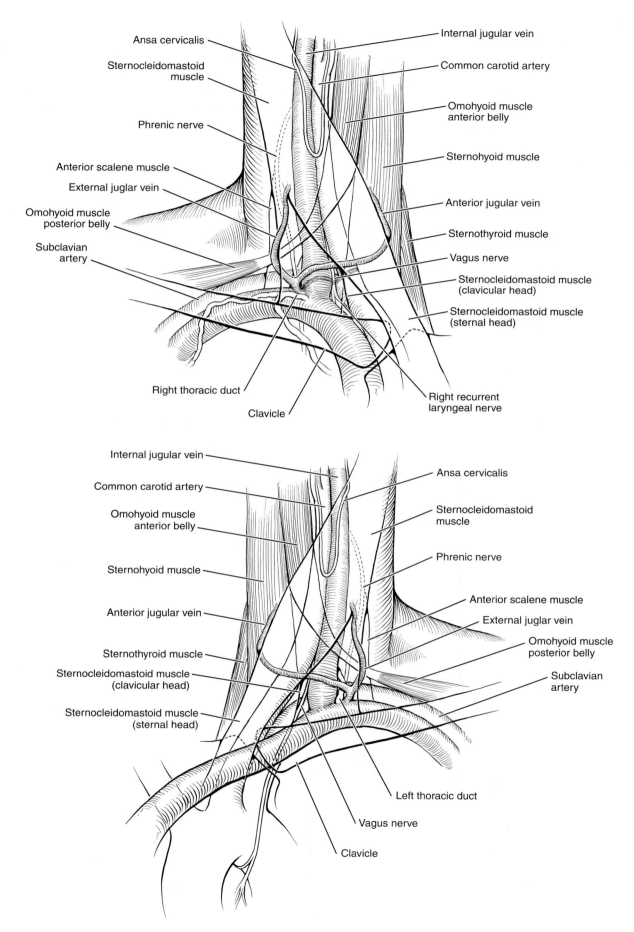

FIGURE 92–1

STEP 2: PREOPERATIVE CONSIDERATIONS

♦ The patient should be placed supine with the head rotated to the contralateral side from the planned incision. Left or right sides may be used, but care must be taken not to injure the thoracic duct on the left. A roll or bump under the flank may facilitate exposure of the lateral upper abdomen **(Figure 92-2, A).**

♦ If one of the jugular veins has been dissected or catheterized previously, using the other untouched vein may be prudent.

STEP 3: OPERATIVE STEPS

1. INCISION

♦ The patient is placed supine with the head rotated to the side opposite the vein being used. The patient is placed in a Trendelenburg position to engorge the vein by increasing the venous pressures. A roll or bump under the flank may facilitate exposure of the lateral upper abdomen. The venous incision is made approximately 1 fingerbreadth above the clavicle and between the two heads of the sternocleidomastoid muscle. The abdominal incision is made lateral to the rectus muscle, approximately 2 fingerbreadths below the costal margin and transversely for approximately 3 to 5 cm **(Figure 92-2, B).**

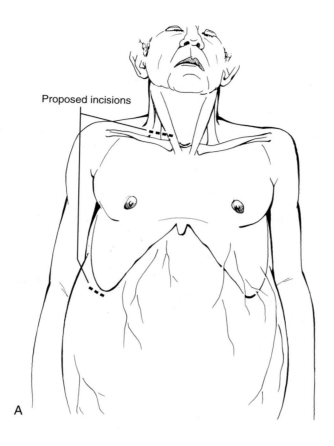

Proposed incisions

A

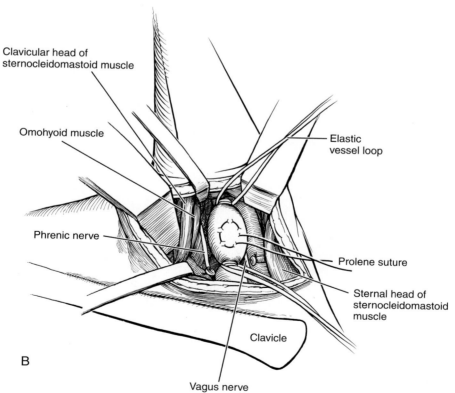

Clavicular head of
sternocleidomastoid muscle

Omohyoid muscle

Phrenic nerve

Elastic
vessel loop

Prolene suture

Sternal head of
sternocleidomastoid
muscle

Clavicle

B

Vagus nerve

FIGURE 92–2

2. DISSECTION

◆ The skin, subcutaneous fat, and platysma muscle are incised. The sternal and clavicular heads of the sternocleidomastoid muscle are split. The jugular vein is located lateral to the carotid artery and can be used as a landmark to facilitate the identification of the vein. The sheath that enwraps the vein keeps the vein from collapsing. This facilitates the circumferential dissection of the vein. If the dissection is close to the vein, damage to adjacent structures is minimal. The vein may have small tributaries coming into it, and disruption of these may cause a moderate amount of bleeding. Identification and ligation with division of these small vessels is advised. Elastic vessel loops are used proximally and distally to allow occlusion of the blood flow and control of the vessel in the operative field (see Figure 92-2, B).

◆ After the skin incision is made, the subcutaneous fat is incised to the muscle. A 0.5% to 1% solution of lidocaine is injected into the subcutaneous tract from the abdominal incision to the jugular incision. The tract should run laterally on the chest wall, outside the area of the breast and over the clavicle. Marking the route of the tract on the skin will help you stay on course when passing the catheter/shunt. Push a vascular tunneling device through the subcutaneous tissues deep to the skin but above the muscle fascia, following the tract that was injected with the anesthetic. Pull the shunt from the bottom up, taking care to orient the shunt correctly. Denver shunts have a one-way pump that should fit over the ribs. The LeVeen shunts have a multiperforated abdominal end and a venous end that can be cut to appropriate length **(Figure 92-3)**.

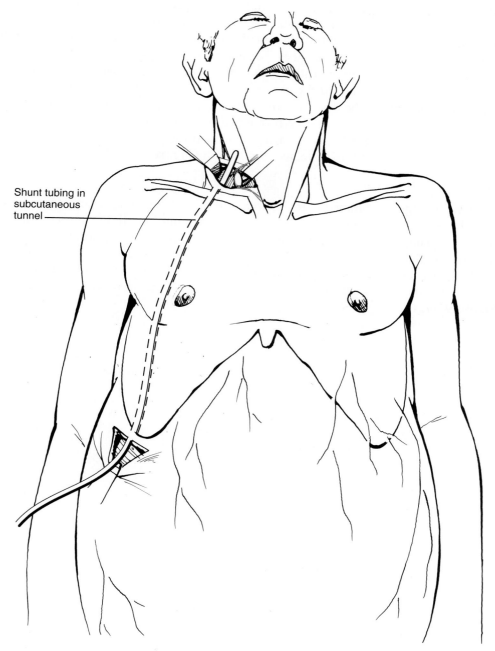

Shunt tubing in
subcutaneous
tunnel

FIGURE 92–3

◆ The muscle in the abdomen should be split to expose the peritoneum. A purse-string with a radius of 1 cm should be made in the peritoneum. Permanent suture is advised. Incision of the peritoneum within the purse-string is made with electrocautery or scissors. While the ascites is draining, place the intra-abdominal end of the shunt into the opening and thread the tubing into the peritoneal cavity. Secure the purse-string around the shunt. If using the LeVeen shunt, thread the entire catheter in until the disc is flush with the peritoneum. Connect the tubing running toward the neck incision to the port on the side of the abdominal disc. Secure the tube to the disc with a large tie. If using the Denver shunt, thread the catheter in until the "valve/pump" can be positioned over ribs 9 to 11. The subcutaneous tissue will have to be dissected to create a cavity to support the pump. The pump should be secured to the underlying tissue to avoid migration **(Figure 92-4, A).**

◆ Prime the tubing by aspirating at the venous end until there are no bubbles in the tubing. If using the Denver shunt, press the pump several times until the fluid comes out the end of the shunt. Clamp the tubing at the site where it enters the neck incision from below. Estimate the length of the venous end of the shunt by placing the tubing onto the sternum. Cut the tube at the point where it crosses the manubrium. Do not cut the tube at an angle, because the tube may push against the side wall of the vein and obstruct the fluid flow **(Figure 92-4, B).**

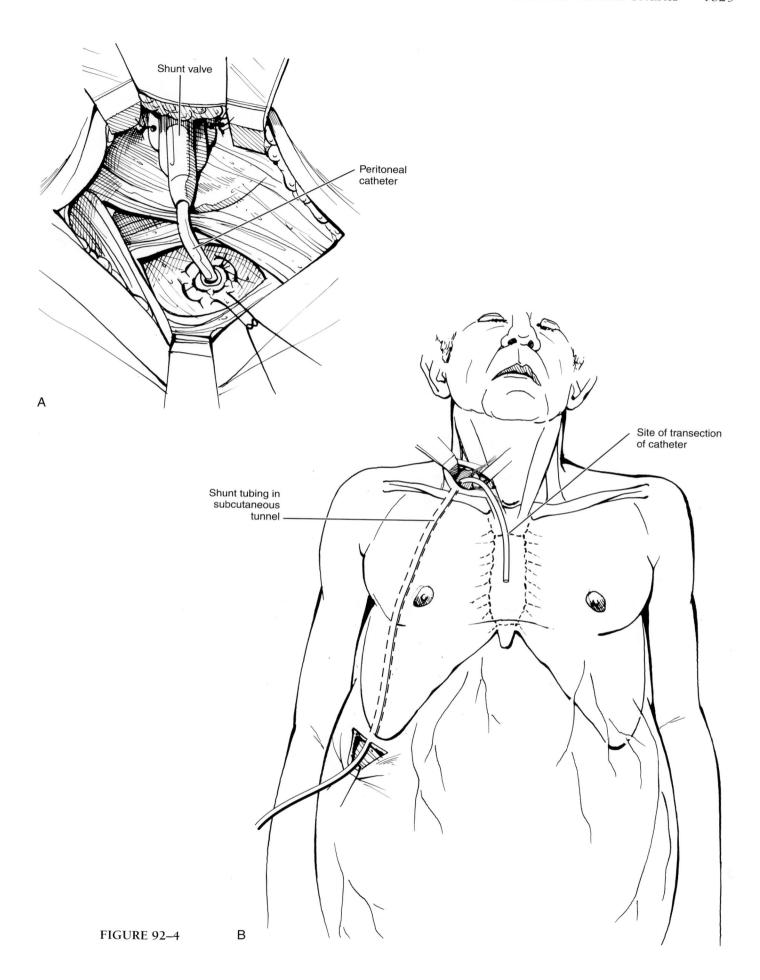

Shunt valve

Peritoneal catheter

Site of transection of catheter

Shunt tubing in subcutaneous tunnel

A

B

FIGURE 92–4

◆ Place a purse-string suture in the anterior wall of the jugular vein with Prolene suture (3-0 or 4-0). Occlude the vein with the elastic loops. Incise the vein within the purse-string. Raise the head of the patient to approximately 35 degrees. Keep the tubing clamped at skin level and tubing distal to the clamp filled with the ascitic fluid or heparinized saline (2500 U heparin in 250 mL normal saline).

◆ Hold the edge of the incised vein and insert the tubing. Take tension off the lower elastic loop to allow the tube to be advanced into the thorax. Secure the purse-string around the tubing **(Figure 92-5).**

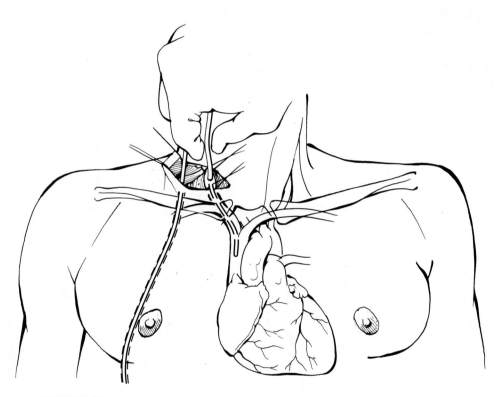

FIGURE 92–5

3. CLOSURE

◆ The course of the shunt should be from the peritoneal cavity, exiting out the abdomen and coursing along the lateral chest wall, across the clavicle to enter into the internal jugular vein, ending at the junction of the superior vena cava and right atrium. All wounds should be closed in two layers over the foreign body (the shunt) **(Figure 92-6)**.

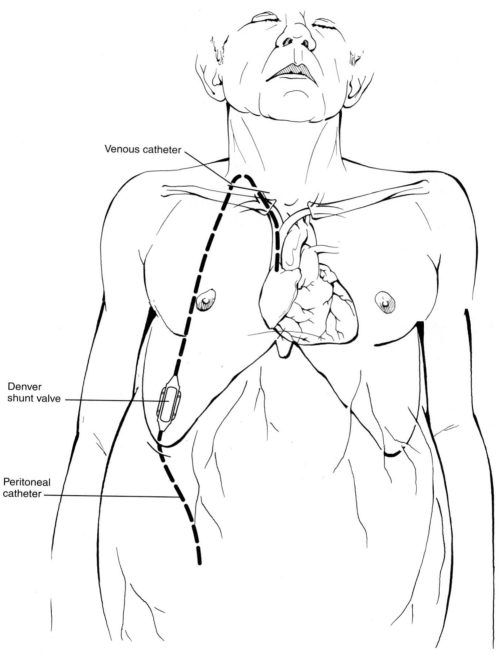

FIGURE 92–6

STEP 4: POSTOPERATIVE CARE

◆ The patient should be admitted for an overnight stay. The potential problems are fever, fluid overload, and disseminated intravascular coagulation (DIC). Fever is usually transient and treated symptomatically. The identification of infection occurs in approximately 5% of those patients with fever and warrants treatment. Pulmonary edema occurs in approximately 10% of the patients but usually can be handled with diuretics. DIC is usually subclinical and can be treated expectantly. The worst case scenario is fulminant bleeding, which requires removal of the shunt. The bleeding may be related to exposure of the systemic circulation to fibrin split products (FSP)–rich ascitic fluid that may activate the coagulation mechanism. Bleeding complications do not appear to be related to the severity of the post-shunt coagulopathy but rather to the severity of liver dysfunction and presence of preoperative DIC, probably caused by the liver disease.

STEP 5: PEARLS AND PITFALLS

◆ The contraindications for shunt insertion should include pseudomyxoma peritonei, recent or current infection, preoperative coagulopathy, liver failure, and loculated ascites. Relative contraindications include positive cytologic findings in ascitic fluid and concurrent cardiac failure. Bloody ascites and ascitic fluid protein content greater than 4.5 g/L are also considered contraindications to shunting, secondary to increased risk of shunt blockage from clot or fibrin plugs.

◆ If a patient has had episodes of variceal bleeding, the risk of rebleeding postshunt is great secondary to the risk of postshunt coagulopathy and increased intravascular volume.

SELECTED REFERENCES

1. Smith EM, Jayson GC: The current and future management of malignant ascites. Clin Oncol (R Coll Radiol) 2003;15:59-72.
2. Becker G, Galandi D, Blum HE: Malignant ascites: Systematic review and guideline for treatment. Eur J Cancer 2006;42:589-597.
3. Suzuki H, Stanley AJ: Current management and novel therapeutic strategies for refractory ascites and hepatorenal syndrome. QJM 2001;94:293-300.

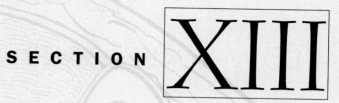
AMPUTATIONS

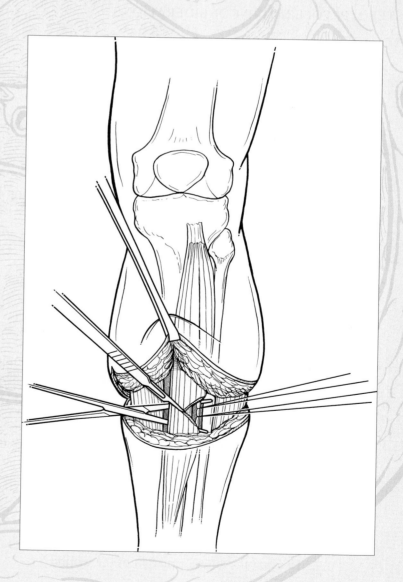

CHAPTER 93

BELOW-KNEE AMPUTATION

Arthur P. Sanford

STEP 1: SURGICAL ANATOMY

- Cross-sectional anatomy of the lower leg is shown in **Figure 93-1, A.**

STEP 2: PREOPERATIVE CONSIDERATIONS

- Selection of level for amputation depends on the underlying pathology and the need to ascertain efficient wound healing of the amputation stump.

- Below-knee amputation stumps do not rely on a symmetrical flap closure, but rather the posterior flap with extensive musculature is to be brought anteriorly.

- Use of a tourniquet is at the discretion of the surgeon.

STEP 3: OPERATIVE STEPS

1. INCISION

- Planning the level of incision begins by determining the bony structures to preserve, typically 2 to 3 fingerbreadths below the tibial tuberosity **(Figure 93-1, B).**

- From this landmark, skin flaps are developed, typically the midpoint of the leg in an anterior to posterior plane is identified, just below this level.

- The anterior flap is incised anteriorly.

- The posterior flap is incised as a semicircle, at its apex with a length equal to the distance to reach the anterior margin of the wound.

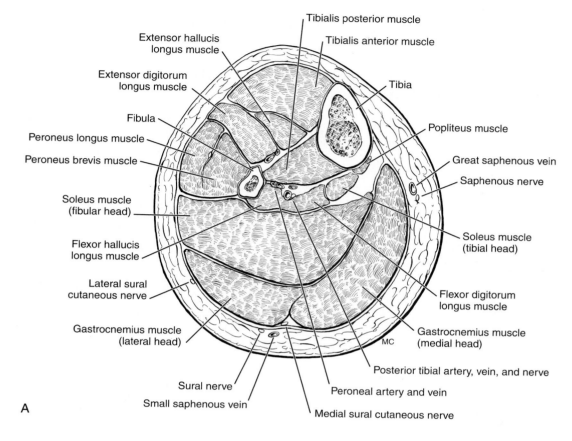

Tibialis posterior muscle

Extensor hallucis
longus muscle

Tibialis anterior muscle

Extensor digitorum
longus muscle

Tibia

Fibula

Popliteus muscle

Peroneus longus muscle

Peroneus brevis muscle

Great saphenous vein

Saphenous nerve

Soleus muscle
(fibular head)

Soleus muscle
(tibial head)

Flexor hallucis
longus muscle

Lateral sural
cutaneous nerve

Flexor digitorum
longus muscle

Gastrocnemius muscle
(lateral head)

Gastrocnemius muscle
(medial head)

MC

Posterior tibial artery, vein, and nerve

Sural nerve

Peroneal artery and vein

Small saphenous vein

Medial sural cutaneous nerve

A

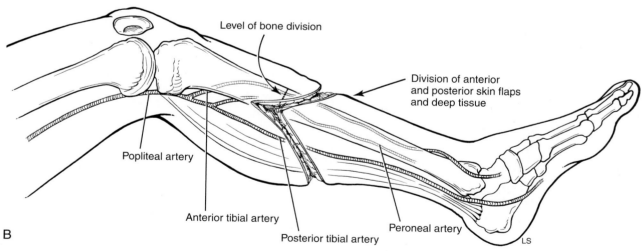

Level of bone division

Division of anterior
and posterior skin flaps
and deep tissue

Popliteal artery

Anterior tibial artery

Peroneal artery

Posterior tibial artery

LS

B

FIGURE 93–1

2. DISSECTION

◆ Divide the anterior compartment with an amputation knife, down to the interosseous membrane, taking care to ligate the anterior tibial artery **(Figure 93-2).**

◆ Expose minimal lengths of tibia and fibula with periosteal elevation, because this compromises the blood supply to bony segments.

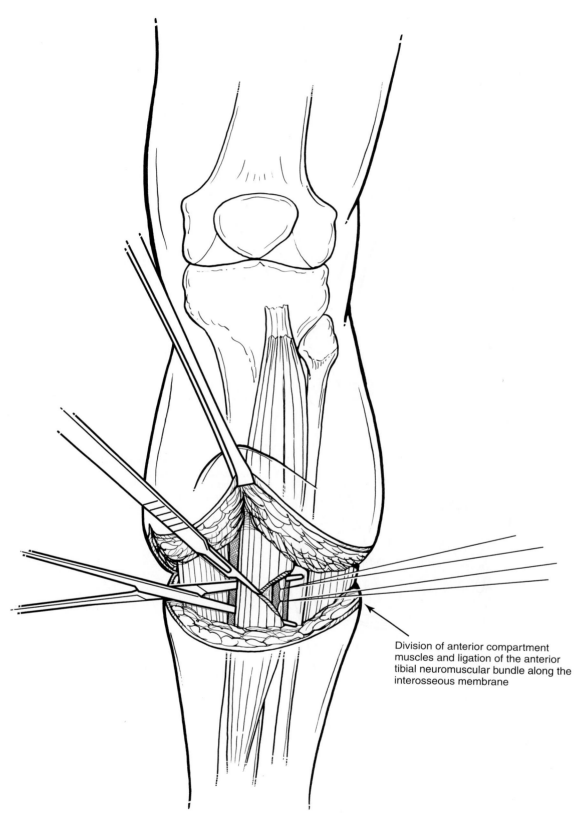

Division of anterior compartment muscles and ligation of the anterior tibial neuromuscular bundle along the interosseous membrane

FIGURE 93–2

◆ Divide the tibia and fibula using a bone saw and beveling the anterior surface, taking the fibula more proximally, because this will not be a weight-bearing component of the amputation stump **(Figures 93-3 through 93-6).**

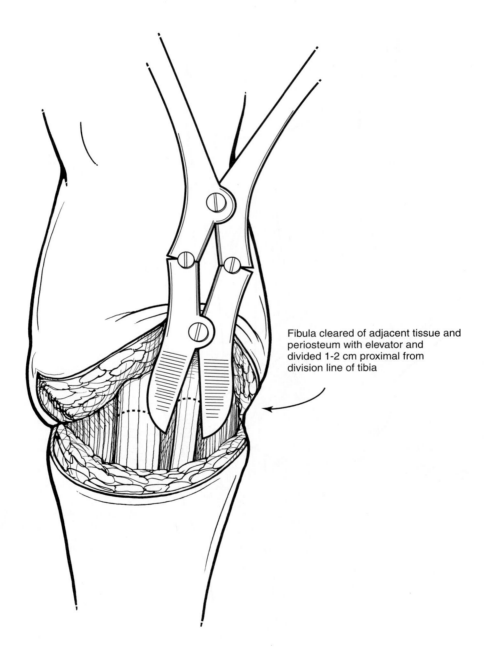

Fibula cleared of adjacent tissue and periosteum with elevator and divided 1-2 cm proximal from division line of tibia

FIGURE 93–3

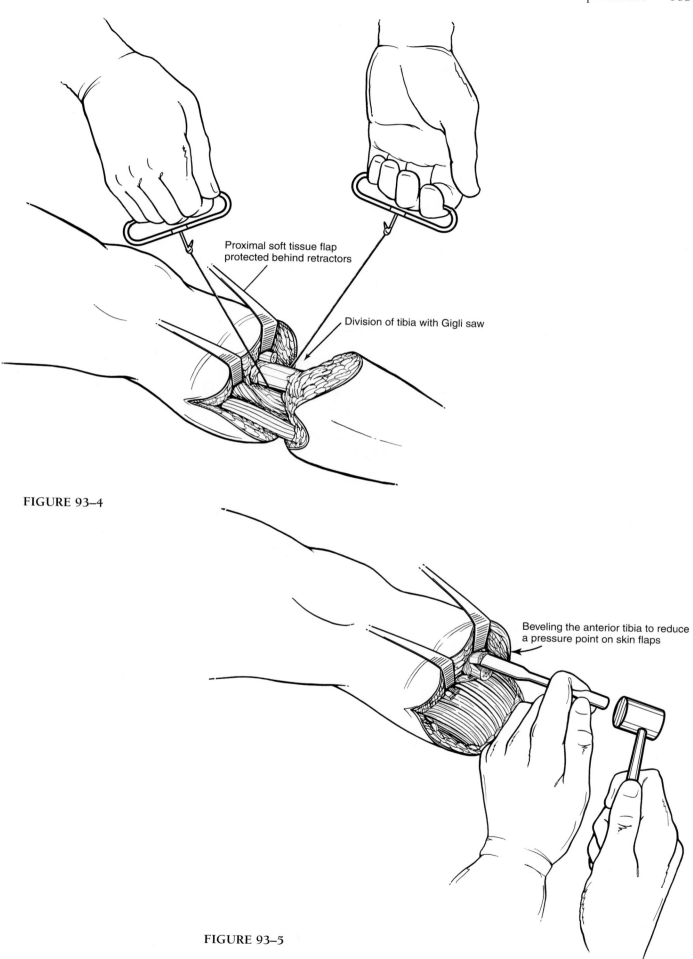

Proximal soft tissue flap
protected behind retractors

Division of tibia with Gigli saw

FIGURE 93–4

Beveling the anterior tibia to reduce
a pressure point on skin flaps

FIGURE 93–5

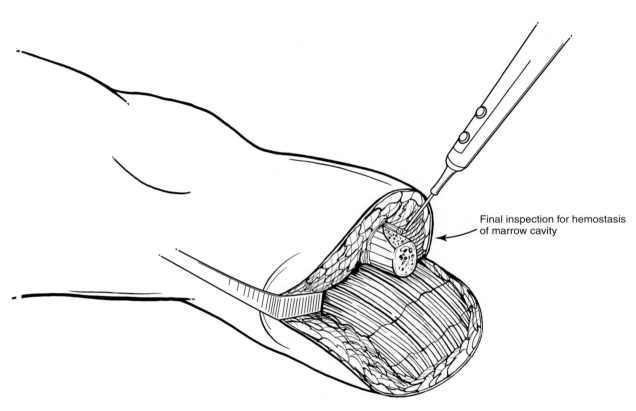

Final inspection for hemostasis of marrow cavity

FIGURE 93–6

◆ Identify and ligate posterior compartment vessels short of the wound (**Figure 93-7**).

◆ Similarly, identify and strip nerves short, and allow retraction to prevent neuromas in the closed wound.

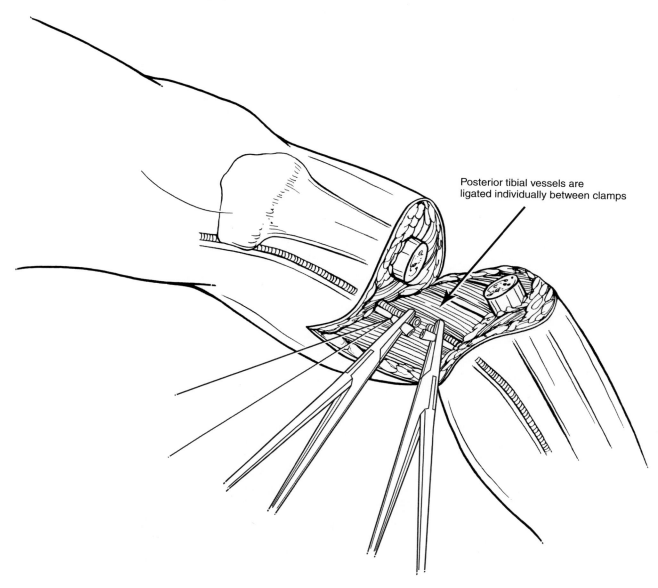

Posterior tibial vessels are ligated individually between clamps

FIGURE 93–7

◆ Use the amputation knife to divide the posterior compartment between the level of dissection and the tip of the posterior flap **(Figure 93-8)**.

3. CLOSING

◆ Use absorbable sutures to approximate the fascia of the muscle posteriorly to the pretibial fascia, closing the deep structures **(Figure 93-9)**.

◆ Close the skin with either surgical staples or nonabsorbable sutures **(Figure 93-10)**.

◆ Closed-suction drains may be used at the discretion of the surgeon.

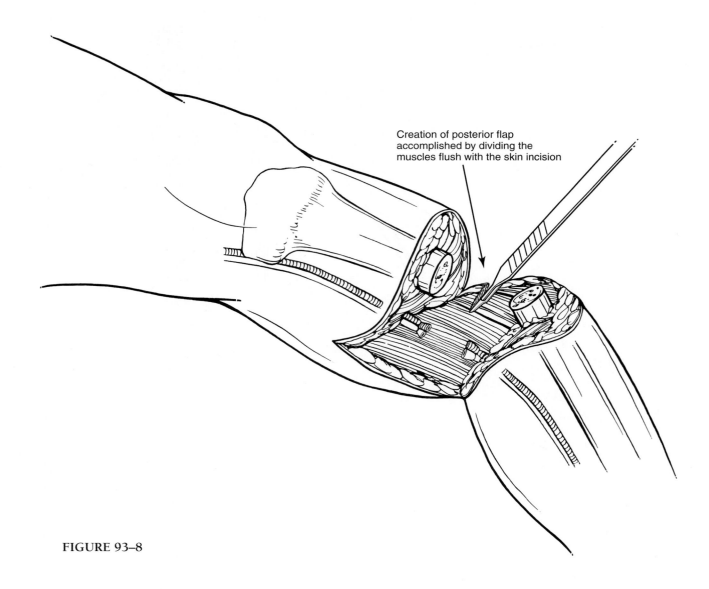

Creation of posterior flap accomplished by dividing the muscles flush with the skin incision

FIGURE 93–8

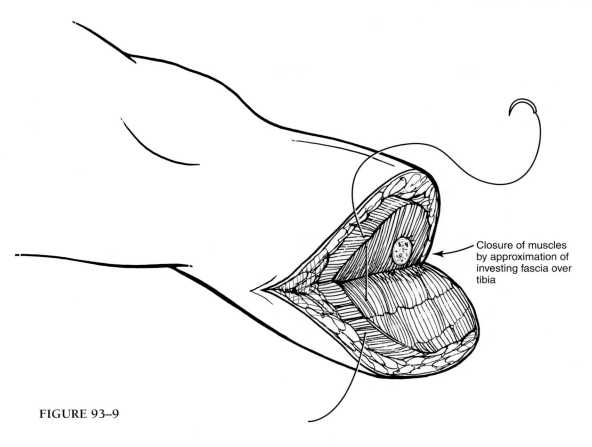

Closure of muscles by approximation of investing fascia over tibia

FIGURE 93–9

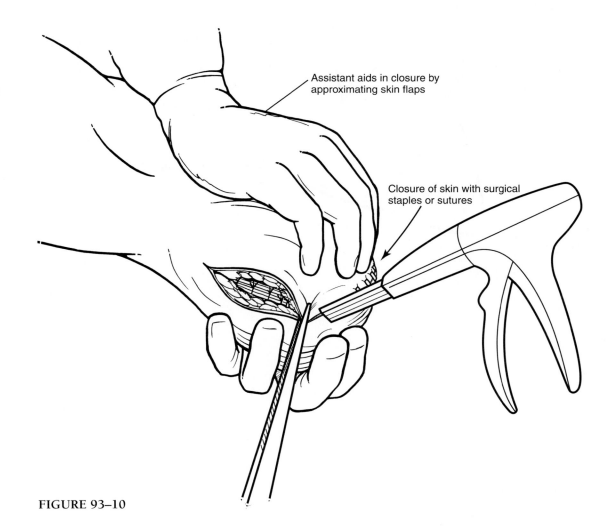

Assistant aids in closure by approximating skin flaps

Closure of skin with surgical staples or sutures

FIGURE 93–10

STEP 4: POSTOPERATIVE CARE

◆ Use posterior knee extension splints to keep the knee joint in extension for use in prosthesis **(Figure 93-11).**

◆ Use "stump shapers" or elastic wraps to shape the amputation stump into a cone shape to facilitate prosthetic socket fitment.

◆ Skin sutures or staples are typically left in place for extended periods of time to allow the wound to adequately heal.

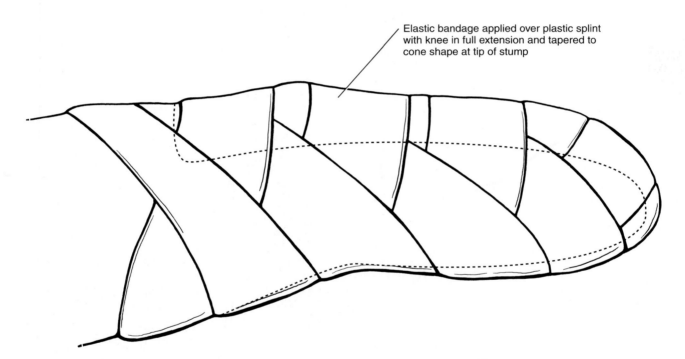

Elastic bandage applied over plastic splint with knee in full extension and tapered to cone shape at tip of stump

FIGURE 93–11

STEP 5: PEARLS AND PITFALLS

- Creation of a posterior flap initially with excess tissue allows the surgeon to trim and tailor the flap, removing redundant tissue and providing adequate soft tissue coverage.

- When the patient is ambulating on the below-knee amputation stump, the socket is typically designed to not bear weight on the distal tip of the tibia but to distribute the load over a large area below the knee.

SELECTED REFERENCE

1. Lower-extremity amputation for ischemia. In Wilmore D, Cheung LY, Harken AH, et al (eds): ACS Surgery Principles & Practice. New York, WebMD, 2002, pp 934-956.

CHAPTER 94

SUPRACONDYLAR AMPUTATION

Jong O. Lee

STEP 1: SURGICAL ANATOMY

- ◆ A comprehensive understanding of the anatomy of the thigh and knowledge of the pre-existing level of circulation is critical before undertaking amputation of the leg.

- ◆ **Figure 94-1** demonstrates key anatomic structures that must be considered with supracondylar amputation, including the relationship of the femur with the surrounding vessels.

STEP 2: PREOPERATIVE CONSIDERATIONS

- ◆ Select the level of amputation that will optimize healing and preserve as much function as possible.

- ◆ The indications for supracondylar amputations include the following:
  - ◆ Nonambulatory, debilitated patient with indication for amputation with high risk for developing flexion contracture of the knee after below-knee amputation.
  - ◆ Debilitated patients with knee joint contracture and/or nonviable calf muscle or skin for creation of the below-knee flap.
  - ◆ Failure of a bypass graft.
  - ◆ Failure of below-knee amputation.
  - ◆ Severe ischemia, necrosis, infection, joint contractures, neoplasm, trauma, and crush injuries involving the calf or distal thigh may preclude performing below-knee amputation.

- ◆ A vascular study should be obtained to determine whether below-knee amputation can be attempted.

- ◆ Objective evidence that the selected level is one at which primary healing is likely to occur should be established.

- ◆ The most common level for supracondylar amputation is at the midfemur. Objective evidence that the selected level is one at which primary healing is likely to occur should be established.

- ◆ Preservation of the length of the femur results in better function.

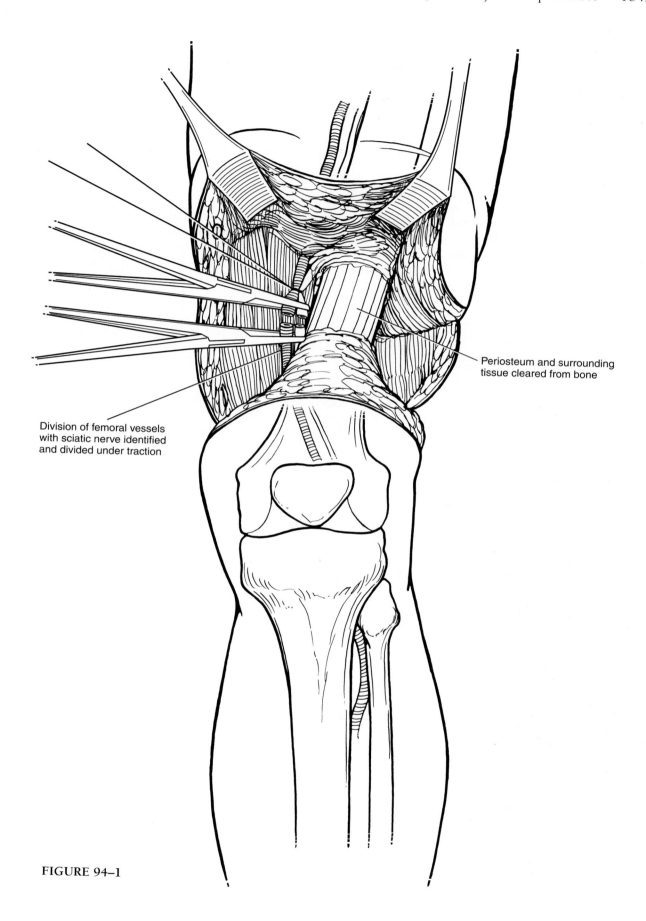

Periosteum and surrounding
tissue cleared from bone

Division of femoral vessels
with sciatic nerve identified
and divided under traction

FIGURE 94–1

STEP 3: OPERATIVE STEPS

1. INCISION

◆ Proper positioning of the patient is supine. A roll can be placed under the thigh to position the leg.

◆ The incision must be carefully planned to allow optimal skin flap for closure. The fish-mouth–shaped incision is made using equal length posterior and anterior flaps. The corners of the fish-mouth incision should be at the level of the amputation of the femur. The length of the flaps should be approximately two thirds of the diameter of the thigh at that level **(Figure 94-2)**.

◆ The length of the flaps should be sufficient to provide secure, tension-free closure over the femoral stump.

◆ The skin incision is made and extended through the subcutaneous tissue and the fascia over the underlying muscle at the same level of the skin incision. The muscles are divided using electrocautery at least 5 cm distal to the intended site of femur amputation and are allowed to retract.

◆ The anterior femoral muscles are divided first followed by the medial femoral muscles. The posterior femoral muscles are divided last.

◆ A clamp can be used under the muscles to retract them and place them under traction.

◆ The muscle flaps should be longer if myodesis/myoplasty is planned.

2. DISSECTION

◆ As muscles are divided, the nerves and vessels are identified.
  ◆ The femoral artery and vein are found deep in the anterior medial thigh, lying adjacent to the femur.
  ◆ The femoral artery and vein are isolated, double clamped, suture ligated, and divided (see Figure 94-1).
  ◆ The sciatic nerve is identified between the adductor magnus and biceps femoris muscles. The nerve is placed on a gentle traction, ligated proximately, sharply divided, and allowed to retract.
  ◆ The sciatic nerve contains relatively large arteries and therefore should be ligated.

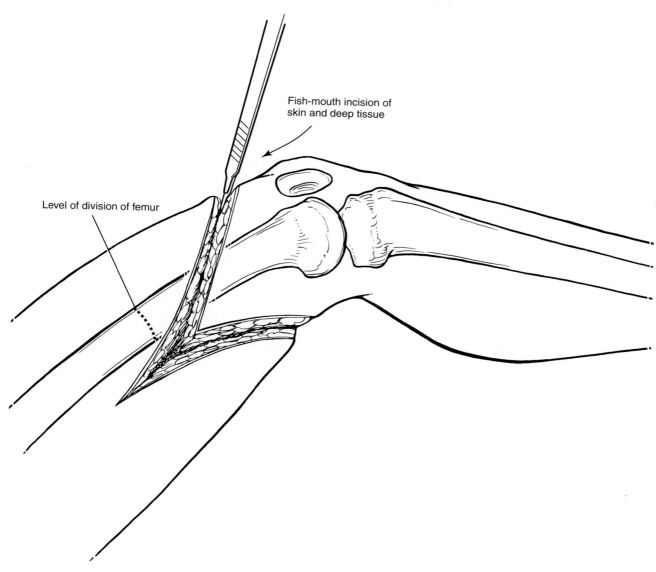

FIGURE 94–2

- The femur is divided using a saw.
  - After anterior muscles are divided, the periosteum of the femur is incised circumferentially and is cleared approximately 2 cm distally. The femur is divided immediately distal to the periosteal incision.
  - The level of the femur resection is identified by cutting the periosteum, but periosteum should not be stripped from the femur. Stripping periosteum from the femur may result in loss of blood supply to the exposed bone.
  - The femur is divided at least 3 to 5 cm proximal to the line of skin incision.
  - The edges of the bone should be rasped to form a smooth contour.
  - Divided muscles are retracted superiorly for better exposure during resection **(Figure 94-3).**
  - An oscillating power saw or Gigli saw is used to divide the femur (see Figure 94-3).

3. MYODESIS/MYOPLASTY

- A long quadriceps flap with its fascia can be sutured to the posterior fascia and major muscle groups.

- Several small holes ($\frac{7}{64}$ inch) are placed through the cortex of the distal end of the femur $\frac{3}{8}$ inch from the distal cut end of the femur. Loop mattress sutures are placed through the major muscle groups and drawn through the holes.

- The adductor and hamstring muscles are sutured to and across the end of the femur through the drill holes. The femur is kept in adduction as the adductors are tied down.

- The femur should be in full extension as the quadriceps are secured to avoid hip flexion contracture.

- Myodesis or myoplasty is performed in a nonischemic limb. It is avoided in ischemic limbs because of increased risk of wound breakdown.

- If myodesis is planned, the posterior muscle flaps are left 2 inches longer than the level of bony transection. If both myodesis and myoplasty are planned, all muscle groups are left long.

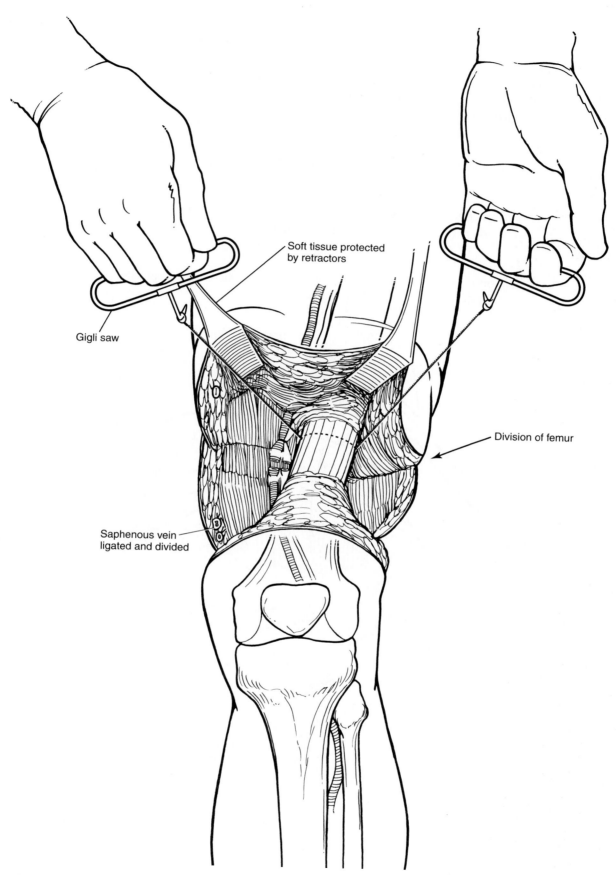

Soft tissue protected by retractors

Gigli saw

Division of femur

Saphenous vein ligated and divided

FIGURE 94–3

4. CLOSING

◆ The wound is irrigated. Once hemostasis is achieved, closure is performed by first approximating the fascias of the anterior and posterior flaps using interrupted 2-0 Vicryl sutures **(Figure 94-4).**

◆ If there is persistent oozing, a drain is placed.

◆ The skin edges of the two flaps are approximated with 3-0 nylon sutures in interrupted fashion or with staples **(Figure 94-5),** which are left in for 3 weeks.

◆ After soft dressings are applied, splints may be applied. To prevent flexion contracture of the hip, pillows are not used for support.

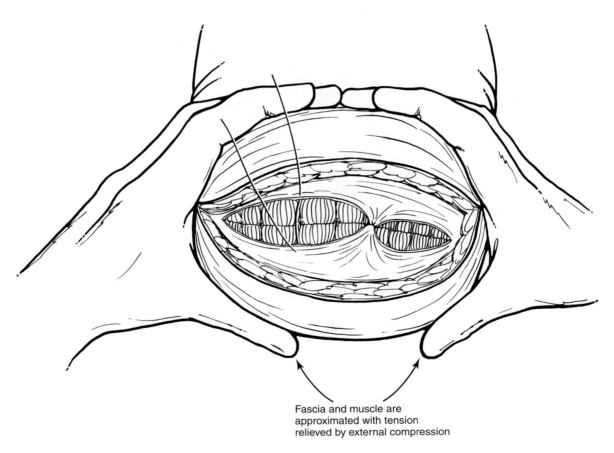

Fascia and muscle are
approximated with tension
relieved by external compression

FIGURE 94–4

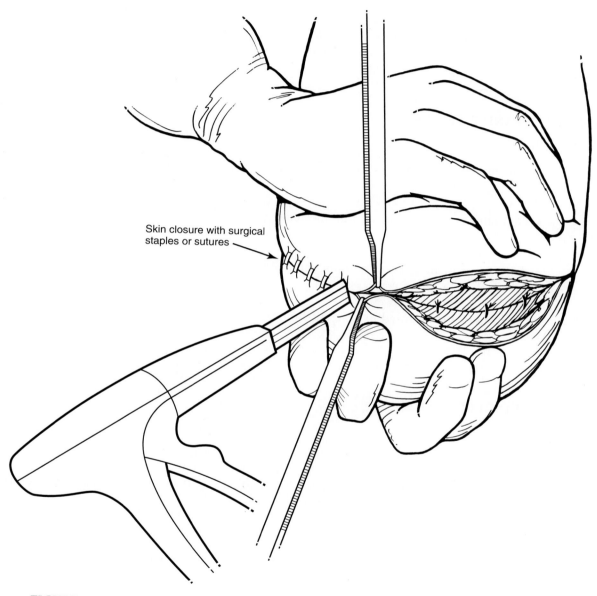

Skin closure with surgical staples or sutures

FIGURE 94–5

STEP 4: POSTOPERATIVE CARE

- Complications include hematoma, infection, wound necrosis, and contractures.

- A drain may be used if there is persistent oozing.

- One of the most immediate postoperative complications can be wound hematoma, which occurs in a small percentage of patients.
  - Small hematomas can be observed.
  - Large hematomas may need to be drained.

STEP 5: PEARLS AND PITFALLS

- It is imperative to handle tissues gently and attain absolute hemostasis.

- Guillotine amputation is used in infected leg or sepsis.

- A tourniquet can be used in nonischemic limbs.

- A tourniquet is not used in ischemic limbs.

SELECTED REFERENCES

1. Fisher DF: Lower extremity amputations. In Baker RJ, Fischer JE (eds): Mastery of Surgery, 4th ed. Philadelphia, Lippincott Williams & Wilkins, 2001, pp 2191-2198.
2. Carnesale PG: Amputations of lower extremity. In Carnale ST (ed): Campbell's Operative Orthopaedics, 10th ed. Philadelphia, Mosby, 2002, pp 575-586.
3. Anderson KM: Knee disarticulation and above-knee amputation. Oper Tech Gen Surg 2005;7:90-95.

CHAPTER 95

TRANSMETATARSAL AMPUTATION

Michael D. Trahan

INTRODUCTION

- Transmetatarsal amputation may be indicated for ischemic tissue loss and/or infection of the great toe or several toes. Infection that extends proximal to the metatarsophalangeal crease or involving the deep tissues of the foot will likely need a higher level of amputation.

STEP 1: SURGICAL ANATOMY

- The pertinent anatomy of the foot and lower leg is illustrated in **Figure 95-1**.

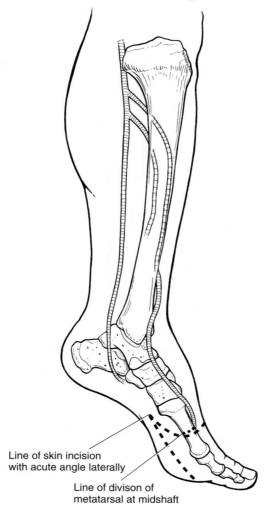

Line of skin incision
with acute angle laterally

Line of divison of
metatarsal at midshaft

FIGURE 95–1

STEP 2: PREOPERATIVE CONSIDERATIONS

♦ General, spinal, or regional anesthesia may be selected when appropriate.

STEP 3: OPERATIVE STEPS

1. INCISION

♦ The proposed incision is mapped on the foot. Dorsally, the incision is slightly curved just distal to the midshaft of the metatarsal bones. The plantar flap extends to the metatarsophalangeal crease (**Figure 95-2**).

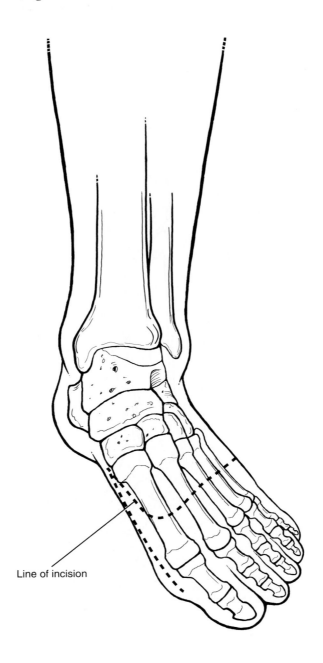

Line of incision

FIGURE 95–2

2. DISSECTION

♦ The incision is begun on the dorsal surface of the foot directly down to the level of the bone without undermining the flaps. As the medial and lateral extents of the dorsal flap are reached, the plantar incision is begun, leaving an acute angulation to avoid dog ears with closure. Soft tissue coverage of the metatarsals will be provided by the long plantar flap.

♦ Once hemostasis has been achieved, the small-bladed oscillating saw is used to divide the metatarsal bones approximately 1 cm proximal to the dorsal skin flap, starting with the first metatarsal **(Figure 95-3)**. The second metatarsal shaft is cut at the same level as the first, and the remaining metatarsals are cut 3 mm shorter than the first two. The oscillating saw is used to avoid splintering of the bones. The cut edges are smoothed with a rasp.

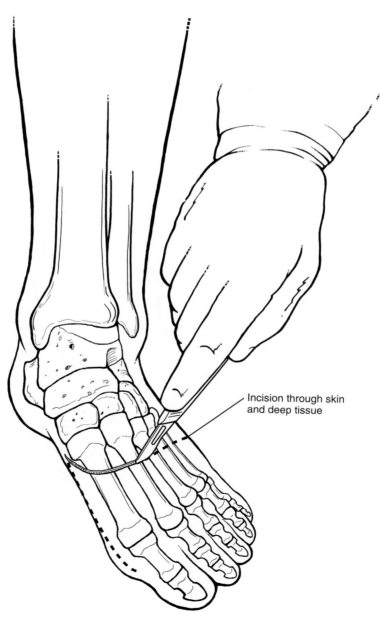

Incision through skin and deep tissue

FIGURE 95–3

◆ The plantar soft tissues are divided to release the amputated segment. The tendons are placed on stretch and cut short so that they retract into the stump **(Figure 95-4)**.

◆ Redundant and devitalized soft tissues of the planter flap are trimmed and hemostasis is ensured. An estimation of the tension on the closed flap is made, and if necessary, the metatarsal bones are trimmed further **(Figure 95-5)**.

3. CLOSING

◆ The superficial fascia may be approximated with 2-0 interrupted absorbable sutures.

◆ Skin staples or 2-0 vertical mattress permanent sutures are placed to close the wound and are left in place until complete healing is certain **(Figure 95-6)**.

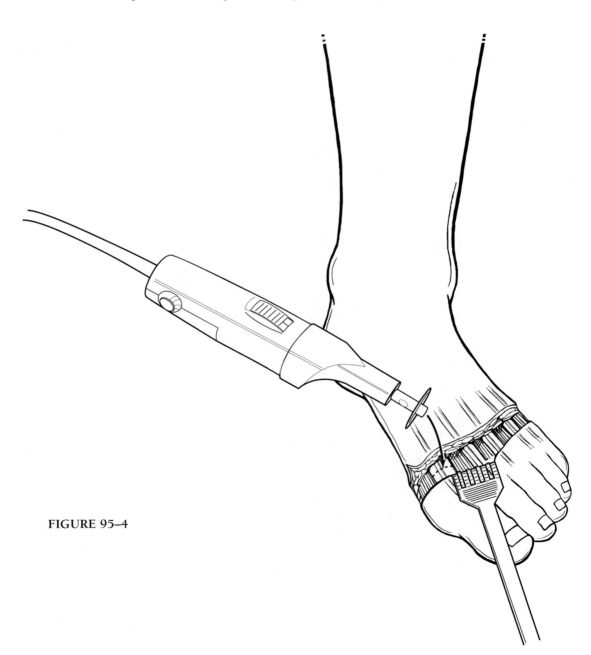

FIGURE 95–4

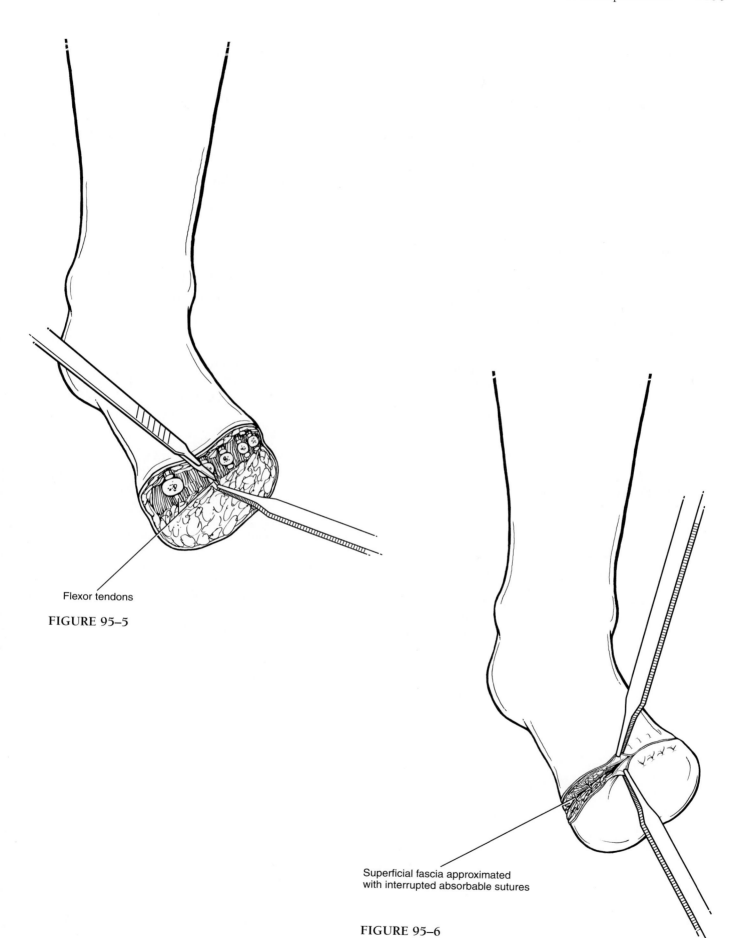

Flexor tendons

FIGURE 95–5

Superficial fascia approximated
with interrupted absorbable sutures

FIGURE 95–6

STEP 4: POSTOPERATIVE CARE

- A sturdy dressing such as a well-padded cast will help limit postoperative edema and protect the stump. The stump should be inspected at least weekly to assess for viability and infection.

- The patient should avoid weight bearing on the extremity until the wound is safely healed.

STEP 5: PEARLS AND PITFALLS

- Careful attention to hemostasis, debridement of devitalized tissue, and tension-free closure will help ensure the optimal outcome.

- In the setting of a contaminated wound, the stump may be left open to heal by secondary intention or subsequent grafting. Premature closure of a contaminated stump will likely result in further soft tissue loss and necessitate a higher level of amputation.

SELECTED REFERENCES

1. Durham JR, McCoy DM, Sawchuk AP, et al: Open transmetatarsal amputation in the treatment of severe foot infections. Am J Surg 1989;158:127-130.
2. Dwars BJ, van den Broek TA, Rauwerda JA, Bakker FC: Criteria for reliable selection of the lowest possible level of amputation in peripheral vascular disease. J Vasc Surg 1992;15:536-542.
3. McKittrick LS, McKittrick JB, Risley TS: Transmetatarsal amputation for infection or gangrene in patients with diabetes mellitus. Ann Surg 1949;130:826-842.
4. Effeney DJ, Lim RC, Schecter WP: Transmetatarsal amputation. Arch Surg 1977;112:1366-1370.

CHAPTER 96

HIP DISARTICULATION

Celia Chao and Courtney M. Townsend, Jr.

INDICATION

- Hip disarticulation is performed for malignant soft tissue or bony tumors of the proximal thigh region (below the lesser trochanter of the femur) in which negative margins cannot be achieved without a less radical operation. Most sarcomas can be treated with limb-sparing procedures and the use of adjuvant or neoadjuvant therapies. In general, bone and vessels can be resected and replaced with grafts. Sacrifice of a single nerve, either the femoral nerve or the sciatic nerve, would result in some neuromuscular dysfunction but is preferable to amputation. This operation may be appropriate in locally recurrent cases of extensive (unresectable) tumor involvement (usually when adjuvant radiotherapy options have already been exhausted).

- This procedure can also be considered for massive trauma and crush injury to the lower extremity or following multiple failed vascular procedures and distal amputations.

STEP 1: SURGICAL ANATOMY

- See Figure 96-2 for illustration of key anterior structures. See Figures 96-4 and 96-5 for the posterior lateral anatomy, which must be considered with hip disarticulation.

STEP 2: PREOPERATIVE CONSIDERATIONS

- Magnetic resonance imaging of soft tissue tumors of the proximal thigh can delineate the extent of tumor involvement relative to muscular compartments, neurovascular bundles, and bony structures. A bone scan is useful to ensure that the acetabulum and pelvis are not involved with tumor. A Tru-Cut needle biopsy or an open biopsy should have already been performed to confirm the malignant nature of the tumor and the necessity of such a radical operation.

- A complete neurologic examination of the involved extremity may reveal significant loss of function and intractable pain preoperatively.

- General anesthesia is used.

STEP 3: OPERATIVE STEPS

1. INCISION

◆ A Foley catheter is placed in the bladder. The patient is positioned in the lateral decubitus position to provide adequate exposure for both anterior and posterior aspects of the thigh **(Figure 96-1)**. A bean bag may be used to help maintain this position. The skin is prepped from midchest down to the toes. The extremity below the thigh can be covered with a stockinette, such that the entire leg can be manipulated and repositioned intraoperatively to facilitate the resection.

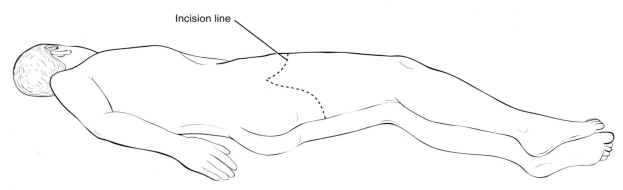

Incision line

FIGURE 96–1

◆ Anteriorly, a skin incision is made approximately 3 cm below the inguinal ligament. The posterior skin flap is much longer. It is approximately 6 to 8 cm below the anterior incision to facilitate a fish-mouth closure at the lateral and medial corners (**Figure 96-2**; see also Figure 96-1).

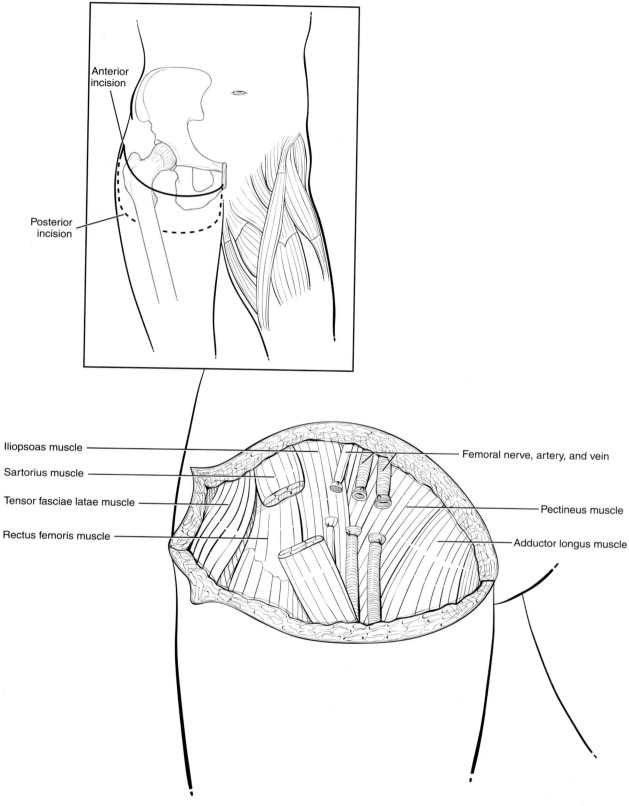

FIGURE 96–2

2. DISSECTION

◆ After dissecting past Scarpa's fascia, the surgeon creates the anterior flap. The femoral vessels are identified below the inguinal ligament and are serially divided and suture ligated. The femoral nerve and the sartorius muscles, lateral to the vessels, are also divided. The femoral nerve should be on gentle traction and ligated just as it exits the inguinal ligament. The residual nerve will retract beneath the external oblique aponeurosis. If a neuroma forms, it should be well away from the weight-bearing portion of the stump. Muscles lateral to the vessels are identified and include the iliopsoas and the rectus femoris. The insertion of the iliopsoas onto the less trochanter is divided with electrocautery, preserving most of the proximal aspects of the muscle **(Figure 96-3)**.

◆ Medially, a finger is passed beneath the pectineus muscle, and the muscle can be released from its origin on the pubis using electrocautery. Continuing medially, the surgeon transects the adductor magnus and brevis muscles and the gracilis muscles at their origin on the symphysis pubis, exposing the obturator externus muscle **(Figures 96-4 and 96-5)**. Beneath the pectineus and adductor muscles, branches of the obturator nerve and vessels are identified and ligated. The tendinous insertion of the obturator externus muscle is cut at its insertion into the lesser trochanter.

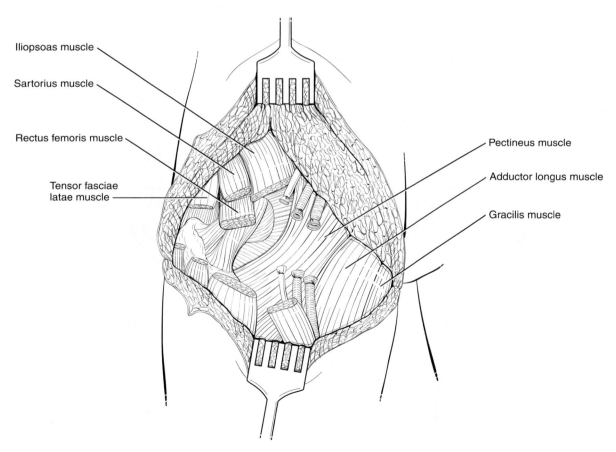

FIGURE 96–3

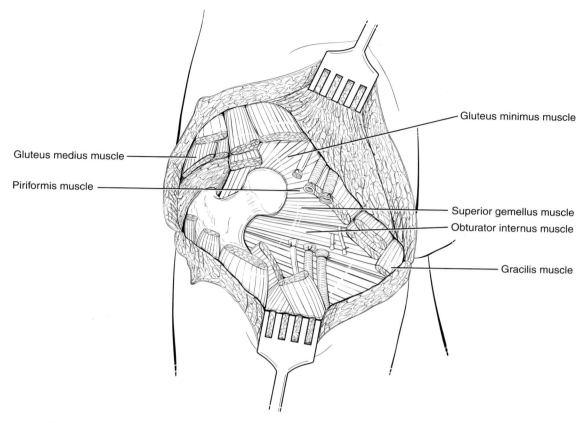

Gluteus minimus muscle

Gluteus medius muscle

Piriformis muscle

Superior gemellus muscle

Obturator internus muscle

Gracilis muscle

FIGURE 96–4

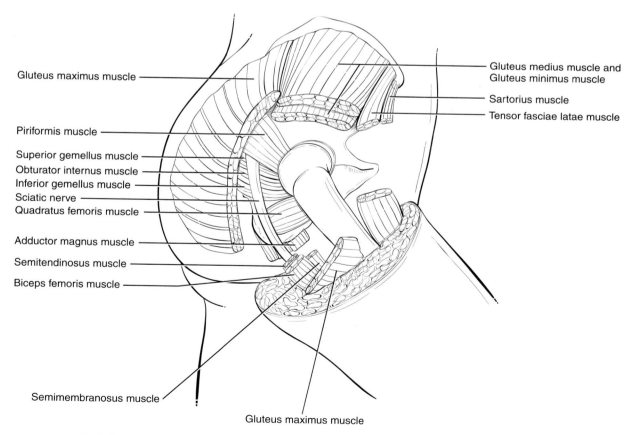

Gluteus maximus muscle

Gluteus medius muscle and
Gluteus minimus muscle

Sartorius muscle

Tensor fasciae latae muscle

Piriformis muscle

Superior gemellus muscle

Obturator internus muscle

Inferior gemellus muscle

Sciatic nerve

Quadratus femoris muscle

Adductor magnus muscle

Semitendinosus muscle

Biceps femoris muscle

Semimembranosus muscle

Gluteus maximus muscle

FIGURE 96–5

◆ Posterior laterally, the tensor fasciae latae muscle is incised below the anterior aspect of the gluteus maximus. This muscle is divided at its insertion to the gluteal tuberosity. The gluteus medius and minimus, piriformis, gemellus, and obturator externus muscles are divided near their insertion to the greater trochanter. The capsule of the hip joint is opened to expose the neck and head of the femur (see Figure 96-5).

◆ The sciatic nerve is transected high, just below the piriformis muscle, and allowed to retract beneath this muscle (**Figure 96-6**). The insertions of the obturator internus and quadratus femoris to the greater trochanter are divided. The origins of the hamstring muscles are divided off the ischial tuberosity: semimembranosus, semitendinosus, and long head of the biceps. The extremity can be removed once the ligamentum capitis femoris is divided between the head of the femur and the acetabulum (**Figure 96-7**).

◆ The wound is irrigated and a suction drainage catheter is positioned in the resection bed.

Resection Bed

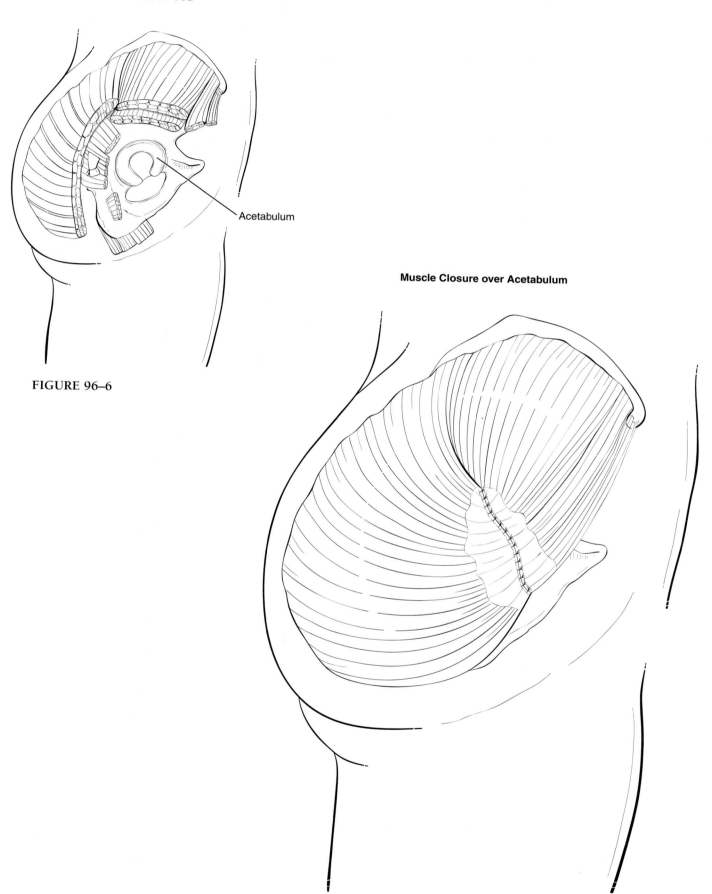

Acetabulum

FIGURE 96–6

Muscle Closure over Acetabulum

FIGURE 96–7

3. CLOSING

◆ The posterior muscles (quadratus femoris) can be approximated to anterior muscles (iliopsoas) to cover the exposed acetabulum using 2-0 Vicryl interrupted absorbable sutures (see Figure 96-7).

◆ The residual obturator externus and gluteus muscles can be reapproximated together. The posterior flap is longer so that the flap can be brought anteriorly and sutured to the anterior flap.

◆ The deeper subcutaneous tissues are first reapproximated, and then the skin can be sutured or stapled **(Figure 96-8).** This closure should be tension free to minimize flap necrosis.

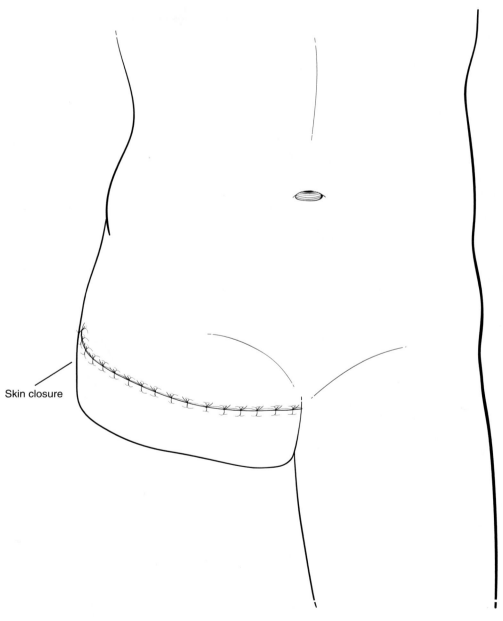

Skin closure

FIGURE 96–8

STEP 4: POSTOPERATIVE CARE

- ◆ After the closed-suction drain and sutures are removed, the patient should be fitted for a prosthetic limb and referred to physical therapy for early ambulation.

STEP 5: PEARLS AND PITFALLS

- ◆ When possible, all muscles are transected at their origin or insertion to minimize blood loss. Viable muscles are used to cover the exposed acetabulum. Phantom limb pain may be managed in conjunction with experts in pain management and rehabilitation medicine.

SELECTED REFERENCES

1. Boyd HB: Anatomic disarticulation of the hip. Surg Gynecol Obstet 1947;84:346-349.
2. Slocum DB: An Atlas of Amputations. St. Louis, Mosby, 1949.
3. Sugarbaker PH, Nicholson TH: Atlas of Extremity Sarcoma Surgery. Philadelphia, JB Lippincott Company, 1984.

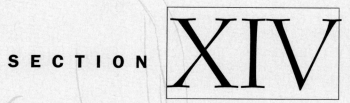

SECTION XIV

GYNECOLOGY

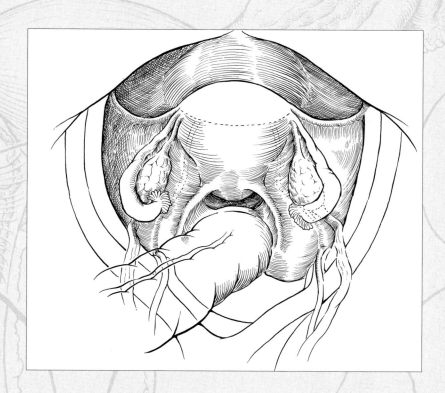

CHAPTER 97

ABDOMINAL HYSTERECTOMY

Concepcion Diaz-Arrastia

STEP 1: SURGICAL ANATOMY

- **Figures 97-1 and 97-2** demonstrate the anatomy of the female pelvis as it pertains to gynecologic surgery.
  - The bladder is attached to the anterior lower uterine segment and cervix at the anterior reflection of the visceral peritoneum.
  - The uterine arteries insert into the uterus laterally at the level of the internal cervical os.
  - The ureters cross over the bifurcation common iliac arteries and are found inferior to the infundibulopelvic ligament on the medial leaf of the broad ligament. As the ureter continues on its course to the bladder, it passes under the uterine artery 1 to 2 cm lateral to the insertion of the uterine artery at the level of the internal cervical os (see Figure 97-1).

- Figure 97-2 demonstrates the key ligaments of the uterus.
  - The infundibulopelvic ligament carries the blood supply to the ovaries.
  - The utero-ovarian ligament attaches the uterus to the adnexal structures, fallopian tubes, and ovaries.
  - Round ligaments are insubstantial anterior lateral attachments of the uterine fundus that help maintain the normal uterine position.
  - Cardinal ligaments attach the entire length of the cervix to the pelvic sidewall. These sturdy ligaments supply most of the uterine support.
  - Uterosacral ligaments attach the cervix to the sacrum.

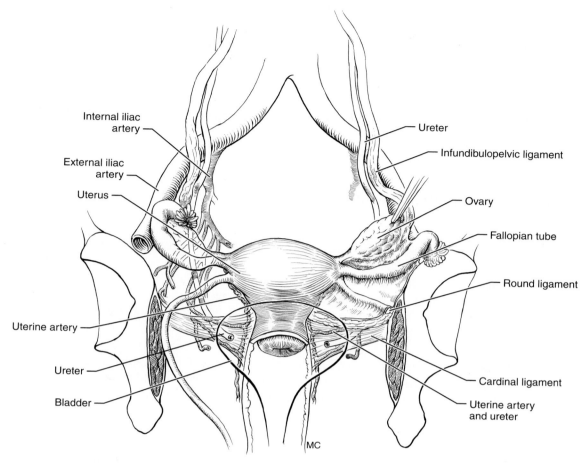

FIGURE 97–1

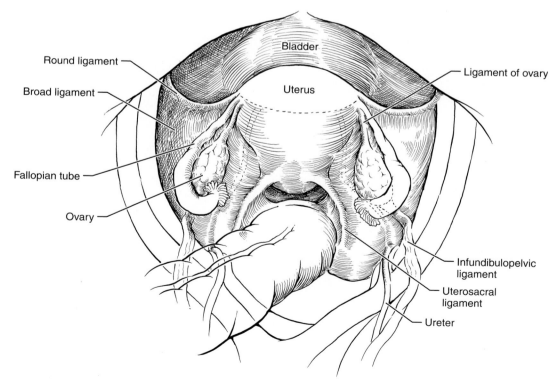

FIGURE 97–2

- **Figure 97-3** demonstrates the parts of the uterus.
  - The uterine corpus has two horns laterally.
  - The internal cervical os is where the uterine arteries enter the uterine body.
  - The external cervical os is at the junction with the vagina.

- **Figure 97-4** demonstrates the cervicovesical potential space that separates the bladder from the cervix.

STEP 2: PREOPERATIVE CONSIDERATIONS

- Several laboratory tests should be documented as part of the preoperative evaluation for a hysterectomy.
  - Pap smear to exclude invasive cervical carcinoma
  - Negative pregnancy test in women of reproductive age
  - Endometrial biopsy revealing no malignancy in a woman with abnormal uterine bleeding

- Indications for concomitant bilateral salpingo-oophorectomy (BSO) should be discussed with the patient. In general, BSO is recommended in any woman older than the age of 40 to 45 years or in a younger woman with familial or hereditary breast or ovarian cancer risk or severe endometriosis.

- Prophylactic antibiotics are indicated because the peritoneal cavity is contaminated by the vaginal incision to remove the cervix.

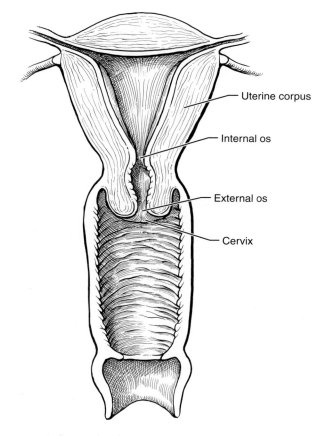

FIGURE 97–3

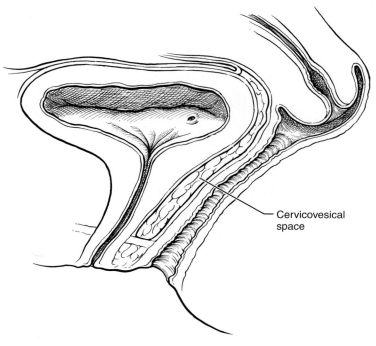

FIGURE 97–4

STEP 3: OPERATIVE STEPS

1. INCISIONS

◆ A vertical skin incision allows for excellent exposure, as well as the ability to extend the incision to the upper abdomen, at the expense of cosmetic result and an increased rate of wound complications.

◆ A transverse skin incision allows for adequate exposure in the pelvis. Three transverse incisions are available to the pelvic surgeon, depending on the body habitus of the patient and the uterine pathology. **Figure 97-5, A,** depicts the skin incision for all transverse incisions, 1 to 2 cm above the symphysis pubis extending approximately 6 cm to both sides of the rectus abdominis muscles. This incision is carried down to the anterior rectus sheath or fascia **(Figure 97-5, B).** The fascia is then incised, also transversely, for the length of the incision. After the fascial incision, the procedures diverge.

◆ The Pfannenstiel skin incision is the most popular transverse skin incision and is appropriate for removal of a normal-sized uterus. The rectus muscles are dissected from the anterior rectus sheath in both the cephalad and caudad directions **(Figure 97-5, C).** The posterior rectus sheath is then opened vertically at the midline **(Figure 97-5, D),** the rectus muscles are retracted laterally, and the exposed peritoneum is opened the length of the incision to expose the pelvis.

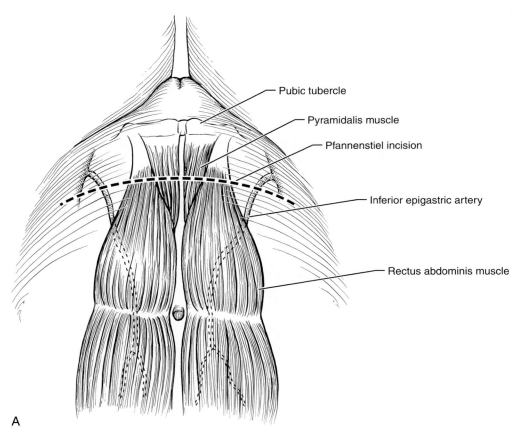

Pubic tubercle

Pyramidalis muscle

Pfannenstiel incision

Inferior epigastric artery

Rectus abdominis muscle

A

FIGURE 97–5

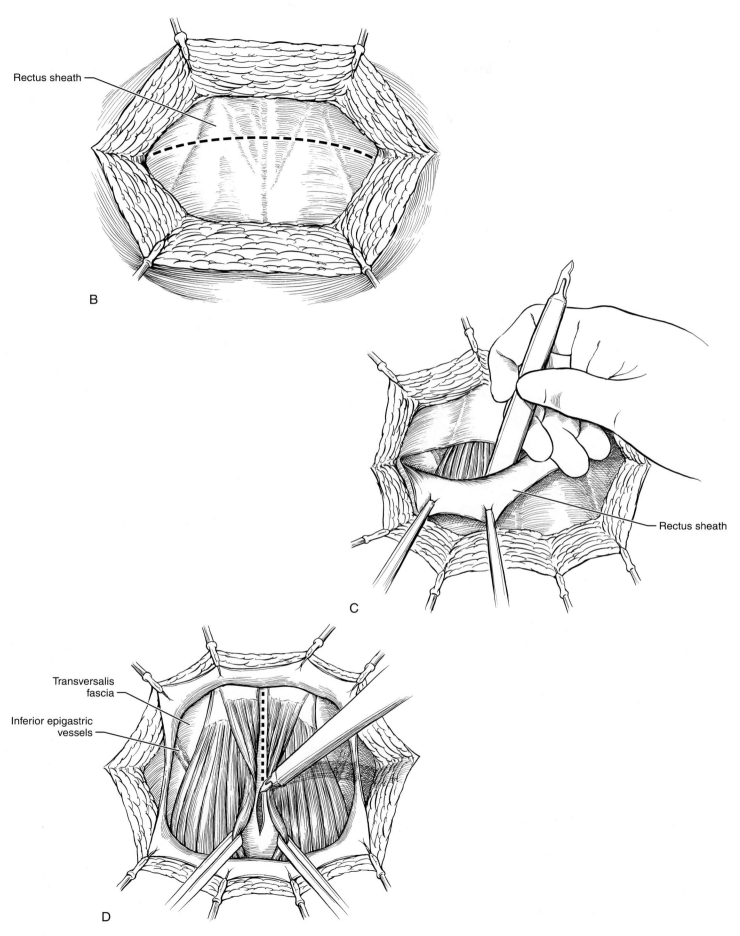

Rectus sheath

B

Rectus sheath

C

Transversalis fascia

Inferior epigastric vessels

D

FIGURE 97–5, cont'd

- ◆ The Maylard and Cherney transverse incisions are used when a larger opening in required than that allowed by the Pfannenstiel. In comparison with the Pfannenstiel incision the rectus muscles must not be separated from the anterior fascia or rectus sheath in either incision.
    - ◆ For the Maylard incision, after the transverse skin incision, the inferior epigastric vessels are ligated bilaterally, lateral to the rectus muscles **(Figure 97-6)**. After the blood supply has been secured, the rectus muscles are transected. To avoid retraction of the muscles cephalad, the anterior sheath must remain attached. The posterior fascia and peritoneum are then incised the length of the incision. For the closure, because the muscles were not separated from the anterior rectus sheath, they are reapproximated by the fascial closure.

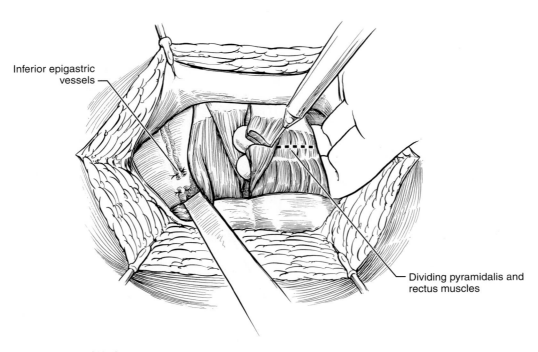

Inferior epigastric vessels

Dividing pyramidalis and rectus muscles

FIGURE 97–6

◆ For the Cherney incision, after the transverse skin incision, the rectus muscle is transected at its tendon, near its insertion to the pubic bone **(Figure 97-7)**. As with the Maylard, to avoid retraction of the muscles cephalad, the anterior sheath must remain attached. The posterior fascia and peritoneum are then incised the length of the incision. For the closure, the tendons are reapproximated with 0 interrupted absorbable sutures. A limitation to the Cherney incision is that many women do not have a well-demarcated rectus abdominis tendon. In these cases, the Maylard incision is a better option.

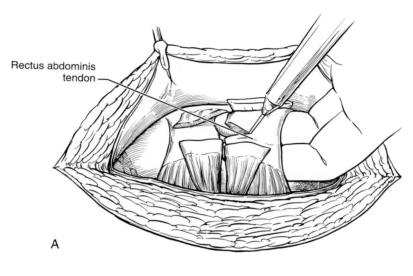

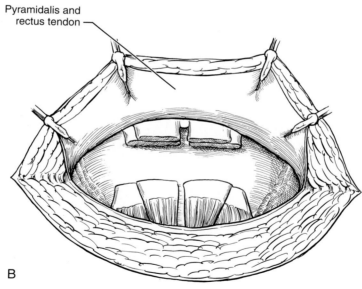

FIGURE 97–7

2. DISSECTION

- The operative field is prepared by placing the patient in Trendelenburg position, inserting a self-retaining retractor to expose the pelvis, and packing the intestines away from the operative field with moist laparotomy pads.

- The uterus is grasped with atraumatic curved clamps placed on the uterine horns bilaterally for traction. Each of the next steps is performed on each side of the uterus before advancing to the next step. Delayed absorbable suture of the appropriate caliber for the size of the pedicles (2-0 or 0) is used throughout.

- The broad ligament is opened, starting with the round ligament ligation bilaterally **(Figure 97-8)**.

- If the adnexal structures are not to be removed, they are separated from the uterus by ligation of the utero-ovarian ligament **(Figure 97-9)**.

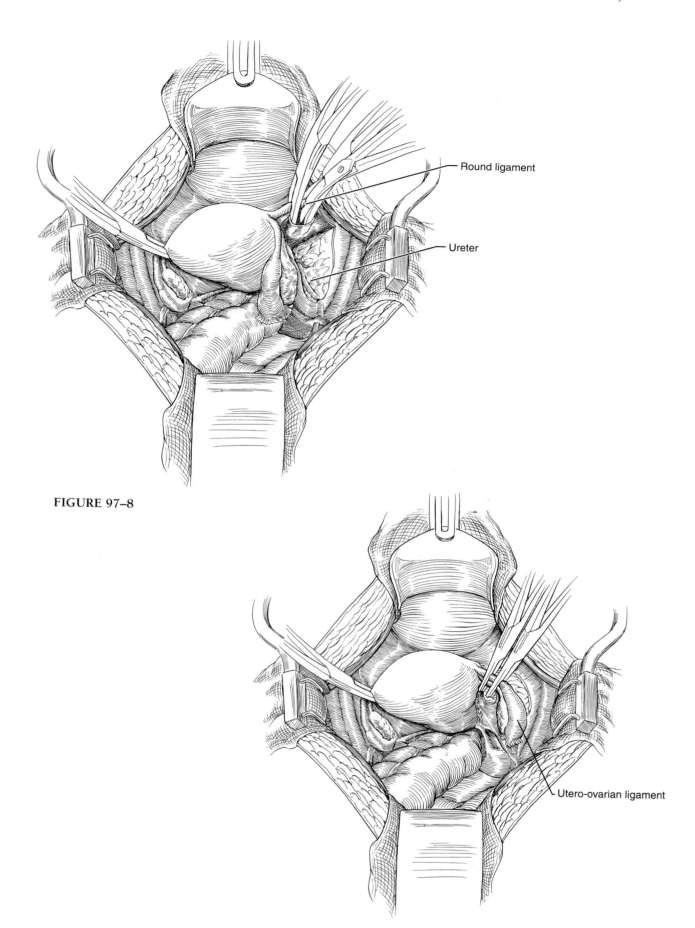

Round ligament

Ureter

FIGURE 97–8

Utero-ovarian ligament

FIGURE 97–9

◆ The incised peritoneal incision is extended anteriorly across the midline to the loosely attached peritoneum of the bladder reflection **(Figure 97-10)**. The bladder flap or cervico-vesical space is developed by placing traction on the incised bladder peritoneum and sharply dissecting the vesicocervical fascia at the midline for 3 to 4 cm until the level of the vagina is reached **(Figure 97-11)**. At the completion of this step, the bladder and ureter have been displaced caudad, as upward traction is placed on the uterus, resulting in increasing the distance between the uterine arteries and the ureters in preparation for ligation of the uterine arteries.

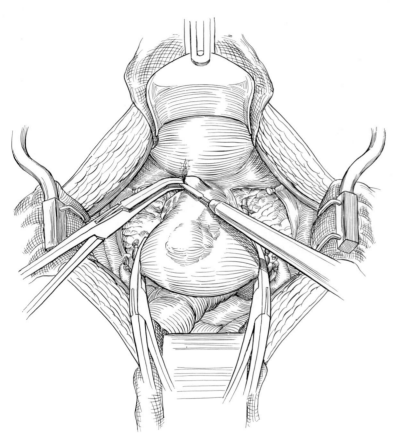

FIGURE 97–10

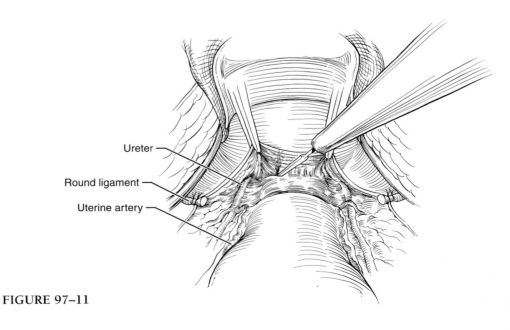

Ureter —

Round ligament —

Uterine artery —

FIGURE 97–11

◆ In preparation for ligation of the uterine artery, the surgeon cleans the retroperitoneal areo-lar tissue at the level of the internal cervical os to skeletonize the uterine vessels. The uter-ine vessels are clamped at the level of the internal cervical os, at a right angle to the cervix **(Figure 97-12).** For bleeding from the pedicle to be avoided, the tips of the heavy curved hysterectomy clamps should approximate and slide off the cervix. The pedicle is incised around the tip of the clamp to separate the ligated pedicle from the specimen and expose the cardinal ligaments.

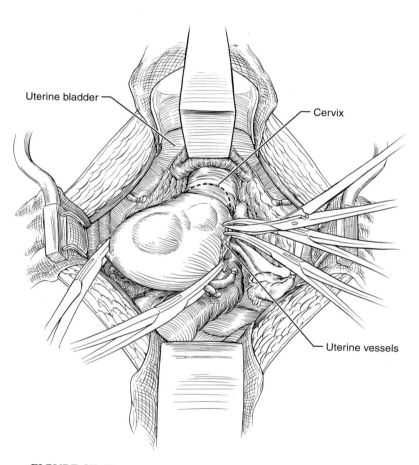

FIGURE 97–12

◆ After the uterine arteries have been ligated bilaterally, attention is brought to the cardinal ligament. Serial bites of this dense ligament are incised at its insertion on the cervix down to the vagina **(Figure 97-13)**. To avoid retraction of this thick pedicle, use a straight hysterectomy clamp and incise a wedge-shaped pedicle, stopping 1 to 2 mm short of the tip of the clamp.

◆ The uterosacral ligament is ligated at its insertion on the posterior cervix **(Figure 97-14)**. These pedicles may be tagged for incorporation into the vaginal closure for added vaginal support.

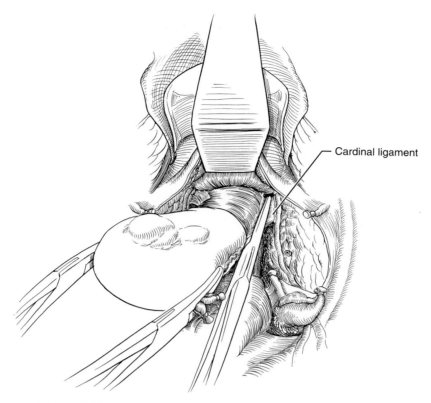

Cardinal ligament

FIGURE 97–13

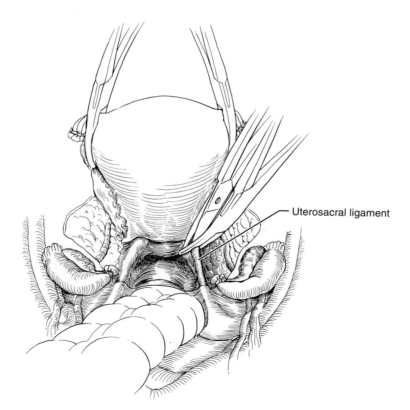

Uterosacral ligament

FIGURE 97–14

◆ Identify the upper vagina by palpating the hollow organ at the end of the cervix **(Figure 97-15)**. Incise across the upper vagina circumferentially, clamping to decrease spillage of uterine contents into the operative field **(Figures 97-16 and 97-17)**.

3. CLOSING

◆ The vagina is closed with interrupted figure-of-eight sutures. To avoid injury to the bladder, suture from anterior to posterior **(Figure 97-18)**. The pelvis is copiously irrigated.

◆ The abdominal wall is closed in layers. The anterior rectus fascia is closed in a continuous mass closure.

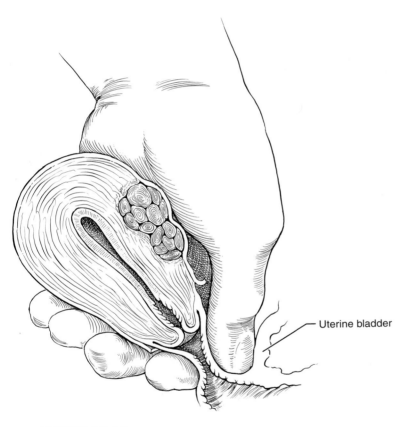

Uterine bladder

FIGURE 97–15

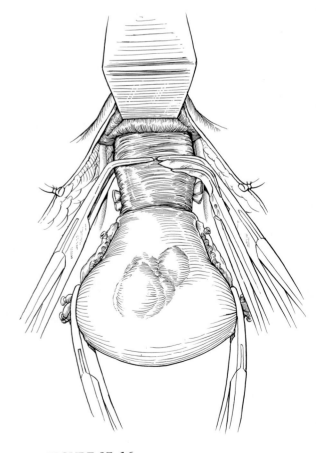

FIGURE 97–16

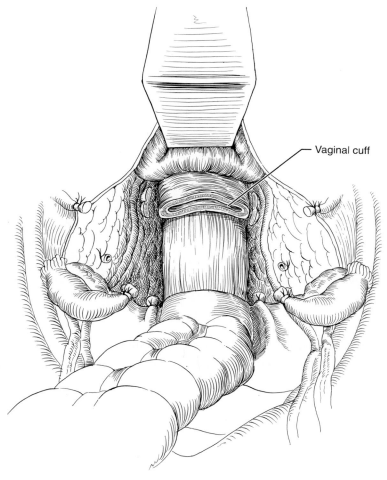

FIGURE 97–17

Vaginal cuff

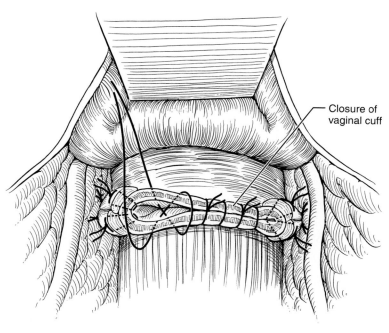

Closure of
vaginal cuff

FIGURE 97–18

STEP 4: POSTOPERATIVE CARE

- Bladder drainage is maintained until the first postoperative day.

- Diet is advanced as tolerated.

- Early ambulation is encouraged.

STEP 5: PEARLS AND PITFALLS

- Avoid suturing through the middle of the uterine pedicle, because a vessel may be easily pierced, leading to a retroperitoneal hematoma.

- In a patient with previous pelvic surgery or history of endometriosis or pelvic inflammatory disease, a mechanical bowel preparation should be ordered to prepare for extensive bowel lysis of adhesions.

- Use the appropriate-length instruments and sutures based on the depth of pelvis and weight of the patient.

SELECTED REFERENCE

1. Rock JA, Jones HW (eds): TeLinde's Operative Gynecology, 10th ed. Philadelphia, Lippincott Williams & Wilkins, 2008.

CHAPTER 98

BILATERAL SALPINGO-OOPHORECTOMY

Concepcion Diaz-Arrastia

STEP 1: SURGICAL ANATOMY

♦ **Figure 98-1** demonstrates the key anatomy of the uterus, fallopian tube, and ovary (adnexa) as it pertains to the removal of the adnexa.
  ♦ The infundibulopelvic ligament carries the blood supply to the adnexa.
  ♦ Round ligaments are insubstantial anterior lateral attachments of the uterine fundus that help maintain the normal uterine position. They are an important landmark in the opening of the retroperitoneum for identification of the ureters.
  ♦ Utero-ovarian ligaments connect the uterus to the adnexa.
  ♦ The ureters cross over the bifurcation of the common iliac arteries and are found inferior to the infundibulopelvic ligament on the medial leaf of the broad ligament. The ureter must be identified before ligation of the infundibulopelvic ligament.

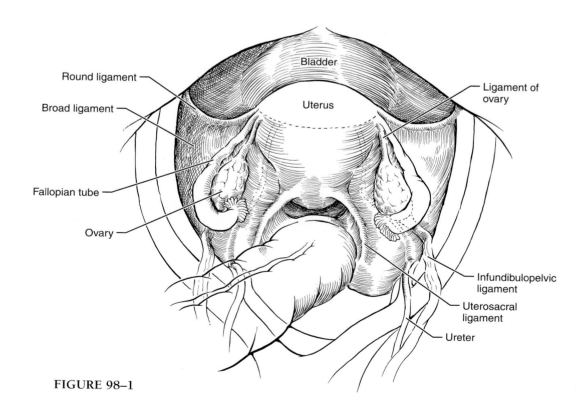

FIGURE 98–1

STEP 2: PREOPERATIVE CONSIDERATIONS

- The indications for salpingo-oophorectomy include excision of an ovarian mass or ovarian cancer prophylaxis.

- Frozen section surgical consultation should be available for all cases of ovarian mass. If intraoperative diagnosis of ovarian cancer is made, the surgeon and patient should be prepared to proceed with ovarian cancer surgical staging or cytoreductive surgery as indicated.

STEP 3: OPERATIVE STEPS

1. INCISION

- In cases of a suspected ovarian mass, a vertical skin incision is recommended to allow for excellent exposure, as well as the ability to extend the incision to the upper abdomen for exploration, surgical staging, or cytoreductive surgery.

- A transverse Pfannenstiel incision or laparoscopic approach is acceptable for prophylactic salpingo-oophorectomy. (See Chapter 97 for discussion of transverse incisions.)

2. DISSECTION

- The operative field is prepared by placing the patient in Trendelenburg position, inserting a self-retaining retractor to expose the pelvis, and packing the intestines away from the operative field with moist laparotomy pads.

- The uterus is grasped with atraumatic curved clamps placed on the uterine horns bilaterally for upward traction.

- An L-shaped incision is made on the peritoneum of the posterior leaf of the broad ligament, parallel and posterior to the round ligament and lateral to the infundibulopelvic ligament **(Figure 98-2)**. This avascular retroperitoneal space is developed by blunt dissection. The external iliac artery is identified on the lateral leaf, and the ureter is identified on the medial leaf, inferior to the infundibulopelvic ligament **(Figure 98-3)**.

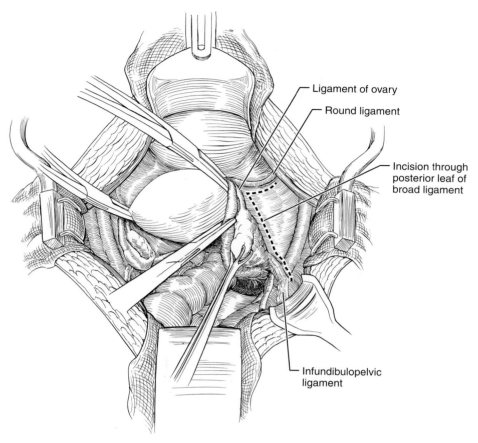

Ligament of ovary

Round ligament

Incision through posterior leaf of broad ligament

Infundibulopelvic ligament

FIGURE 98–2

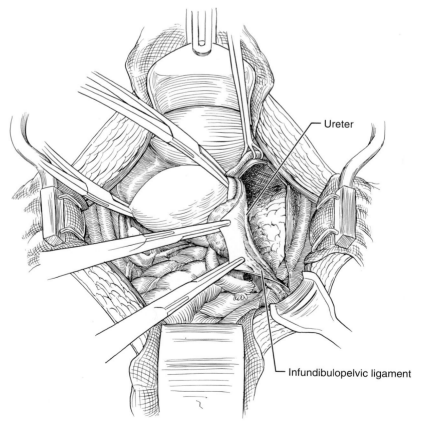

Ureter

Infundibulopelvic ligament

FIGURE 98–3

◆ Under visualization of the ureter, the surgeon makes a window in the medial leaf of the broad ligament, between the vascular infundibulopelvic ligament and the ureter, then clamps and incises the infundibulopelvic ligament **(Figure 98-4)**.

◆ Because of the vascularity of the infundibulopelvic ligament and the risk of an ascending retroperitoneal hematoma, the surgeon first ligates the pedicle with a free tie then transfixes the pedicle with suture ligation **(Figure 98-5)**.

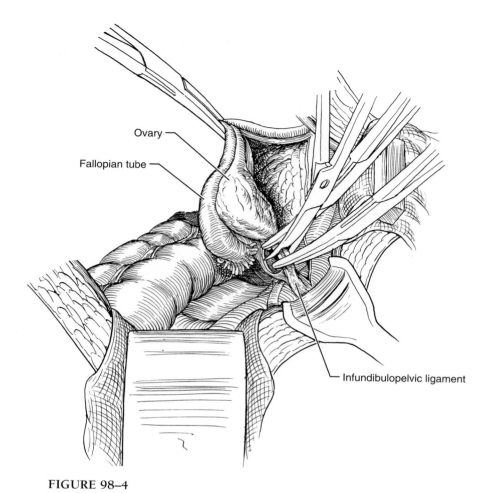

Ovary

Fallopian tube

Infundibulopelvic ligament

FIGURE 98–4

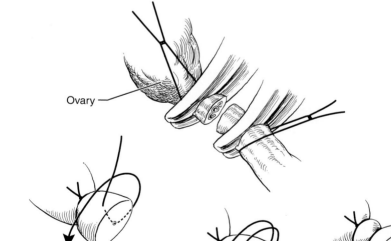

Ovary

FIGURE 98–5

◆ Under full visualization of the ureter, incise the medial leaf of the peritoneum/broad ligament from the infundibulopelvic pedicle to the uterus **(Figure 98-6)**. Ligate the utero-ovarian ligament, which is the remaining attachment of the adnexa **(Figures 98-7 and 98-8)**.

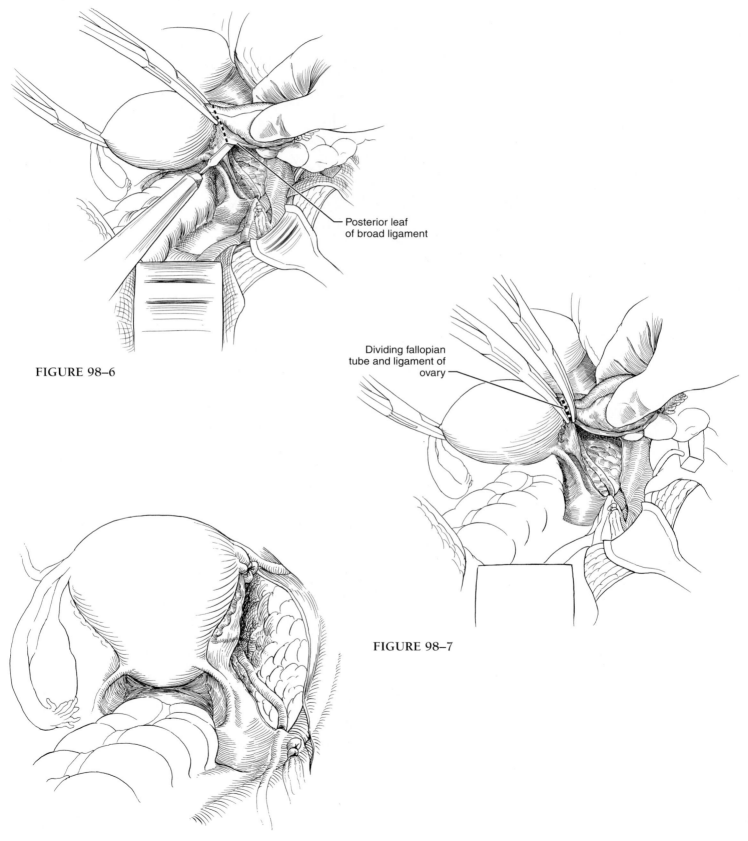

Posterior leaf
of broad ligament

FIGURE 98–6

Dividing fallopian
tube and ligament of
ovary

FIGURE 98–7

FIGURE 98–8

3. CLOSING

◆ The abdominal wall is closed in layers. The anterior rectus fascia is closed in a continuous mass closure.

STEP 4: POSTOPERATIVE CARE

◆ Bladder drainage is maintained until the first postoperative day.

◆ Diet is advanced as tolerated.

◆ Early ambulation is encouraged.

STEP 5: PEARLS AND PITFALLS

◆ Salpingo-oophorectomy in a menstruating woman will effect a surgical menopause, which may cause severe hot flashes and other sequelae of premature menopause.

◆ Mechanical bowel preparation is advised in patients undergoing surgery for an ovarian mass.

SELECTED REFERENCE

1. Rock JA, Jones HW (eds): TeLinde's Operative Gynecology, 10th ed. Philadelphia, Lippincott Williams & Wilkins, 2008.

CHAPTER 99

REPAIR OF RECTOVAGINAL FISTULAE

Margie A. Kahn

STEP 1: SURGICAL ANATOMY

- Although rectovaginal fistulae may spontaneously arise from Crohn's disease or malignancy, most cases result from failed obstetric repairs and complications of posterior vaginal prolapse repair operations.

- Successful repair requires a wide enough dissection to obtain a tension-free layered closure of viable, well-vascularized tissue, using a pedicled Martius bulbocavernosus graft if necessary.

- Although successful early secondary repair has been described, repair after postpartum dehiscence is traditionally delayed for 3 months to allow maximal reinnervation and vascularization of the wound.

- Numerous failed repairs may require a diverting colostomy before and 3 months following reoperation to ensure adequate healing.

- Fistulae superior to the levator muscles may require an abdominal approach to achieve adequate mobilization of tissue. In the pre-antibiotic era, the rectal advancement and vaginal flap operations had the advantage of avoiding a suture line in the rectum. However, the use of these operations may make overlapping the retracted muscle of the anal sphincter more difficult.

- Preoperatively, all patients receive a bowel preparation and prophylactic antibiotics.

- Infiltration of the operative field with 20 U of vasopressin in 100 mL of normal saline or a local anesthetic with epinephrine reduces blood loss and helps hydrodissect scarred tissue planes.

STEP 2: PREOPERATIVE CONSIDERATIONS

◆ Most postpartum fistulae are accompanied by two quadrant anal sphincter defects identifiable by perineal dimples at the 3 o'clock and 9 o'clock positions.

◆ In the worst cases, the vaginal mucosa directly abuts the rectal mucosa. If gross inspection and palpation are equivocal, endoanal ultrasonography and anorectal manometry may be used to identify the anatomic and functional significance of the defects. In the following figure, the normal sphincter is on the right.

◆ Extensive dissection to achieve anal overlapping sphincteroplasty can interfere with the neurovascular bundles at the 4 o'clock and 8 o'clock positions **(Figure 99-1)**.

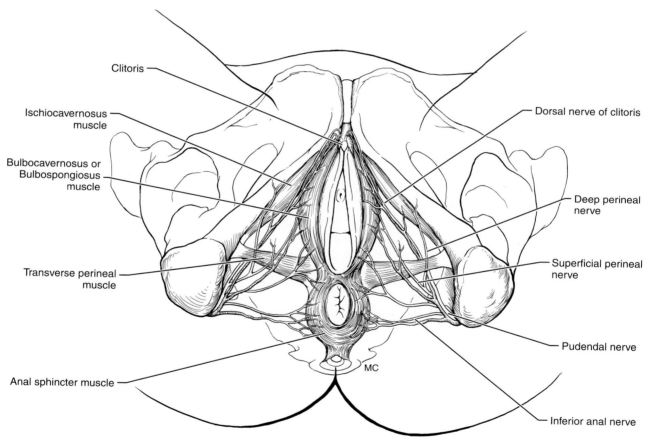

FIGURE 99–1

STEP 3: OPERATIVE STEPS

1. INCISION

- The Lone Star Retractor and stays are applied, and the proposed surgical field is injected with vasopressin.

- The perineal incision line is marked at the junction of the vagina and perineum **(Figure 99-2)**. (If there is deficient perineum, a modified cruciate incision will allow a Z-plasty.)

- The initial incision is made with needle-tip electrocautery set on a pure cutting current **(Figure 99-3)**.

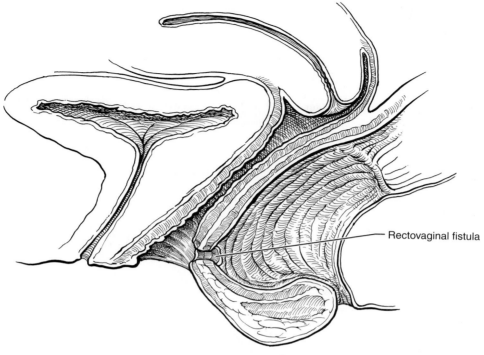

FIGURE 99–2

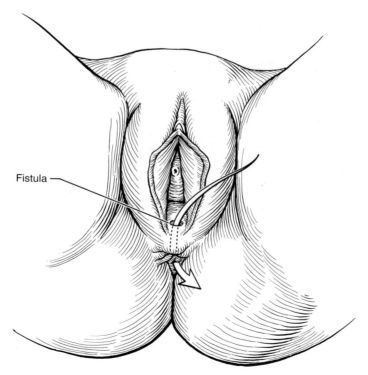

FIGURE 99–3

2. DISSECTION

◆ The rectovaginal space is dissected sharply to the fistula tract.

◆ Sharp dissection against a finger in the rectum helps avoid inadvertently buttonholing the rectum.

◆ After a plane is developed, Sklar Pratt clamps often supply a better grasp of the tissue than Allis clamps **(Figures 99-4 and 99-5)**.

◆ For further ease of dissection, the vagina is incised in the midline and the dissection is continued.

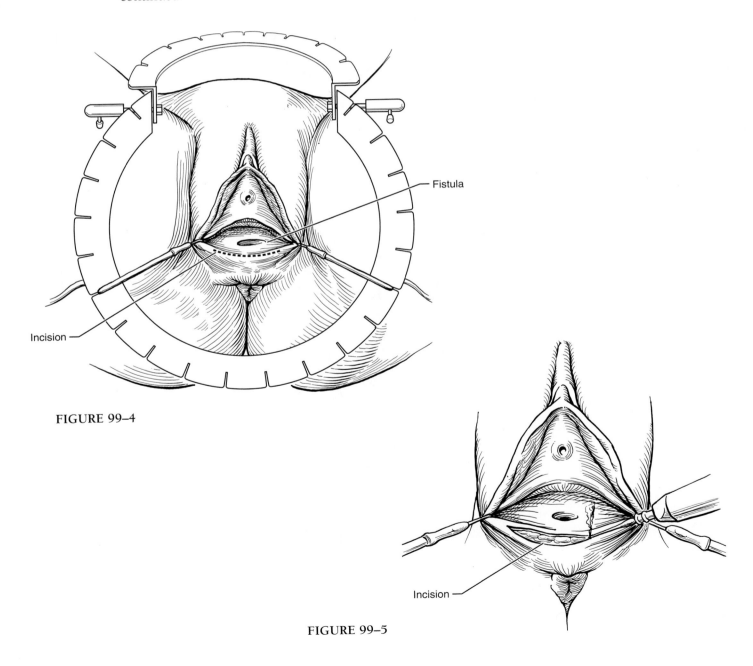

FIGURE 99–4

FIGURE 99–5

◆ The fistula edges may be trimmed to ensure well-vascularized tissue.

◆ However, care must be taken on the rectal side to avoid removing excessive tissue (**Figures 99-6 and 99-7**).

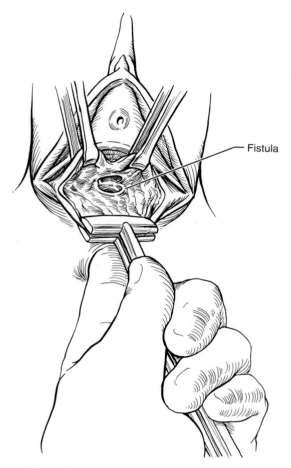

Fistula

FIGURE 99–6

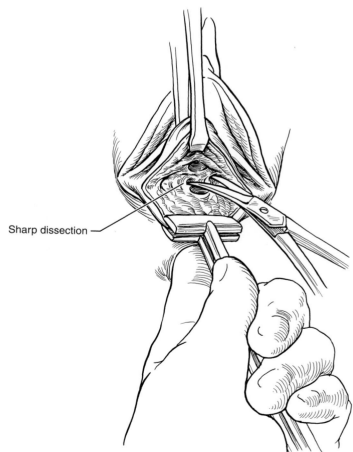

Sharp dissection

FIGURE 99–7

◆ As the dissection continues, the smooth shiny rectovaginal fascia (the fibromuscular layer of the vagina) is identified, and the separation of the planes becomes easier **(Figure 99-8).**

◆ The dissection continues to the posterior fornix **(Figures 99-9 and 99-10).**

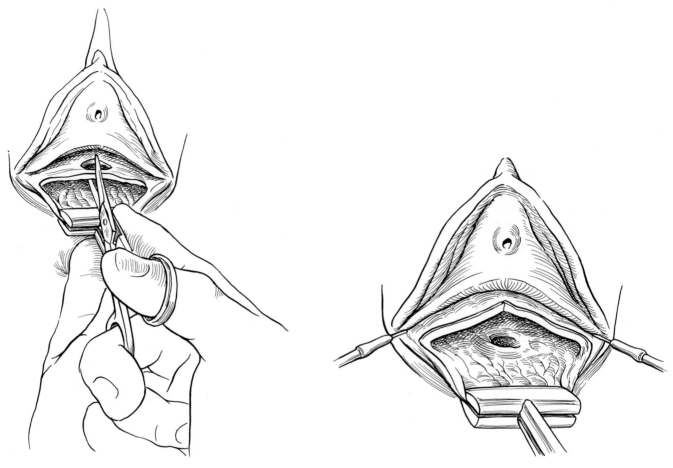

FIGURE 99–8

FIGURE 99–9

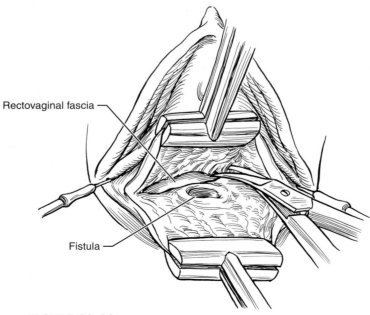

Rectovaginal fascia —

Fistula —

FIGURE 99–10

◆ The retracted ends of the anal sphincter are sharply dissected from the surrounding scar, with care given to avoid the posterior lateral neurovascular bundles **(Figure 99-11)**.

◆ Extension of the initial incision into the ischioanal fat can aid in identifying the outer margin of the anal sphincter **(Figure 99-12)**.

◆ Both ends of the anal sphincter are identified.

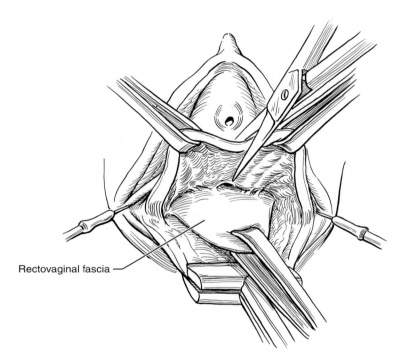

Rectovaginal fascia —

FIGURE 99–11

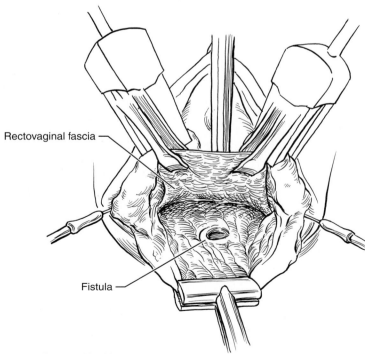

Rectovaginal fascia —

Fistula —

FIGURE 99–12

◆ The labium majus is incised to obtain the Martius bulbocavernosus fat pad **(Figure 99-13)**.

◆ In this case, the blood supply from the external pudendal artery is ligated.

◆ The internal pudendal artery provides the blood supply inferiorly.

◆ The flap is largely composed of adipose tissue, because the muscle is not very prominent **(Figure 99-14)**.

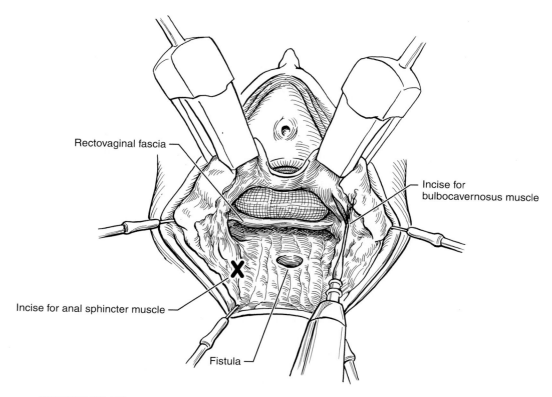

Rectovaginal fascia

Incise for
bulbocavernosus muscle

Incise for anal sphincter muscle

Fistula

FIGURE 99–13

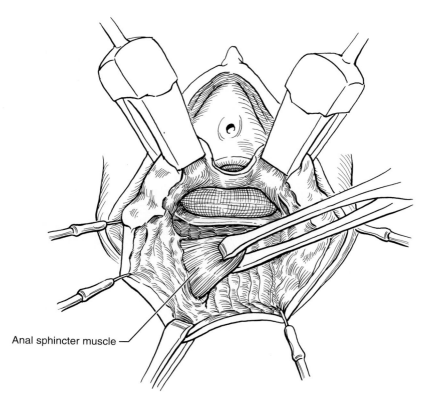

Anal sphincter muscle

FIGURE 99–14

3. CLOSURE

◆ The rectal mucosa is closed with an absorbable, monofilament 000 continuous suture from inside the rectum so that the knots are expelled out of the rectum **(Figure 99-15)**.

◆ In this case, there is insufficient internal anal sphincter to imbricate as a second layer, so the pedicled graft is applied to improve the integrity of the repair **(Figure 99-16)**.

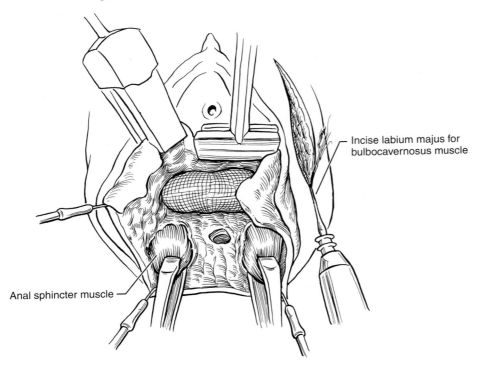

Incise labium majus for bulbocavernosus muscle

Anal sphincter muscle

FIGURE 99–15

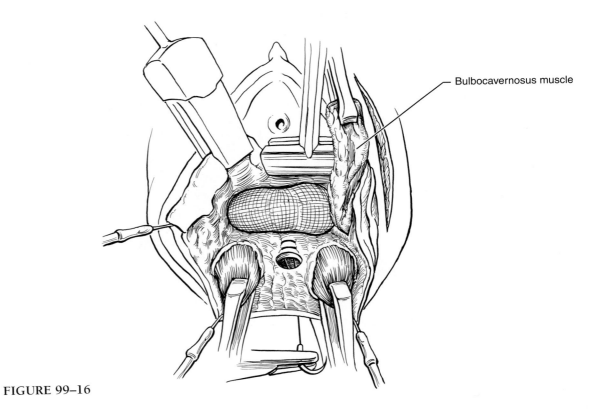

Bulbocavernosus muscle

FIGURE 99–16

◆ Overlapping sphincteroplasty is performed with 000 delayed absorbable monofilament sutures (**Figures 99-17 and 99-18**).

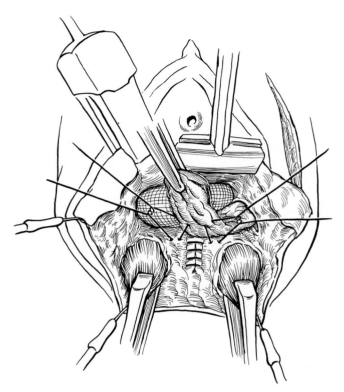

FIGURE 99–17

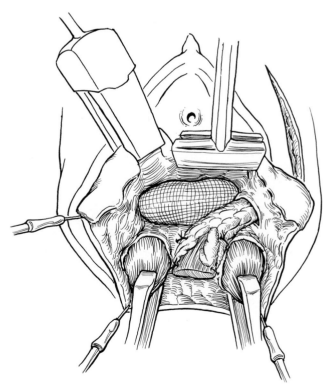

FIGURE 99–18

- The rectovaginal fascia is sutured to the center of the perineal body **(Figures 99-19 and 99-20)**.

- The transverse perineal and bulbocavernosus (also called bulbospongiosus) muscles join the anal sphincter and rectovaginal septum at the perineal body.

- If these muscles are not inextricably bound together, they may be joined end-to-end. If there is excessive perineal laxity, the perineal muscles may also be overlapped, but such overlap may require extensive lateral dissection of the transverse perineal muscles toward the ischial tuberosities **(Figure 99-21)**.

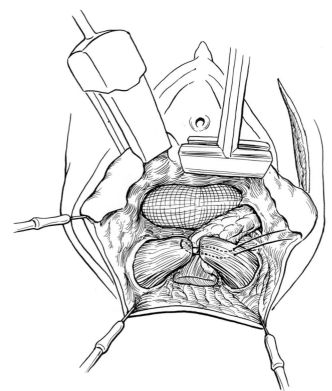

FIGURE 99–19

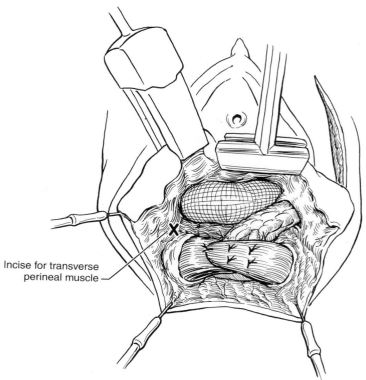

Incise for transverse
perineal muscle

FIGURE 99–20

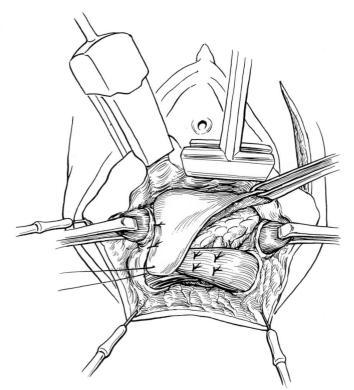

FIGURE 99–21

◆ A 00 or 000 rapid absorbable suture is used to close the vaginal mucosa and perineal skin (**Figures 99-22 through 99-24**).

STEP 4: POSTOPERATIVE CARE

◆ The most common short-term complication is urinary retention, so a urinary catheter may be necessary until the normal micturition reflex recovers.

◆ Postoperative management consists of careful perineal hygiene and stool softeners.

◆ Excessive antibiotic use in the absence of infection may lead to diarrhea and impaired wound healing of the rectal mucosal suture line, in addition to the increased risk of infection with resistant organisms.

◆ Although perineal skin breakdown is common, it does not seem to affect the ultimate success of the repair.

STEP 5: PEARLS AND PITFALLS

◆ Long-term functional outcome of overlapping anal sphincteroplasty may be disappointing, with anal continence rates as low as 50%.

◆ Patients should be counseled that restoration of anatomy does not guarantee restoration of function.

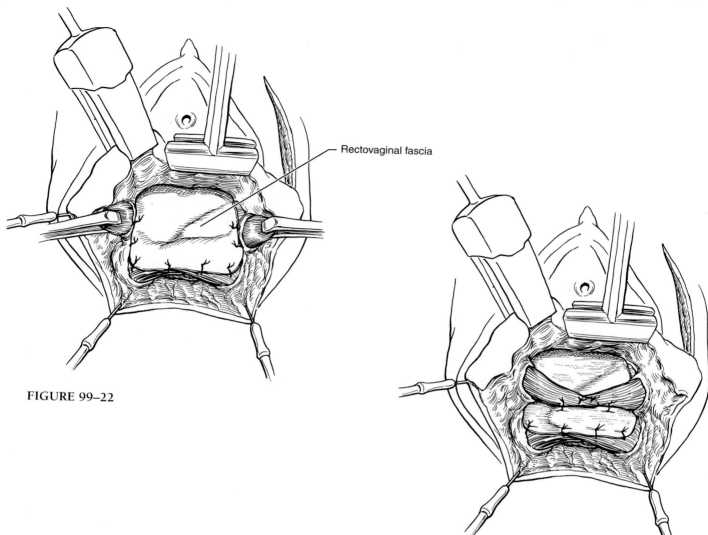

Rectovaginal fascia

FIGURE 99–22

FIGURE 99–23

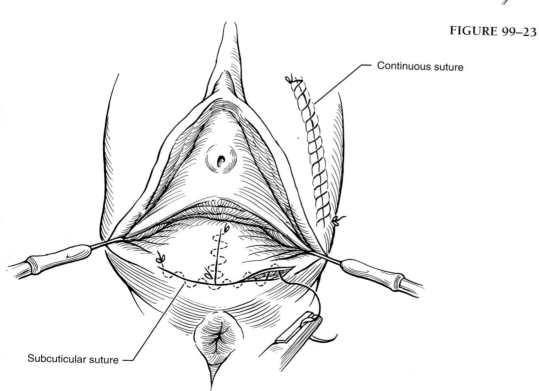

Continuous suture

Subcuticular suture

FIGURE 99–24

SELECTED REFERENCES

1. Martius H: Die Gynäkologischen Operationen. Leipzig, Georg Thieme, 1949.
2. Hankins GDV, Hauth JC, Gilstrap LC, et al: Early repair of episiotomy dehiscence. Obstet Gynecol 1990;75:48-51.
3. Mengert WF, Fish SA: Anterior rectal wall advancement. Technique for repair of complete perineal laceration and rectovaginal fistula. Obstet Gynecol 1955;3:262-267.
4. Noble GH: A new operation for complete laceration of the perineum designed for the purpose of eliminating danger of infection from the rectum. Trans Am Gynecol Soc 1902;27:357-363.
5. Sultan AH, Kahn MA: Perineal and primary anal sphincter repairs. In Cardozo L, Staskin D (eds): Textbook of Female Urology and Urogynecology. London, Isis Medical Media, 2001, pp 628-642.

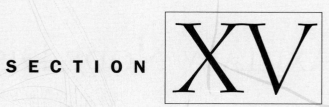
MISCELLANEOUS PROCEDURES

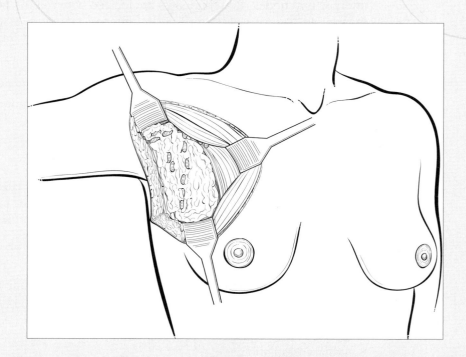

CHAPTER 100

AXILLARY NODE DISSECTION

Baiba J. Grube

STEP 1: SURGICAL ANATOMY

- ◆ A comprehensive understanding of the location of the lymph nodes in relation to the chest wall musculature, fascial boundaries, lymphatic drainage pathways, vascular supply supporting structures, and innervation of surrounding tissues is essential for appropriate surgical management.

- ◆ **Figure 100-1** demonstrates the breast gland and its rich intraparenchymal lymph channels coursing toward the deeper major nodal reservoirs.

- ◆ **Figure 100-2** illustrates the supporting structure of the chest wall musculature, the major blood vessels, and the location of the lymph nodes.

- ◆ The lymph nodes lateral to the pectoralis minor muscle constitute level I nodes; those immediately beneath the muscle, the level II nodes; and those medial to it, level III nodes. The interpectoral nodes (Rotter's nodes) are located between the pectoralis major and minor muscles and are part of level III nodes. Internal mammary nodes are located medially along internal mammary vessels beneath the sternum. Unnamed intramammary lymph nodes can be present in all quadrants of the breast.

- ◆ The boundaries of the axilla are defined by the pectoral minor muscle medially, the latissimus dorsi muscle laterally, the axillary vein superiorly, and the subscapularis and teres major muscles posteriorly.

- ◆ Axillary lymph node dissection removes the lymph nodes lateral to the pectoralis minor muscle (level I nodes) and posterior to the pectoralis minor muscle (level II nodes). In some cases, the lymph nodes medial to the pectoralis (level III nodes) and the interpectoral nodes (Rotter's nodes) are also removed.

- ◆ Other types of lymph node procedures or treatments include the following:
  - ◆ Sentinel node biopsy
  - ◆ Lymph node sampling
  - ◆ Excision of a palpable lymph node
  - ◆ Axillary irradiation

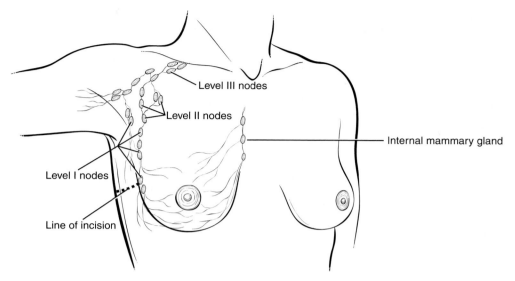

Level III nodes

Level II nodes

Internal mammary gland

Level I nodes

Line of incision

FIGURE 100-1

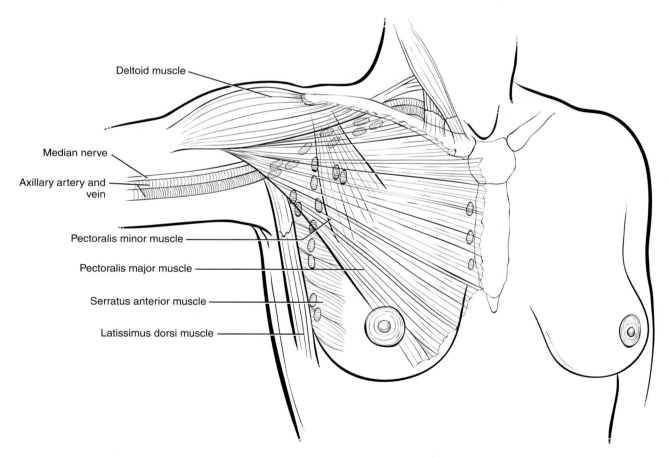

Deltoid muscle

Median nerve

Axillary artery and vein

Pectoralis minor muscle

Pectoralis major muscle

Serratus anterior muscle

Latissimus dorsi muscle

FIGURE 100-2

STEP 2: PREOPERATIVE CONSIDERATIONS

- Selection of a surgical option for local control of breast cancer is a complex decision based on the tumor features, the body habitus, and individual choice. Interdisciplinary discussion with radiation oncologists, medical oncologists, and plastic surgeons, in addition to the oncologic surgeon, provides a comprehensive understanding of the options available to the patient.

- Lumpectomy with axillary lymph node dissection may be an alternative procedure to a modified radical mastectomy for many women, especially in the current era of mammographic screening and identification of early stage disease and with the use of induction chemotherapy to reduce the size of the primary tumor.

- Discussion of the planned procedure with the anesthesiologist is critical.
  - Long-acting paralytic agents should be avoided when an axillary dissection is planned to detect intact motor nerve function.

STEP 3: OPERATIVE STEPS

1. INCISION

- The patient is placed in the supine position, close to the edge of the operating table for ease of exposure of the axilla, with the arm extended on a padded arm board with or without a wedge. The arm may be prepped out separately and covered in a sterile stockinette to allow free rotation of the arm medially to relax the pectoralis major and minor muscles.

- Many incisions have been used for axillary dissection. The transverse incision approximately 1 cm below the hair-bearing area extending from the latissimus dorsi to the pectoralis major medially results in the most cosmetically attractive incision. Other incisions may be perpendicular to the axilla or S-shaped incisions.

- A marking pen is used to draw the planned incision. The skin is incised and extended through the dermis into the subcutaneous adipose tissue to expose the investing fascia of the axilla **(Figure 100-3).** The thickness of the flaps will vary according to body mass index. In heavyset individuals, the flaps will be thick and may cave into the axilla, making dissection difficult. Adequate exposure is essential to avoid injury to important structures.

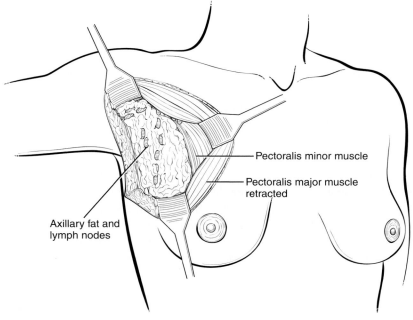

Pectoralis minor muscle

Pectoralis major muscle
retracted

Axillary fat and
lymph nodes

FIGURE 100–3

2. DISSECTION

- Dissection is initiated by elevating the skin flaps with skin hooks or Freeman face lift retractors with electrocautery.

- As the flaps are elevated, the assistant holds upward tension on the skin flaps while the surgeon uses countertraction on the axillary fat pad.

- The skin flaps are raised circumferentially and retracted with medium Richardson retractors to expose the axillary fat and lymph nodes (see Figure 100-3).

- Dissection is initiated along the pectoralis major muscle medially from superior to inferior. Care must be exercised to avoid injury to the medial anterior thoracic nerve (medial pectoral nerve), which may penetrate both pectoral muscles and emerge medially or may course along the lateral aspect of the pectoralis minor. Injury to this nerve may lead to atrophy of part of the pectoralis major muscle.

- The fascia along the pectoralis major is incised and retracted medially with a small or medium Richardson retractor, exposing the underlying pectoralis minor. The clavipectoral fascia along the pectoralis minor is then incised and the retractor is replaced, exposing the level II nodes posterior to the pectoralis minor. The arm may now be rotated medially to take tension off the pectoral muscles and expose the axillary contents. Care must be taken to avoid traction of the extremity and the brachial plexus in the anesthetized patient.

- The inferior reflection of the axillary fascia is identified, and dissection is continued from medial to lateral on the serratus anterior muscle to the latissimus dorsi muscle laterally.

- Dissection is continued along the lateral aspect of the latissimus dorsi muscle to the level of its tendinous insertion **(Figure 100-4).** This marks the location of the overlying axillary vein. Dissection along the ventral aspect of the latissimus dorsi should be avoided until the thoracodorsal nerve, artery, and vein are identified, visualized, and maintained in view during dissection.

- Dissection from the tendinous insertion of the latissimus dorsi proceeds medially, inferior to the axillary vein.

- The superior extent of the axillary dissection should begin approximately 5 mm below the axillary vein to preserve the lymphatics of the arm and reduce the likelihood of upper extremity lymphedema (see Figure 100-4). This tissue is rich in lymphatics and blood vessels, which should be ligated with fine silk ties or Weck Hemoclips.

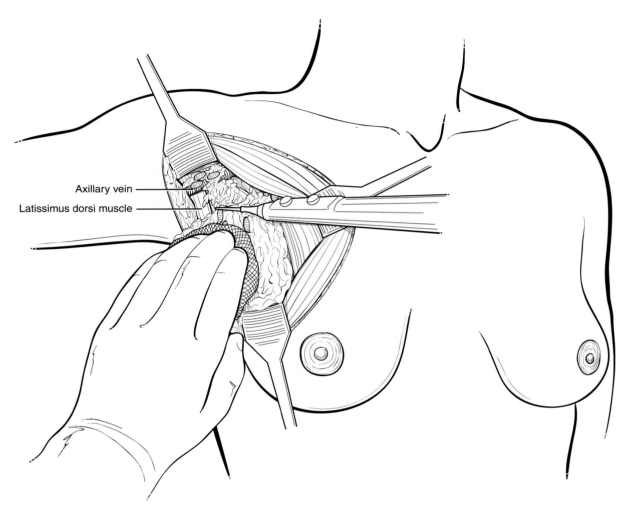

Axillary vein

Latissimus dorsi muscle

FIGURE 100–4

◆ The thoracodorsal artery and vein with the thoracodorsal nerve medially will be identified in the lateral third of the axillary artery **(Figure 100-5).** The thoracodorsal trunk courses on the medial aspect of the latissimus dorsi. Transection of the thoracodorsal nerve leads to weakened shoulder adduction.

◆ Once the thoracodorsal trunk is identified, lateral dissection is safe as long as the intercostalbrachial cutaneous nerve is visualized as it emerges from the axillary fat pad approximately halfway up the latissimus dorsi muscle, coursing toward the arm.

◆ The intercostalbrachial cutaneous nerve may be identified coursing transversely below the axillary vein and should be preserved if free of matted tumor-laden nodes to prevent bothersome sensory dysesthesias along the medial aspect of the upper arm.

◆ Dissection medially should be cautious, with attention to the long thoracic nerve, which lies on the serratus anterior muscle beneath the fascia (see Figure 100-5). Retraction of the fascia off the chest wall will pull the long thoracic nerve off the chest wall and place it at risk of injury. The nerve can be identified deep to the intercostalbrachial nerve or higher, inferior to the axillary vein on the chest wall, where it is less likely to have been pulled away from the serratus anterior into the axillary fat. The nerve should be protected and preserved. The function can be confirmed by very gentle compression and demonstration of contraction of the serratus muscle in the unparalyzed individual. Injury to the long thoracic nerve causes a winged scapula.

◆ After the axillary boundaries and important structures are identified, resection of the axillary contents is carried out from superior to inferior, maintaining visualization of the nerves at risk. As the fatty tissue is swept inferiorly, lymphatics and blood vessels are ligated or clipped and transected.

◆ The axillary contents are oriented to identify the apex of the axilla.

◆ The axilla devoid of lymphatics and the chest wall are visualized (see Figure 100-5). The cavity is irrigated with warm saline. Any residual bleeding vessels are cauterized or ligated.

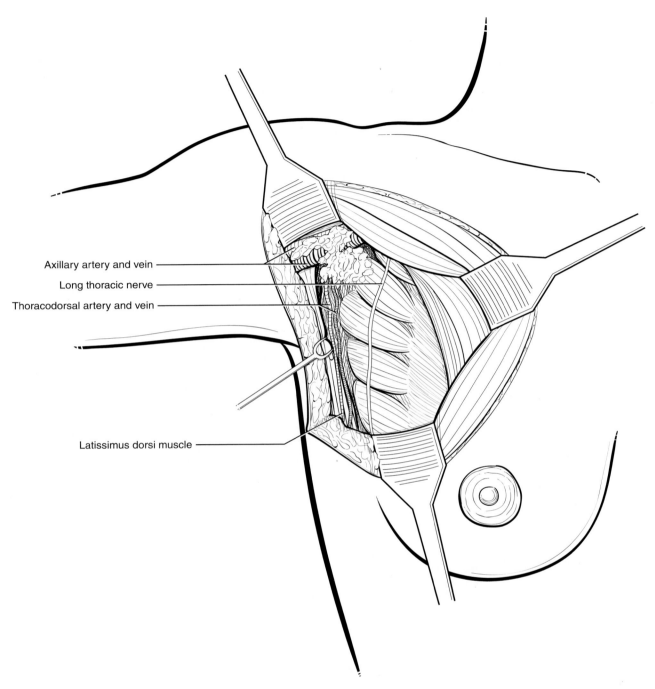

Axillary artery and vein

Long thoracic nerve

Thoracodorsal artery and vein

Latissimus dorsi muscle

FIGURE 100–5

3. CLOSING

◆ A closed-suction drain, such as a 10-mm Jackson-Pratt drain, is inserted through a separate small stab incision inferior laterally and oriented toward the apex of the axilla **(Figure 100-6).** The drain is secured with a 2-0 silk suture.

◆ The skin is closed in two layers with absorbable sutures, a deep layer of 3-0 Vicryl and a subcuticular closure with 4-0 Monocryl (see Figure 100-6). Steri-Strips or Dermabond may be used for skin approximation. A light dressing or special mastectomy bra is applied with loose fluff gauze dressings.

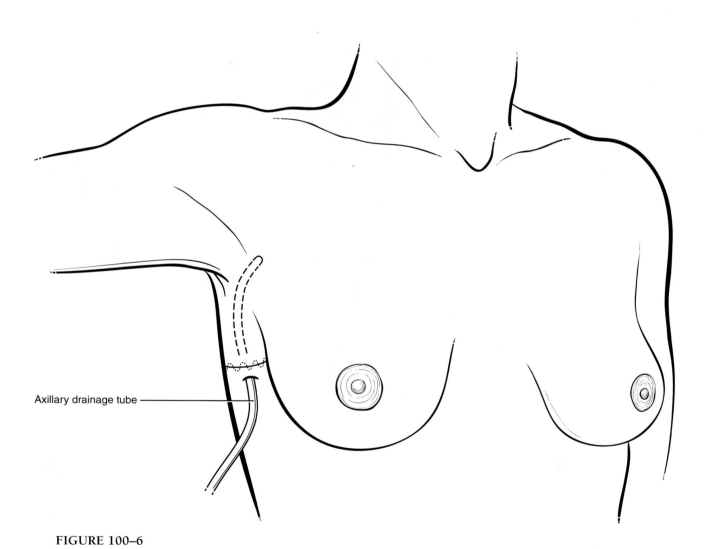

Axillary drainage tube

FIGURE 100–6

STEP 4: POSTOPERATIVE CARE

- The drain is emptied 2 to 3 times per day, and drain output is recorded on a log.
  - Drainage may be sanguinous immediately postoperatively but should be dilute.
  - Continued postoperative frank bloody output indicates ongoing bleeding and warrants return to the operating room.
  - Drainage clears to serosanguinous, then clear and straw-colored.
  - Cloudy fluid may indicate bacterial infection and should be cultured.

- Drains are removed when the output is less than 30 mL for 2 consecutive days. Drains usually remain for 7 to 10 days.

- Seroma may form after drain removal.
  - Aspirate it in clinic if it is large, suspicious for infection, or uncomfortable.
  - Multiple aspirations may be required.
  - Compression dressing may reduce the likelihood of reaccumulation.
  - Some seromas are reabsorbed without aspiration if they are small.

- Dressings are removed after 48 hours.
  - Pain out of proportion to the procedure may indicate a significant hematoma, for which dressings should be removed sooner.
  - Other indications include fever and excessive drainage.

- Taking a shower may be acceptable after 48 hours when dressings are removed.
  - The surgical site is bathed with mild soap and water, patted dry, and re-dressed around the drain site.
  - The incision may be left open according to individual preference.

- Tub baths are usually not advised while drains are in place.

- Antibiotics are usually not needed but may be considered on an individual basis for the following:
  - Previous surgical biopsy
  - Immunocompromised individuals
  - Local wound conditions

- Limited exercises are initiated on postoperative day 1 and increased to range-of-motion and strengthening exercises after the drains are removed.
  - Consultation with American Cancer Society for Reach to Recovery is helpful.
  - Consultation with occupational therapy for rehabilitation is useful.

- Individuals are monitored for lymphedema.

- Patient education about long-term precautions for protection of the affected extremity include the following:
  - Avoidance of blood pressure measurements and phlebotomy sticks on the affected extremity
  - No intravenous infusion lines
  - No constrictive clothing
  - Use of electric razors for shaving
  - Protective gloves for tasks that may lacerate the skin and lead to infection
  - Early intervention with antibiotics for a hand or arm infection, often requiring hospitalization for parenteral antibiotics

- Compression sleeve and glove may be indicated for cases of extensive nodal disease, combination surgery and radiotherapy, and evidence of lymphedema, as well as for prophylaxis for air travel.

- Postoperative radiotherapy or chemotherapy is not initiated for 2 to 3 weeks.

- Scarring maybe reduced with application of a silicone sheet such as Biodermis.

STEP 5: PEARLS AND PITFALLS

- Discussion with the interdisciplinary team will sequence treatment in the most appropriate manner.

- Preservation of the fascia of the serratus anterior muscle on the chest wall and identification of the long thoracic nerve underlying it on the chest wall will reduce the risk of transection and the winged scapula deformity.

- Dissection along the lateral aspect of the latissimus dorsi muscle reduces the likelihood of injury to the thoracodorsal trunk and weakened shoulder adduction.

- Preservation of the medial pectoral nerve prevents atrophy of the pectoralis major muscle and chest wall contour.

- Preservation of the intercostal brachial cutaneous nerves maintains sensation to the medial aspect of the upper extremity and prevents bothersome dysesthesias.
  - Preservation of fatty tissue and lymphatic channels from the arm around the axillary vein reduces the risk of lymphedema.
  - In obese patients, anatomic boundaries may be more difficult to identify and require time and patience during the procedure.
  - The pulse in the axillary artery is a landmark that can help orient the surgeon to stay inferior.

SELECTED REFERENCES

1. Fisher B, Anderson S, Bryant J, et al: Twenty-year follow-up of a randomized trial comparing total mastectomy, lumpectomy, and lumpectomy plus irradiation for the treatment of invasive breast cancer. N Engl J Med 2002;347:1233-1241.
2. Grube BJ, Rose CM, Giuliano AE: Local management of invasive breast cancer: Axilla. In Harris JR, Lippman ME, Morrow M (eds): Diseases of the Breast. Philadelphia, Lippincott Williams & Wilkins, 2004, pp 745-784.
3. Iglehart JD, Kaelin CM: Diseases of the breast. In Townsend C Jr, Beauchamp R, Evers B, Mattox K (eds): Sabiston Textbook of Surgery. Philadelphia, Elsevier Saunders, 2004, pp 867-927.
4. Lyman GH, Giuliano AE, Somerfield MR, et al: American Society of Clinical Oncology guideline recommendations for sentinel lymph node biopsy in early-stage breast cancer. J Clin Oncol 2005;23:7703-7720.
5. Veronesi U, Cascinelli N, Mariani L, et al: Twenty-year follow-up of a randomized study comparing breast-conserving surgery with radical mastectomy for early breast cancer. N Engl J Med 2002;347:1227-1232.

CHAPTER 101

SUPERFICIAL INGUINAL NODE DISSECTION

Celia Chao

STEP 1: SURGICAL ANATOMY

- The surgical anatomy of the groin is depicted in **Figure 101-1.**

STEP 2: PREOPERATIVE CONSIDERATIONS

- Accurate nodal staging may be accomplished by applying the techniques of sentinel lymph node biopsy. The current recommendation for treatment of a histologically positive sentinel lymph node is completion superficial inguinal node dissection. This operation is also indicated for bulky groin disease, because this procedure is very effective treatment for local disease control.

- Anesthesia: Either general anesthesia or epidural anesthesia may be used.

- Operative preparation: The patient is placed supine and prepared from 3 cm above the umbilicus and groin, down to the ipsilateral toes and the perineum. The extremity is prepped in its entirety and is externally rotated at the hip. A stack of sterile towels may be placed behind the lateral aspect of the knee to facilitate a frog-leg position.

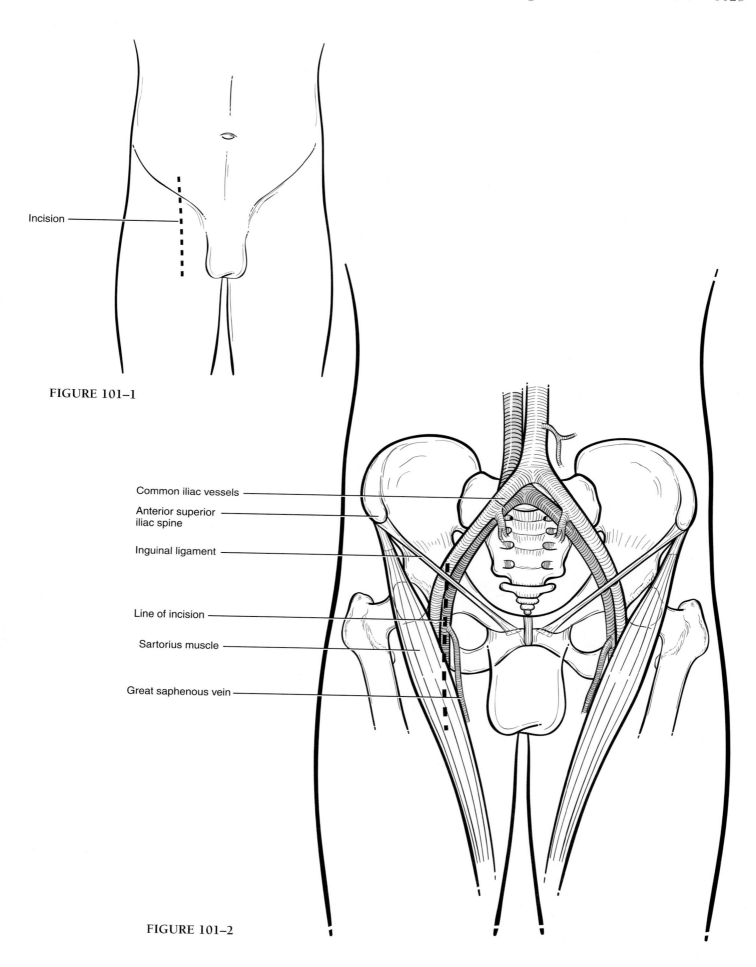

Incision

FIGURE 101–1

Common iliac vessels

Anterior superior iliac spine

Inguinal ligament

Line of incision

Sartorius muscle

Great saphenous vein

FIGURE 101–2

STEP 3: OPERATIVE STEPS

1. INCISION

- A longitudinal incision **(Figures 101-2 and 101-3)** is made overlying the groin, incorporating any previous biopsy scars (such as that from a sentinel lymph node biopsy) with an elliptical incision. Superiorly, the incision starts approximately 3 cm superior medial to the anterior superior iliac spine, extends past the inguinal ligament, and ends at the femoral triangle (the point at which the sartorius muscle crosses over the superficial femoral vessels; see Figures 101-2 and 101-3). A scalpel is used to incise the skin down to dermis.

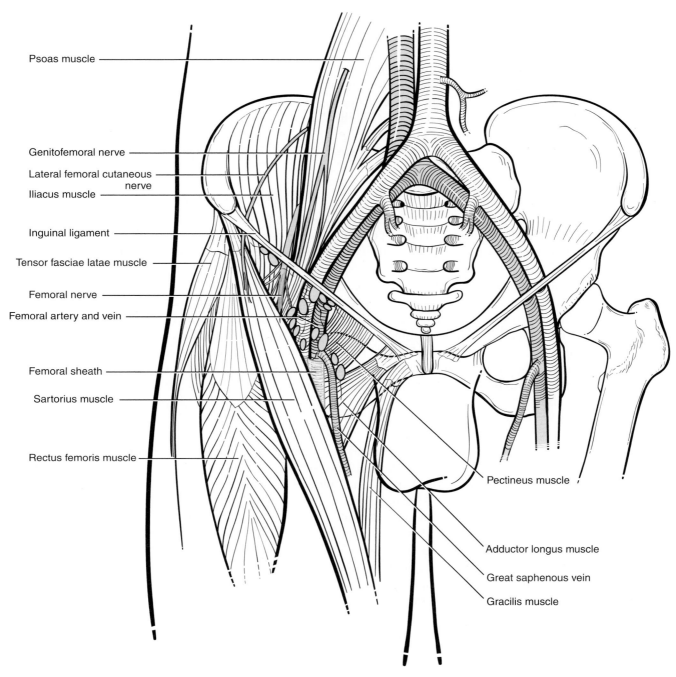

Psoas muscle

Genitofemoral nerve

Lateral femoral cutaneous
nerve

Iliacus muscle

Inguinal ligament

Tensor fasciae latae muscle

Femoral nerve

Femoral artery and vein

Femoral sheath

Sartorius muscle

Rectus femoris muscle

Pectineus muscle

Adductor longus muscle

Great saphenous vein

Gracilis muscle

FIGURE 101–3

2. DISSECTION

◆ Electrocautery is used to dissect down to subcutaneous tissue. Medial and lateral skin flaps are created. Superiorly, the skin flaps should be thinner because nodal-bearing tissue may be more superficial; as the dissection moves inferiorly toward the midthigh, the flap can become thicker. The medial aspect of the dissection extends to the pubic tubercle and extends laterally to include the entire length of the inguinal ligament. The boundaries of the dissection include the medial border of the adductor magnus muscle and the lateral border of the sartorius muscle.

◆ All fatty tissues, which include lymph node–bearing tissue (see Figure 101-1) both above and below the inguinal ligament, down to the external oblique fascia and the inguinal ligament are swept inferiorly. Medially, fatty nodal tissue is reflected away from the spermatic cord or round ligament, and all tissues overlying the femoral vessels, including the femoral sheath, are carefully dissected en bloc into the specimen. Laterally, tissue anterior to the sartorius fascia are swept toward the specimen. Distally, as the saphenous vein dives behind the sartorius muscle at the apex of the femoral triangle, the vein is divided (approximately 4 cm beyond the saphenofemoral junction). The tissue is swept superiorly until the foramen ovalis is encountered. Using a right-angled clamp, the surgeon ligates the saphenous vein at the saphenofemoral junction and secures the vein with a 2-0 silk ligature. Posteriorly, the limits of dissection include tissue anterior to the fascia of the adductor muscles and pectineus.

◆ The origin of the sartorius is identified and divided off the anterior superior iliac spine. The sartorius muscle is mobilized medially and transposed to cover the femoral vessels **(Figures 101-4 and 101-5).** The lateral femoral cutaneous nerve arises underneath the lateral aspect of the inguinal ligament and extends obliquely over the origin of the sartorius. Care should be taken to identify and preserve this sensory nerve to the lateral thigh. Blood vessels entering the sartorius muscle are preserved as the muscle is mobilized medially to cover the exposed femoral vessels in a tension-free manner. The proximal aspect of the muscle has to be rotated for the coverage to be tension free. The tendinous end of the muscle is sutured to the inguinal ligament with 3-0 absorbable sutures using interrupted vertical mattress stitches. The sartorius muscle will protect the femoral vessels from exposure and subsequent bleeding, in case of skin edge necrosis, wound infection, and tissue breakdown, especially after adjuvant radiotherapy.

3. CLOSING

◆ The wound is irrigated and two closed-suction drains are placed, one exiting medially and one exiting laterally. If the blood supply to the skin edges appears marginal, the edges should be trimmed back to healthy tissue. The incision is closed in two layers. The deeper fascial layer is reapproximated with 2-0 or 3-0 interrupted absorbable sutures, and the skin can be closed using skin staples.

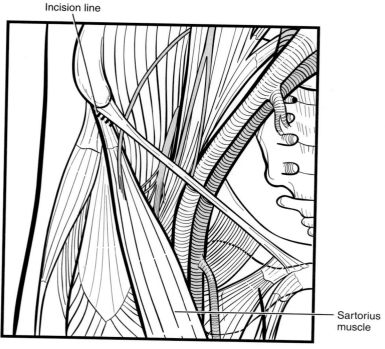

Incision line

Sartorius
muscle

FIGURE 101–4

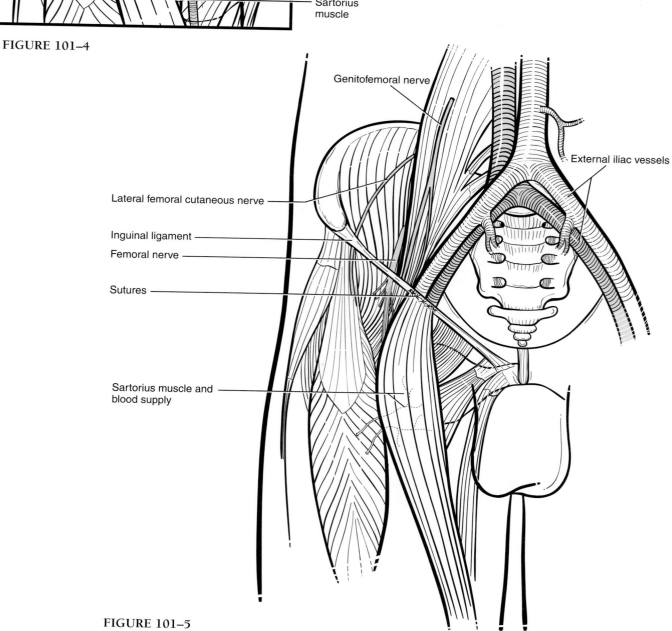

Genitofemoral nerve

External iliac vessels

Lateral femoral cutaneous nerve

Inguinal ligament

Femoral nerve

Sutures

Sartorius muscle and
blood supply

FIGURE 101–5

STEP 4: POSTOPERATIVE CARE

- Postoperatively, the patient may ambulate with elastic support on the leg, as tolerated. However, when the patient is at rest, the extremity should be elevated to decrease limb edema. The drains can be removed when the drainage decreases to 30 mL or less per 24 hours.

- Lymphedema can occur in more than 50% of patients who have undergone superficial lymph node dissection. Prophylactic measures, such as elevating the leg and wearing elastic stockings, are important means to decrease the severity and incidence of this potential complication.

STEP 5: PEARLS AND PITFALLS

- The most common acute postoperative complication is cellulitis and/or wound infection. Although prophylactic preoperative antibiotics are recommended, the infection rates can range up to 30%.

- The rate of lymphocele or seroma formation ranges from 3% to 23%. The use of closed-suction drains for a longer period of time can decrease the incidence of fluid formation under the flaps; however, prolonged use has to be balanced with the increased potential for wound infection.

- The incidence of extremity lymphedema can be decreased with the use of elastic stockings, limb elevation, and exercise.

- The incidence of thromboembolic events, such as deep vein thrombosis and pulmonary embolus, was reported to be 13.6% in a study of patients who underwent inguinal node dissection for melanoma. Prophylaxis with intermittent pneumatic compression devices and low-dose anticoagulants may minimize this complication.

SELECTED REFERENCES

1. Karakousis CP, Heiser MA, Moore RH: Lymphedema after groin dissection. Am J Surg 1983;145:205-208.
2. Arbeit JM, Lowry SF, Line BR, et al: Deep venous thromboembolism in patients undergoing inguinal lymph node dissection for melanoma. Ann Surg 1981;194:648-655.
3. Johnson TM, Sondak VK, Bichakjian CK, et al: The role of sentinel node biopsy for melanoma: evidence assessment. J Am Acad Dermatol 2006;54:19-27.
4. Health Care Center for the Homeless. Available on the Internet: www.hcch.org

CHAPTER 102

DONOR NEPHRECTOMY

Jacqueline A. Lappin

STEP 1: SURGICAL ANATOMY

- ◆ The left kidney is most commonly procured for live donor kidney transplantation because of its longer vein and greater ease of access. However, given the basic tenet of live kidney donation, "leaving the best kidney in the donor," the donor surgeon should be familiar with right and left donor nephrectomy. There are many donor nephrectomy surgical techniques available and include pure laparoscopic; hand-assisted laparoscopic; robot-assisted pure laparoscopic; robot-assisted and hand-assisted, using either a transabdominal or retroperitoneal approach; and of course, open nephrectomy. The donor surgeon and operating room should be equipped to convert from a laparoscopic to an open approach at short notice. Regardless of technique used, understanding the three-dimensional relationships of both kidneys is essential.

- ◆ **Figure 102-1** illustrates some of the important anterior relationships of the right and left kidney. Both kidneys are positioned high up in the retroperitoneum under cover of the costal margin. The body of the kidney is oriented obliquely on the diaphragm and quadratus lumborum muscle in the long axis of the psoas. The hilum of the kidney and its contents are angled forward. Although the position of the kidneys is altered with movement of the diaphragm, the hilum of the right kidney (pushed down by the liver) lies just below the level of the transpyloric plane, whereas that of the left kidney lies just above the level of the transpyloric plane, approximately 5 cm from the midline. With such intimate association with the pancreas and duodenum, it is easy to see how injuries can occur.

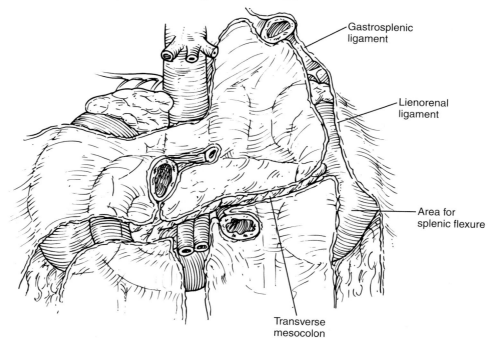

FIGURE 102–1

Gastrosplenic ligament

Lienorenal ligament

Area for splenic flexure

Transverse mesocolon

- **Figure 102-2, A** (anterior view) **and Figure 102-2, B** (posterior view) illustrate the relationship of each kidney to the pleura and rib cage. The parietal pleura reaches all the way down to the spinous process of the 12th vertebra posteriorly and the 10th rib in the mid-axillary line. This relationship becomes more important with a posterior approach to the kidney.

STEP 2: PREOPERATIVE CONSIDERATIONS

- Each kidney donor must undergo an extensive examination to determine physiologic, psychological, immunologic, and anatomic suitability.

- The best kidney must be left in the donor.

- Surgical experience of the donor team will determine the surgical technique used in each individual case.

- A preoperative bowel preparation, although not essential, can facilitate intraoperative and postoperative management of the donor.

- Care should be taken to prevent dehydration of the donor as is apt to occur with preoperative imaging, bowel preparation, and travel from out of town.

- Although donor evaluation is similar for both open and laparoscopic nephrectomy, it is important to be familiar with the sensitivities and specificities of preoperative imaging techniques used in your facility.

Anterior View

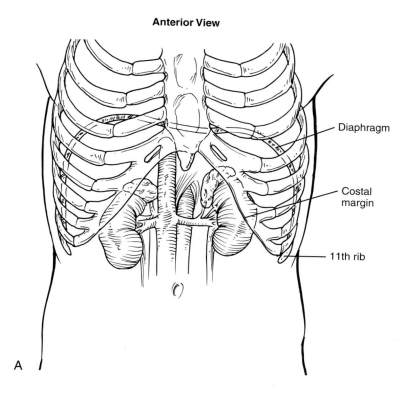

Diaphragm

Costal margin

11th rib

A

Posterior View

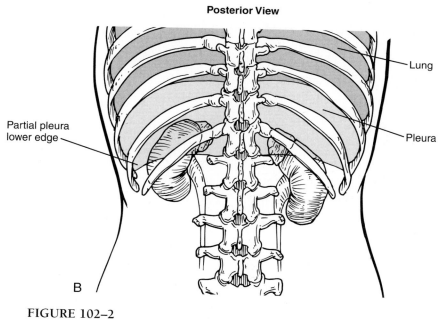

Lung

Partial pleura lower edge

Pleura

B

FIGURE 102–2

STEP 3: OPERATIVE STEPS

LAPAROSCOPIC TRANSABDOMINAL LEFT DONOR NEPHRECTOMY

♦ What follows is a description of a laparoscopic transabdominal left donor nephrectomy. Differences in technique for pure laparoscopic and hand-assisted approaches are described.

♦ Position of the patient is shown in **Figure 102-3.** An alternate position is supine with rotation toward a right lateral decubitus position. Addition of Trendelenburg can also be helpful.

♦ After induction of general anesthesia, preoperative antibiotics are given; an orogastric tube and Foley catheter are placed. Thromboembolic-deterrent (TED) stockings and sequential compression devices are applied to the lower extremities. The patient is carefully positioned in a modified lateral decubitus position with the hips rotated posteriorly. An axillary roll is placed and the arms are flexed at the elbow and padded. A second roll is placed between the patient's knees with the lower limb flexed at the knee. The kidney rest is elevated and the patient is secured. Additional padded support may be applied to the patient's right shoulder, lower abdomen, and buttocks to facilitate intraoperative rotation of the table.

♦ The position of all the participants are illustrated **(Figure 102-4).** The surgeon stands on the right side of the patient, and the camera operator, more caudad. The scrub nurse and additional assistant stand on the patient's left side. There are two video towers placed at the top of the table on either side of the patient.

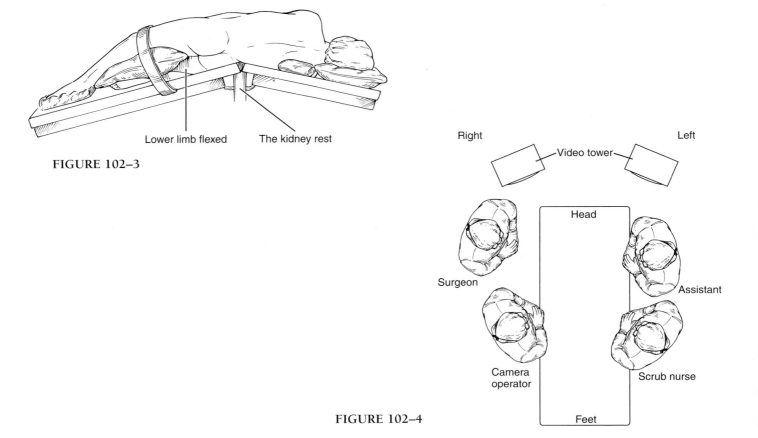

Lower limb flexed   The kidney rest

FIGURE 102–3

FIGURE 102–4

1. INCISION

◆ Placement of trochars is shown in **Figure 102-5.** There are, however, many variations for trochar and hand-port placement.

◆ Before placement of the pneumoperitoneum, the abdomen is marked for placement of tro-chars and extraction incision. Each port site is infiltrated with local anesthesic, which can facilitate a reduction in narcotic use postoperatively. The ports are placed as illustrated. A 10- or 12-mm port that is primarily used for dissection is placed at the level of the umbili-cus, a second 10- or 12-mm camera port is placed lateral to the rectus muscle, halfway between the umbilicus and the anterior superior iliac spine. Transillumination of the abdo-men can be used to prevent injury to the inferior epigastric artery with this latter trochar placement. A third 5-mm port is placed in the midline, halfway between the umbilicus and the xiphoid process, and a fourth 5-mm port can be placed in the flank for retraction. As the operation progresses, the camera port and dissection ports can be interchanged to obtain optimal exposure. Once the pneumoperitoneum is established, the zero-degree lens camera is replaced with a 30-degree angled scope.

◆ For hand-assisted laparoscopic left nephrectomy, the umbilical port is lengthened in the midline to facilitate placement of a pneumatic cuff or GelPort **(Figure 102-6).** At least two laparotomy sponges can be introduced at this time.

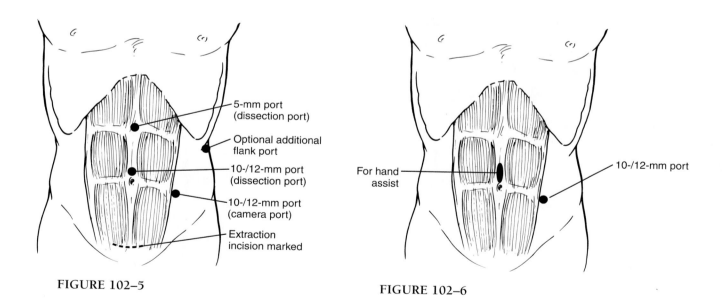

5-mm port
(dissection port)

Optional additional
flank port

10-/12-mm port
(dissection port)

10-/12-mm port
(camera port)

Extraction
incision marked

FIGURE 102–5

For hand
assist

10-/12-mm port

FIGURE 102–6

2. DISSECTION

◆ The Harmonic scalpel or Bovie electrocautery, or both, can be used for the dissection. Because pneumoperitoneum affects renal blood flow, a pneumoperitoneum of 12 to 14 mm Hg is maintained. The dissection proceeds with an incision placed along the white line of Toldt. This is extended superiorly to include takedown of the splenocolic and lienorenal ligaments and inferiorly to the sigmoid colon and iliac vessels **(Figure 102-7).** The superior and lateral attachments of the kidney helps suspend and fix the kidney to facilitate hilar dissection. The analogy of taking the sheet off the bed has been used to describe this reflection of the colon medially to expose Gerota's fascia and the kidney. As with open surgery, maintaining the correct plane is essential. There is a perceptible difference in the appearance of the mesenteric and retroperitoneal fat (mesenteric fat is a brighter yellow).

◆ Next, the gonadal vein is identified and traced superiorly to the renal vein, which is then dissected out **(Figure 102-8).**

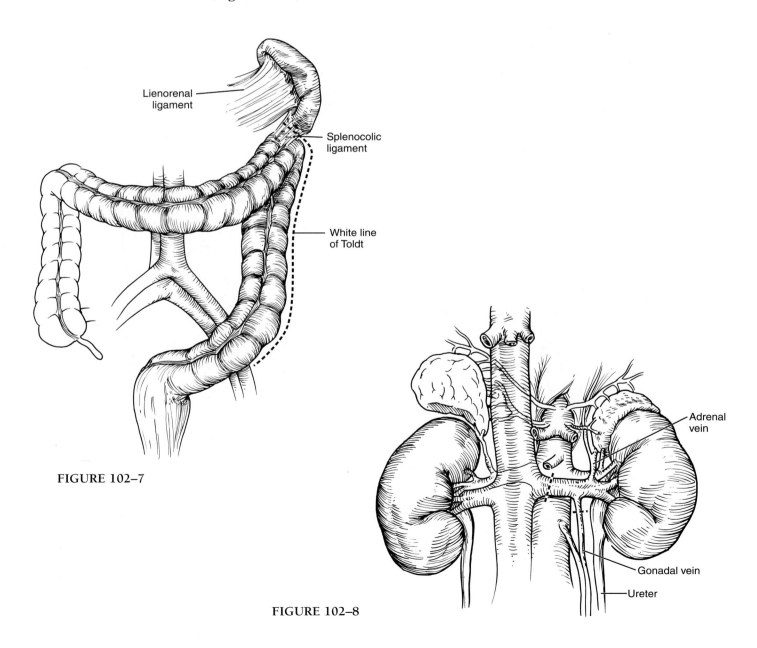

FIGURE 102–7

FIGURE 102–8

◆ The adrenal vein can also be divided at this time. It is always assumed (although present only approximately a third of the time) that there are posterior lumbar veins present and if not readily dissected at this juncture, they can be taken when the kidney is further mobilized. The gonadal vein can also be used to facilitate dissection of the ureter. Tracing the vein to the lower pole of the kidney, the ureter is mobilized with its essential periureteral fat down to the iliac vessels **(Figure 102-9)**.

◆ The gonadal vein can be divided at this time. The surgeon can now proceed with probably one of the more technically demanding parts of the operation—dissection of the adrenal gland from the upper pole of the kidney **(Figure 102-10)**.

◆ The presence of an adrenal artery is less consistent than the vein but should be looked for. Next, the renal artery is dissected to the level of the aorta. If there are any lumbar veins, they may be divided at this time as necessary **(Figure 102-11)**.

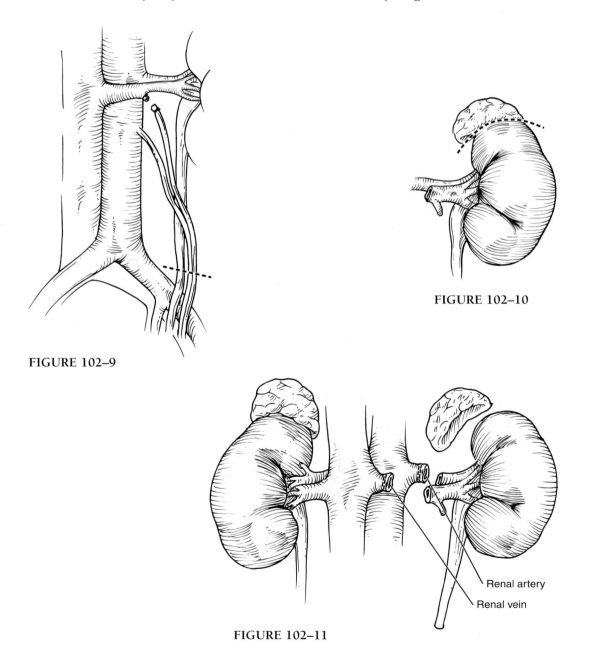

FIGURE 102–9

FIGURE 102–10

Renal artery

Renal vein

FIGURE 102–11

◆ It is only at this time that the kidney is further mobilized with takedown of the lateral attachments of the kidney. Throughout the procedure, the patient should be well hydrated and actively excreting urine. Once the kidney is completely free, a 6- to 8-cm Pfannenstiel incision is made without entrance into the peritoneum. This incision is unnecessary, of course, with a hand-assisted laparoscopic approach. The ureter can now be transected (see Figure 102-9).

◆ Mannitol (12.5 g) or furosemide (Lasix) (10 to 20 mg), or both, is administered before clamping the renal artery and vein in some centers, but I prefer volume loading to promote natriuresis.

◆ Communication between the donor and recipient team is essential to streamline the sequence of events. If the recipient room is not yet ready for implantation, the pneumoperitoneum can be released in the donor and the nephrectomy can be delayed. When both rooms are synchronized, systemic heparinization of the donor (also optional) can be performed.

◆ An Endocatch bag is now placed through the peritoneum via the Pfannenstiel incision, and the kidney is loaded. It is important that the donor is completely relaxed to minimize trauma as the kidney is removed. The renal artery and renal vein are then transected (see Figure 102-11) with a vascular linear stapler or clip device, or both, and the kidney is removed to the back table by one of the senior assistants or implanting surgeon.

◆ The staple lines of the donated kidney vessels and ureter are excised and the renal artery is flushed with ice-cold preservation solution.

3. CLOSING

◆ The time from intracorporeal vessel clamping to vessel flushing with ice-cold solution is defined as warm ischemia time and is usually approximately 2 to 4 minutes. The time from vessel clamping to reperfusion in the recipient is cold ischemia time. The donor surgeon, in the interim, is ensuring hemostasis in the donor with reestablishment of the pneumoperitoneum, so that all staple lines can be reevaluated and confirmed to be intact. The use of a linear staple device or clip on the renal artery is a matter of surgeon preference. There is some evidence to support the improved safety of stapling devices versus clips, which can fall off. Reversal of heparin is optional once the donor kidney artery and vein are transected.

◆ Once hemostasis is ensured, the pneumoperitoneum is released and the fascia is closed.

OPEN LEFT DONOR NEPHRECTOMY

◆ Although most donor nephrectomies are performed laparoscopically, there will always be occasion to perform open donor nephrectomy electively or with laparoscopic failure. Similar to patient positioning for a laparoscopic procedure, the patient is placed in a modified lateral decubitus position with the hips rotated posteriorly. An axillary roll is placed and the arms are flexed at the elbow and padded. A second roll is placed between the patient's knees, with the lower limb flexed at the knee. The kidney rest is elevated and the patient is secured. The operating table is flexed in the middle so that the patient's flank is taut **(Figure 102-12)**.

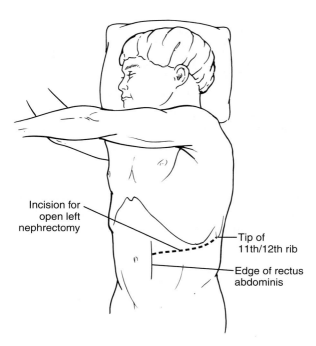

FIGURE 102–12

- The incision is placed over the distal end of the 11th or 12th rib, extending from the mid-axillary line posteriorly to the lateral edge of the rectus abdominis muscle anteriorly at the level of the umbilicus. The latissimus dorsi muscle posteriorly and external oblique muscle anteriorly are first incised, followed by the internal oblique and transversus abdominis muscles to expose the peritoneum and its contents **(Figure 102-13)**.

- Although well described, taking the tip of the 12th rib is not usually necessary. Care is taken not to enter the peritoneal cavity medially or the pleural space anterior laterally. The peritoneum and its contents are bluntly reflected medially to expose Gerota's fascia and the retroperitoneal space **(Figure 102-14)**.

- A fixed retractor greatly facilitates exposure. The gonadal vein and ureter are first identified and traced inferiorly to the iliac artery and superiorly to Gerota's fascia, which can now be opened.

- The upper pole of the kidney is then dissected from the adrenal gland, with care given not to injure the pancreas. As with the laparoscopic nephrectomy, the renal vein is identified, and the gonadal, adrenal, and lumbar veins can be divided at this time.

- The renal artery is dissected to the aorta, avoiding injury to small polar branches. The surgeon should also try to avoid traction on the kidney, because this can lead to vasospasm and acute tubular necrosis in the recipient postoperatively.

- The proximity of the diaphragm and pleural space should be kept in mind to prevent pneumothorax. Just as in laparoscopic nephrectomy, volume loading and saline natriuresis of the donor remains an important component of renal protection and cannot be overemphasized.

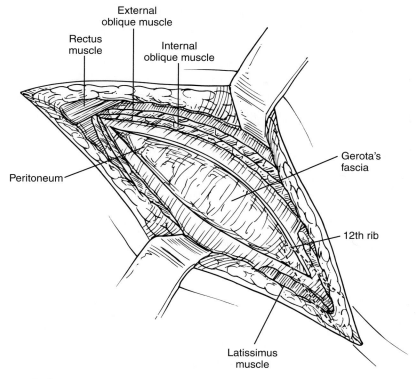

FIGURE 102–13

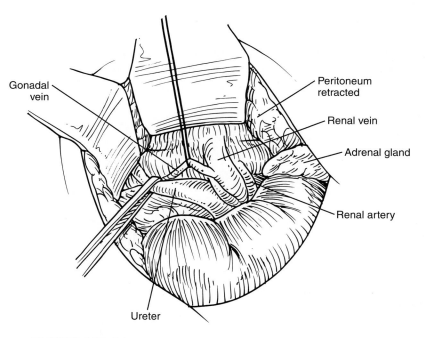

FIGURE 102–14

RIGHT LAPAROSCOPIC DONOR NEPHRECTOMY

◆ Several modifications to the left donor nephrectomy can be made to counter the technical challenges posed by a right nephrectomy. The patient is placed in a modified lateral decubitus position with the right side up. Port sites are placed on the opposite side of the body but in a more cephalad position as for left nephrectomy, with an additional liver retractor port (**Figure 102-15**).

◆ Either of these upper ports can be used to retract the right lobe of the liver superiorly to facilitate dissection of the upper pole of the right kidney.

◆ Alternatively, the upper midline port can be placed more superiorly as for a left nephrectomy.

◆ This port site and the liver retractor site can be incorporated into a subcostal incision following complete laparoscopic dissection to retrieve the kidney. Some authors have also suggested using this mini incision to place a Satinsky clamp across the base of the right renal vein so that the inferior vena cava (IVC) can be sutured closed, because stapling devices can significantly shorten an already short right renal vein.

◆ It is essential to mobilize the duodenum medially to expose the IVC to access the right renal vein. There are occasional small anterior branches on the renal vein that can be easily avulsed. The right renal artery can also be identified at this time and dissected out.

◆ The kidney is then mobilized medially, and the vascular dissection is completed. It is important to remember that the right gonadal vein drains directly into the IVC and is unavailable as a guide to the ureteric dissection.

◆ For hand-assisted laparoscopic right nephrectomy, the port sites are as illustrated in **Figure 102-16**.

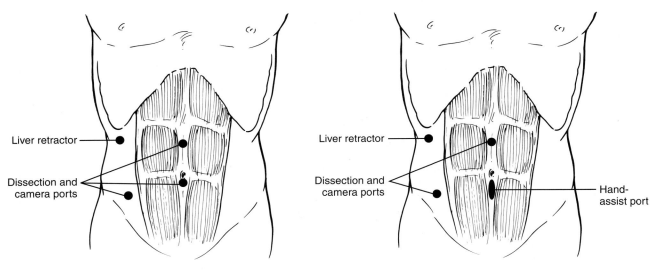

FIGURE 102–15   **FIGURE 102–16**

OPEN RIGHT DONOR NEPHRECTOMY

◆ For open right nephrectomy, the patient is set up as for a left nephrectomy, with the right side up. The main differences with the right nephrectomy are that the kidney is somewhat lower, the renal vein is thinner and shorter, and the gonadal vein drains into the IVC.

RETROPERITONEAL LAPAROSCOPIC APPROACH TO THE KIDNEY

◆ Some centers advocate a retroperitoneal approach to right and left nephrectomy; the main advantages appear to be avoidance of the peritoneal cavity, decreased risk of ileus, and lesser hemodynamic effects with unilateral pneumoperitoneum.

◆ The disadvantages of a laparoscopic retroperitoneal approach are a smaller working space, a steeper learning curve, and some reports of more prolonged warm ischemia times.

USE OF THE ROBOT

◆ The robot can be used for either pure laparoscopic or hand-assisted nephrectomy. The advantages include retention of binocular vision and greater flexibility of the operating head.

◆ The chief disadvantage is expense.

STEP 4: POSTOPERATIVE CARE

◆ A Foley catheter is left in the donor overnight.

◆ The patient is monitored for bleeding.

◆ Early ambulation (on day of surgery) is encouraged.

◆ The patient should not take food or fluids the first day and should start clear liquids the next day.

STEP 5: PEARLS AND PITFALLS

◆ Success of the live donor kidney transplant begins with optimal hemodynamic management of the donor. Adequate hydration of the donor preoperatively and intraoperatively cannot be overemphasized.

◆ Ensure diuresis before clamping of the vessels to counter the effects of renal artery traction and the effect of the pneumoperitoneum on renal blood flow.

◆ Coordinate between the donor and recipient operating rooms to minimize cold ischemia time.

SELECTED REFERENCES

1. Potter SR, Buell JF, Hanaway M, Woodle ES: Laparoscopic live donor nephrectomy: Rationale, techniques and implications. Semin Dial 2001;14:365-372.
2. Ratner LE, Fabrizio M, Chavin K, et al: Technical considerations in the delivery of the kidney during laparoscopic live-donor nephrectomy. J Am Coll Surg 1999;189:427-430.
3. Bolte SL, Chin LT, Moon TD, et al: Maintaining urine production and early allograft function during laparoscopic donor nephrectomy. Urology 2006;68:747-750.

CHAPTER 103

SKIN GRAFT—SPLIT THICKNESS AND FULL THICKNESS

James J. Gallagher and David N. Herndon

STEP 1: SURGICAL ANATOMY

◆ **Figure 103-1** shows a detailed cross-section of the skin.

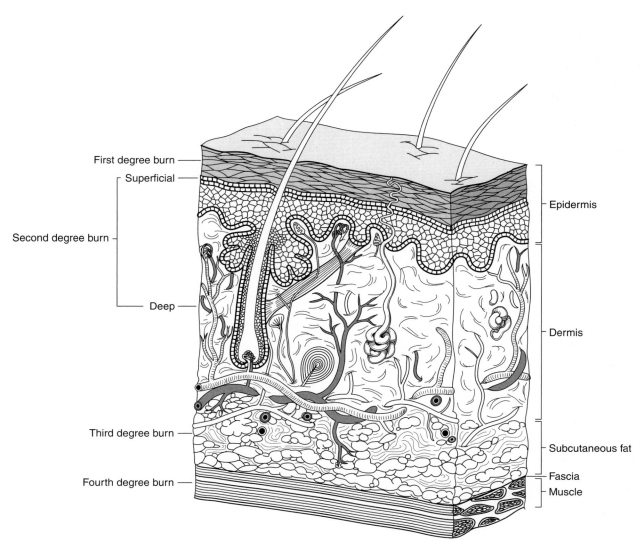

FIGURE 103–1

INDICATIONS

- The most common reason for skin grafting is a deep second- or third-degree burn (see Figure 103-1).

- Other causes include infection, cancer, reconstruction, and trauma.

- Burn injury that is clearly third degree should be surgically excised and grafted promptly unless it is small enough to allow healing by secondary intention.

- Second-degree burns are either superficial or deep partial thickness. This distinction can be difficult to determine clinically.

- As a general rule, burns that will heal within 2 to 3 weeks with good wound care should be allowed to do so without grafting. During this period, the clinician has a number of choices to manage the second-degree wound: removal of blisters and tangential excision of dead tissue followed by the application of homograft, xenograft, Biobrane, or other artificial skin. Alternatively, these burns may be treated with serial dressing changes with a topical antimicrobial, typically silver sulfadiazine. Clinical judgment is the best guide as to burns that will heal and those that will not.

- The following is a review of debridement and grafting strategies for burns, as well as modern techniques of skin grafting for all skin defects.

- Free skin grafts will take to (in order of declining take rate) healthy dermis, fascia, fat, muscle, periosteum, and peritenon. Granulation tissue growth indicates a healthy bed for grafting; the granulation tissue maybe removed before the graft is placed, or it may be left in place depending on physician judgment. Removal improves topographic irregularities, as well as the biofilm of bacterial colonization that may decrease graft take. Removal is associated with increased operative blood loss.

- Modern dermatomes come in a variety of types. Most are powered by compressed air or electricity (Figure 103-2).

- Calibration for depth of harvest is in the thousandths of an inch. Typically, a graft is taken between 8 and 15 thousandths of an inch; the choice of depth varies with the area to be grafted and the overall needs of the patient. We have found that the calibrations can be inaccurate, and we routinely use the sharp edge of a scalpel to act as a mechanical check of cutting depth. Reharvesting of donor sites is limited by the healing rates of the donor sites, with thinner harvest sites obviously healing quicker. Each time the donor is harvested, the epithelium is taken with some amount of dermis. The epithelium regrows, but the underlying dermis does not. Deeper donor sites have the potential to produce more scarring. Defects to the head and neck area are best covered with skin from above the clavicles. The shaved head provides a reliable donor site with excellent healing potential; a caution is in order to avoid areas of alopecia (senescent or autoimmune). Donor site placement should be mindful of normally exposed areas in conventional dress patterns. Full-thickness grafts require either the donor site to be closed or that a split-thickness graft be placed for healing. Depth greater than 15 to 20 thousandths of an inch with the dermatome may near full thickness and require the donor site to be autografted. It is common to harvest small amounts of skin to cover areas of the palm or the eyelids. These small full-thickness donor sites are usually closed primarily.

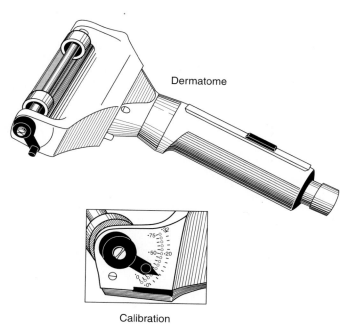

Dermatome

Calibration

FIGURE 103–2

STEP 2: PREOPERATIVE CONSIDERATIONS

- ◆ Burn and skin defect closure operations are elective or semielective operations.

- ◆ Preoperative antibiotics are chosen to cover gram-positive organisms in smaller burns. Patients with larger burns, residents of the intensive care unit, or patients with other history of contamination should have broader antibiotic coverage to include gram-negative organisms, as well as institutional-specific coverage of resistant organisms.

- ◆ Most of the preoperative dressings used provide some topical antimicrobial. Blood loss of 0.5 to 1.0 mL/cm^2 area (depending on the timing of surgery) that is prepared can guide the surgeon as to the need for perioperative blood transfusion.

ANESTHESIA

- ◆ Burn and wound surgery is performed with the patient under a combination of local anesthesia, conscious sedation, and general anesthesia depending on the extent of the area involved.

- ◆ Efforts at minimizing blood loss during surgery may involve tourniquets in extremity burns; topical epinephrine; topical thrombin; and possibly, tumescence of the tissue with balanced salt solution, with or without epinephrine.

- ◆ The need for large access will best be judged by the area to be treated. Clear communication with the anesthesia care team is critical, because blood loss is mainly into the laparotomy pads and can easily be underestimated.

- ◆ Volume replacement during surgery in patients with burns over more than 40% of the body is largely with blood and fresh frozen plasma. Maintenance of temperature is critical; this can be accomplished by warming the operating room and fluids and using blankets and radiant heaters.

POSITION

- ◆ The patient's position on the operating table is determined by the area to be treated and the choice of donor site. We routinely use a specially designed operating room for larger burns, which allows for an on-table bath and hanging of an extremity to facilitate circumferential work.

STEP 3: OPERATIVE STEPS

- Begin by preparing the wound bed. This will allow a clear estimation of the size of the defect and will allow for hemostasis to occur while the surgeon's attention is directed at the harvesting of autograft.

- For adequate wound bed preparation, the surgeon must remove the eschar down to healthy tissue to ensure a bed that will accept the skin. There are many choices to accomplish this goal. Most commonly, tangential excision is chosen. Tangential excision is achieved by serially cutting through the eschar until viable dermis or other viable tissue is reached. Specialized knives have been invented for this purpose **(Figure 103-3)**.

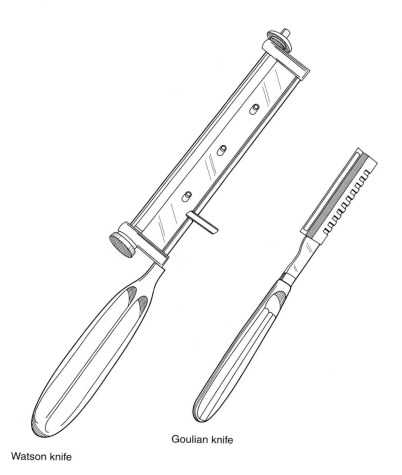

Goulian knife

Watson knife

FIGURE 103–3

◆ Living dermis is characterized by punctate bleeding points and the pearly white appearance of the healthy dermis. Tangential excision is the ideal for a partial-thickness burn of small to moderate size. With larger and deeper burns, the surgeon may choose fascial excision. Often, Bovie electrocautery is used to excise the eschar with its underlying fat. Although underlying fat is often viable, it is removed down to fascia because of its susceptibility to infection from a poor blood supply. Fascial excision in the care of the most extensive burns is often necessary for survival. Once excision is complete, lap pads wet with saline and epinephrine are placed over the wound. Point areas of bleeding are controlled with the Bovie. On an extremity, an elastic bandage wrap can be used to aid in hemostasis.

◆ The donor site is then prepared, often with oil to aid in the smooth movement of the dermatome over the skin. If a bony prominence or other irregularity is noted, it can prevent the smooth movement of the dermatome.

◆ A balanced salt solution with epinephrine can be infused via a spinal needle to swell the tissue. This allows easier passage of the dermatome to harvest a wider, more uniform, and better quality skin graft. This is a routine practice when harvesting the head as a donor. The dermatome is held steady at a 45-degree angle with some pressure on the skin. Traction and countertraction is very helpful in achieving the best result. It also can be helpful to withdraw the skin out of the dermatome as it is being harvested. This can allow evaluation and adjustment of the depth of skin depending on the need (**Figure 103-4**).

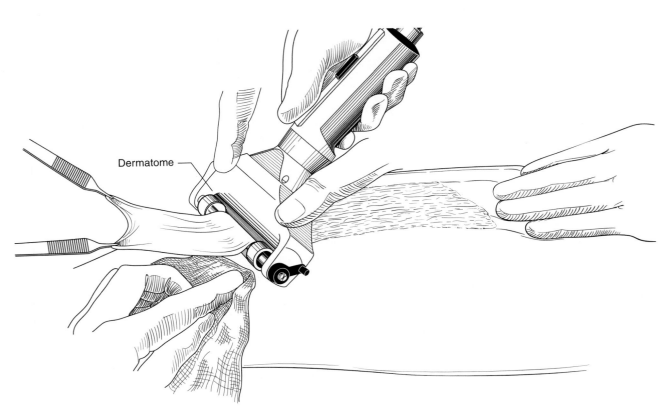

FIGURE 103–4

◆ The donor site is covered with a dressing. The choice of donor site dressing is based on experience and available options. There are clearly many choices and no clear standard.

◆ The skin is then left as a sheet, or meshed to increase its size and to allow drainage, depending on the surgeon's choice and the clinical situation. A variety of meshers are available.

◆ **Figure 103-5** demonstrates a carrierless mesher.

◆ If a wide area is to be covered, 4:1 meshed autograft may be used. This will require an overlay of 2:1 homograft, which will be lost as the autograft underneath heals (see Figure 103-5).

◆ If 2:1 autograft is used, it is placed in the prepared bed, trimmed to fit, and secured with staples or sutures (see Figure 103-5).

◆ Whenever possible, sheet autograft should be consistent to improve the cosmetic result.

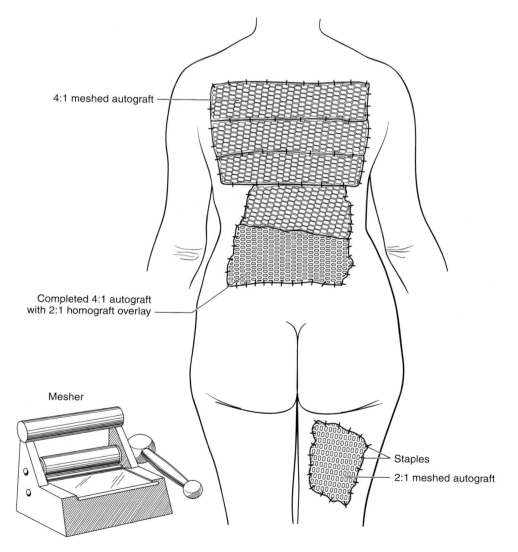

FIGURE 103–5

◆ The goal of the dressing chosen is to provide a humid environment with elimination of shear forces for 3 to 5 days. During this period, the graft adheres to the bed underneath. Our routine dressing after skin grafting is as follows: fine mesh gauze impregnated with Bacitracin/polymyxin single layer followed by dry bulky gauze dressing secured by Kerlix wrap. Often, a splint to immobilize the joints proximal and distal to the graft is placed followed by an elastic bandage wrap. In areas where an elastic bandage wrap is impractical and shear a realistic concern, a bolster dressing can be placed. The bolster is made of a sheet of impregnated fine mesh gauze with bulky dressing and tie-over silk sutures **(Figure 103-6)**.

◆ Facial grafts are left open to air with a layer of Bacitracin/polymyxin ointment.

STEP 4: POSTOPERATIVE CARE

◆ The amount of time varies as to when the dressing is removed. Typically in a clean elective case, the dressing can be safely left in place for 4 to 5 days. At this time, the skin should be adherent. If a sheet graft has been placed, often it will be checked on postoperative day 1 or 2 to evaluate for seroma or blood clot. When identified, these are removed by a small hole in the graft created with a no. 11 blade and tip or vacuum extraction using a fine pediatric respiratory suction catheter. If the dressings are removed early, then they are replaced until postoperative day 4 to 5. The donor site treated with Scarlet Red should be dried postoperatively with open air desiccation or, occasionally, careful use of a hair dryer. The donor site should be checked routinely. Healing should be complete in nearly all cases by postoperative day 10. If healing has not occurred, consider removing any remaining donor site coverage material and change to daily care washing with topicals to treat colonization or infection.

◆ Once the skin has taken, application of moisturizer and protection from the sun to both the donor and recipient sites are recommended. The patient should be given exercises to aggressively regain full use of any involved joint. Immobilization beyond what is required for the graft to take promotes contractures and limited return of function. The surgical sites should be monitored closely for evidence of scar hypertrophy and contracture. This typically will present within the first few months postoperatively. The treated areas are monitored until complete healing has taken place, often over a year. A good measure of a mature wound is the absence of hyperemia in the scar. A coordinated effort with a physical therapist with burn experience is highly recommended. It is our practice to fit most grafted areas with custom-made garments for pressure application. Silicone gel pads can be of help with scar hypertrophy in localized areas.

STEP 5: PEARLS AND PITFALLS

FACE GRAFTS

◆ It is recommended when applying skin grafts to the face that aesthetic units are respected. This will achieve the best cosmetic result over time as the face grafts mature **(Figure 103-7)**.

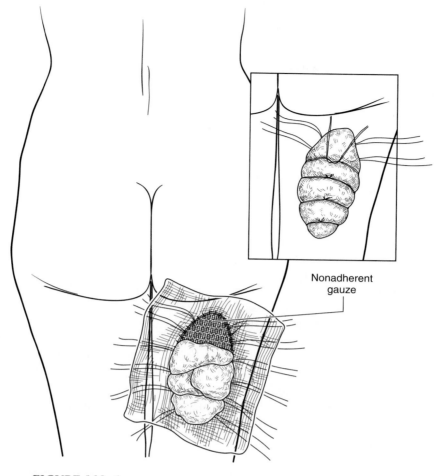

Nonadherent
gauze

FIGURE 103–6

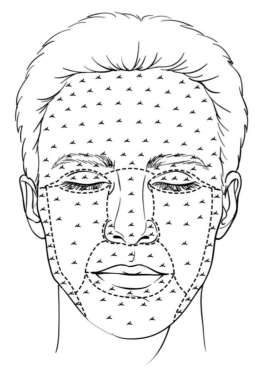

FIGURE 103–7

ESCHAROTOMIES

STEP 1: SURGICAL ANATOMY

◆ See Figure 103-1 for cross-section of skin.

INDICATIONS

◆ In burn resuscitation, recognition of pathology related to increased tissue pressure is critical to complete care and limiting secondary tissue injury. Skin, particularly skin burned to full thickness, can become a constricting element to tissue swelling and cause a tourniquet-like effect. Key to proper decompression is recognizing the potential, knowing the clinical signs and symptoms, and when necessary, having the ability to test the pressure within the compartment. A circumferential burn that is on an extremity of full thickness is particularly at risk for increased tissue pressure even if the percent of the burn is small, such as an isolated burn to fingers and hand. Clinically, the signs of compartment syndrome are paresthesia, pallor, pulselessness, paralysis, and pain. In the hand, in addition to the usual signs of elevated compartment pressure outlined, delayed or absent capillary refill, resistance to passive stretch, and a claw position at rest are clues to the need for decompression. The large burn may require monitoring of the abdominal compartment pressures and consideration of the fascial compartments in the extremities as possibly in need of decompression. Electrical injury presents one of the most difficult challenges, because there maybe extensive damage within deep muscular compartments with intact overlying skin. The surgical exploration, fascial decompression, and removal of dead muscle should not be delayed, because the resultant myoglobin in the serum is nephrotoxic.

STEP 2: PREOPERATIVE CONSIDERATIONS

◆ Escharotomies are usually completed safely at the bedside with sedation and electrocautery. The possibility of significant blood loss must be considered by the surgeon, and blood should be available if needed. Positioning should be based on exposure of the area to be decompressed, with arms supinated into anatomic position.

STEP 3: OPERATIVE STEPS

◆ Included are diagrams of properly placed incisions for decompressive escharotomies of various body regions **(Figure 103-8)**.

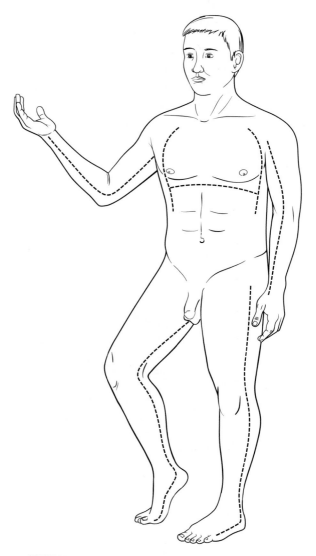

FIGURE 103–8

◆ To obtain an adequate release, the incisions should be mid-axial and completely through the eschar. Avoid deep penetration of the subcutaneous tissue below. Deep penetration can cause excessive bleeding and damage to underlying nerves and blood vessels. However, if there is clinical suspicion of fascial compartment hypertension, an escharotomy can be combined with a fasciotomy for diagnostic and therapeutic purposes. Escharotomy of the upper extremity should begin on the radial side down to the wrist. Details of hand and finger decompressions are represented in **Figure 103-9.**

◆ A special consideration is the circumferentially deeply burned thorax. Thoracic compartment is manifest by difficulty with ventilation and increased peak airway pressures. Recognition and decompressive escharotomy can be life-saving. Incision lines for thoracic decompression are outlined in Figure 103-8.

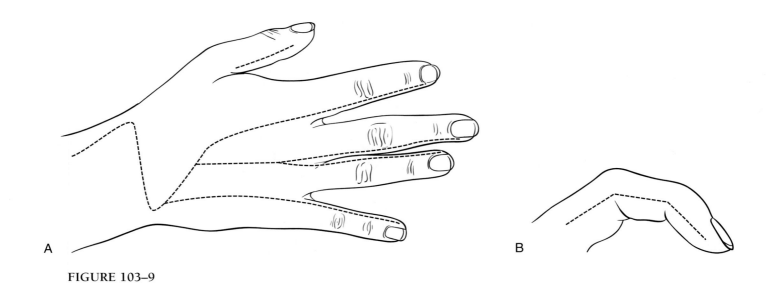

FIGURE 103–9

STEP 4: POSTOPERATIVE CARE

- Wounds that result from decompression should be kept moist and wrapped with the burn. Elevation should be routine to help decrease edema whenever possible.

STEP 5: PEARLS AND PITFALLS

- Keep in mind that all circumferential burns do not need to have decompression.

- In a moderate burn with an awake patient, you can follow closely with a clinical examination.

SELECTED REFERENCES

1. Herndon DN: Total Burn Care. London, Saunders, 2002.
2. Barret JP, Herndon DN: Color Atlas of Burn Care. London, Saunders, 2001.
3. Sood R, Achauer BM: Achauer and Sood's Burn Surgery: Reconstruction and Rehabilitation. Philadelphia, Elsevier, 2006.
4. Green DP, Hotchkiss RN, Pederson WC, Wolfe S: Green's Operative Hand Surgery, 5th ed. Amsterdam, Elsevier, 2005.

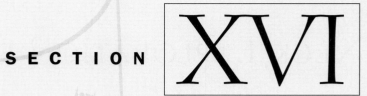

OPERATIONS—ELECTIVE AND TRAUMA

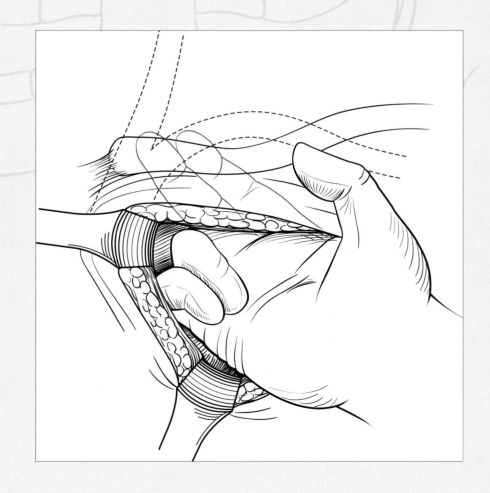

CHAPTER 104

NECK EXPLORATION FOR TRAUMA

William J. Mileski

STEP 1: SURGICAL ANATOMY

The following anatomic features must be observed:

◆ Mastoid muscle

◆ Sternocleidomastoid muscle

◆ Thyroid cartilage

◆ Trachea

◆ Esophagus

◆ Carotid sheath
  ◆ Carotid artery (common, internal, external) **(Figure 104-1)**
  ◆ Jugular vein (facial vein)
  ◆ Vagus nerve and ansa cervicalis

◆ Angle of mandible (see Figure 104-1)

◆ Platysma muscle

◆ Hypoglossal nerve

◆ Digastric muscle (see Figure 104-1)
  ◆ Zone I: Inferior to cricothyroid cartilage
  ◆ Zone II: Cricothyroid to angle of mandible
  ◆ Zone III: Superior to angle of mandible

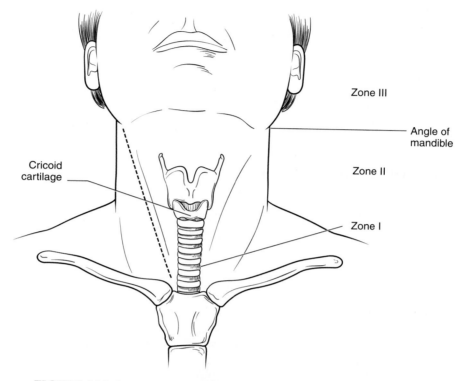

FIGURE 104–1

- ◆ Omohyoid muscle

- ◆ Inferior thyroid artery

- ◆ Middle thyroid vein

- ◆ Thyroid gland

- ◆ Parotid gland

- ◆ Cross-sectional view **(Figure 104-2)**
  - ◆ Investing layer of deep cervical fascia
  - ◆ Carotid sheath
  - ◆ Prevertebral fascia
  - ◆ Retropharyngeal space

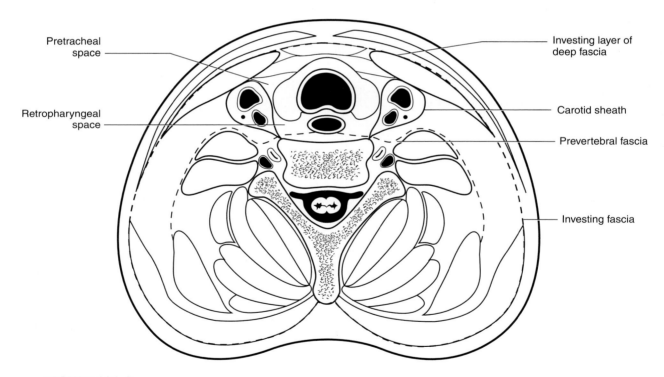

FIGURE 104–2

STEP 2: PREOPERATIVE CONSIDERATIONS

- The most common indication for neck exploration is penetrating trauma, although blunt trauma may also present with vascular and aerodigestive tract injury requiring treatment, identified by hard signs on examination (active hemorrhage, expanding hematoma) or by diagnostic study, computed tomography (CT), or ultrasound.

STEP 3: OPERATIVE STEPS

1. POSITIONING AND PREPARATION

- The patient is placed supine with a 3-inch towel roll beneath the shoulder, and the head is rotated to the contralateral side.

- The field is prepared from the base of the skull to include the entire chest, abdomen, and both groins (for possible vein graft).

2. INCISION AND DISSECTION

◆ The skin incision is made along the anterior border of the sternocleidomastoid muscle from the mastoid to the clavicle. The platysma muscle is incised (using electrocautery), the sternocleidomastoid is retracted lateral, and the carotid sheath is opened from proximal to distal. Transection of the omohyoid muscle proximally and digastric muscle distally may improve exposure **(Figure 104-3)**. Ligation of the facial vein, the inferior thyroid artery, and the middle thyroid vein and transection of the ansa cervicalis allow exposure of the trachea and esophagus by permitting easy lateral mobilization of the carotid sheath contents and medial retraction of the thyroid gland **(Figure 104-4, A)**.

◆ Tracheal injury may be primarily repaired with interrupted 3-0 polydioxanone (PDS) sutures. Esophageal injuries are best repaired in two layers with an inner layer of 3-0 Vicryl and an outer layer of 3-0 silk.

◆ When very distal exposure of the internal carotid is required, the mandible may be subluxed anteriorly and medially using temporary wire fixation (26 gauge) between the lower bicuspids and anterior incisors **(Figure 104-4, B)**. As the dissection on the anterior aspect of the internal carotid is carried distally, transection of the digastric muscle will be necessary, and care must be taken to avoid injury to the hypoglossal nerve.

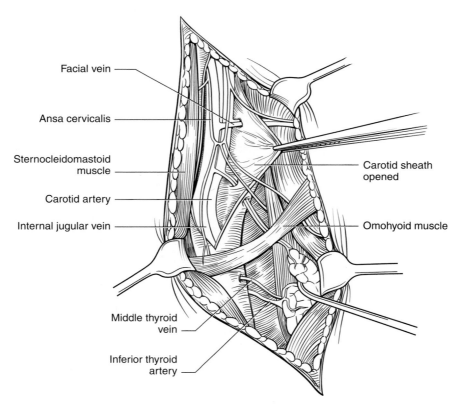

FIGURE 104–3

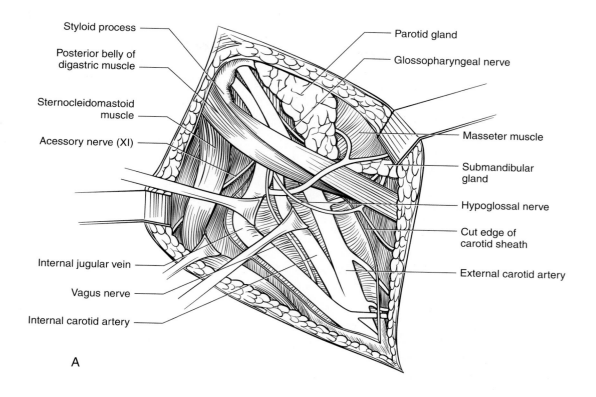

Styloid process

Posterior belly of
digastric muscle

Sternocleidomastoid
muscle

Acessory nerve (XI)

Internal jugular vein

Vagus nerve

Internal carotid artery

Parotid gland

Glossopharyngeal nerve

Masseter muscle

Submandibular
gland

Hypoglossal nerve

Cut edge of
carotid sheath

External carotid artery

A

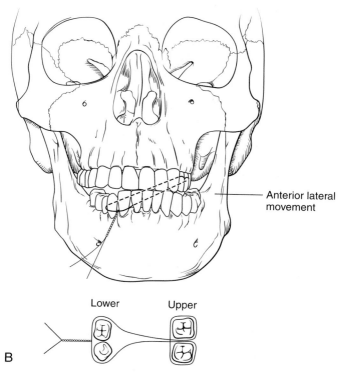

Anterior lateral
movement

Lower   Upper

B

FIGURE 104–4

3. CLOSING

◆ A closed-suction drain is placed in the deep space between the investing fascia **(Figure 104-5)** and closed with absorbable suture (3-0 Vicryl), and the skin is closed with subcuticular 4-0 Monocryl.

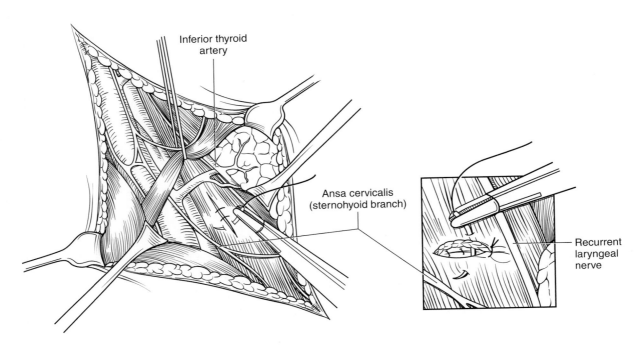

FIGURE 104–5

STEP 4: POSTOPERATIVE CARE

- Elevate head, and maintain close observation for hematoma formation.

STEP 5: PEARLS AND PITFALLS

- Selective use of closed suction drainage may be indicated in aerodigestive injuries.

SELECTED REFERENCE

1. Thal ER, Weigelt JA, Carrico CJ: Operative Trauma Management: An Atlas, 2nd ed. New York, McGraw Hill, 2002, pp 75-90.

CHAPTER 105

SUBCLAVIAN ARTERY STAB

William J. Mileski

STEP 1: SURGICAL ANATOMY

The following structures must be observed (**Figure 105-1**):

- Clavicle

- Sternum

- Sternoclavicular junction

- Deltopectoral groove

- Right subclavian artery

- Right subclavian vein

- Innominate artery

- Innominate vein

- Aorta

- Left subclavian artery

- Left subclavian vein

- Thoracic duct (left)

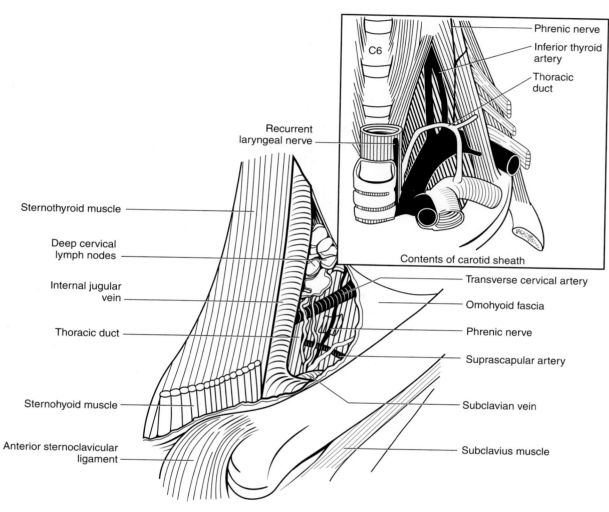

FIGURE 105–1

STEP 2: PREOPERATIVE CONSIDERATIONS

- Operative approach to stab wounds of the subclavian vessels is based on the patient's clinical (i.e., hemodynamic) status. In patients who present with massive bleeding in extremis, initial attempts at digital compression through the wound or a limited second intercostal anterior thoracotomy with compression of the vessels by insertion of two fingers may allow temporary control, permitting resuscitation and surgical exposure.

- In patients with near normal vital signs or who stabilize with initial resuscitation, imaging studies, either angiogram or computed tomography (CT) angiogram that provides anatomic definition, can guide decisions on surgical approach. Both the right and left subclavian vessels can be approached by medial clavicular resection. If it is suspected that proximal control at either the innominate or aortic junction will be needed, a median sternotomy may be required.

STEP 3: OPERATIVE STEPS

- The incision is at the second interspace.
  - A curvilinear incision 5 to 7 cm in length is rapidly created, beginning at the lateral border of the sternum through the pectoralis into the pleura (**Figure 105-2**).
  - The right second and third fingers are inserted and used to apply pressure superiorly and medially to compress the subclavian artery and vein against the clavicle (**Figure 105-3**).
  - After the hemorrhage is controlled, the subclavian vessels can be exposed by resecting the medial clavicle.

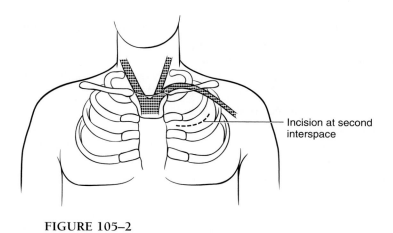

FIGURE 105–2

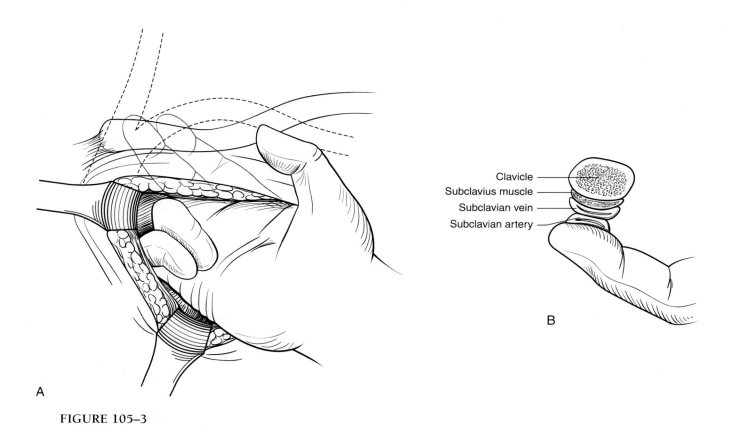

FIGURE 105–3

◆ Clavicular resection
  ◆ The incision is begun at the midline and extended laterally, directly over the clavicle to the deltopectoral groove **(Figure 105-4, A)**. Subcutaneous tissue and the anterior periosteum can be quickly dissected with electrocautery.
  ◆ The periosteum is separated from the clavicle circumferentially using periosteal elevators **(Figure 105-4, B)**.
  ◆ The clavicle is then transected at the lateral aspect of the exposure using a Gigli saw **(Figure 105-4, C)**.
  ◆ The medial aspect is retracted medially and superiorly, allowing separation of the sternoclavicular joint with sharp dissection or electrocautery.
  ◆ The posterior periosteum is incised at the lateral aspect of the incision and extended medially **(Figure 105-4, D)**.
  ◆ Placing two self-retaining retractors beneath the incised periosteum will allow dissection of the subclavian artery and vein, permitting proximal and distal vascular control in preparation for vascular repair **(Figure 105-4, E-F)**.

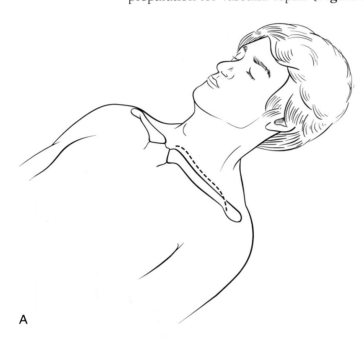

A

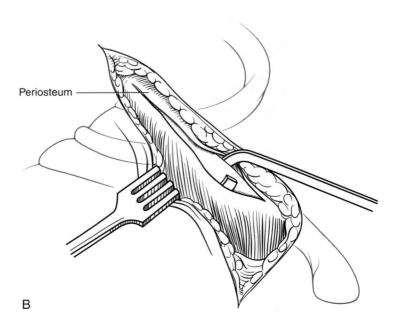

Periosteum

FIGURE 105–4   B

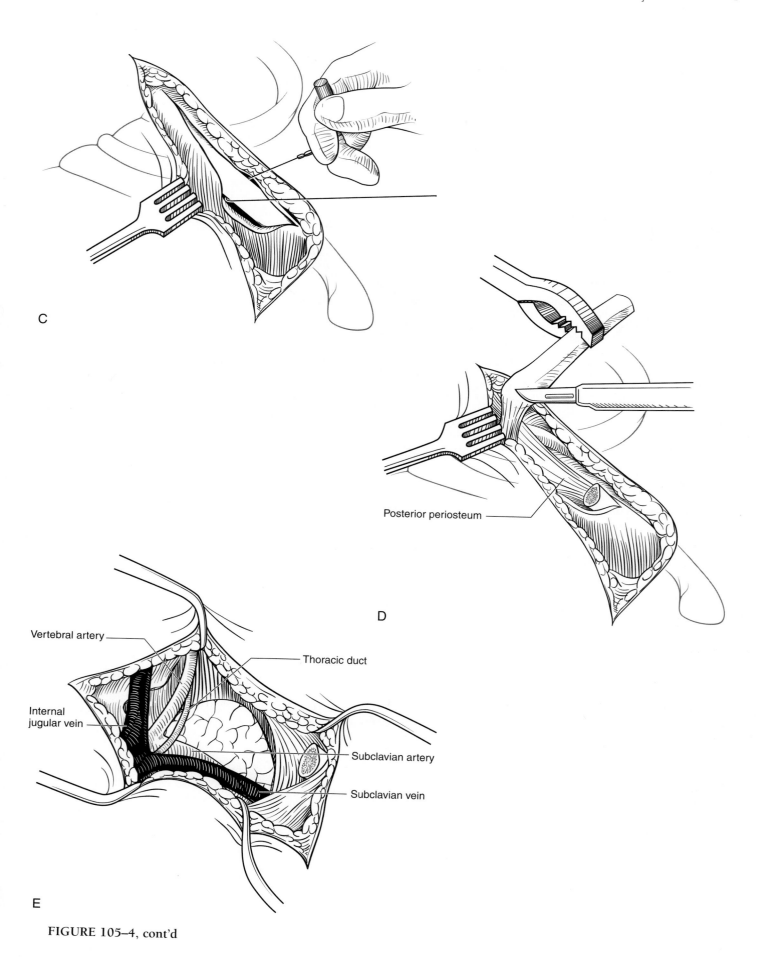

C

D

Posterior periosteum

E

Vertebral artery

Internal
jugular vein

Thoracic duct

Subclavian artery

Subclavian vein

FIGURE 105–4, cont'd

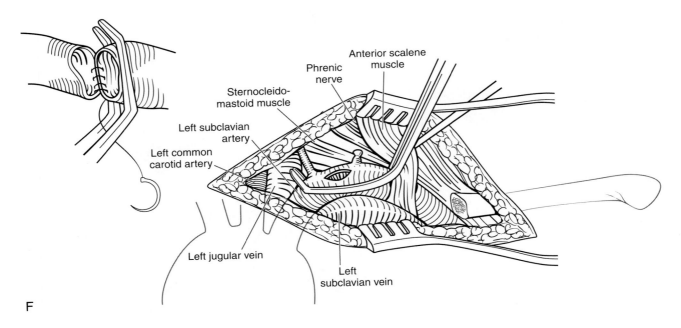

Anterior scalene muscle

Phrenic nerve

Sternocleido-mastoid muscle

Left subclavian artery

Left common carotid artery

Left jugular vein

Left subclavian vein

F

FIGURE 105–4, cont'd

STEP 4: POSTOPERATIVE CARE

- Patient should wear a shoulder immobilizer.

STEP 5: PEARLS AND PITFALLS

- Although numerous references suggest replacement and reconstruction of the clavicle, it may be unnecessary. If the patient's condition allows, replacement of the medial clavicle with internal fixation should be attempted to reduce long-term morbidity.

SELECTED REFERENCE

1. Thal ER, Weigelt JA, Carrico CJ: Operative Trauma Management: An Atlas, 2nd ed. New York, McGraw Hill, 2002, pp 110-114.

CHAPTER 106

THORACOTOMY FOR TRAUMA

William J. Mileski

STEP 1: SURGICAL ANATOMY

The following structures must be observed:

- Xiphoid process

- Fifth intercostal space

- Latissimus dorsi muscle

- Sternum

- Clavicles

- Pericardium

- Phrenic nerves

- Lungs

- Intercostal muscles

- Intercostal vessels

- Internal mammary vessel

STEP 2: PREOPERATIVE CONSIDERATIONS

- Patients with combined cardiac and pulmonary injuries or bilateral thoracic injuries may require a bilateral anterior lateral thoracotomy, or "clamshell thoracotomy," which provides exposure of bilateral hemithoraces, the pulmonary hila, and the mediastinum.

- Emergent thoracotomy requiring extension from left anterior lateral thoracotomy to right thoracotomy is infrequently needed but may be necessary when penetrating injuries unexpectedly require exposure of both right and left hemithoraces. Median sternotomy would be preferred for treating penetrating cardiac injuries.

- There is generally insufficient time for formal preparation. Rapid painting with povidone-iodine (Betadine) is generally performed. The neck, entire thorax, abdomen, and upper thighs should be included. The incision of the thigh may facilitate use of mechanical cardiopulmonary support.

STEP 3: OPERATIVE STEPS

1. INCISION

- The incision begins at the junction of the xiphoid process and sternum and is extended laterally in a curvilinear fashion to the anterior border of the latissimus dorsi (**Figure 106-1**).

- The incision should be carried down to the intercostal muscles on the superior aspect of the fifth or sixth rib, with care given not to cut through the intercostals into the underlying pulmonary parenchyma (**Figure 106-2**).

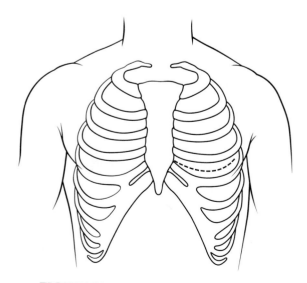

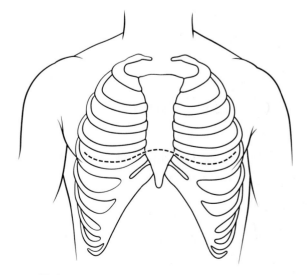

FIGURE 106–1

FIGURE 106–2

2. DISSECTION

- The intercostal muscles and pleura are best taken down using a curved Mayo scissors, partially opened, pressed on the superior aspect of the rib, and advanced lateral to medial. At the medial aspect, the internal mammary vessels are often transected and require ligation if resuscitation is successful.
  - A rib spreader is inserted and retracted.
  - The pericardium is inspected if indicated, and pericardiotomy is performed in a longitudinal fashion, anterior to the phrenic nerve.

- In the absence of a source of hemorrhage in the left hemithorax or a cardiac injury and suspected hemorrhage in the right hemithorax, the incision may be rapidly extended to the right hemithorax in a mirrored fashion.

- The xiphisternal junction may be transected with an osteotome, Lebsche knife, or sternal saw.
  - Again, the internal mammary vessels are transected and ligated **(Figure 106-3)**.
  - The superior thoracic cage can then be retracted cephalad, exposing the anterior mediastinum and bilateral hemithoraces and the pulmonary hila **(Figure 106-4)**.

3. CLOSING

- If resuscitation is successful and a treatable injury is identified and repaired, thoracic closure should be rapidly accomplished.
  - Bilateral 36F thoracostomy tubes are placed, the ribs are approximated with interrupted #1 Vicryl suture, the subcutaneous tissue is reapproximated with absorbable suture, and the skin is closed with staples.

STEP 4: POSTOPERATIVE CARE

- Pain control and respiratory therapy are critical to recovery.

STEP 5: PEARLS AND PITFALLS

- Care must be exercised to avoid damage to the phrenic nerve when pericardiotomy is performed.

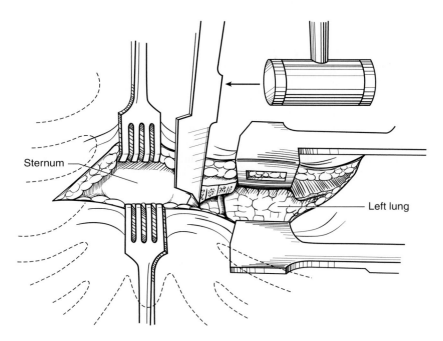

FIGURE 106–3

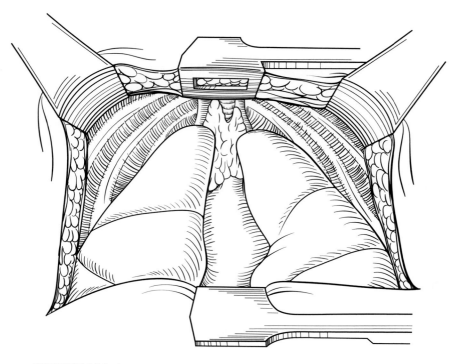

FIGURE 106–4

SELECTED REFERENCES

1. Wright C: Transverse sternothoracotomy. Chest Surg Clin N Am 1996;6:149-156.
2. Working Group, Ad Hoc Subcommittee on Outcomes, American College of Surgeons, Committee on Trauma: Practice management guidelines for emergency department thoracotomy. J Am Coll Surg 2001;193:303-309.
3. Baxter BT, Moore EE, Moore JB, et al: Emergency department thoracotomy following injury: Critical determinants for patient salvage. World J Surg 1988;12:671-675.
4. Biffl WL, Moore EE, Harken AH: Emergency department thoractomy. In Mattox KL, Feliciano DV, Moore EE (eds): Trauma, 4th ed. New York, McGraw-Hill, 2000, p 245.
5. Feliciano DV, Mattox KL: Indications, technique and pitfalls of emergency center thoracotomy. Surg Rounds 1981;4:32.

CHAPTER 107

RETROPERITONEAL EXPOSURE

William J. Mileski

STEP 1: SURGICAL ANATOMY

- ◆ Exposure of the retroperitoneal structures—duodenum, pancreas, kidneys, ureters, vena cava, and aorta—may be required to address injury of these structures or other emergent conditions.

STEP 2: PREOPERATIVE CONSIDERATIONS

- ◆ For trauma, wide preparation of the torso is necessary, including neck and groins.

STEP 3: OPERATIVE STEPS

♦ A full midline incision is made.

♦ Beginning on the right, the surgeon exposes the retroperitoneal structures by mobilization of the cecum and ascending colon, releasing the lateral peritoneal reflection, the white line of Toldt, from caudad and lateral to the cecum and extending the release cephalad, combining with mobilization of the lateral attachments of the duodenum **(Figure 107-1)**.

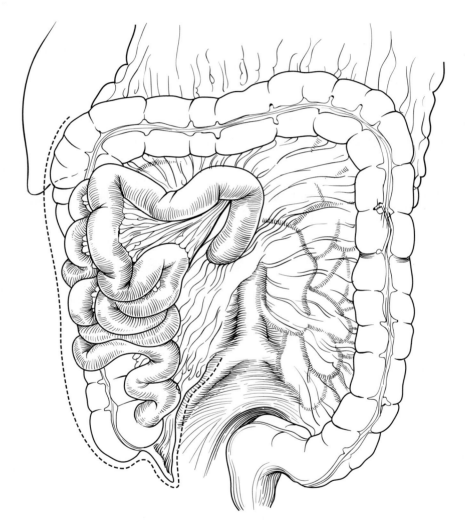

FIGURE 107–1

♦ This extended Kocher maneuver allows medial rotation of the colon and duodenum. It can be further extended by mobilization of the mesentery of the small intestine to the ligament of Treitz, the Cattell maneuver includes retraction of the entire right side of the colon, most of the transverse colon, and the small intestine and left cephalad, which exposes the right kidney, right adrenal gland, right ureter, entire duodenum, head of the pancreas, inferior vena cava, and infrarenal aorta **(Figure 107-2)**.

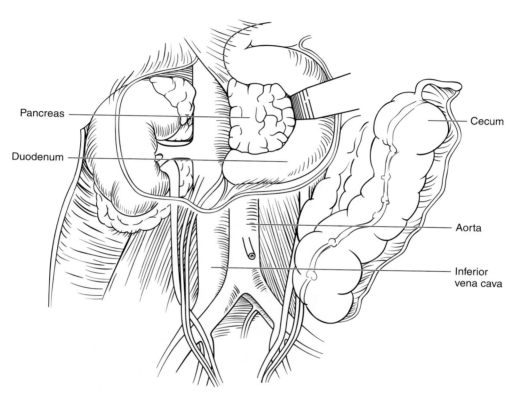

FIGURE 107–2

◆ Exposure of the retroperitoneal attachments on the left can be accomplished in a mirrored fashion, incising the left retroperitoneum from the lateral aspect of the sigmoid colon and extending cephalad to incise the splenorenal ligament and splenophrenic attachments **(Figure 107-3)**.

◆ A plane of dissection is then bluntly developed between the spleen, pancreas, and colonic mesentery anterior to Gerota's fascia **(Figure 107-4)**. With the left colon, spleen, and tail of the pancreas retracted to the right, the left kidney, left adrenal gland, left ureter, and aorta—from celiac axis to bifurcation—can be visualized.

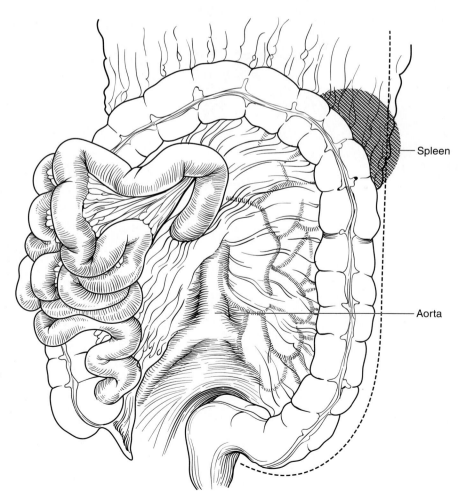

FIGURE 107–3

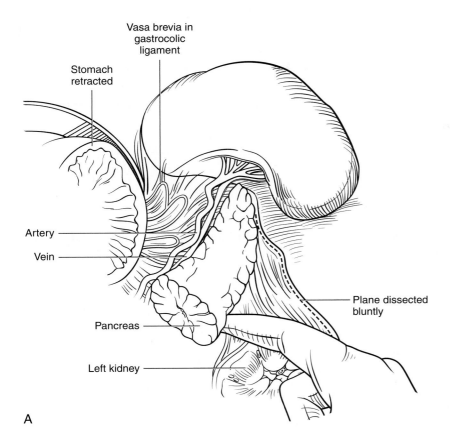

Stomach retracted

Vasa brevia in gastrocolic ligament

Artery

Vein

Pancreas

Left kidney

Plane dissected bluntly

A

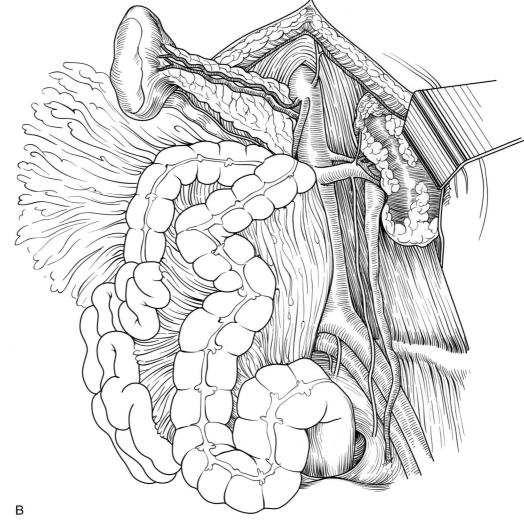

FIGURE 107–4   B

STEP 4: POSTOPERATIVE CARE

- Nasogastric decompression may be required for a prolonged period following this extensive retroperitoneal dissection.

STEP 5: PEARLS AND PITFALLS

- Steady rotation and countertraction with blunt dissection (a sponge stick is often helpful) is critical to maintaining the plane of dissection.

SELECTED REFERENCE

1. Cattell RB, Braasch JW: A technique for the exposure of the third and fourth portions of the duodenum. Surg Gynecol Obstet 1960;111:378-379.

INDEX